Sports Endocri.

CONTEMPORARY ENDOCRINOLOGY

P. Michael Conn, SERIES EDITOR

23. *Sports Endocrinology,* edited by *MICHELLE P. WARREN AND NAAMA W. CONSTANTINI,* 2000
22. *Gene Engineering in Endocrinology,* edited by *MARGARET A. SHUPNIK,* 2000
21. *Hormones and the Heart in Health and Disease,* edited by *LEONARD SHARE,* 1999
20. *Endocrinology of Aging,* edited by *JOHN E. MORLEY AND LUCRETIA VAN DEN BERG,* 1999
19. *Human Growth Hormone: Research and Clinical Practice,* edited by *ROY G. SMITH AND MICHAEL O. THORNER,* 1999
18. *Menopause: Endocrinology and Management,* edited by *DAVID B. SEIFER AND ELIZABETH A. KENNARD,* 1999
17. *The IGF System: Molecular Biology, Physiology, and Clinical Applications,* edited by *RON G. ROSENFELD AND CHARLES ROBERTS,* 1999
16. *Neurosteroids: A New Regulatory Function in the Nervous System,* edited by *ETIENNE-EMILE BAULIEU, PAUL ROBEL, AND MICHAEL SCHUMACHER,* 1999
15. *Autoimmune Endocrinopathies,* edited by *ROBERT VOLPÉ,* 1999
14. *Hormone Resistance Syndromes,* edited by *J. LARRY JAMESON,* 1999
13. *Hormone Replacement Therapy,* edited by *A. WAYNE MEIKLE,* 1999
12. *Insulin Resistance: The Metabolic Syndrome X,* edited by *GERALD M. REAVEN AND AMI LAWS,* 1999
11. *Endocrinology of Breast Cancer,* edited by *ANDREA MANNI,* 1999
10. *Molecular and Cellular Pediatric Endocrinology,* edited by *STUART HANDWERGER,* 1999
9. *The Endocrinology of Pregnancy,* edited by *FULLER W. BAZER,* 1998
8. *Gastrointestinal Endocrinology,* edited by *GEORGE H. GREELEY,* 1998
7. *Clinical Management of Diabetic Neuropathy,* edited by *ARISTIDIS VEVES,* 1998
6. *G Protein-Coupled Receptors and Disease,* edited by *ALLEN M. SPIEGEL,* 1997
5. *Natriuretic Peptides in Health and Disease,* edited by *WILLIS K. SAMSON AND ELLIS R. LEVIN,* 1997
4. *Endocrinology of Critical Diseases,* edited by *K. Patrick Ober,* 1997
3. *Diseases of the Pituitary: Diagnosis and Treatment,* edited by *Margaret E. Wierman,* 1997
2. *Diseases of the Thyroid,* edited by *Lewis E. Braverman,* 1997
1. *Endocrinology of the Vasculature,* edited by *James R. Sowers,* 1996

SPORTS ENDOCRINOLOGY

Edited by

MICHELLE P. WARREN, MD
Columbia University College of Physicians and Surgeons, New York, NY

and

NAAMA W. CONSTANTINI, MD
Ribstein Center for Sport Medicine Sciences and Research, Wingate Institute, Netanya, Israel

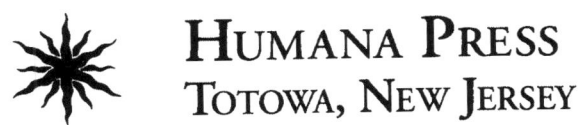

HUMANA PRESS
TOTOWA, NEW JERSEY

© 2010 Humana Press Inc.
999 Riverview Drive, Suite 208
Totowa, New Jersey 07512

For additional copies, pricing for bulk purchases, and/or information about other Humana titles, contact Humana at the above address or at any of the following numbers: Tel: 973-256-1699; Fax: 973-256-8341; E-mail: humana@humanapr.com or visit our Website at http://humanapress.com

All rights reserved. No part of this book may be reproduced, stored in a retrieval system, or transmitted in any form or by any means, electronic, mechanical, photocopying, microfilming, recording, or otherwise without written permission from the Publisher.

All articles, comments, opinions, conclusions, or recommendations are those of the author(s), and do not necessarily reflect the views of the publisher.

Due diligence has been taken by the publishers, editors, and authors of this book to assure the accuracy of the information published and to describe generally accepted practices. The contributors herein have carefully checked to ensure that the drug selections and dosages set forth in this text are accurate and in accord with the standards accepted at the time of publication. Notwithstanding, as new research, changes in government regulations, and knowledge from clinical experience relating to drug therapy and drug reactions constantly occurs, the reader is advised to check the product information provided by the manufacturer of each drug for any change in dosages or for additional warnings and contraindications. This is of utmost importance when the recommended drug herein is a new or infrequently used drug. It is the responsibility of the treating physician to determine dosages and treatment strategies for individual patients. Further it is the responsibility of the health care provider to ascertain the Food and Drug Administration status of each drug or device used in their clinical practice. The publisher, editors, and authors are not responsible for errors or omissions or for any consequences from the application of the information presented in this book and make no warranty, express or implied, with respect to the contents in this publication.

Cover design by Patricia F. Cleary.

Photocopy Authorization Policy:
Authorization to photocopy items for internal or personal use, or the internal or personal use of specific clients, is granted by Humana Press Inc., provided that the base fee of US $10.00 per copy, plus US $00.25 per page, is paid directly to the Copyright Clearance Center at 222 Rosewood Drive, Danvers, MA 01923. For those organizations that have been granted a photocopy license from the CCC, a separate system of payment has been arranged and is acceptable to Humana Press Inc.

Printed in the United States of America.   10 9 8 7 6 5 4 3 2 1

ISBN 978-1-61737-085-4   e-ISBN 978-1-59259-016-2

PREFACE

Since the observation in the 19th century that an extract of the suprarenal bodies injected into the circulation caused a rise in blood pressure, the endocrine system has become a major component in our understanding of human physiology. The introduction of radioimmunoassay techniques and the ability to measure minimal amounts of hormones (a term derived from the Greek "to excite") have shown that acute exercise causes a release of a large number of hormones and that chronic exercise may further lead to long-term alterations in endocrine homeostasis. Actually, almost every organ and system in the body is affected by physical activity and exercise, much of it through the endocrine and neuroendocrine system.

Investigation of the effect of acute or chronic physical activity on the endocrine system is a complex matter since the stimulus called "exercise" has many components, such as mode, intensity, duration, and others. In addition, several other factors, such as age, gender, training status, body temperature, circadian rhythm, metabolic state, menstrual cycle, and various external conditions as well as psychological factors, can modify the effect of physical activity on hormonal secretion. Moreover, the physiological stimulus of exercise often provokes several and parallel cascades of biochemical and endocrine changes. It is therefore often extremely difficult to distinguish between primary and secondary events and between cause and effect. These limitations will be discussed in Chapter 1.

In this volume we have tried to cover the various hormonal pathways that are known to be altered by exercise and how these changes affect different organs and systems of the body. Other subjects are the hormonal regulation of fluid homeostasis, substrate metabolism, and energy balance. A substantial part of the book is devoted to the exercising female in view of certain unique features, e.g. menstrual cycle, use of contraceptives, pregnancy, menopause, and others. Another important issue is the effect of exercise on puberty and growth. Although investigated for many years, it would be premature to draw final conclusions regarding the precise amount of exercise needed to achieve positive effects without compromising growth and puberty. Exercise has also been observed in altering mood. The role of hormones in the development of "exercise euphoria" is discussed in a separate chapter.

The final chapter will not deal with the effect of physical activity on the endocrine system, but rather with its opposite: the effect of exogenous hormones on performance. Unfortunately, the manipulation of physiological stimuli by the use of hormones has become common practice at all levels of sport, from fitness rooms to elite world events. The International Olympic Committee is engaged in what seems to be a lost battle against the increasing sophistication of the use of hormones, such as anabolic steroids, hGH, HGC, and EPO to enhance performance.

The editors hope that this volume will not only reflect the present state of our knowledge, but also stimulate further study.

Michelle P. Warren, MD
Naama W. Constantini, MD

CONTENTS

Preface
List of Contributors

1. Hormonal Response to Exercise: *Methodological Considerations* 1
   Mark S. Tremblay and Samuel Y. Chu

2. Exercise and Endogenous Opiates 31
   Tim Meyer, Lothar Schwarz, and Wilfried Kindermann

3. The Effect of Exercise on the Hypothalamo–Pituitary–Adrenal Axis 43
   Gary Wittert

4. Impact of Chronic Training on Pituitary Hormone Secretion in the Human 57
   Johannes D. Veldhuis and Kohji Yoshida

5. Exercise and the Growth Hormone–Insulin-Like Growth Factor-1 Axis 77
   Alon Eliakim, Jo Anne Brasel, and Dan M. Cooper

6. Thyroid Function and Exercise 97
   Victor J. Bernet and Leonard Wartofsky

7. The Male Reproductive System, Exercise, and Training 119
   David C. Cumming

8. Exercise and the Hypothalamus: *Ovulatory Adaptions* 133
   Moira A. Petit and Jerilynn C. Prior

9. Exercise Training in the Normal Female: *Effects of Exercise Stress and Energy Availablility on Metabolic Hormones and LH Pulsatility* 165
   Anne B. Loucks

10. Adrenergic Regulation of Energy Metabolism 181
    Michael Kjær and Kai Lange

11. Energy Balance and Weight Control: *Endocrine Considerations* 189
    Gilbert W. Gleim and Beth W. Glace

12. Hormonal Regulation of Fluid Homeostasis During and Following Exercise 207
    Charles E. Wade

13. Diabetes and Exercise 227
    Stephen H. Schneider and Pushpinder S. Guleria

14	Hormonal Regulations of the Effects of Exercise on Bone: *Postive and Negative Effects* 239
	Philip D. Chilibeck
15	The Role of Exercise in the Attainment of Peak Bone Mass and Bone Strength 253
	Shona L. Bass and Kathryn H. Myburgh
16	Interrelationships Between Acute and Chronic Exercise and the Immune and Endocrine Systems 281
	Valéria M. Natale and Roy J. Shephard
17	Exercise and the Developing Child: *Endocrine Considerations* 303
	Sita M. Sundaresan, James N. Roemmich, and Alan D. Rogol
18	Exercise and the Female Reproductive System: *The Effect of Hormonal Status on Performance* 321
	David M. Quadagno
19	Exercise and Pregnancy: *Hormonal Considerations* 335
	Fred K. Lotgering
20	The Endocrine System in Overtraining 347
	Axel Urhausen and Wilfried Kindermann
21	The Effects of Altitude on the Hormonal Responses to Exercise 371
	Roland J. M. Favier
22	Exercise, Circadian Rhythms, and Hormones 391
	Thomas Reilly, Greg Atkinson, and Jim Waterhouse
23	Physical Activity and Mood: *The Endocrine Connection* 421
	Gal Dubnov and Elliot M. Berry
24	Hormones as Performance-Enhancing Drugs 433
	Mark Myhal and David R. Lamb
Index 477	

CONTRIBUTORS

GREG ATKINSON • *Research Institute for Sport and Exercise Sciences, Liverpool John Moores University, Liverpool, UK*
SHONA L. BASS • *School of Health Sciences, Deakin University, Victoria, Australia*
VICTOR J. BERNET, MD • *Endocrinology and Metabolic Service, Walter Reed Army Medical Center, Washington, DC*
ELLIOT M. BERRY, MD, FRCPS • *Department of Human Nutrition and Metabolism, Hadassah Medical School, The Hebrew University, Jerusalem, Israel*
JO ANNE BRASEL, MD • *Division of Endocrinology and Metabolism, Harbor-UCLA Medical Center, Torrance, CA*
PHILIP D. CHILIBECK, PHD • *College of Physical Education, University of Saskatchewan, Saskatoon, SK, Canada*
SAMUEL Y. CHU, PHD • *Biochemistry Department, Dr. Everett Chalmers Hospital, Fredericton, NB, Canada*
NAAMA W. CONSTANTINI, MD • *Ribstein Center for Sport Medicine Sciences and Research, Wingate Institute, Netanya, Israel*
DAN M. COOPER, MD • *Department of Pediatrics, UCI Medical Center, Orange, CA*
DAVID C. CUMMING, MBCHB, FRCSC • *Department of Obstetrics and Gynaecology, University of Alberta, Edmonton, AB, Canada*
GAL DUBNOV, MD, MSc • *Department of Human Nutrition and Metabolism, Hadassah Medical School, The Hebrew University, Jerusalem, Israel*
ALON ELIAKIM, MD • *Department of Pediatrics, Meir Hospital, Kfar-Saba, Israel, and Ribstein Center for Sport Medicine Sciences and Research, Wingate Institute, Netanya, Israel*
ROLAND J. M. FAVIER, DR. ES SCI • *Laboratoire de Physiologie, Faculté de Médecine, Lyon, France*
BETH W. GLACE, MS • *Nicholas Institute of Sports Medicine and Athletic Trauma, Lenox Hill Hospital, New York, NY*
GILBERT W. GLEIM, PHD • *Nicholas Institute of Sports Medicine and Athletic Trauma, Lenox Hill Hospital, New York, NY*
PUSHPINDER S. GULERIA, MD • *Department of Endocrinology, University of Medicine and Dentistry of New Jersey and Robert Wood Johnson Hospital, New Brunswick, NJ*
WILFRIED KINDERMANN, MD, PHD • *Institute of Sports and Preventive Medicine, Department of Clinical Medicine, University of Saarland, Saarbrücken, Germany*
MICHAEL KJÆR, MD, PHD • *Sports Medicine Research Unit, Department of Rheumatology, Bispebjerg Hospital, Copenhagen, Denmark*
DAVID R. LAMB, PHD • *School of Physical Activity and Educational Services, The Ohio State University, Columbus, OH*
KAI LANGE • *Sports Medicine Research Unit, Department of Rheumatology, Bispebjerg Hospital, Copenhagen, Denmark*
FREDERIK K. LOTGERING, MD, PHD • *Department of Obstetrics and Gynaecology, Erasmus University and Academic Hospital, Rotterdam, The Netherlands*
ANNE B. LOUCKS, PHD • *Department of Biological Sciences, Ohio University, Athens, OH*
TIM MEYER, MD, PHD • *Department of Clinical Medicine, Institute of Sports and Preventive Medicine, University of Saarland, Saarbrücken, Germany*

KATHRYN H. MYBURGH, PHD • *Department of Human and Animal Physiology, University of Stellenbosch, Mastieland, South Africa*
MARK MYHAL, PHD • *School of Physical Activity and Educational Services, The Ohio State University, Columbus, OH*
VALÉRIA M. NATALE, MD • *Hospital das Clínicas da Faculdade de Medicina da Universidade de São Paulo, Brazil*
MOIRA A. PETIT, BA, MS • *School of Human Kinetics, University of British Columbia, Vancouver, BC, Canada*
JERILYNN C. PRIOR, MA, MD, FRCPC • *Division of Endocrinology, Department of Medicine, University of British Columbia, Vancouver, BC, Canada*
DAVID QUADAGNO, PHD • *Department of Biological Science, Florida State University, Tallahassee, FL*
THOMAS REILLY • *Research Institute for Sport and Exercise Sciences, Liverpool John Moores University, Liverpool, UK*
JAMES N. ROEMMICH, PHD • *Department of Pediatrics, Division of Endocrinology, University of Virginia Health Sciences Center, Charlottesville, VA*
ALAN D. ROGOL, MD, PHD • *Department of Pediatrics, Division of Endocrinology and Department of Pharmacology, University of Virginia Health Sciences Center, Charlottesville, VA*
STEPHEN H. SCHNEIDER, MD • *Department of Endocrinology, University of Medicine and Dentistry of New Jersey and Robert Wood Johnson Hospital, New Brunswick, NJ*
LOTHAR SCHWARZ • *Institute of Sports and Preventive Medicine, University of Saarland, Saarbrücken, Germany*
ROY J. SHEPHARD, MD, PHD, DPE • *Department of Applied Physiology, Faculty of Physical Education and Health, University of Toronto, ON, Canada; Defence and Civil Institute of Environmental Medicine, North York, ON, Canada; and Health Sciences Program, Brock University, St. Catharines, ON, Canada*
SITA M. SUNDARESAN, BA • *Department of Pediatrics, Division of Endocrinology, University of Virginia Health Sciences Center, Charlottesville, VA*
MARK TREMBLAY, PHD • *Faculty of Kinesiology, University of New Brunswick, Fredericton, NB, Canada*
AXEL URHAUSEN, MD, PHD • *Institute of Sports and Preventive Medicine, Department of Clinical Medicine, University of Saarland, Saarbrücken, Germany*
JOHANNES VELDHUIS, MD • *Division of Endocrinology and Metabolism, Department of Internal Medicine, University of Virginia Health Sciences Center, Charlottesville, VA*
CHARLES E. WADE, PHD • *Life Sciences Division, NASA Ames Research Center, Moffett Field, CA*
MICHELLE P. WARREN, MD • *Columbia University College of Physicians and Surgeons, New York, NY*
LEONARD WARTOFSKY, MD • *Department of Medicine, Washington Hospital Center, Washington, DC*
JIM WATERHOUSE • *Research Institute for Sport and Exercise Sciences, Liverpool John Moores University, Liverpool, UK*
GARY WITTERT, MD, FRACP • *Department of Medicine, University of Adelaide and Royal Adelaide Hospital, Adelaide, South Australia, Australia*
KOHJI YOSHIDA • *Department of Obstetrics and Gynecology, University of Occupational and Environmental Health, Kitakyushu, Japan*

1 Hormonal Response to Exercise
Methodological Considerations

Mark S. Tremblay, PhD and Samuel Y. Chu, PhD

CONTENTS
    INTRODUCTION
    SOURCES OF VARIATION
    SUBJECT PROFILE
    STANDARDIZED CONDITIONS
    SPECIMEN COLLECTION
    ANALYTICAL PROCEDURE
    EXERCISE VARIABLES
    SECULAR TRENDS AND EVOLUTION
    DATA PRESENTATION AND ANALYSIS
    SUMMARY
    REFERENCES

INTRODUCTION

The importance of hormones in regulating physiological functions and processes has intrigued scientists since they were first characterized by Baylis and Starling in 1904 *(1)*. Research advances in endocrinology have led to an improved understanding of the intricate and diverse functions of the endocrine system. In addition, advances in technology and analytical procedures have facilitated the convenience and accuracy of hormone measurements. These advancements have facilitated the proliferation of endocrine research in exercise and sport science over the past 30 years (Fig. 1). This relative explosion in research related to exercise endocrinology has contributed greatly to the understanding of the physiological consequences of exercise and physical training. Nevertheless, the emerging research is often inconsistent, contradictory, and difficult to interpret. In some cases, research discrepancies may be explained by methodological or analytical inconsistencies.

From: *Contemporary Endocrinology: Sports Endocrinology*
Edited by: M. P. Warren and N. W. Constantini © Humana Press Inc., Totowa, NJ

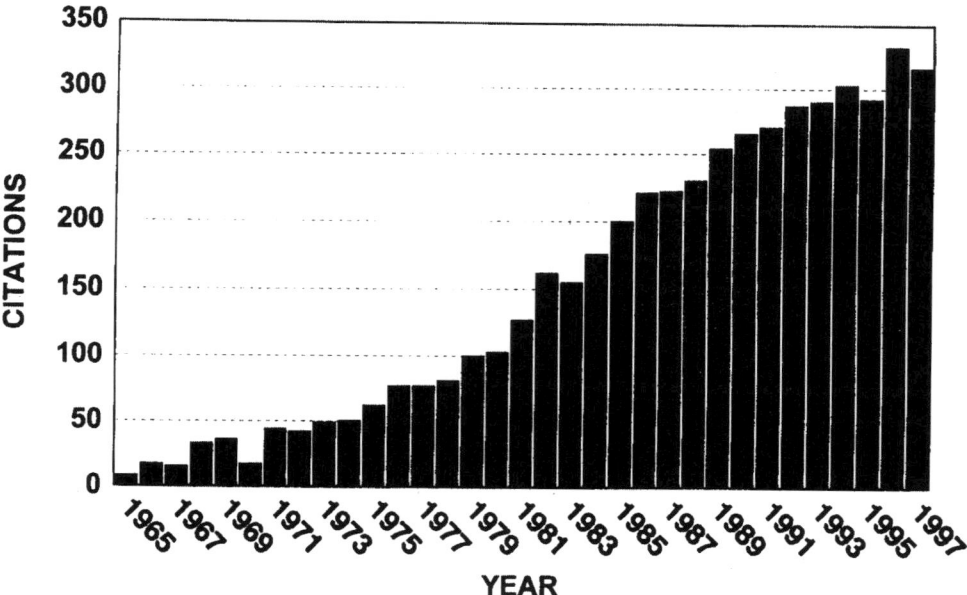

Fig. 1. Historical progression of MEDLINE citations searching "exercise and hormones."

To minimize confusion, ensure valid experimental outcomes, and accelerate progress in exercise and sports endocrinology, researchers must be cognizant and vigilant of the methods and procedures necessary to minimize experimental interference by confounding variables. Meticulous control of confounding variables and careful attention to analytical procedures will facilitate the isolation of an experimental effect being investigated. The purpose of this chapter is to acquaint the reader with some of the many variables that should be considered when interpreting the results of hormonal analyses, particularly as they relate to exercise or sport situations. The chapter will also serve as a helpful "checklist" for researchers and clinicians interested in designing experiments intended to isolate the effect of a specific intervention variable (notably exercise) on endocrine function. This chapter will review systematically the potential influence of variables related to subject profile, pretesting conditions, specimen collection, analytical procedures, exercise protocol, and data analysis. A brief discussion regarding the sources of variation and their acceptable limits will also be presented. Much of the information presented in this chapter represents an updated and expanded version of a previous review article written by the authors (2).

It must be recognized that circulating levels of hormones do not necessarily directly reflect changes in physiological function at the cellular or subcellular level. The biological impact of a change in circulating hormones is not realized until it has initiated a cellular response. The presence and magnitude of the response are dependent on the availability and sensitivity of hormone receptors, the responsiveness of the cellular or nuclear environment to a stimulus from a hormone–receptor complex, the genetic characteristics of the cell, and the availability of substrates and materials for adaptive responses. Although studying exercise and sports endocrinology primarily through changes in circulating hormone levels is overly simplistic, the methods and procedures related to the acquisition of valid circulating hormone concentrations will be the focus of this chapter.

SOURCES OF VARIATION

Biological Variation

Variations in the results of chemical analyses of samples taken from the same individual over a period of time have been observed, despite efforts to standardize measurement conditions. The variances observed are the result of a combination of analytical and biological variation (3,4). To assess exercise-induced hormone effects properly, the variability of hormone measurement must be taken into consideration. The biological variation of an individual (intraindividual) refers to the differences in the true level of the substance within an individual over a time period. This variation occurs as a result of differences in seasonal activity, emotional state, internal hormonal control, short-term health, and the genetic makeup of the individual (5). Other factors that also contribute to the biological variation are posture, stress level, cyclical variation, diet, and environmental effects. These preanalytical sources of biological variation to a certain extent are controllable with proper preparation of the individual prior to the specimen collection. Such factors as genetics, endogenous hormonal regulation, and other long-term effects are difficult to control, and their influence on intraindividual variation should be acknowledged in the evaluation of the study data. Biological variation is normally expressed by the standard deviation (SD_b) of the analyte value around the homeostatic set point of that subject, or by the coefficient of variation (CV_b) expressed as (SD_b/mean × 100). In the case that the CV_b of a particular hormone analyte is not known, the researcher should determine its value by performing multiple pre-exercise assessments of the basal hormone levels under controlled conditions over a 1- to 2-wk period. It has been reported that the within-subject biological variation is smaller in a short time interval than a longer-term period (months) (6,7). Valid estimates of the biological variation, therefore, could be obtained from relatively small numbers of specimens collected over a short time (8), but under well-controlled conditions.

Analytical Variation

Analytical variation refers to the differences in the analytical measurements of a sample after it has been prepared for analysis (5). Analytical procedures are subject to inaccuracy or bias from a variety of sources. In addition, laboratory analysis is also subject to imprecision or random error. Analytical bias is systemic in nature, and the sources of variation are related to assay method, instrumentation, reagents and standards, and the skill of the staff used to perform the test. Imprecision, which relates to the reproducibility and repeatability of the assay, is an inherent limitation of the procedure, whereas random errors are accidental and indeterminate. The analytical variation, similar to the biological variation, is expressed as the standard deviation (SD_a) and/or coefficient of variation (CV_a) of the assay. In a long-term study of an analyte, the extent of the analytical imprecision poses a far greater impact than the assay bias on the outcome of the study (9). For an analytical procedure, one will experience intra-assay (within-run) and interassay (between-run) imprecision. In general, the interassay variance is greater than the intra-assay variance. In repeated measures or repeated design studies, wherever possible, samples from the same individual should be batched and assayed together to reduce or eliminate the influence of interassay variance.

Impact of Biological and Analytical Variation on Study Data

Both analytical and biological variation are important to consider when interpreting significant results from a longitudinal study. Chu *(9)* in his enzyme inhibition studies showed that for a method with 3% CV_a and a biological variation of 4.3%, a total change of 16.5% was required in order to conclude that the magnitude of change between two consequent events was meaningful, and not just a result of the natural variation. Furthermore, if the imprecision of the test increased to 10%, the experimental effect necessary to indicate a significant outcome increased to 33.9%. This illustrates how the precision of a test impacts on the study result. The minimum difference between two successive measurements obtained from samples in the same individual (one-tailed test, p 0.05; i.e., significant difference [d_s]) is given by the formula:

$$[d_s (\%) = 2.3 \times (cv_a^2 + cv_b^2)^{1/2}] \quad (1)$$

Thus, to detect exercise-induced hormone changes, one should select an assay design that minimizes the assay imprecision. The within-subject CV_b for follicle-stimulating hormone (FSH), luteinizing hormone (LH), sex hormone binding globulin (SHBG), and testosterone reported by Valero-Politi et al. *(10)* are 17.3, 24, 12.1, and 10.9%, respectively. It is best to employ an experimental protocol where, during the experimental sampling time, the intraindividual biological variation not related to exercise is minimized. This could be achieved by minimizing or standardizing the influence of many preanalytical factors described later in the chapter.

Acceptable Variation and Internal Validity

The maximum allowable analytical variation (CV_a) for repeated testing on an individual should be less than or equal to half of the within-subject (intraindividual) biological variation (CV_b) *(11)*, such that [CV_a 1/2 CV_b]. By adhering to this guideline, the total assay imprecision will not exceed 12% of the biological variation *(12)*. Unfortunately, not many hormone assays achieve such an analytical precision goal. Valero-Politi and Fuentes-Arderiu *(10)*, based on the biological variation data, reported a maximum allowable CV_a of 8.7% for FSH, 12.0% for LH, 5.4% for testosterone, and 6.0% for SHBG. However, the hormone assays they used had an imprecision of 10.3% for FSH, 6.8% for LH, 14.6% for testosterone, and 6.3% for SHBG. The acceptable analytical precision for hormone analysis, therefore, at present, shall be that achievable by the "state-of-the-art" procedures. The "state-of-the-art" precision, defined here as the mean precision for the hormone analyses obtained by the participants in the national proficiency quality assurance programs, is listed in Table 1. To be confident when interpreting exercise- and sport-related hormone analyses, researchers should ensure that their analytical precision is at least close to, if not better than, those that are cited in Table 1.

Laboratories performing hormone analyses must ensure that their assay performance is reliable. This measure of internal validity should include a quality-control program to monitor and maintain both the accuracy and the precision of the hormone assay results. The use of commercially available controls (low, medium, high) can be used to monitor interassay variance and, when used throughout an individual assay, can be used to moni-

Table 1
Analytical Precision for Selected Hormones
and Other Immunoassay Tests

Analyte	State-of-the-art[a] analytical precision, CV%
Aldosterone	11.0
α-feto protein	6.5
Androstenedione	10.0
Cortisol	9.0
Dehydroepiandrosterone sulfate (DHEA-S)	6.0
Estradiol	15.5
FSH	6.5
Gastrin	13.0
Growth hormone (GH)	11.0
Human chorionic gonadotropin (hCG)	10.0
17 Hydroxy Progesterone	12.0
Insulin	7.0
LH	7.0
Progesterone	10.5
Prolactin	7.5
PTH	13.0
Renin	17.0
SHBG	9.0
Testosterone	10.5
Thyroxine binding globulin (TBG)	9.0
Triiodothyronine (T3)	11.0
T4	7.0
Free thyroxine	8.0
TSH	7.0

[a] Estimated from the mean precision obtained from participants of various quality-control programs with analyte levels at reference range.

tor analytical drift. There should also be a strict protocol set for the selection and validation of the commercial assay methodology. There must be criteria set for rejection of individual data (i.e., acceptable intraindividual CV_a limits) or the entire assay results (i.e., acceptable variation on control sample measures taken at the beginning, middle, and end of an assay). Meaningful conclusions can only be drawn from research findings if confidence in the assay results is assured. More discussion of experimental design procedures to ensure internal validity is available from standard research design texts.

SUBJECT PROFILE

Species

It is beyond the scope of this chapter to discuss the details of endocrinological differences among various species. However, inherent differences in the anatomy and physiology of various animals could be expected to influence the adaptive responses observed in response to a physical overload, like exercise. For example, the overload, and subsequent endocrine response, may differ between herbivores and primary carnivores, hibernators and nonhibernators, or even quadrupedal vs bipedal animals. Though there have been some reviews that discuss various differences in exercise metabolism and hormone response between species *(13–16)*, there is only a very superficial body of knowledge available on comparative exercise endocrinology. Given this, researchers should be cautious before making generalizations from species-specific research. A good understanding of comparative physiology is a prerequisite if research conducted on a variety of animals is being used to compare endocrine responses to exercise or physical stress.

Gender

Until puberty, there are few differences in laboratory hormone data between boys and girls. After puberty, the production of testosterone and dihydrotestosterone is much higher in healthy men than women. Salivary testosterone levels, for example, are five-fold higher in men than in women *(17)*. Progesterone in conjunction with estrogen regulates the accessory organs during the menstrual cycle. A surge in LH and FSH occurs to stimulate ovulation in midcycle. Following ovulation, the production of progesterone by the corpus luteum increases rapidly reaching a concentration of 10–20 ng/mL in 4–7 d *(18,19)*. These and other gender-specific endocrine profiles associated with puberty, pregnancy, menstrual cycle, and menopause make direct comparisons between genders difficult. In support of this, several gender differences in hormonal response to an exercise bout have been identified *(15,20–22)*. These include an earlier *(20,21)* and greater *(22)* exercise-induced rise in testosterone in men compared with women and a higher pre-exercise growth hormone level in women *(22)*. It has been speculated that gender differences in steroid responses to exercise may reflect differences in secretion from the gonads vs the adrenals *(21)*. Ruby and Robergs recently discussed the role of several hormones in explaining the gender differences in substrate utilization during exercise *(23)*.

Age and Maturation Status

When designing an experiment to evaluate hormonal responses to exercise or physical training, it is essential that the group used for comparison are matched for age or maturation level. Prepubertal individuals exhibit higher levels of plasma growth hormone when compared to adults *(18)*. During childhood, the circulating levels of sex steroids and gonadotropins are low and gradually rise to adult levels when full sexual maturity is reached *(18)*. Because of these and other hormone variations that occur with age, careful evaluation of maturation level must be performed when matching control and experimental individuals in the circumpubertal years or during menopause. Many hormones also demonstrate an aging effect *(15,19,24,25)*. For example, androgen excretion decreases with advancing age, whereas serum testosterone level does not decline with age in healthy men until the seventh decade *(26,27)*. Dehydroepiandrosterone (DHEA) and its sulfated conjugate (DHEAS) show a clear and substantial age-related decline *(25)*. Gonadotropins, FSH, and LH, on the other hand, increase as one ages *(28)*. Accurate indicators of maturation or biological age should be made and reported when examining hormone responses to exercise or physical training, particularly for circumpubertal or circumenopausal subjects.

Racial Background

Racial differences in certain biochemical constituents have been identified *(24)*. Serum total protein is higher in Blacks than Whites. Glucose tolerance is less in Blacks,

Polynesians, American Indians, and Eskimos than in comparable age- and sex-matched Whites *(24)*. An elevation in parathyroid hormone (PTH) level has been reported in Black compared to White individuals *(29)*. Also, higher estrogen production has been demonstrated in Caucasian women compared to Asian women *(30)*, possibly elevating the risk of breast cancer. Median human chorionic gonadotropin (hCG), unconjugated estriol, and α-fetoprotein levels at various gestational ages are quite different among White, Black, Hispanic, and other women with the highest levels in Asians and Indians *(31)*. Ethnic-specific differences in hormone responses to exercise and training, however, have not been studied.

Pregnancy

Few studies have examined the hormonal responses to exercise in pregnant subjects *(32,33)*. The anatomical and physiological changes associated with pregnancy will affect endocrine responses to exercise. Pregnancy has been described as a diabetogenic state *(32)* and consequently impacts on glucose regulatory and counterregulatory hormones *(32,33)*. Hormonal responses to exercise in pregnant subjects will likely differ between stages of pregnancy and may be different between nulliparous and multiparous subjects. This topic will be addressed in detail in a subsequent chapter.

Body Composition

If exercise workload has been calculated according to body mass (e.g., Wingate anaerobic test), then the muscular overload per unit muscle will be greater in obese individuals. This variation in muscular overload may elicit varying endocrine responses to exercise. Depending on the exercise environment, the thermoregulatory challenge (and subsequent hormonal response) to individuals of different body composition could be profound. Exercise endocrinology research done on individuals with wide variations in body fat should carefully consider how to match exercise demands across subjects.

In addition to the direct effects of differing body composition on the demands of exercise, some differences in resting hormone levels have been identified between obese and nonobese individuals. Johannsson et al. *(34)* demonstrated that growth hormone binding protein was dependent on body fat in humans. Horswill et al. *(35)* provided an interesting discussion on the potential mediating role exercise may have on insulin's contribution to growth in children. In their discussion, Horswill et al. contrast insulin profiles between children with cystic fibrosis (undernourished) and those characterized as obese (overnourished). The tendency for obese individuals to be somewhat insulin-resistant may be an important consideration when designing or interpreting exercise endocrinology research.

Mental Health

Psychological stress stimulates the hypothalamic–pituitary–adrenal axis and the adrenal medulla to secrete stress hormones *(19)*. In most exercise-related hormone studies, blood sampling is required. Venipuncture is a stressful procedure for most individuals. When testing for stress-related hormones (e.g., adrenocorticotropic hormone, cortisol, catecholamines), it is important to get the blood sample before the hormone surge related to the venipuncture has circulated to the vein where the sample is being gathered. Both the acute and chronic stress levels of an individual, whether related to the exercise intervention or to other events in the person's life, could interfere with experimental outcomes.

Altered hormone profiles have also been seen in depressed individuals. For example, lower free thyroxine levels have been observed in depressed adolescents when compared to matched controls *(36)*.

Disease, Surgery, and Medications

The presence of any endocrine or related disease or disorder can interfere with exercise-related hormone changes. This point may appear obvious. However, undetected endocrine disorders often exist. The potential for this to occur provides motivation to inspect individual data visually. During an experiment in our laboratory *(37)* examining DHEAS levels, an otherwise healthy subject was found to have levels 300% higher than the clinical reference range. Simply pooling these results with those from other subjects would have significantly altered the absolute mean level. On the other hand, the relative changes seen in response to certain exercise stimuli were perfectly normal. Most standard texts of endocrinology *(19)* delineate the specific endocrine changes observed with various pathological conditions.

When screening potential candidates for participation in exercise endocrinology research studies, it is essential that a comprehensive medical history is obtained, which includes a summary of any surgery. Any surgery that involved the removal of endocrine tissue (e.g., hysterectomy and ovariectomy) could obviously affect subsequent responses and/or adaptations to exercise.

The use of medications and pharmaceutical interventions can significantly alter endocrine responses to exercise. In many cases, pharmaceutical interventions are used to create a physiologic environment conducive to the experimental question. For example, blocking agents are often used to examine the relative importance of the hormone being blocked to the physiological response being examined. In some cases, the extent of the blocking agent's influence is not clearly known and is influenced by the dose administered *(38)*. Less obvious effects of medications and pharmacological interventions also need to be considered. For example, women using certain oral contraceptives have been shown to have reduced glucose tolerance and insulin sensitivity without a concomitant increase in pancreatic β-cell function *(39)*. Phosphate supplementation can ameliorate the reduction in triiodothyronine observed during low-calorie diets *(40)*. Careful recording and examination of any dietary or pharmaceutical supplements should be made prior to an investigation trying to isolate an endocrine response to exercise.

STANDARDIZED CONDITIONS

Testing Environment: Temperature, Humidity, Altitude, Hypoxia

Conventional guidelines for both applied and clinical exercise testing recommend that standardized testing conditions prevail *(41,42)*. Wherever possible, researchers should ensure that exercise testing be performed at 22°C or less and a relative humidity of 60% or less *(42)*. Failure to standardize these conditions can lead to unnecessary hormonal changes. It is well established that sympathoadrenal activity is augmented at environmental extremes *(15)*. If catecholamines are being measured, the standardization of environmental conditions is essential. Less obvious is the potential impact of varying catecholamine levels on other hormones. For example, an increase in catecholamine level has been speculated to stimulate β-receptors in the testis *(43)* and alter testicular blood flow *(44–46)*, thereby influencing exercise-induced changes in testicular androgens. The effects of altitude *(47)*, hypoxia, and temperature *(15)* on endocrine responses to exercise can be profound. In addition, high levels of humidity will place a proportionately greater challenge on the volume and pressure regulating hormones.

Substance Use

Consistent guidelines with respect to substance use prior to an experimental assessment should be established and enforced. Testing should be performed at least 2 h after subjects have eaten, smoked, or ingested caffeine *(41)*, at least 6 h after subjects have consumed any alcohol *(41)*, and at least 6 h after any previous exercise *(41)*.

Alcohol intoxication has been associated with the suppression of testosterone in a dose-related fashion *(48)*. In contrast, cigaret smoking has been positively correlated with testosterone levels *(49)*. Caffeine ingestion stimulates the central nervous system and the release of epinephrine from the adrenal gland *(50)*. The variable elimination of caffeine further complicates catecholamine research, because the half-life of caffeine ranges from approx 3 to 10 h in different individuals *(51)*. Graham and Spriet have demonstrated that the effect of caffeine on epinephrine levels during exercise is dose-dependent *(52)*. Careful standardization of laboratory conditions and pretesting behavior can minimize the influence of these variables.

Nutritional Status and Hydration

The acute and chronic nutritional status of experimental subjects can profoundly alter hormone levels, particularly those associated with substrate utilization and mobilization (e.g., insulin, glucagon, growth hormone, epinephrine). Clinical blood sampling procedures suggest that specimens be collected in a fasted state. This is often not possible in an applied sport setting, so investigators are required to control or standardize pretesting diets. The influence of diet on hormone levels is not always obvious. For example, steroid hormone levels may be influenced by precursor (cholesterol) availability *(53)*. In fact, a lacto-ovo vegetarian diet can cause minor decreases in testosterone compared to a mixed diet *(54)*. Glucose availability has been shown to have a significant impact on catecholamine responses to exercise *(15)*.

Acid/Base Balance

Changes in tissue pH provoke many physiological responses. Purposeful alterations in the buffering capacity of blood, as with bicarbonate or phosphate loading, may delay or prevent normal changes in pH associated with high-intensity exercise *(55)*. Changes in the buffering capacity of the blood can alter hormonal responses to exercise. Gordon et al. demonstrated that administration of sodium bicarbonate reduced the decrease in pH following high-intensity exercise and also lowered the growth hormone response to exercise *(56)*. It is also known that individuals with compromised or deprived buffer systems show endocrinological changes *(57)*.

Stress Level and Sleep Deprivation

Changes in emotional stress and sleep deprivation can affect hormonal responses to exercise. Studies that have investigated resting or basal testosterone levels pre- and postendurance training, or between endurance-trained and untrained subjects, typically have not measured changes in emotional stress fluctuations, yet this has been shown to influence steroid levels *(58–61)*. Certainly in the studies by Aakvaag et al. *(62,63)* and others *(64,65)*, psychological stress, caloric deficit, and perhaps sleep deprivation contributed to the dramatic change observed in basal testosterone levels. Aakvaag et al. *(63)* demonstrated that sleep rapidly reversed the depressed levels of testosterone and prolactin observed during prolonged physical strain and sleep deprivation. The effect of sleep *(16)* and sleep deprivation *(16,66)* on the hormonal response to exercise has been reviewed elsewhere.

Menstrual Cycle

Much attention and research have been directed toward "The Female Athlete Triad" issues in recent years *(67)*. The potential effects of disordered eating, amenorrhea, and osteoporosis on endocrine function are numerous. Menstrual cycle irregularities can alter both resting hormone levels and hormonal responses to exercise (for reviews, *see* refs. *67–69*). Also, hormonal responses to exercise may be different during different phases of the menstrual cycle *(70,71)*. When evaluating hormonal responses to exercise in females, the absence or presence and phase of menstruation should be considered.

Previous Activity

The proximity of a previous exercise session may affect exercise-related hormone results. Fry et al. *(72)* investigated the hormone changes after intense interval training and found that recovery values were depressed even 24 h later. Lutoslawska et al. *(73)* found decreases in plasma testosterone and testosterone/cortisol ratio 18 h after a 42-km kayak race. Recovery testosterone, cortisol, and SHBG levels have indicated an anabolic deficit for several days after an Olympic distance triathlon *(74)*. These examples suggest that particular attention must be given to experimental conditions when comparing resting hormone measurements from different exercise sessions.

SPECIMEN COLLECTION

Posture

The blood concentrations of body compounds change as one changes posture. In an upright position, an individual's blood volume is 600–700 mL less when compared to a recumbent position. When one goes from supine to standing posture, water and filterable substances move from the intravascular space to the interstitial fluid space, and a reduction of about 10% in blood volume occurs *(24)*. Because only protein-free fluid passes through the capillaries to the tissue, blood concentrations of nonfilterable substances, such as protein and protein-bound steroids, for instance, will increase. The free nonprotein-bound fractions, however, are not affected. Testosterone, for example, is 98–99% protein-bound with 60–75% bound to SHBG and 20–40% to serum albumin. Only 1–2% is unbound. About 10% of cortisol is unbound with 75% bound to transcortin and about 15% bound to albumin. Circulating androstenedione and DHEA are less protein-bound and only bound to albumin.

In general, the shift of body water in a healthy individual will result in an approx 10% increase in total protein and other nonfilterable substances. The normal decrease in blood volume from lying to standing is completed in 10 min, whereas the increase in blood volume from standing to lying is completed in approx 30 min *(24)*.

Apart from the effect of the efflux of intravascular fluid, the action of going from the supine to the standing position also affects a number of hormones, including a dramatic increase in plasma norepinephrine. Increased secretion of other hormones (aldosterone, angiotensin II, renin, antidiuretic hormone [ADH]) is also seen with this change in posture. The increase in catecholamines can be seen within 10 min, whereas plasma aldosterone levels will double within an hour. The plasma atrial natriuretic peptide (ANP) level, on the other hand, decreases as posture is changed from a supine to an upright position *(75)*. Cumming et al. *(76)* speculated that postural differences may explain the discrepancy between the decreased testosterone levels they observed following maximal swimming exercise and the typical increase seen following maximal upright exercise. When one is evaluating the effect of exercise on hormone levels, the condition of specimen collection related to posture must be explicitly stated and controlled.

Circadian and Rhythmic Variation

Throughout the day, most blood hormones fluctuate and exhibit cyclical variation *(16,77)*. The cause of such rhythmic variation may be related to postural changes, activity level, food ingestion, stress, daylight and darkness, and wakefulness and sleep. These fluctuations make it necessary to control the timing of specimen collection strictly. Most hormones are also secreted in a pulsatile fashion and consequently limit the reliability of measurements based on single-sample evaluations.

There is a profound diurnal variation in cortisol secretion with values in the evening being about half those in the morning *(78)*. Adrenocorticotropic hormone (ACTH) secretion is affected by cortisol with the highest concentration occurring between 8 and 10 AM and the lowest values near midnight. The difference between maximum and minimum level may be as high as fivefold. Thyrotropin (TSH) has a diurnal variation in the order of 50% with highest levels occurring at about 2–4 AM and lowest levels between 6 and 10 PM. However, the variation in TSH between 9 AM and 4 PM usually does not exceed 10% *(79–81)*. There is a diurnal variation of total thyroxine (T4) likely related to the binding protein changes brought by postural change. No significant diurnal change in free T4 are seen *(81)*. Plasma testosterone is relatively stable in individuals, showing a small but very consistent diurnal change with peaks occurring at 6–7 AM *(78,82–84)*. However, de Lacerda et al. *(82)* reported that only 20% of the testosterone within subject variation was diurnally related, whereas 80% was random. LH shows no significant circadian rhythm in men, but is secreted intermittently in pulses occurring every 1–6 h, with a mean period of 100 min, in response to pulses of LH-releasing hormone from the hypothalamus *(85)*. Growth hormone secretion is greatest after sleep, and plasma insulin is higher in the morning than late in the day.

A circannual variation pattern has also been established for plasma testosterone with peak levels observed during the summer and a nadir in the winter *(86)*. Controlling for rhythmical variations is essential and is often overlooked in exercise and sport endocrinology research. Thuma et al. *(87)* provide an example and good discussion of the importance of examining hormonal changes relative to the circadian baseline for a given time of day. The relationship between biological rhythms and exercise has been reviewed in more detail elsewhere *(16)*.

Specimen Collection and Storage

Proper precautions must be taken in the collection, transportation, and storage of hormone samples. Blood for hormone analysis may be obtained from veins, arteries, or capillaries. Venous blood is, however, the specimen of choice. Venous occlusion by the use of a tourniquet will cause fluid and low-mol-wt compounds to pass through the capillary wall similar to the postural effect. Small changes in the blood concentration of the substance occurs if the tourniquet use is less than a minute, but marked changes may be seen after 3 min *(24)*. For example, an increase of protein-bound compound by 15% after 3 min of stasis has been seen *(24)*. This stasis effect is particularly important for peptides and protein hormones that do not equilibrate with the interstitium. A uniform procedure for blood collection must be used throughout an investigation.

Many protein hormones are thermally labile and serum or plasma samples should be stored frozen. Examples of these are ACTH, ADH, calcitonin, gastrin, glucagon, growth hormone, insulin, PTH, prolactin, and renin. ACTH, glucagon and renin are required to be separated from the blood cells immediately after collection at 4°C.

Except for free testosterone, steroids are very stable, and no special precautions are necessary during collection and storage. However, if analysis cannot be performed within a short time period, freezing the separated serum or plasma is necessary. Repeated freezing and thawing of serum, plasma, or urine samples should be avoided, since hydrolysis of the conjugates may occur and will yield falsely high values for the unconjugated steroid. Nonpolar steroids, such as progesterone and androstenedione, are very unstable when stored at −20°C in aqueous solution without protein (i.e., in urine sample). As much as 80% of the steroid may be lost after 6 mo of storage, unless an inert protein at a concentration of 0.1–0.5 g/L is added for preservation *(18)*.

Studies have shown that the results of biochemical analyses are similar when samples are collected in plastic or glass containers *(88)*. Steroid hormones, however, are hydrophobic and may interact differently with glass and plastic tubes *(89,90)*. A recent study indicated that for commonly measured hormones, no statistical differences were found between serum-separator glass and serum-separator plastic tubes *(91)*. Statistically significant (but probably not clinically significant) differences were found between plain glass tubes and serum-separator glass tubes for DHEAS and estradiol *(91)*.

Choice of Specimen

Although 24-hr urinary hormone assays are considered to reflect the secretory activity of the endocrine glands, blood samples are the preferred specimen for most exercise-induced hormone studies. Both serum and plasma samples give similar steroid hormone results. Rapid separation of red cells from the blood sample is important, since red cells at room temperature can alter the plasma concentration of active steroid hormones. Red cells degrade estradiol to estrone and cortisol to cortisone, and absorb testosterone. Plasma has an advantage over serum, since it can be removed from the red cells faster and subsequently put in cold storage. For plasma, heparin is the preferred anticoagulant over ethylenediaminetetra-acetic acid (EDTA), since it causes the least interference with most tests. EDTA causes up to a 25, 15, and 10% decrease in TSH, LH, and estradiol, respectively, and erratic changes in progesterone. In comparison, heparin causes a 10, 8, 8, and up to 15% decrease in T4, LH, estradiol, and progesterone, respectively *(92)*. Furthermore, samples collected with EDTA yield high free testosterone results *(93)*. Plasma samples also allow fibrin clot formation if stored for prolonged periods after collection. Consequently, serum is the preferred sample for most radioimmunoassay (RIA) hormone evaluations.

Recently, there has been great interest in measuring free steroid hormones with saliva specimens *(94–96)*. Saliva steroid levels appear to correlate well with the concentration of free steroid in serum *(95,97–99)*. The use of salivary samples for protein hormones is limited. Halimi et al. *(100)* reported that the measurement of insulin-like growth factor-1 (IGF-1) in saliva is less reliable than the determination in serum in the evaluation of the disease activity in acromegaly. Saliva sampling allows for frequent and easy specimen collection, and is noninvasive. This approach is stress-free, which is particularly important when assessing adrenal steroid hormones. Cook et al. *(97)* have used the saliva-sampling technique to assess the adrenal and testicular hormone activity of marathon runners. Judging by the missed sample rate of <10%, they concluded the collection of saliva samples on run and test days was well accepted by marathon runners and that salivary sampling is of value in monitoring acute and rhythmic changes in endocrine function in marathon runners. Although the saliva cortisol parallels the plasma cortisol during controlled study *(101)*, recent reports have cautioned the interpretation of dynamic hormone results obtained from saliva samples.

Despite all the advantages that saliva offers for measuring steroid hormones, there are limitations. Because only the free fraction enters the salivary gland, the steroid concentration is 50- to 100-fold lower in saliva than in serum. Therefore, methods with high sensitivity must be used. The contamination of saliva with traces of blood owing to small lacerations of the gum and the mucosa would falsely increase the saliva hormone level. Schramm et al. *(102)* have shown a 9% increase in testosterone levels in whole saliva after toothbrushing, but with no changes in the ultrafiltrate of saliva. They attribute this to the blood protein contamination resulting from toothbrushing. Between 20 and 50% of people have hemoglobin from blood in saliva *(103)*. Furthermore, there is the presence of a steroid-metabolizing enzyme in the salivary gland *(104,105)*. Swinkels et al. *(106)* have shown an in vivo conversion of androstenedione to testosterone by 17-hydroxysteroid oxidoreductase activity in the salivary gland. The other potential problem associated with salivary hormone measurement is that the salivary protein or cellular debris from the mucosa can interfere with the processing of saliva samples, and may produce a disproportionately high binding of steroid hormones *(107)*. Hofreiter et al. *(108)* and Silver et al. *(109)* have shown that saliva samples exhibited fractional decreases in cortisol concentration as a function of time at room temperature. Preservation of saliva is therefore necessary if sample analytes are not determined within a short period. Chen et al. *(110)* have successfully preserved salivary cortisol by adding citric acid at a concentration of 10 g/L. The stability of other saliva steroid samples remains to be studied.

To overcome some of the problems with salivary sampling, Schramm's group *(103)* reported the development of a device for the *in situ* collection of an ultrafiltrate of saliva and used the device to determine free progesterone. The possible drawback of such sampling is the longer time required for saliva collection (15 min). Similarly, a device designed to produce samples representing the average tissue availability of steroids over known periods of time has also been developed *(111,112)*. It is used to obtain saliva samples in a defined time interval rather than at a particular moment, and thus may be used in studies of hormones that are secreted episodically and rapidly cleared. The suitability of these sampling devices for exercise-induced hormone studies needs further evaluation.

Hemolysis

Hemolysis is common in blood specimens, occurring when blood contacts foreign surfaces. Visible hemolysis is seen when hemoglobin concentration is >0.2 g/L *(113,114)*.

In general, only a negligible analytical effect is seen with slight hemolysis, but severe hemolysis introduces a dilutional effect in addition to the leakage of cell constituents. Yucel and Dalva *(115)* found that most common biochemical tests are unaffected by hemolysis. The effect of hemolysis on hormones has not been well studied. Since erythrocytes metabolize steroid hormones, hemolysis can affect results and should be avoided. For most protein hormone assays, grossly hemolyzed specimens should not be used, because the protein binding effect of the RIA may be altered. To avoid in vitro hemolysis, small-bore needles are preferred to large-bore needles for blood collection *(116)*.

Experimental Intrusion and Sampling Frequency

Depending on the details of the experimental protocol (e.g., clothing, environment, physical confinement, invasive probes, mouthpiece/nose clips, presence of technicians, exercise protocol), the physical and emotional stress between individuals may vary greatly. Though this is inherent in research of this type, attention to the magnitude of experimental intrusion is necessary when interpreting the experimental outcomes, and particularly when trying to generalize to nonlaboratory situations.

The frequency of blood sampling can introduce small errors in hormone measurements. Because blood volume is changed (although slightly) with each sample removed, the probability of blood removal impacting on the level of hormone being measured increases with each subsequent sample. Under normal circumstances, the ethical review process will prevent experimental protocols that require large volumes of blood to be removed, thereby minimizing the effect of sampling frequency.

ANALYTICAL PROCEDURE

A wide range of assay techniques are available for hormone measurements. From the early use of bioassay and chemical colorimetric methods, the methodologies now have advanced to include chromatographic techniques and immunoassays, with each having its distinct application.

Bioassay

Bioassays are based on a specific physiological response on a tested animal or mammalian cell or tissue section induced by the hormone contained in the sample. Using a reference preparation or standard, the physiological response of the unknown sample is graded, and the hormone level estimated. Owing to the impurity of the sample and the variability of animal response, bioassays are fairly imprecise and lack sensitivity *(18)*. Bioassays are also labor-intensive. There may also be problems in obtaining sufficient amounts of standard material for testing. Nevertheless, bioassays still play an important role in basic and pharmaceutical research *(117–119)*.

Colorimetric and Fluorometric Assays

Many steroids have chemical functional groups that react with particular chemical reagents to produce specific color products. For instance, the keto group at the 17 position of steroids reacts with *m*-dinitrobenzene to produce a purplish color *(18)*. The intensity of this color can be measured by a photometer and is proportional to the amount of steroid present. Similarly, some steroid compounds (e.g., estrogens) produce fluorescence in concentrated sulfuric acid or phosphoric acid. The emitted light can be measured.

The colorimetric method is nonspecific, and many other compounds may interfere and give similar-colored products. The assay is not sensitive enough to measure hormones present in minute amounts. Fluorometric assay, although more specific and sensitive than the colorimetric assay, has problems with nonspecific background fluorescence and the quenching effect caused by the solvent or impure reagents. Both colorimetric and fluorometric assays require relatively inexpensive equipment and are therefore used for measuring some hormones when absolute accuracy of the assay may not be required.

Chromatographic Assays

The common chromatographic techniques employed for hormone determination are gas chromatography (GC) and high-performance liquid chromatography (HPLC). GC has been used for steroid measurement, and the technique is accurate, specific, and sensitive. Recently, HPLC assay, owing to its speed and increased sensitivity, has become increasingly used in steroid and some low-mol-wt hormone measurements. In contrast to GC, derivitization is not normally required. HPLC can also be used to measure nonvolatile and thermal labile hormones, which GC is not capable of handling.

One specific advantage of chromatographic assays is that a family of related compounds can be measured simultaneously, and thus, they are especially useful in steroid determination and in the study of hormone synthesis, transformation, and metabolism. Because chromatographic assays can have high degrees of discrimination between chemical structures, they are often used for specific hormone analysis prior to the development of its immunoassay method.

Receptor Assays

Radioreceptor assays are based on the displacement of the radioactively labeled hormone from the cell receptor site by the sample hormone. Specific protein hormone receptors from cellular plasma membrane or steroid receptors from nuclei proteins are used. This assay technique has been applied to the determination of many hormones, such as insulin, glucagon, growth hormone, prolactin, and T4. This assay procedure has the advantage of measuring the active hormone. It is much more sensitive and specific than the bioassay. The problems with this technique are the impurity of the receptor material, interference by other compounds, and the instability of the receptor preparation in the absence of the hormone or stabilizing agent. The lack of sufficient quantity of stable receptor preparation limits its present use. With the advancement of recombinant technology and more receptor proteins being cloned *(120,121)* leading to the production of high-affinity receptors, the application of receptor assays may be expanded in the future, particularly in basic research.

Immunoassays

Immunoassay is an analytical technique that depends on the reaction of the analyte (e.g., hormone) of interest (the antigen) and its binding protein (the antibody). Immunoassays that use a radioactive labeled tracer are described as an RIA. During the past two decades, there have been major advances in RIA technology. Because of its speed, simplicity, and specificity, RIA has been used for nearly all types of hormones. The technique eliminates specimen purification, hydrolysis, or extraction required by colorimetric, fluorometric, GC, and HPLC assays. RIA offers very high analytical sensitivity, making the measurement of many free hormones possible.

Although RIA has been widely used, the biohazardous nature of radioactive tracers is a concern. Recently, newer nonradioactive labeled immunoassays have become available. These assays include the fluorescence immunoassay (FIA), enzyme immunoassay (EIA), chemiluminescent immunoassay (CLIA), and the latest electrochemiluminescent immunoassay (ECIA). FIA uses a fluorescent substance as the tagging agent. In EIA, an enzyme substrate color-forming system is employed. Similarly, a light-generating chemical reaction system with a flurophor (acridinum ester or luminol) is used in CLIA. In ECIA, the emission of light from a ruthenium label is initiated by electricity, thus eliminating the adding and mixing of the chemical reagents and, hence, improved precision.

The use of nonisotopic labels also facilitates the introduction of automation for hormone measurements. CLIA assays are more sensitive than EIA and are equal to or better than the RIA method in terms of sensitivity *(122)*. CLIA is able to measure analytes to the femtogram (10^{-15} g)/mL level. With the improved features, such as reagent stability, high sensitivity, relatively cheap reagent cost, and being environmentally friendly, CLIA is now becoming the technique of choice for most hormone determinations.

Specificity and Crossreactivity

The specificity of a method relates to the ability of the method to measure one specific compound of interest and no other compounds. For immunoassays, this is mainly determined by the antibody used. Polyclonal antibodies, where the antiserum is raised in an animal host in response to the immunogen administration, are derived from different plasma cell lines and thus possess diverse specificities in their reaction to the immunogen. Monoclonal antibodies (MAbs), on the other hand, are derived from a single clone or plasma cell line in response to immunization, and as such are more specific than polyclonal antibodies.

Specificity of the antiserum is normally represented by the degree of crossreactivity of the antiserum with other structurally similar compounds. Crossreactivity is expressed in terms of the mass of the analyte required to displace 50% of the tracer from the label-bound analyte. Thus, percent crossreactivity of a substance Y with respect to the antibody produced against a substance Z is equal to $[(a/b) \times 100]$ where a = mass of substance Z required to displace 50% of bound labeled Z; and b = mass of substance Y required to displace 50% of bound labeled Z. One other method of estimating the percent crossreactivity of an antiserum is by direct spiking of the sample with the interference compound to detect the apparent increase in the concentration of the analyte of interest.

The problem with crossreactivity is considerable in steroid assays as a result of the small structural differences among various classes of steroids. In protein hormone assays, because of prohormones and metabolized fragments, crossreactivity may still exist. Some hormones have similar antigen binding sites, such as the α-subunit of glycoprotein hormones—LH, FSH, TSH, and hCG. Polyclonal antibodies raised against any of these hormones may crossreact to other hormones having similar α-subunits. Immunoassay kits supplied by different suppliers may have antisera with different specificities and crossreactivities. It is paramount to note what crossreacts with the particular assay that one uses when interpreting the experimental results. Most manufacturers provide crossreactivity data of potential interfering compounds. Any compound that is not listed, but is important to a particular study in the manipulation of the experimental data should have its crossreactivity checked.

It is also possible to increase the analytical specificity of immunoassays by adjusting the kinetic or equilibrium conditions, by sample purification or extraction and by modifying the thermodynamic conditions of the assays (123). If RIA methodologies are used, researchers must also not use expired tracers, since radioactivity drift influences the performance of the assay.

Future Development

The future development of immunoassays for hormone measurement will likely include: producing homogenous assays for automation, simplifying assay procedures, development of recombinant proteins with specific binding epitopes on hormones, advancement of detection techniques with the use of immunosensors (124), and measuring hormones *in situ* for continuous monitoring. In the nonimmunoassay area, advancements will be made in detecting small mol-wt hormones, in chromatographic techniques combined with high-resolution mass spectrometry, particularly in the determination of performance enhancing compounds, such as synthetic steroids and recombinant peptide hormones (125).

EXERCISE VARIABLES

The subsequent chapters in this text will review in detail the effects of exercise on the specific hormones. Consequently, this section will merely introduce the various exercise variables that have been shown to influence hormonal responses to exercise.

Intensity

Exercise intensity has a profound influence on hormone dynamics with plasma levels of most hormones being elevated after a bout of intense exercise (a notable exception is insulin) (15). For example, Yoon and Park (126) showed a clear dose–response relationship between exercise intensity and plasma levels of β-endorphin, ACTH, and cortisol. There is also evidence that lactate production associated with intense exercise directly or indirectly affects the hormone response to exercise (127,128).

The endocrine changes observed with changes in exercise intensity are intricately linked to exercise duration. Kuoppasalmi et al. (129) demonstrated that LH and testosterone did not change in response to maximal short-term running, whereas both hormones were depressed following a moderate intensity run of 90 min. Using heavy-resistance exercise protocols, Hakkinen and Pakarinen found similar results, showing that 20 sets of 1 repetition maximum (RM) lifts produced no change in testosterone, cortisol, or growth hormone, whereas 10 sets of 10 RM lifts produced significant increases in all three hormones (130). It has also been demonstrated that significant changes in training duration vs training intensity produce significantly different hormonal changes (131). The quantification of intensity is further complicated by the findings of Kraemer et al. (132), who identified the length of the rest period between exercise sets during resistance exercise as an important factor influencing postexercise hormone levels.

Duration

Most hormones show distinct time-related changes during exercise. The effect of varying exercise duration on reproductive hormone function in males has been reviewed by

Cumming et al. *(133)* and generally demonstrates an initial rise in testosterone during exercise of relatively short duration, but prolonged exercise of >2 h typically results in reduced levels. Similar findings have been reported elsewhere *(129)*. Growth hormone rises sharply during short-term exercise after an initial delay of about 10 min, but plateaus after about 30 min of exercise *(134)*. Glucagon and cortisol do not increase significantly during submaximal exercise until after 60 min or more *(134)*. Norepinephrine levels, in contrast, show significant increases within minutes of initiating exercise *(134)*.

Volume

The product of exercise intensity and exercise duration is exercise volume. Kraemer et al. *(132)* suggested that exercise volume (sets × repetitions × intensity) is an important determinant of hormonal response in men, whereas Mulligan et al. demonstrated a resistance exercise volume effect in women *(135)*. In support of a volume effect, Guezennec et al. *(136)* found no changes in testosterone levels following moderate intensity (70% 1 RM) low-volume (1 exercise, 7 sets) exercise, but Weiss et al. *(137)* showed significant elevations in serum testosterone following moderate intensity (80% 1 RM) and moderate volume (4 exercises, 3 sets) exercise. Furthermore, those hormones related to energy substrate availability (e.g., insulin, glucagon, epinephrine, growth hormone) will be influenced by exercise volume. Tremblay matched the volume of exercise completed during a weight training session with a treadmill running session based on caloric expenditure values *(37)*. Cortisol, DHEAS, and testosterone levels were significantly higher following the weight training session. These findings likely demonstrate the effect of differing exercise intensities and suggest that the influence of exercise volume as an independent variable is not as important as the combination of exercise intensity and duration. Jezova et al. *(138)* have also suggested that hormonal responses to physical effort depend more on exercise intensity than total work output. After controlling for external work output, exercise duration, and work–rest intervals during vertical leg lifts, VanHelder et al. *(139)* found that growth hormone responses varied depending on the external load and number of repetitions.

Mode/Type

The mode of exercise under examination can affect exercise-related hormone changes. For example, in contrast to the literature on running *(140)*, cycling *(141)*, and resistance exercise *(142)*, Cumming et al. observed a decrease in testosterone levels following intense swimming exercise *(76)*. These authors speculated that changes in hepatic blood flow resulting from the horizontal posture and/or immersion-related hemodilution may explain these contrasting results. Tremblay *(37)* directly compared steroid hormone results between moderate intensity treadmill running (50–55% VO_2 max) and circuit weight training (8–10 RM), and found testosterone, cortisol, and DHEAS values to be higher following resistance exercise. In contrast to these findings, Jensen et al. *(143)* observed no difference in testosterone concentrations following intense endurance exercise compared to strength exercise. Jensen et al. noted that despite profound interindividual differences, individual subjects tended to respond similarly to each type of exercise *(143)*. Kraemer *(142)* suggested that some hormonal responses to exercise are dependent on exceeding a certain threshold intensity, volume, and muscle mass activation. Clearly, different modes of exercise will influence these factors. Kindermann et al. *(144)* demonstrated different hormone responses when comparing anaerobic to aerobic exercise.

Finally, the environmental conditions existing during any activity (e.g., open water swimming in cool water vs running a tropical marathon) can influence the hormonal response to exercise, as previously discussed.

Initial Training Status

In general, if subjects perform an exercise bout at an absolute exercise intensity, untrained subjects will elicit more profound endocrine changes than their trained counterparts *(145)*. A blunted hormone response is particularly evident in endurance-trained athletes *(146)* even when relative exercise intensities are used *(37)*. Catecholamine levels during submaximal exercise are lower in trained subjects than untrained subjects *(15)*. The postexercise elevation of cortisol frequently seen following intense or prolonged exercise has been shown to be persistently elevated in untrained subjects, but not trained subjects *(147)*. Luger et al. *(145)* also concluded that physical conditioning is associated with a reduction in pituitary–adrenal activation in response to an absolute workload. In contrast to these findings, Pyka et al. found no differences in growth hormone or IGF-1 response to exercise between resistance-trained and untrained older adults *(148)*, indicating a potential age–hormone response interaction effect. Some studies have demonstrated changes in basal levels of hormones in response to regular training programs *(149,150)* (see refs. *15,133,134* for reviews), whereas others have not *(151,152)*. In addition, resting testosterone and cortisol levels appear to be unresponsive to a reduction in training *(153)*. Remes et al. *(154)* and Schmid et al. *(155)* have also observed modifications in androgen responses to physical exercise with changes in fitness level. Hackney et al. *(156)* speculated that depressed testosterone levels found subsequent to 4–6 wk of intensive training may be related to elevated prolactin levels simultaneously observed. Because testosterone and prolactin levels rebounded to near pretraining levels after 8 wk of training, the altered levels noticed after 4–6 wk may have represented a relative overtraining period.

Frequency of Training and Overtraining

The frequency of exercise bouts has been demonstrated to impact on subsequent hormone concentrations *(157–159)*. Hakkinen et al. found that two successive strength-training sessions in one day elicited different hormone responses *(157)*. Furthermore, these endocrine differences change as several double workout days are linked together *(158)*. In this latter study, the authors suggested that the progressive decrease in testosterone during the training period was indicative of the magnitude of the physiologic stress of training *(158)*. If a high volume of training persists, the threat of overtraining symptoms increases. Because characteristics of overtraining include changes in endocrine function, including hypothalamic dysfunction *(159,160)*, a decrease in plasma-free testosterone/cortisol ratio *(161)*, and a decrease in nocturnal catecholamine excretion *(131)*, attention must be given to the training regimen of subjects prior to testing. Other indicators of overtraining (weight loss, reduced appetite, reduced quality of sleep, lethargy), which may influence hormone levels, should also be monitored. The effects of overtraining on the endocrine system are discussed in detail in Chapter 20.

Length of Training Intervention

There is a lack of research that provides time-course changes in basal or resting hormone levels in response to exercise training. Because information in this area is lacking, it is difficult to interpret research results from short-term intervention studies. For example, if no changes in resting hormones levels were observed after 8 wk of training, should the conclusion be that training does not affect the resting levels of hormones? Perhaps the adaptation requires a longer period. In some cases, resting levels of hormones may not change until structural adaptations have occurred and relatively short-term studies would fail to observe these results. When possible, study results should be compared to findings from studies with similar design and protocol characteristics.

SECULAR TRENDS AND EVOLUTION

Secular trends suggest that the average age at mortality is increasing, children and adolescents are larger and more mature than their same-aged peers of previous generations *(162)*, and North American children are becoming fatter *(163)*. These and other secular trends could modify basal hormone levels at any particular age and may also influence the hormonal response to exercise. Correction for, or at least acknowledgment of, important secular trends is necessary, particularly when making data comparisons across extended time periods. It is also important to consider the sensitivity and specificity of the analytical procedure used to derive hormone levels when comparing research results from different decades or generations. Although there is no research available, it is also conceivable that rapid changes in the environment (e.g., ozone depletion, deforestation, increased CO_2 emissions, climatic variations) and lifestyle behaviors (e.g., sedentary living, more electronic interaction, changes in the preparation of food, increased reliance on medications) could change the amount and pattern of hormone circulation. Any resultant adaptations from changes in basal hormone levels that occur as we evolve as a species will likely alter the bodies response to an exercise stimulus. The potential influence of any such variation is likely exceedingly small across a researcher's career and any effects from recent evolutionary adaptations remain only speculation.

DATA PRESENTATION AND ANALYSIS

Data Manipulation

Depending on the experimental situation, sampling procedures, and analytical methods employed, some data manipulation may be required before performing statistical analyses. Two particular data manipulation procedures are relevant in exercise endocrinology research: adjustments for changes in plasma volume and data transformation to reflect either net change or relative change in hormone concentration.

The issue of correcting for exercise-induced changes in plasma volume has been discussed repeatedly. For example, the increase in testosterone seen following an acute bout of exercise has been explained by many as a mere reflection of hemoconcentration *(137,144,164–166)*. If the question being addressed relates to hormone secretion or clearance, then concern over changes in plasma volume is warranted. If, however, the question relates to biological responses dependent on plasma hormone concentrations, then the issue of correcting for plasma volume changes is moot. Kraemer submits that when the blood concentration of hormones increases, regardless of the mechanism, increased interaction with receptors is possible *(166)*.

Exercise-induced plasma volume shifts may complicate the interpretation of changes in plasma hormone concentrations. If, for example, free testosterone is the only biologically active fraction, then the plasma volume shift from vascular to extravascular compartments that is typical during exercise will likely confound plasma levels since unbound testosterone passively exits the capillary. This shift of fluid out of the plasma should result in a proportional quantity of free testosterone leaving the plasma, and therefore, subsequent plasma measurements may not demonstrate an increase associated with hemoconcentration. This could be misinterpreted as a reduction in free hormone availability, since the extravascular free testosterone may enter the target cell or return to the plasma for further circulation. If target tissue stimulation is of interest, it may be inappropriate to correct hormone concentrations for changes in plasma volume.

The process of normalization has been used in several investigations *(43,76,87,143,147,167,168)*. The appropriateness of such transformations depends on the research question being addressed. In some cases, failure to transform data can mask existing differences. For example, a change in LH from 4.0 to 4.5 IU/L may not produce the same biological response as a change from 1.0 to 1.5 IU/L. In this case, the net change is the same (0.5 IU/L), but the relative change is very different (12 vs 50%). Because of the typical downregulation response of hormone receptors to an increase in hormone exposure, it would seem that changes in hormone concentrations are important in terms of biological impact. In fact, changes in hormone levels have been correlated with changes in sport performance indicators. For example, Alen and Hakkinen *(169)* concluded that serum-free testosterone played an important role during intensive strength training because of the significant correlation between changes in maximal strength and changes in testosterone/SHBG ratio. The relevance of this change depends on what is actually important to the target tissues. If the tissues only respond to absolute concentration levels, then this finding is unimportant. If the cells respond according to a change in concentration, then these findings are relevant. It may be that the relative change is most important.

Sometimes it is necessary to transform hormone results to achieve a distribution of data points that accommodates the assumptions required to conduct the statistical test being used properly. This requires some knowledge of the underlying situation generating the data. Finally, transformation of the data may actually simplify the statistical analysis. When baseline values are used in an analysis of variance (ANOVA) to account for values observed later in the subject, the baseline value is often included as a covariate. In order for the baseline to be properly taken into account, the relationship between the response and the baseline value should be linear. However, an analysis of the change (relative or absolute) may be simpler and require fewer assumptions. Thuma et al. *(87)* demonstrated recently the importance of adjusting exercise-induced hormone changes for pre-exercise hormone levels and diurnal hormone variations during the testing period.

If an experimental design employs sequential specimen sampling, the statistical analyses can be performed by using repeated measures and/or area under the curve (AUC). The latter technique has been successfully used in bioavailability studies *(170)*. If comparisons between any time-points are of interest, or if potential interactions between time and any of the main effects are important, then a repeated measures analysis is necessary. If the physiological impact of a series of measurements, irrespective of whether specific time-related variations is of concern, then the AUC analyses may be simpler and better. Both analytical methods can be used for group and session comparisons; however, the results may differ somewhat owing to differences in degrees of freedom and error terms. The repeated measures analysis includes more information; however, it also

Table 2
Summary of Potential Confounding or Interfering Variables
for Exercise Endocrinology Research

Potential confounding variable	Relative impact on hormone measurement
Subject profile	
Species	+
Gender	++
Age and maturation status	+++
Racial background	+
Pregnancy	++
Body composition	+
Mental health	+
Disease, surgery, medications	+++
Standardized conditions	
Temperature and humidity	++
Altitude and hypoxia	++
Substance use	+
Nutritional status	++
Hydration	++
Acid/base balance	+
Emotional stress	+
Sleep deprivation	++
Menstrual cycle	+
Previous activity	+++
Specimen collection	
Posture	++
Rhythmical variations	+++
Specimen collection	++
Specimen storage	++
Choice of specimen	++
Hemolysis	++
Experimental intrusion	+
Analytical procedure	
Assay type	++
Specificity and crossreactivity	+++
Exercise variables	
Exercise intensity	+++
Exercise duration	+++
Exercise volume	+
Exercise type	++
Initial training status	++
Overtraining	++
Length of training intervention	+

places greater stress on the assumptions required in the more complex repeated measures design. The AUC has the stability of a time-weighted average and carries the information of overall hormone level differences between groups.

Finally, studies in which conclusions are based on small sample sizes are obligated to disclose individual responses, since grouped data may not be indicative of individual responses *(171)*, and may be significantly influenced by random biological variation. The consistency of hormone response, both within and between subjects, should be considered and where possible individual data should be presented.

Statistical Considerations

Inappropriate statistical analyses can lead to incorrect conclusions. Addressing the problems identified in the previous section will help to reduce problems with data analyses. For a summary of some of the statistical issues related to exercise endocrinology, the reader is referred to a previous review article by Tremblay et al. *(2)* and standard statistical references *(172–175)*.

SUMMARY

This chapter has attempted to provide a brief review of some of the issues to consider when designing research experiments in exercise endocrinology. It is hoped that the methodological considerations examined in this chapter will assist researchers and clinicians in making informed and critical interpretations of published work in this area. The methodological considerations in this chapter have been presented in a "checklist" fashion to accommodate subsequent referrals to particular methodological issues. The confounding variables discussed in this chapter rarely manifest their effect in isolation, but rather present themselves as some composite reflecting the interaction of many of the variables presented here. The complicated integration of the various confounding effects discussed in this chapter is important to recognize and consider.

Table 2 provides a summary of the potential confounding variables discussed in this chapter, including the authors' evaluation of their relative importance. Other review articles in this area are also available *(2,176)*.

REFERENCES

1. Stryer L. Biochemistry. W.H. Freeman and Company, New York, 1988.
2. Tremblay MS, Chu SY, Mureika R. Methodological and statistical considerations for exercise-related hormone evaluations. Sports Med 1995;20:90–108.
3. William GZ, Young DS, Stein MR, Cotlove E. Biological and analytic components of variation in long-term studies of serum constituents in normal subjects: I. Objective, subject, selection of laboratory procedure and estimation of analytic derivation. Clin Chem 1970;16:1016–1021.
4. Harris EK, Kanefsky P, Shakarji G, Cotlove E. Biological and analytic components of variation in long-term studies of serum constituents in normal subjects: II. Estimating biological component of variation. Clin Chem 1970;16:1022–1027.
5. Kingle RD, Johnson GF. Statistical procedure. In: Tietz NW, ed. Textbook of Clinical Chemistry. Saunders, Philadelphia, 1986, pp. 287–355.
6. Rotterdam EP, Katan MB, Knuiman JT. Importance of time interval between repeated measurements of total or high-density lipoprotein cholesterol when estimating an individual's baseline concentration. Clin Chem 1987;33:1913–1915.
7. Choudhury N, Lyons-Wall PM, Truswell AS. Effect of time between measurements on within-subject variability for total cholesterol and high-density lipoprotein cholesterol in women. Clin Chem 1994;40:710–715.
8. Fraser CG, Harris EK. Generation and application of data on biological variation in clinical chemistry. Crit Rev Clin Lab Sci 1989;27:409–437.
9. Chu SY. Depression of serum cholinesterase activity as an indicator of insecticide exposure—consideration of the analytical and biological variation. Clin Biochem 1985;18:323–326.

10. Valero-Politi J, Fuentes-Arderiu X. Within and between subject biological variation of FSH, LH, Testosterone and sex hormone binding globulin in men. Clin Chem 1993;39:1723–1725.
11. Harris EK. Statistical principles underlying analytical goal setting in clinical chemistry. Am J Clin Pathol 1979;72:274–282.
12. Fraser CG, Harris EK. Generation and application of data on biological variation in clinical chemistry. Crit Rev Clin Lab Sci 1989;27:409–437.
13. Hargraves M, ed. Exercise Metabolism. Human Kinetics, Champaign, 1995.
14. Graham TE, MacLean DA. Ammonia and amino acid metabolism in skeletal muscle: human, rodent and canine models. Med Sci Sports Exerc 1998;30:34–36.
15. Galbo H. Hormonal and Metabolic Adaptation to Exercise. Georg Thieme Verlag, New York, 1983.
16. Reilly T, Atkinson G, Waterhouse J. Biological Rhythms & Exercise. Oxford University Press, New York, 1997.
17. Dabbs JM Jr, Campbell BC, Galdue BA, Midgley AR, Navarro MA, Read GF, et al. Reliability of salivary testosterone measurement: a multicenter evaluation. Clin Chem 1995;41:1581–1584.
18. Chattoraj SC, Watts NB. Endocrinology. In: Tietz NW, ed. Textbook of Clinical Chemistry. Saunders, Philadelphia, 1986, pp. 997–1171.
19. Wilson JD, Foster DW, eds. Williams Textbook of Endocrinology, 8th ed. Saunders, Philadelphia, 1992.
20. Webb ML, Wallace JP, Hamill C, Hodgson JL, Mashaly MM. Serum testosterone concentration during two hours of moderate intensity treadmill running in trained men and women. Endocrinol Res 1984;10:27–38.
21. Bunt JC, Bahr JM, Bemben DA. Comparison of estradiol and testosterone levels during and immediately following prolonged exercise in moderately active males and females. Endocrinol Res 1987;13:157–172.
22. Kraemer WJ, Gordon SE, Fleck SJ, Marchitelli LJ, Mello R, Dziados JE, et al. Endogenous anabolic hormonal and growth factor response to heavy resistance exercise in males and females. Int J Sports Med 1991;12:228–235.
23. Ruby BC, Robergs RA. Gender differences in substrate utilisation during exercise. Sports Med 1994;17:393–410.
24. Young DS, Bermes EW. Specimen collection and processing: source of biological variation. In: Tietz NW, ed. Textbook of Clinical Chemistry. Saunders, Philadelphia, 1986, pp. 478–518.
25. Orentreich N, Brind JL, Rizer RL, Vogelman JH. Age changes and sex differences in serum dehydroepiandrosterone sulfate concentrations throughout adulthood. J Clin Endocrinol Metab 1984;59:551–555.
26. Vermeulen A. Testosterone excretion, plasma levels and testosterone production in health and disease. In: Tamm J, ed. Testosterone. Hafner, New York, 1967, pp. 170–175.
27. Purifoy FE, Koopmars LH, Tatum RW. Steroid hormones and aging: free testosterone, testosterone and androstenedione in normal females age 20–87 years. Hum Biol 1980;52:181–191.
28. Isurugi K, Fukutani K, Takayasu H, Wakabayashi K, Tamaoki B. Age related changes in serum LH and FSH level in normal men. J Clin Endocrinol Metab 1974;39:955–957.
29. Fuleihan E, Gundberd CM, Gleason R. Racial differences in parathyroid hormone dynamics. J Clin Endocrinol Metab 1994;76:1642–1647.
30. Adlercreutz H, Goldin BR. Estrogen metabolism and excretion in Oriental and Caucasian women. J Natl Cancer Inst 1994;86:1076–1082.
31. Benn PA, Clive JM, Collins R. Medians for second trimester maternal serum AFP, unconjugated estriol, and hCG: difference between race or ethnic groups. Clin Chem 1997;43:333–337.
32. Mittelmark RA. Hormonal responses to exercise in pregnancy. In: Mittelmark RA, Wiswell RA, Drinkwater BL, eds. Exercise in Pregnancy. Williams and Wilkins, Baltimore, 1991, pp. 175–184.
33. McMurray RG, Mottola MF, Wolfe LA, Artal R, Millar L, Pivarnik JM. Recent advances in understanding maternal and fetal responses to exercise. Med Sci Sports Exerc 1993;25:1305–1321.
34. Johannsson G, Bjarnason R, Bramnert M, Carlsson LM, Degerblad M, Manhem P, et al. The individual responsiveness to growth hormone (GH) treatment in GH-deficient adults is dependent on the level of GH-binding protein, body mass index, age, and gender. J Clin Endocrinol Metab 1996;81:1575–1581.
35. Horswill CA, Zipf WB, Kien CL, Kahle EB. Insulin's contribution to growth in children and the potential for exercise to mediate insulin's action. Pediatr Exerc Sci 1997;9:18–32.
36. Dorn LD, Burgess ES, Dichek HL, Putnam FW, Chrousos GP, Gold PW. Thyroid hormone concentrations in depressed and nondepressed adolescents: Group differences and behavioural relations. J Am Acad Child Adolesc Psychiatry 1996;35:299–306.

37. Tremblay MS. The effects of training status, exercise mode, and exercise duration on endogenous anabolic and catabolic steroid hormones in males [dissertation]. University of Toronto, Toronto, 1994.
38. Alexander SL, Irvine CHG. The effect of Naloxone administration on the secretion of corticotropin-releasing hormone, arginine vasopressin, and adrenocorticotropin in unperturbed horses. Endocrinology 1995;136:5139–5147.
39. Watanabe RM, Azen CG, Roy S, Perlman JA, Bergman RN. Defects in carbohydrate metabolism in oral contraceptive users without apparent metabolic risk factors. J Clin Endocrinol Metab 1994;79:1277–1283.
40. Nazar K, Kaciuba-Uscilko H, Szczepanik J, Zemba AW, Kruk B, Chwalbinska-Moneta J, et al. Phosphate supplementation prevents a decrease of triiodothyronine and increases resting metabolic rate during low energy diet. J Physiol Pharmacol 1996;47:373–383.
41. Ministry of Fitness and Amateur Sport. Canadian Standardized Test of Fitness Operations Manual, 3rd ed. Minister of Supply and Services, Canada, 1986.
42. American College of Sports Medicine. Guidelines for Exercise Testing and Prescription, 5th ed. Williams and Wilkins, Baltimore, 1995.
43. Jezova D, Vigas M. Testosterone response to exercise during blockade and stimulation of adrenergic receptors in man. Horm Res 1981;15:141–147.
44. Galbo H, Hummer L, Petersen I, Christensen N, Bie N. Thyroid and testicular hormone responses to graded and prolonged exercise in man. Eur J Appl Physiol 1977;36:101–106.
45. Webb ML, Wallace JP, Hamill C, Hodgson JL, Mashaly MM. Serum testosterone concentration during two hours of moderate intensity treadmill running in trained men and women. Endocrinol Res 1984;10:27–38.
46. Hackney AC. Endurance training and testosterone levels. Sports Med 1989;8:117–127.
47. Milledge JS. High altitude. In: Harries M, Williams C, Stanish WD, Micheli LJ, eds. Oxford Textbook of Sports Medicine. Oxford University Press, New York, 1994, pp. 217–230.
48. Mendelson JH, Mello NK, Ellingboe J. Effects of acute alcohol intake on pituitary-gonadal hormones in normal human males. J Pharmacol Exp Ther 1977;202:676–682.
49. Dotson LE, Robertson LS, Tuchfeld B. Plasma alcohol, smoking, hormone concentrations and self-reported aggression. J Stud Alcohol 1975;36:578–586.
50. Williams MH. Nutrition for Fitness and Sport, 3rd ed. W.C. Brown, Dubuque, 1992.
51. Parsons WD, Neims AH. Effect of smoking on caffeine clearance. Clin Pharmacol Ther 1978;24:40–45.
52. Graham TE, Spriet LL. Metabolic, catecholamine, and exercise performance responses to various doses of caffeine. J Appl Physiol 1995;78:867–874.
53. Carr BR, Parker CR, Ohashi M, MacDonald PC, Simpson ER. Regulation of human fetal testicular secretion of testosterone: low-density lipoprotein-cholesterol and cholesterol synthesized de novo as steroid precurser. Am J Obstet Gynecol 1983;146:241–247.
54. Raben A, Kiens B, Richter EA, Rasmussen LB, Svenstrup B, Micic S, et al. Serum sex hormones and endurance performance after a lacto-ovo vegetarian and a mixed diet. Med Sci Sports Exerc 1992;24:1290–1297.
55. Horswill CA. Effects of bicarbonate, citrate, and phosphate loading on performance. Int J Sport Nutr 1995;5(suppl):S111–S119.
56. Gordon SE, Kraemer WJ, Vos NH, Lynch JM, Knuttgen HG. Effect of acid-base balance on the growth hormone response to acute high-intensity cycle exercise. J Appl Physiol 1994;76:821–829.
57. Dominguez JH, Gray RW, Lemann J Jr. Dietary phosphate deprivation in women and men: effects on mineral and acid balances, parathyroid hormone and the metabolism of 25-OH-vitamin D. J Clin Endocrinol Metab 1976;43:1056–1068.
58. Kreuz L, Rose R, Jennings J. Suppression of plasma testosterone levels and psychological stress. Arch Gen Psychiatry 1972;26:479–482.
59. Dai WS, Kuller LH, LaPorte RE, Gutai JP, Falvo-Gerard L, Caggiula A. The epidemiology of plasma testosterone levels in middle-aged men. Am J Epidemiol 1981;114:804–816.
60. Vaernes R, Ursin H, Darragh A, Lambe R. Endocrine response patterns and psychological correlates. J Psychosom Res 1982;26:123–131.
61. Diamond P, Brisson GR, Candas B, Peronnet F. Trait anxiety, submaximal physical exercise and blood androgens. Eur J Appl Physiol 1989;58:699–704.
62. Aakvaag A, Bentdal O, Quigstad K, Walstad P, Ronningen H, Fonnum F. Testosterone and testosterone binding globulin (TeBG) in young men during prolonged stress. Int J Androl 1978;1:22–31.

63. Aakvaag A, Sand T, Opstad P, Fonnum F. Hormonal changes in serum in young men during prolonged physical strain. Eur J Appl Physiol 1978;39:283–291.
64. Schurmeyer T, Jung K, Nieschlag E. The effect of an 1100 km run on testicular, adrenal and thyroid hormones. Int J Androl 1984;7:276–282.
65. Dressendorfer RH, Wade CE. Effects of a 15-d race on plasma steroid levels and leg muscle fitness in runners. Med Sci Sports Exerc 1991;23:954–958.
66. VanHelder T, Radomski MW. Sleep deprivation and the effect on exercise performance. Sports Med 1989;7:235–247.
67. American College of Sports Medicine. The female athlete triad. Med Sci Sports Exerc 1997;29:i–ix.
68. Loucks AB. Physical activity, fitness, and female reproductive morbidity. In: Bouchard C, Shephard RJ, Stephens T, eds. Physical Activity, Fitness, and Health: International Proceedings and Consensus Statement. Human Kinetics, Champaign, 1994, pp. 943–954.
69. Constantini NW, Warren MP. Physical activity, fitness, and reproductive health in women: clinical observations. In: Bouchard C, Shephard RJ, Stephens T, eds. Physical Activity, Fitness, and Health: International Proceedings and Consensus Statement. Human Kinetics, Champaign, 1994, pp. 955–966.
70. Keizer HA, Kuipers H, de Haan J, Janssen GME, Beckers E, Habets L, et al. Effect of a 3-month endurance training program on metabolic and multiple hormonal responses to exercise. Int J Sports Med 1987;8:154–160.
71. Keizer HA, Kuipers H, de Haan J, Beckers E, Habets L. Multiple hormonal responses to physical exercise in eumenorrheic trained and untrained women. Int J Sports Med 1987;8:139–150.
72. Fry RW, Morton AR, Garcia-Webb P, Keasy D. Monitoring exercise stress by changes in metabolic and hormonal responses over a 24-h period. Eur J Appl Physiol 1991;63:228–234.
73. Lutoslawska G, Obminski Z, Krogulski A, Sendecki W. Plasma cortisol and testosterone following 19-km and 42-km kayak races. J Sports Med Phys Fit 1991;31:538–542.
74. Urhausen A, Kindermann W. Behaviour of testosterone, sex hormone binding globulin (SHBG), and cortisol before and after a triathlon competition. Int J Sports Med 1987;8:305–308.
75. Westendorp RG, Roos AN, Riley LC, Walma S, Frolich M, Meinders AE. Chronic stimulation of atrial natriuretic peptide attenuates the secretory response to postural changes. Am J Med Sci 1993; 306:371–375.
76. Cumming DC, Wall SR, Quinney HA, Belcasto AN. Decrease in serum testosterone levels with maximal intensity swimming exercise in trained male and female swimmers. Endocrinol Res 1987;13:31–41.
77. Weitzman ED. Circadian rhythms and episodic hormone secretion. Ann Rev Med 1976;27:225–243.
78. Rose R. Kreutz L, Holoday J, Sulak K, Johnson C. Diurnal variation of plasma testosterone and cortisol. J Endocrinol 1972;54:177,178.
79. Rose SR, Nisula BC. Circadian variation of thyrotropin in childhood. J Clin Endocrinol Metab 1989;68:1086–1089.
80. van Coevorden A, Laurent E, Decoster C, Kerkhofs M, Neve P, van Cauter E, et al. Decreased basal and stimulated thyrotropin secretion in healthy elderly men. J Clin Endocrinol Metab 1989;69:177–185.
81. Fisher DA. Physiological variation in thyroid hormones: physiological and pathphysiological considerations. Clin Chem 1996;42:135–139.
82. de Lacerda L, Kowarski A, Johanson AJ, Athanasiou R, Migeon CJ. Integrated concentration and circadian variation of plasma testosterone in normal men. J Clin Endocrinol Metab 1973;37:366–371.
83. Rosenfield RL, Helke JC. Small diurnal and episodic fluctuation of plasma free testosterone level in normal woman. Am J Obstet Gynecol 1974;120:461–465.
84. Yie SM, Wang R, Zhu YX, Liu GY, Zheng FX. Circadian variation of serum sex hormone binding globulin binding capacity in normal men and women. J Steroid Biochem 1990;36:111–115.
85. Santen RJ, Bardin LW. Episodic luteinizing hormone secretion in man: pulse analysis, clinical interpretation, physiologic mechanisms. J Clin Invest 1973;52:2617–2628.
86. Smals AGH, Kloppenberg PWC, Benraad THJ. Circannual cycle in plasma testosterone level in man. J Clin Endocrinol Metab 1976;42:979–982.
87. Thuma JR, Gilders R, Verdun M, Loucks AB. Circadian rhythm of cortisol confounds cortisol responses to exercise: implications for future research. J Appl Physiol 1995;78:1657–1664.
88. Hill BM, Laessig RH, Koch DD, Hassemer DJ. Comparison of plastic vs glass evacuated serum-separator (SST) blood drawing tubes for common clinical chemistry determination. Clin Chem 1992;38:1474–1478.

89. Brunning PF, Jonker KM, Boereman-Baan AW. Absorption of steroid hormones by plastic tubing. J Steroid Biochem 1981;14:553–555.
90. Diagnostic Productions Corporation. Progesterone package, prescribary information. Los Angeles, DPC, 1991.
91. Reinartz JJ, Ramay ML, Fowler MC, Killeen AA. Plastic vs glass SST evacuated serum-separator blood-drawing tube for endocrinologic analytes. Clin Chem 1993;39:2535,2536.
92. CIBA Corning Diagnostics. Information on ACS:180 sample type. Medfield MA, 1994.
93. Diagnostic Products Corporation. Coat-a-count free testosterone. Prescribary information. Los Angeles, DPC, 1990.
94. Riad-Fahmy D, Read GF, Walker RF, Griffiths K. Steroids in saliva for assessing endocrine function. Endocrinol Rev 1982;3:367–395.
95. Vining RF, McGinley RA. The measurement of hormones in saliva: possibility and pitfalls. J Steroid Biochem 1987;27:81–94.
96. Walker RF, Riad-Fahmy D, Read GF. Adrenal status assessed by direct RIA of cortisol in whole saliva or parotid saliva. Clin Chem 1978;24:1460–1463.
97. Cook NJ, Read GF, Walker RF, Harris B, Riad-Fahmy D. Changes in adrenal and testicular activity monitored by salivary sampling in male throughout marathon runs. Eur J Appl Physiol 1986;55:634–638.
98. Bolaji II. Sero-salivary progesterone correlation. Int J Gynecol Obstet 1994;45:125–131.
99. Rilling JK, Worthman CM, Campbell BC, Stallings JF, Mbizva M. Ratio of plasma and salivary testosterone throughout puberty: production versus availability. Steroid 1996;61:374–378.
100. Halimi S, Tepavcevic D, Suchanek D, Giljevic Z, Palvsic V, Korsic M. Measurement of salivary insulin-like growth factor I in acromegaly: comparison with serum insulin-like growth factor I and growth hormone concentrations. Eur J Clin Chem Clin Biochem 1994;32:705–707.
101. Vining RF, McGinley RA, Makavytis JJ, Ho KY. Salivary cortisol: a better measurement of adrenal cortisol function than serum cortisol. Ann Clin Biochem 1983;20:329–335.
102. Schramm W, Smith RH, Craig PA, Grates HE. Testosterone concentration is increased in whole saliva, but not in ultrafiltrate after toothbrushing. Clin Chem 1993;39:519–521.
103. Schramm W, Smith RH, Craig PA, Paek SH, Kuo HH. Determination of free progesterone in an ultrafiltrate of saliva collected in situ. Clin Chem 1990;36:1488–1493.
104. Meulenberg P, Ross HA, Swinkels L, Benraad TJ. The effect of oral contraceptives on plasma free and salivary cortisol and cortisone. Clin Chem Acta 1987;165:379–385.
105. Ferguson NM, MacPhee GB. Kinetic study of 11-hydroxysteroid dehydrogenase in rat submandibular salivary gland. Arch Oral Biol 1975;20:241–245.
106. Swinkels L, van Hoof H, Ross HA, Smals AG, Benraad TJ. Low ratio of androstenedione to testosterone in plasma and saliva of Hirsute women. Clin Chem 1992;38:1814–1823.
107. Fulton A, Chan S, Coleman G. Effect of salivary proteins on binding curves of three RIA kits. Amerlex-M-progesterone, Amerlex cortisol and Biodata testosterone. Clin Chem 1989;35:641–644.
108. Hofreiter BT, Mizera AC, Allen JP, Masi AM, Hicok WC. Solid-state extraction of cortisol from plasma or serum for liquid chromatography. Clin Chem 1983;29:1808,1809.
109. Silver AC, Landon J, Smith DS, Perry LA. RIA of cortisol in saliva with "gamma coat" kit. Clin Chem 1983;29:1869,1870.
110. Chen YM, Cintron NM, Whitson PA. Long term storage of salivary cortisol samples at room temperature. Clin Chem 1992;38:304.
111. Wade SE. Less-invasive measurement of tissue availability of hormone and drugs. Diffusion-sink sampling. Clin Chem 1992;38:1639–1644.
112. Wade SE. An oral-diffusion sink device for extended sampling of multiple steroid hormone from saliva. Clin Chem 1992;38:1878–1882.
113. Caraway WT. Chemical and diagnostic specificity of laboratory tests. Am J Clin Pathol 1961;37:445–464.
114. Sanntag O. Hemolysis as interference factor in clinical chemistry. J Clin Chem Clin Biochem 1986;24:127–139.
115. Yucel D, Dalva K. Effect of in vitro hemolysis on 25 common biochemical tests. Clin Chem 1992;38:575–577.
116. Calam RR. Reviewing the importance of specimen collection. J Am Med Technol 1977;38:297.
117. Veldhuis JD, Danfan ML. Steroidal regulation of biologically active luteinizing hormone secretion in men and women. Hum Reprod 1993;suppl 2:84–96.

118. Mire-Sluis AR, Roger L, Thorpe R. Quantitative cell line based bioassay for human cytokine. J Immunol Method 1995:187:191–199.
119. Thiery JC, Martin GB. Neurophysiological control of the secretion of gonadotrophin-releasing hormone and luteinizing hormone in the sheep—a review. Reprod Fertil Dev 1991;3:137–173.
120. Straub RE, Frech GC, Joho RH, Gershengorn MC. Expression cloning of a cDNA encoding the mouse pituitary TRH receptor. Proc Natl Acad Sci USA 1990;87:9514.
121. Bieth E, Cahoreau C, Cholin S, Molinas C, Cerutti C, Rochiccioli P, et al. Human growth hormone receptor: cloning and expression of full-length complementary DNA after site directed inactivation of a cryptic bacterial promoter. Gene 1997;194:97–105.
122. Dudley RF. Chemiluminescence Immunoassay; an alternative to RIA. Lab Med 1990;21:216–222.
123. Miller JJ, Valders R Jr. Approaches to minimizing interference by cross reacting molecules in immunoassays. Clin Chem 1991;37:144–153.
124. Morgan CL, Newman DJ, Price CP. Immunosensors: technology and opportunities in laboratory medicine. Clin Chem 1996;42:193–209.
125. Bowers LD. Analytical advances in detection of performance enhancing compounds. Clin Chem 1997;43:1299–1304.
126. Yoon J, Park S. Exercise intensity-related responses of β-endorphin, ACTH, and cortisol. Korean J Sport Sci 1991;3:21–32.
127. Obminski Z, Klusiewicz A, Stupnicki R. Changes in salivary and serum cortisol concentrations in junior athletes following exercises of different intensities. Biol Sport 1994;11:49–57.
128. Lu S, Lau C, Tung Y, Huang S, Chen Y, Shih H, et al. Lactate and the effects of exercise on testosterone secretion: evidence for the involvement of a cAMP-mediated mechanism. Med Sci Sports Exerc 1997;29:1048–1054.
129. Kuoppasalmi K, Naveri H, Harkonen M, Adlercreutz H. Plasma cortisol, androstenedione, testosterone and luteinizing hormone in running exercise of different intensities. Scand J Clin Lab Invest 1980;40:403–409.
130. Hakkinen K, Pakarinen A. Acute hormonal responses to two different fatiguing heavy-resistance protocols in male athletes. J Appl Physiol 1993;74:882–887.
131. Lehmann M, Gastmann U, Petersen KG, Bachl N, Seidel A, Khalaf AN, et al. Training—overtraining: performance, and hormone levels, after a defined increase in training volume versus intensity in experienced middle- and long-distance runners. Br J Sports Med 1992;26:233–242.
132. Kraemer WJ, Marchitelli L, Gordon SE, Harman E, Dziados JE, Mello R, et al. Hormonal and growth factor responses to heavy resistance exercise protocols. J Appl Physiol 1990;69:1442–1450.
133. Cumming DC, Wheeler GD, McColl EM. The effects of exercise on reproductive function in men. Sports Med 1989;7:1–17.
134. Richter EA, Sutton JR. Hormonal adaptation to physical activity. In: Bouchard C, Shephard RJ, Stephens T, eds. Physical Activity, Fitness, and Health. Human Kinetics, Champaign, 1994, pp. 331–342.
135. Mulligan SE, Fleck SJ, Gordon SE, Koziris LP, Triplett-McBride NT. Influence of resistance exercise volume on serum growth hormone and cortisol concentrations in women. J Strength Cond Res 1996;10:256–262.
136. Guezennec Y, Leger L, Lhoste F, Aymonod M, Pesquies PC. Hormone and metabolite response to weight-lifting training sessions. Int J Sports Med 1986;7:100–105.
137. Weiss L, Cureton K, Thompson F. Comparison of serum testosterone and androstenedione responses to weight lifting in men and women. Eur J Appl Physiol 1983;50:413–419.
138. Jezova D, Vigas M, Tatar P, Kvetnansky R, Nazar K, Kaciuba-Uscilko H, et al. Plasma testosterone and catecholamine responses to physical exercise of different intensities in men. Eur J Appl Physiol 1985;54:62–66.
139. VanHelder WP, Radomski MW, Goode RC. Growth hormone responses during intermittent weight lifting exercise in men. Eur J Appl Physiol 1984;53:31–34.
140. Kuoppasalmi K, Naveri H, Rehunen S, Harkonen M, Adlercreutz H. Effect of strenuous anaerobic running exercise on plasma growth hormone, cortisol, luteinizing hormone, testosterone, androstenedione, estrone and estradiol. J Steroid Biochem 1976;7:823–829.
141. Cumming DC, Brunsting LA III, Strich G, Ries AL, Rebar RW. Reproductive hormone increases in response to acute exercise in men. Med Sci Sports Exerc 1986;18:369–373.
142. Kraemer WJ. Endocrine responses to resistance exercise. Med Sci Sports Exerc 1988; 20(suppl):S152–S157.

143. Jensen J, Oftebro H, Breigan B, Johnsson A, Ohlin K, Meen HD, et al. Comparison of changes in testosterone concentrations after strength and endurance exercise in well trained men. Eur J Appl Physiol 1991;63:467–471.
144. Kindermann W, Schnabel A, Schmitt W, Biro G, Cassens J, Weber F. Catecholamines, growth hormone, cortisol, insulin, and sex hormones in anaerobic and aerobic exercise. Eur J Appl Physiol 1982;49:389–399.
145. Luger A, Deuster PA, Kyle SB, Gallucci WT, Montgomery LC, Gold PW, et al. Acute hypothalamic-pituitary–adrenal responses to the stress of treadmill exercise: physiologic adaptations to physical training. N Engl J Med 1987;316:1309–1315.
146. Vasankari TJ, Kujala UM, Heinonen OJ, Huhtaniemi IT. Effects of endurance training on hormonal responses to prolonged physical exercise in males. Acta Endocrinol 1993;129:109–113.
147. Mathur DN, Toriola AL, Dada OA. Serum cortisol and testosterone levels in conditioned male distance runners and nonathletes after maximal exercise. J Sports Med 1986;26:245–250.
148. Pyka G, Taaffe DR, Marcus R. Effect of a sustained program of resistance training on the acute growth hormone response to resistance exercise in older adults. Horm Metab Res 1994;26: 330–333.
149. Remes K, Kuoppasalmi K, Adlercreutz H. Effect of long-term physical training on plasma testosterone, androstenedione, luteinizing hormone and sex-hormone- binding globulin capacity. Scand J Clin Lab Invest 1979;39:743–749.
150. Gulledge TP, Hackney AC. Reproducibility of low resting testosterone concentrations in endurance trained men. Eur J Appl Physiol 1996;73:582–583.
151. Young RJ, Ismail AH, Bradley A, Corrigan DL. Effect of prolonged exercise on serum testosterone levels in adult men. Br J Sports Med 1976;10:230–235.
152. Fellmann N, Coudert J, Jarrige J-F, Bedu M, Denis C, Boucher D, et al. Effects of endurance training on the androgenic response to exercise in man. Int J Sports Med 1985;6:215–219.
153. Houmard JA, Costill DL, Mitchell JB, Park SH, Fink WJ, Burns JM. Testosterone, cortisol, and creatine kinase levels in male distance runners during reduced training. Int J Sports Med 1990;11: 41–45.
154. Remes K, Kuoppasalmi K, Adlercreutz H. Effect of physical exercise and sleep deprivation on plasma androgen levels: modifying effect of physical fitness. Int J Sports Med 1985;6:131–135.
155. Schmid P, Pusch HH, Wolf W, Pilger E, Pessenhofer H, Schwaberger G, et al. Serum FSH, LH, and testosterone in humans after physical exercise. Int J Sports Med 1982;3:84–89.
156. Hackney AC, Sharp RL, Runyan WS, Ness RJ. Relationship of resting prolactin and testosterone in males during intensive training. Br J Sports Med 1989;23:194.
157. Hakkinen K, Pakarinen A, Alen M, Kauhanen H, Komi PV. Neuromuscular and hormonal responses in elite athletes to two successive strength training sessions in one day. Eur J Appl Physiol 1988;57:133–139.
158. Hakkinen K, Pakarinen A, Alen M, Kauhanen H, Komi PV. Daily hormonal and neuromuscular responses to intensive strength training in 1 week. Int J Sports Med 1988;9:422–428.
159. Urhausen A, Gabriel HH, Kindermann W. Impaired pituitary hormonal response to exhaustive exercise in overtrained endurance athletes. Med Sci Sports Exerc 1998;30:407–414.
160. Barron J, Noakes T, Levy W, Smith C, Millar R. Hypothalamic dysfunction in overtrained athletes. J Clin Endocrinol Metab 1985;60:803–806.
161. Adlercreutz H, Harkonen M, Kuoppasalmi K, Naveri H, Huhtaniemi I, Tikkanen H, et al. Effect of training on plasma anabolic and catabolic steroid hormones and their response during physical exercise. Int J Sports Med 1986;7(suppl):27,28.
162. Roche AF, ed. Secular trends in human growth, maturation, and development. Monogr Soc Res Child Dev 1979;ser. 179;44(3,4).
163. Pate RR, Shephard RJ. Characteristics of physical fitness in youth. In: Gisolfi CV, Lamb DR, eds. Youth, Exercise, and Sport. Benchmark Press, Indianapolis, 1989, pp. 1–46.
164. Metivier G, Gauthier R, De La Chevrotiere J, Grymala, D. The effect of acute exercise on the serum levels of testosterone and luteinizing hormone in human male athletes. J Sports Med Phys Fitness 1980;20:235–238.
165. Wilkerson J, Horvath S, Gutin B. Plasma testosterone during treadmill exercise. J Appl Physiol 1980;49:249–253.
166. Kraemer WJ. Influence of the endocrine system on resistance training adaptations. Natl Strength Conditioning Assoc J 1992;14:47–53.

167. Bunt JC, Bahr JM, Bemben DA. Comparison of estradiol and testosterone levels during and immediately following prolonged exercise in moderately active males and females. Endocrinol Res 1987;13:157–172.
168. Kuoppasalmi K, Naveri H, Kosunen K, Harkonen M, Adlercreutz H. Plasma steroid levels in muscular exercise. In: Poortmans J, Niset G, eds. Biochemistry of Exercise IV-B. University Park Press, Baltimore, 1981, pp. 149–160.
169. Alen M, Hakkinen K. Androgenic steroid effects on serum hormones and on maximal force development in strength athletes. J Sports Med Phys Fitness 1987;27:38–46.
170. Rodda BE. Bioavailability: designs and analysis. In: Berry DA, ed. Statistical Methodology in the Pharmaceutical Sciences. Marcel Dekker, New York, 1990, pp. 57–81.
171. Viru A, Karelson K, Smirnova T. Stability and variability in hormonal responses to prolonged exercise. Int J Sports Med 1992;13:230–235.
172. Zar JH. Biostatistical Analysis, 2nd ed. Prentice Hall, Englewood Cliffs, 1984.
173. Hicks C. Fundamental Concepts in the Design of Experiments, 3rd ed. Holt, Rinehart and Winston, New York, 1982.
174. Morrison D. Multivariate Statistical Methods, 3rd ed. McGraw-Hill Publishing Co., New York, 1990.
175. Berry DA, ed. Statistical Methodology in the Pharmaceutical Sciences. Marcel Dekker, New York, 1990.
176. Galbo H, Kjaer M, Mikines KJ. Neurohormonal system. In: Skinner J, ed. Future Directions in Exercise and Sport Science Research. Human Kinetics, Champaign, 1989, pp. 329–345.

2 Exercise and Endogenous Opiates

Tim Meyer, MD, Lothar Schwarz, MD, and Wilfried Kindermann, MD, PhD

CONTENTS
> INTRODUCTION
> INFLUENCES OF ACUTE EXERCISE ON PERIPHERAL
>   β-ENDORPHIN LEVELS
> INFLUENCE OF TRAINING STATUS ON β-ENDORPHIN SECRETION
> FACTORS INFLUENCING THE β-ENDORPHIN RESPONSE TO EXERCISE
> IMPLICATIONS OF β-ENDORPHIN LEVELS FOR SPORTS ACTIVITY
> CONCLUSIONS
> REFERENCES

INTRODUCTION

The discovery of endogenous opiates in 1975 *(1)* generated considerable research concerning the effects of exercise on the release of these peptides, particularly on β-endorphin, which represents the main focus of this chapter. Previous research considered changes in peripheral blood concentrations induced by different modes of physical activity, influences of training status on the secretion of endogenous opiates, and the physiological meaning of the β-endorphin release during exercise. Such phenomena as "runner's high," "second wind," or "exercise dependency" were related to endogenous opiate activity.

This chapter summarizes what is known about the stimulation of opioid release by physical activity. Physiological mechanisms responsible for the secretion are highlighted, as well as the consequences of opioid activity. Implications for future research, training, and competition are discussed.

INFLUENCES OF ACUTE EXERCISE ON PERIPHERAL β-ENDORPHIN LEVELS

Different modes of exercise were tested for their impact on opioid/β-endorphin release. Routine incremental graded exercise tests are common in the laboratory and were often chosen as provocative tests for pituitary gland synthesis of endogenous opi-

From: *Contemporary Endocrinology: Sports Endocrinology*
Edited by: M. P. Warren and N. W. Constantini © Humana Press Inc., Totowa, NJ

ates. Endurance competitions of long duration represent another mode of testing opioid reactivity. Thus, aerobic trials and anaerobic exercise bouts were performed to test their effect on endogenous opiates. This leads to a crucial point in hormonal research: accurate determination of exercise intensity—a necessary condition for valid results.

Exercise intensity is usually described using spirometric (maximal oxygen uptake = VO_2max) or metabolic (lactate concentration) parameters. For submaximal exercise, percentages of VO_2max are given. The aerobic range averages intensities up to 60–70% of VO_2max corresponding to blood lactate concentrations of 3–4 mmol/L. Higher intensities include increasing anaerobic components.

Incremental Graded Exercise

Incremental graded exercise tests were found to elevate β-endorphin levels 1.5- to 7-fold *(2–5)*. This wide range appears to be caused by different protocols and—probably even more important—varying degrees of exhaustion. Published data do not always permit a measurement of the participants' exertion. However, some studies suggest that the amount of β-endorphin release depends on exercise intensity *(6–9)*, whereas others report contradictory findings *(10,11)*. De Meirleir et al. *(12)* introduced lactate measurements into opioid research to describe the metabolic demand of exercise more adequately. They reported no significant changes in β-endorphin concentrations with lactate values around 3 mmol/L. Above this level, peptide levels were elevated in parallel to lactate.

Corresponding results stem from Donevan and Andrew *(7)*. No increase in β-endorphin was noted after 8 min of cycling exercise at 25 and 50% of VO_2max, but a 1.5-fold increase after a stage with 75% VO_2max of the same duration and even a 4.4-fold one after 95%. Both of the two higher intensities probably represent anaerobic workloads for the untrained participants. Lactate values were not given.

Nearly the same results are reported for 10 min of cycling exercise in 12 male students whose β-endorphin concentrations did not increase at 40 and 60%, but at 80 and 100% of VO_2max *(13)*. Adrenocorticotropic hormone (ACTH), which is derived from the same precursor as β-endorphin, gave similar reactions to 50, 70, and 90% of VO_2max in 21 subjects at differing endurance training levels *(14)*.

A more precise evaluation of exercise intensity was used by Schwarz and Kindermann *(15)*, who calculated the workload on a bicycle ergometer according to the individual anaerobic threshold (IAT), which describes the beginning of a disproportionate increase in lactate levels during incremental exercise *(16)*. Beyond the IAT β-endorphin, concentrations increased approximately parallel to lactate (schematic illustration in Fig. 1). The highest concentrations were reached 5 min after cessation of exercise (three times the resting value), and there was a correlation between lactate and β-endorphin concentrations. This suggests a link between endorphin levels and exercise intensity. Below the IAT, no changes in β-endorphin levels were detected.

Bouts of Anaerobic Exercise

Short bouts of anaerobic exercise (highly intensive with a duration of a few seconds to several minutes, e.g., the Wingate test) induce a two- to fourfold increase of β-endorphin depending on the duration of exercise stress. Protocols of not more than 1 min of anaerobic activity and maximal lactate values between 12 and 15 mmol/L approximately double the β-endorphin concentration *(9,15,17)*, whereas longer exercise durations result in a more pronounced β-endorphin response *(18)*. Again, a positive correlation between lactate

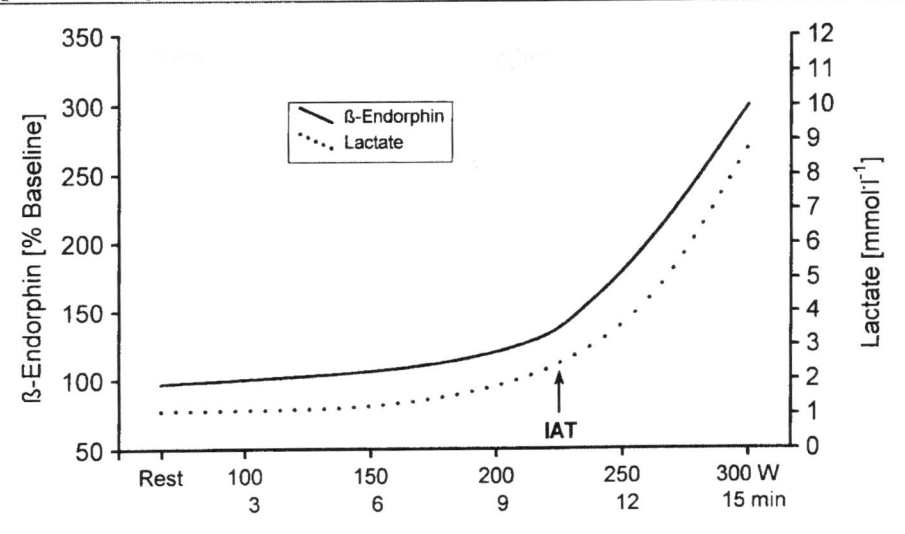

Fig. 1. β-Endorphin lactase during incremental graded exercise (schematic drawing derived from ref. *15*). IAT = individual anaerobic threshold.

and β-endorphin could be established *(15)*, and additionally, catecholamine levels were correlated to maximal lactate concentrations.

Aerobic Exercise of Longer Duration

Longer-lasting exercise for more than 10 min is typically performed at lower intensities that do not induce high lactate concentrations, nor do they regularly fulfill other criteria (concentrations of catecholamines and cortisol) responsible for the release of β-endorphin in incremental or anaerobic exercise. Nevertheless, some investigators reported elevated β-endorphin levels after extensive endurance tasks *(10,19–24)*, whereas others found concentrations unchanged *(12,25–28)*. Two methodological shortcomings limit the generalizability of the older studies: high crossreactivity between β-endorphin and β-lipotropin, low number of subjects. However, the determination of exercise intensity remains crucial, and this may vary considerably even in longer-lasting physical activity, which complicates the assessment of results.

More recent studies tested different intensities expressed as percentages of maximal oxygen uptake for their potential to initiate β-endorphin responses. McMurray et al. *(8)* let subjects cycle for 20 min at 40, 60, and 80% VO_2max and measured the corresponding levels of lactate and β-endorphin. It was shown that only the highest workload induced lactate concentrations above what is considered the anaerobic threshold. In parallel, β-endorphin levels exclusively rose under this condition.

Another investigation by Goldfarb et al. *(29)* used a similar design: 60, 70, and 80% of VO_2max were applied for 30 min on a cycle ergometer. Again only with lactate levels presumably not representing steady-state levels (4.2 and 9.5 mmol/L for the two higher workloads) could β-endorphin increases be detected.

To test if there is a critical exercise duration for a given constant aerobic intensity, Schwarz and Kindermann *(24)* calculated the IAT for each of 10 nonspecifically trained subjects from an incremental cycle ergometry *(16)*. The IAT represents a physiological breakpoint of exercise intensity beyond which lactate concentrations cannot be held constant and is situated at 60–80% of VO_2max, depending on the individual training state. For different modes of exercise (running, cycling), the workload/velocity at the IAT can be maintained for about 1 h. Subjects had to cycle at 100% of the IAT until exhaustion (in this study corresponding to 63% VO_2max; duration on average 80 min), and they reached lactate steady states between 3 and 3.5 mmol/L. The main observation of the study was an elevation of β-endorphin starting after approx 50–60 min (schematic illustration in Fig. 2).

This may explain the results of Heitkamp et al. *(3,4)*, who found 6.9 and 1.4 times the baseline β-endorphin levels after a marathon in men and women (who had much higher baseline values), respectively. Obviously, other factors than lactate or catecholamine increases alone are involved in initiating a β-endorphin release.

On the other hand, exercising beyond a threshold intensity seems to be necessary for elevating endogenous opioids even in long-lasting endurance exercise. Presumably because threshold was not reached, no changes in β-endorphin concentrations were measured after 2 h of cycling at 50% of the maximal oxygen uptake *(26,30)*.

Resistance Exercise

Resistance training is a relatively new field for β-endorphin research. The determination of exercise intensities is often done as a ratio of the so-called 1 repetition maximum (1 RPM), i.e., the weight that can be lifted/pushed/pulled once by a subject with maximal individual effort. Alternatively, intensities are sometimes defined relative to loads that can be lifted more often (5 RPM for a weight that can be lifted exactly five times).

Depending on the exercise protocol, results of different investigators are inconsistent. Decreases in β-endorphin are reported *(31)* as well as no change *(32)* and increases *(33,34)*. A closer look at the applied procedures reveals probable causes for these contradictory findings.

Pierce et al. *(32)* had trained football players lift $3 \times 4 \times 8 \times 80\%$ of 1 RPM with breaks of 3 min between the sets. The highest recorded heart rates were 157 ± 4/min, which would suggest an extensive exercise regimen in terms of cardiocirculatory strain for this young group of subjects (20.5 ± 0.4 yr). Putting these facts together, well-trained athletes were stressed in the average range of their strength capacity with relatively long regeneration periods between the loads. The resulting individual cardiovascular load might be evaluated as moderate, and no β-endorphin response occurred.

A more differentiated study design was applied by Kraemer et al. *(33)*, who tested different heavy-resistance protocols for their capability to raise β-endorphin blood concentrations. Only one of the regimens induced significant elevations in hormone levels. This one was characterized by a high number of repetitions and short resting periods in between. Consequently, the highest heart rates and lactate levels were recorded under these conditions.

The somewhat surprising decline in β-endorphin concentration after $3 \times 4 \times 4 \times 80\%$ 1 RPM observed by McGowan et al. *(31)* cannot be easily commented on, because no information is given about strength-training experience, duration of breaks, and cardiocirculatory strain.

The recent investigations using resistance exercises as stimulus to promote β-endorphin release suggest that—like endurance tasks—the metabolic and cardiocirculatory stress determines the degree of β-endorphin increase. This is in contrast to the traditional way of determining intensity of exercise used by power athletes. At the moment,

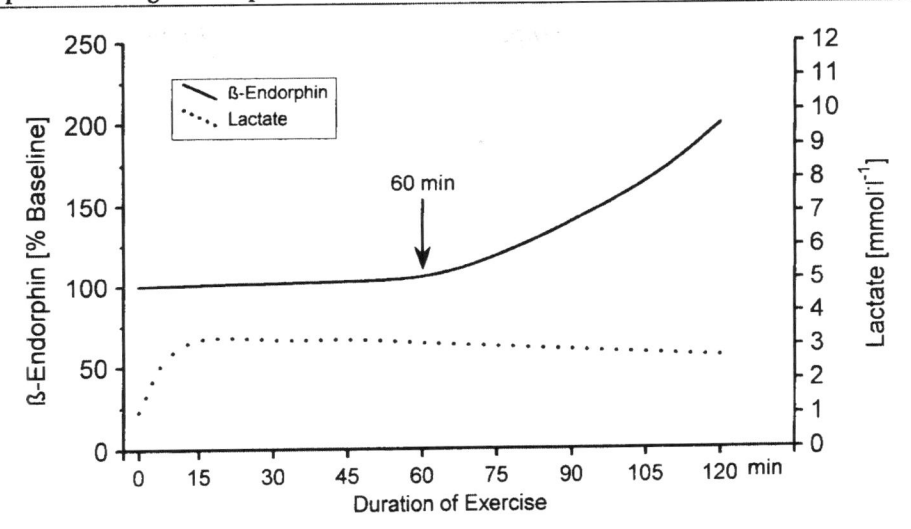

Fig. 2. β-Endorphin and lactase during exercise at the individual anaerobic threshold (schematic drawing derived from ref. *48*).

speculations about a threshold analogous to the anaerobic threshold for endurance exercise seem to be premature.

Summary

β-endorphin increases are induced by anaerobic exercise, and incremental exercise which reaches anaerobic stages. Lactate and—probably—catecholamine concentrations are the main factors being correlated with these responses. Consequently, exceeding the intensity of the individual anaerobic threshold raises β-endorphin levels. Duration of aerobic exercise seems to be an independent factor that stimulates β-endorphin release after about 1 h if a threshold intensity—possibly around 55–60% VO_2max—is reached. For resistance exercises, an evaluation of the metabolic and cardiocirculatory strain is preferable to the classic view of counting repetitions for predicting the β-endorphin response. The involved mechanisms may be the same as in endurance exercise.

INFLUENCE OF TRAINING STATUS ON β-ENDORPHIN SECRETION

Apparently, the training status should influence β-endorphin responses to exercise, because it interferes with the determination of intensity. Well-trained endurance athletes can usually perform work at higher relative workloads than untrained persons. Therefore, at least an individualized intensity determination or, alternatively, a highly homogenous group of subjects seems warranted for research purposes. On the other hand, chronic training stress may alter the hormonal response of the anterior pituitary gland. Theoretically, the capacity to produce β-endorphin may increase, and a chronic suppression of the hypothalamic-pituitary-adrenal (HPA) axis is possible.

Influence of Endurance Training

Resting levels of β-endorphin in endurance-trained individuals were reported to be lowered *(35,36)* or unchanged *(37,40)*. Both studies showing no change were done cross-sectionally and, therefore, susceptible for selection biases, whereas the other two investigations applied an endurance training program. Another cross-sectional investigation *(14)* discovered higher basal values for ACTH and cortisol in trained runners, possibly indicating a parallel behavior of β-endorphin, but trials were executed at an unusual evening time.

The findings under exercise conditions are in slightly better agreement. Only one study showed higher β-endorphin concentrations after 4 mo of mixed aerobic training 6 times a week *(20)*: Cycling at 85% of the individual maximal heart rate induced larger hormonal increases than before the training period. This was evident after 2 mo, and no further significant changes occurred until the end of the training program.

Other investigators did not detect any differences between the trained and untrained state no matter if designed cross-sectionally *(38,39)* or longitudinally/interventionally *(37,40)*. Boineau et al. *(37)* performed their trials, including 10 min of exercise at 70% VO_2max and an incremental test to exhaustion with a considerable number of 39 subjects. Neither influences of training status (which was not exactly specified) nor of gender on the β-endorphin response were observed. The investigation of Berk et al. *(38)* showed higher hormone values after exercise, but a closer look at the data reveals that this conclusion has to be confined to female subjects of which the number is not given. With a total of six untrained participants, one can assume that single outliers have a large influence on the results, which were not tested statistically. Putting this together, no really substantial differences between trained and untrained subjects were documented.

The same is true for the study from Goldfarb et al. *(39)*, who compared six cyclists and six untrained individuals cycling for 20 minutes at 60, 70, and 80% of VO_2max. No significant β-endorphin differences were obtained, despite higher lactate concentrations in the untrained group at the two higher workloads. The authors interpret these findings in opposition to the lactate threshold hypothesis, which states a connection between β-endorphin response and excess of the threshold intensity. This might be misleading, since it is well known that trained athletes very often have lower stress-induced lactate levels compared to untrained persons, even if matched for individualized intensity. Therefore, identical absolute lactate levels do not necessarily indicate the same stress for these groups.

The only interventional investigation available as a detailed publication analyzed data from 13 women before and after a strenuous training program for 2 mo *(40)*. Exercise testing was done in the same manner as in the aforementioned study. The authors reported no differences in β-endorphin release with growing endurance capacity, but met-enkephalin concentrations were reduced in the trained state.

Influence of Resistance Training

Very little is known about effects of resistance training on the release of β-endorphin. The recent studies investigating the influence of resistance training on concentrations of endogenous opioids were mostly conducted with athletes who did resistance training for a few years on a recreational basis or as an adjunct to their routine exercise practice *(32,33)*, but no data from elite power athletes are available. From a theoretical point of view, with growing strength identical external (and presumably even relative) workloads are mastered with reduced exertion and cardiocirculatory stress; this would mean lower β-endorphin levels during resistance exercises. To our knowledge, there is no evidence for changed peptide blood levels under resting conditions in resistance-trained individuals, and no comparison between resistance-trained and untrained persons has been conducted yet.

Summary

It is difficult to come to definitive conclusions about the influences of training on the β-endorphin response to exercise, because study results are rare and inconsistent. Endurance training seems to have a lowering effect on hormone resting levels, but changes in the reaction to exercise stress have not been documented clearly yet. One problem might be intensity determination again, because with growing endurance capacity, even relative workloads (as percentages of VO_2max or of the maximal heart rate) do not indicate the same degree of stress for an individual compared to the untrained state. Consequently, better ways of intensity determination have to be introduced to attain reliable results. The calculation of the individual anaerobic threshold represents a well-validated method feasible for all ergometric testing if lactate measurements are utilized.

No assumptions can be made for effects of the resistance training status, because very few studies have been conducted in this area. On the other hand, individualized intensity determination adequate for hormonal research may be even more difficult than in endurance training.

FACTORS INFLUENCING THE β-ENDORPHIN RESPONSE TO EXERCISE

ACTH and Cortisol

ACTH and β-endorphin are derived from the same precursor molecule in the anterior pituitary gland, and the secretion of both is stimulated by corticotropin-releasing factor (CRF) *(41–43)*. Consequently, the diurnal rhythms of β-endorphin and cortisol are similar as the secretion of cortisol is induced by increasing ACTH levels *(44)*.

Correlations between cortisol and β-endorphin were also reported after a long-distance nordic ski race *(45)*, but other investigators could not replicate these statistical results with incremental graded bicycle exercise and exhaustive work at the individual anaerobic threshold *(15,24)*. The reason for these discrepant findings may be found in the different biological half-lifes of β-endorphin and ACTH (approx 20 and 3 min, respectively). There is a time delay between the ACTH release and the cortisol secretion by the adrenal medulla. Thus, without a causal relationship, there might be an "incidental" correlation between β-endorphin and cortisol.

Catecholamines

As pointed out earlier in this chapter, the individual anaerobic threshold *(16)* probably represents a physiological breakpoint for β-endorphin release. It marks the beginning of the lactate increase in incremental graded exercise, but catecholamine secretion is stimulated overproportionally beyond this intensity, too *(46)*. Consequently, a relationship between both hormones may be assumed, but research is resulting in inconclusive results *(46–48)*. A correlation between endogenous opiates and catecholamines could only be established in short-term anaerobic exercise with considerable lactic acidosis *(15)*, but not in incremental graded exercise and endurance exercise of longer duration until exhaustion *(15,24)*.

Attenuation of adrenergic activity in the central nervous system may be mediated by β-endorphin *(49)*. On the other hand, in animal experiments, an infusion of the adrenoceptor agonist isoprenaline led to elevations in β-endorphin concentrations *(50)*.

Table 1
Exercise-Related Effects of β-Endorphin and Mechanisms Presumably Being Responsible

Proposed effects	Possible mechanisms	References
Euphoria, "runner's high," "second wind"	Stimulation of opiate receptors in the central nervous system	(13,22)
Pain inhibition, increase in acidosis tolerance	Stimulation of central and/or peripheral opiate receptors	(12,44)
Overtraining	Exhaustion of hypophyseal secretion capacity	(7)
Exercise addiction (detraining symptoms)	Downregulation of opiate receptors	(21)
Inhibiting cardiocirculatory effects	Inhibition of catecholamine release	(37,46a,52)
Influence on glucose homeostasis	Inhibition of insulin, stimulation of glucagon	(17,19,38,53)
Influence on fat metabolism	Direct lipolytic effects	(10,25)
Reproductive dysfunction	Feedback inhibition of sex hormones	(6,50)
Immunological effects	Inhibition of natural killer (NK) cell activity	(20)
Anorexia nervosa	Initiation of a self-rewarding system of exercise and starving	(35)

This suggests a physiological inhibition system in which β-endorphin limits the effects of catecholamines and responds to increasing levels of epinephrine and norepinephrine.

Lactate, Acid-Base Status

There is another mechanism that could be involved in inducing β-endorphin release: changes in the acid-base status, which accompany physical activity with a considerable anaerobic component. Recently, it was shown that buffering the lactate acidosis resulting from running on a treadmill at 85% VO_2max leads to reduced levels of β-endorphin *(51)*. In seven subjects, the best correlations with β-endorphin concentrations were observed for base excess and pH. These results correspond well with the findings of Schwarz and Kindermann *(15)* demonstrating a lactate-dependent threshold for raised β-endorphin values. Since lactate is the main agent responsible for declining pH values during high-intensity exercise, it seems tenable that its effect on the anterior pituitary gland is mediated via acidosis.

IMPLICATIONS OF Β-ENDORPHIN LEVELS FOR SPORTS ACTIVITY

There are a few exercise-related phenomena that were connected to levels of endogenous opiates (Table 1). The most obvious one is pain perception, because the main pharmacologic effect of opiates lies in the modulation of pain. There are indications that exercise-induced release of β-endorphin attenuates pain *(53,54)*. At least for strenuous workouts, a point for athletes can be assumed in decreasing the perception of pain. A connection between peripheral blood and brain pools of the peptides that cannot cross the intact blood–brain barrier was considered a necessary condition for this effect. However, peripheral pain receptors are influenced by circulating β-endorphin, too *(52,55)*.

Other proposed—mostly psychological—mechanisms depend on a central action of endogenous opiates, and this research field represents the domain of animal studies and naloxone (opioid antagonist) trials. The most popular hypothesis claims that the so-called runner's high stems from the action of endogenous opiates. Withdrawal symptoms in endurance athletes ("detraining syndrome") are explained by a reduced stimulation of β-endorphin release. Even a resulting exercise dependency is discussed *(53,56)*. Additionally, in the overtraining syndrome, a reduction in β-endorphin levels was observed *(57)*. There is a striking temporal coincidence between the often narratively reported "second wind" in endurance events and the onset of a β-endorphin elevation in aerobic exercise of long duration, i.e., after approx 1 h *(24)*. Altogether, the action of endogenous opiates can be described as a rewarding system that makes the athlete continue physical activity. On the other hand, physiological arousal may be limited to more easily tolerable amounts by attenuating pain and catecholamine action. These assumptions have to be considered speculative, since most of their contents are from indirect deductions via animal trials or psychological reactions to naloxone applications. For obvious reasons, research on humans is difficult, but in the near future, new imaging techniques could be a valuable tool in identifying central nervous system effects of endogenous opiates during exercise.

CONCLUSIONS

The release of β-endorphin during exercise is dependent on intensity and duration of the physical activity. If a threshold intensity is exceeded, rising levels of endogenous opiates can be expected. There seems to be a link to the overproportional increase of lactate and concomitant acidosis. With lower intensities of approx 55–60% of the maximal oxygen uptake, a duration of about 1 h has to be reached before β-endorphin increases. Consequently, common recreational exercise might be too extensive or short-lasting to induce hormone release from the anterior pituitary gland.

In contrast, elite athletes may experience higher levels of endogenous opiates more often—at least in competition. A physiological purpose under these conditions could be the modulation of pain to withstand further exhaustion and the improvement of mood, which may be connected to phenomena like the "second wind" or "runner's high." Sudden cessation of regular training is supposed to induce a depressed mood, which is considered to be part of the "detraining syndrome" by various authors. Some of them even claim the existence of "exercise dependence" partly based on the missing action of endogenous opiates.

At the moment, there is no indication for the introduction of β-endorphin research results into training and competition practice. It is hardly to be expected that the momentary knowledge about this group of hormones can lead to a more precise control of exercise. A more interesting research field seems to be the interrelationship between β-endorphin and other hormones to elucidate the mechanisms into which endogenous opiates are involved in athletes. The actual methods of investigation probably represent too crude tools to discover the basis of psychological exercise effects. An introduction of refined techniques seems necessary.

REFERENCES

1. Hughes J, Smith TW, Kosterlitz HW, Fothergill LA, Morgan BA, Morris HR. Identification of two related pentapeptides from the brain with potent opiate agonist activity. Nature 1975;258: 577–580.
2. Gerra G, Volpi R, Delsignore R, Caccavari R, Gaggiotti MT, Montani G, et al. ACTH and beta-endorphin responses to physical exercise in adolescent women tested for anxiety and frustration. Psychiatry Res 1992;41:179–186.
3. Heitkamp HC, Huber W, Scheib K. β-Endorphin and adrenocorticotrophin after incremental exercise and marathon running—female responses. Eur J Appl Physiol 1996;72:417–424.
4. Heitkamp H-C, Schmid K, Scheib K. β-endorphin and adrenocorticotropic hormone production during marathon and incremental exercise. Eur J Appl Physiol 1993;66:269–274.
5. Oleshansky MA, Zoltick JM, Herman RH, Mougey EH, Meyerhoff JL. The influence of fitness on neuroendocrine responses to exhaustive treadmill exercise. Eur J Appl Physiol 1990;59: 405–410.
6. Colt EW, Wardlaw SL, Frantz AG. The effect of running on plasma beta-endorphin. Life Sci 1981; 28:1637–1640.
7. Donevan RH, Andrew GM. Plasma beta-endorphin immunoreactivity during graded cycle ergometry. Med Sci Sports Exerc 1987;19:229–233.
8. McMurray RG, Forsythe WA, Mar MH, Hardy CJ. Exercise intensity-related responses of beta-endorphin and catecholamines. Med Sci Sports Exerc 1987;19:570–574.
9. Rahkila P, Hakala E, Salminen K, Laatikainen T. Response of plasma endorphins to running exercises in male and female endurance athletes. Med Sci Sports Exerc 1987;19:451–455.
10. Farrell PA, Gates WK, Maksud MG, Morgan WP. Increases in plasma beta-endorphin/beta-lipotropin immunoreactivity after treadmill running in humans. J Appl Physiol 1982;52:1245–1249.
11. Goldfarb AH, Hatfield BD, Sforzo GA, Flynn MG. Serum beta-endorphin levels during a graded exercise test to exhaustion. Med Sci Sports Exerc 1987;19:78–82.
12. de Meirleir K, Naaktgeboren N, Van Steirteghem A, Gorus F, Olbrecht J, Block P. Beta-endorphin and ACTH levels in peripheral blood during and after aerobic and anaerobic exercise. Eur J Appl Physiol 1986;55:5–8.
13. de Vries W, Bernards A, de Rooij M, Thijssen J, van Rijn H, Koppeschaar H. Different responses of stress-related hormones to dynamic exercise. Med Sci Sports Exerc 1996;28:S 76.
14. Luger A, Deuster PA, Kyle SB, Gallucci WT, Montgomery LC, Gold PW, et al. Acute hypothalamic-pituitary-adrenal responses to the stress of treadmill exercise. Physiologic adaptations to physical training. N Engl J Med 1987;316:1309–1315.
15. Schwarz L, Kindermann W. Beta-endorphin, adrenocorticotropic hormone, cortisol and catecholamines during aerobic and anaerobic exercise. Eur J Appl Physiol 1990;61:165–171.
16. Stegmann H, Kindermann W, Schnabel A. Lactate kinetics and individual anaerobic threshold. Int J Sports Med 1981;2:160–165.
17. Brooks S, Burrin J, Cheetham ME. Hall GM, Yeo T, Williams C. The responses of the catecholamines and beta-endorphin to brief maximal exercise in man. Eur J Appl Physiol 1988;57:230–234.
18. Krüger A, Wildmann J. Anstieg des β-Endorphinspiegels bei Wiederholungsbelastungen. D Z Sportmed 1986;245–250.
19. Bortz WM, Angwin P, Mefford IN, Boarder MR, Noyce N, Barchas JD. Catecholamines, dopamine, and endorphin levels during extreme exercise [letter]. N Engl J Med 1981;305:466–467.
20. Carr DB, Bullen BA, Skrinar GS, Arnold MA, Rosenblatt M, Beitins IZ. et al. Physical conditioning facilitates the exercise-induced secretion of beta-endorphin and beta-lipotropin in women. N Engl J Med 1981;305:560–563.
21. de Wet EH, Barnard HC, Luus HG, Oosthuizen JM, Bornman MS. Beta-endorfien—en leusienenkefalienkonsentrasies in marathonatlete. S Afr Med J 1992;81:335.
22. Dearman J, Francis KT. Plasma levels of catecholamines, cortisol, and beta-endorphins in male athletes after running 26.2, 6, and 2 miles. J Sports Med Phys Fitness 1983;23:30–38.
23. Gambert SR, Garthwaite TL, Pontzer CH, Cook EE, Tristani FE, Duthie EH, et al. Running elevates plasma beta-endorphin immunoreactivity and ACTH in untrained human subjects. Proc Soc Exp Biol Med 1981;168:1–4.
24. Schwarz L, Kindermann W. Beta-endorphin, catecholamines, and cortisol during exhaustive endurance exercise. Int J Sports Med 1989;10:324–328.

25. Elias AN, Fairshter R, Pandian MR, Domurat E, Kayaleh R. Beta-endorphin/beta-lipotropin release and gonadotropin secretion after acute exercise in physically conditioned males. Eur J Appl Physiol 1989;58:522–527.
26. Kelso TB, Herbert WG, Gwazdauskas FC, Goss FL, Hess JL. Exercise-thermoregulatory stress and increased plasma beta-endorphin/beta-lipotropin in humans. J Appl Physiol 1984;57:444–449.
27. Kraemer RR, Blair S, Kraemer GR, Castracane VD. Effects of treadmill running on plasma beta-endorphin, corticotropin, and cortisol levels in male and female 10K runners. Eur J Appl Physiol 1989;58:845–851.
28. Langenfeld ME, Hart LS, Kao PC. Plasma beta-endorphin responses to one-hour bicycling and running at 60% VO_{2max}. Med Sci Sports Exerc 1987;19:83–86.
29. Goldfarb AH, Hatfield BD, Armstrong D, Potts J. Plasma beta-endorphin concentration: response to intensity and duration of exercise. Med Sci Sports Exerc 1990;22:241–244.
30. Viru A, Tendzegolskis Z. Plasma endorphin species during dynamic exercise in humans. Clin Physiol 1995;15:73–79.
31. McGowan RW, Pierce EF, Eastman N, Tripathi HL, Dewey T, Olson K. Beta-endorphins and mood states during resistance exercise. Percept Mot Skills 1993;76:376–378.
32. Pierce EF, Eastman NW, Tripathi HT, Olson KG, Dewey WL. Plasma β-endorphin immunoreactivity: Response to resistance exercise. J Sports Sci 1993;11:499–502.
33. Kraemer WJ, Dziados JE, Marchitelli LJ, Gordon SE, Harman EA, Mello R, et al. Effects of different heavy-resistance exercise protocols on plasma β-endorphin concentrations. J Appl Physiol 1993;74:450–459.
34. Walberg Rankin J, Franke WD, Gwazdauskas FC. Response of beta-endorphin and estradiol to resistance exercise in females during energy balance and energy restriction. Int J Sports Med 1992;13:542–547.
35. Belikow J, Starich GH, Lardinois CK. The effect of aerobic conditioning on plasma β-lipotropin and β-endorphin levels in humans. Abstract Med Sci Sports Exerc 1988;20:S 40.
36. Lobstein DD, Rasmussen CL. Decreases in resting plasma beta-endorphin and depression scores after endurance training. J Sports Med Phys Fitness 1991;31:543–551.
37. Boineau RE, Cureton KJ, Hitri A, DeMello JJ, Singh MM. Effects of state of training and gender on plasma beta-endorphin responses to exercise. Abstract Med Sci Sports Exerc 1985;17:209.
38. Berk LS, Tan SA, Anderson CL, Reiss G. β-endorphin response to exercise in athletes and non-athletes. Abstract Med Sci Sports Exerc 1981;13:134.
39. Goldfarb AH, Hatfield BD, Potts J, Armstrong D. Beta-endorphin time course response to intensity of exercise: effect of training status. Int J Sports Med 1991;12:264–268.
40. Howlett TA, Tomlin S, Ngahfoong L, Rees LH, Bullen BA, Skrinar GS, et al. Release of beta endorphin and met-enkephalin during exercise in normal women: response to training. Br Med J Clin Res Ed 1984;288:1950–1952.
41. Mains RE, Eipper BA, Ling N. Common precursor to corticotropins and endorphins. Proc Natl Acad Sci USA 1977;74:3014–3018.
42. Vale W, Rivier C, Yang L, Minick S, Guillemin R. Effects of purified hypothalamic corticotropin-releasing factor and other substances on the secretion of adrenocorticotropin and beta-endorphin-like immunoactivities in vitro. Endocrinology 1978;103:1910–1915.
43. Young EA, Akil H. Corticotropin-releasing factor stimulation of adrenocorticotropin and beta-endorphin release: effects of acute and chronic stress. Endocrinology 1985;117:23–30.
44. Dent RR, Guilleminault C, Albert LH, Posner BI, Cox BM, Goldstein A. Diurnal rhythm of plasma immunoreactive beta-endorphin and its relationship to sleep stages and plasma rhythms of cortisol and prolactin. J Clin Endocrinol Metab 1981;52:942–947.
45. Mougin C, Baulay A, Henriet MT, Haton D, Jacquier MC, Turnill D, et al. Assessment of plasma opioid peptides, beta-endorphin and met-enkephalin, at the end of an international nordic ski race. Eur J Appl Physiol 1987;56:281–286.
46. Urhausen A, Weiler B, Coen B, Kindermann W. Plasma catecholamines during endurance exercise of different intensities as related to the individual anaerobic threshold. Eur J Appl Physiol 1994;69:16–20.
47. Sutton JR, Brown GM, Keane P, Walker WHC, Jones NL. The role of endorphins in the hormonal control and psychological responses to exercise. Int J Sports Med 1982;2:19–24.
48. Thompson DA, Penicaud L, Welle SL, Jacobs LS. Pharmacological evidence for opioid and adrenergic mechanisms controlling growth hormone, prolactin, pancreatic polypeptide, and catecholamine levels in humans. Metabolism 1985;34:383–390.

49. Gold MS, Redmond DEJ, Kleber HD. Clonidine blocks acute opiate-withdrawal symptoms. Lancet 1978;2:599–602.
50. Berkenbosch F, Vermes I, Binnekade R, Tilders FJ. Beta-adrenergic stimulation induces an increase of the plasma levels of immunoreactive alpha-MSH, beta-endorphin, ACTH and of corticosterone. Life Sci 1981;29:2249–2256.
51. Taylor DV. Boyajian JG, James N, Woods D, Chicz-Demet A, Wilson AF, et al. Acidosis stimulates β-endorphin release during exercise. J Appl Physiol 1994;77:1913–1918.
52. Fraioli F, Moretti C, Paolucci D, Alicicco E, Crescenzi F, Fortunio G. Physical exercise stimulates marked concomitant release of beta-endorphin and adrenocorticotropic hormone (ACTH) in peripheral blood in man. Experientia 1980;36:987–989.
53. Arentz T, de Meirleir K, Hollmann W. Die Rolle der endogenen opioiden Peptide während Fahrradergometerarbeit. D Z Sportmed 1986;37:210–219.
54. Kemppainen P, Pertovaara A, Huopaniemi T, Johansson G, Karonen SL. Modification of dental pain and cutaneous thermal sensitivity by physical exercise in man. Brain Res 1985;360:33–40.
55. Allen M. Activity-generated endorphins: a review of their role in sports science. Can J Appl Sport Sci 1983;8:115–133.
56. Janal MN, Colt EW, Clark WC, Glusman M. Pain sensitivity, mood and plasma endocrine levels in man following long-distance running: effects of naloxone. Pain 1984;19:13–25.
57. Urhausen A. Das Übertrainingssyndrom—Ein multifaktorieller Ansatz im Rahmen einer prospektiven Längsschnittstudie bei ausdauertrainierten Sportlern. Postdoctoral Thesis, Institute of Sports and Performance Medicine, Saarbrücken, Germany, 1993.

3 The Effect of Exercise on the Hypothalamo–Pituitary–Adrenal Axis

Gary Wittert, MD, FRACP

CONTENTS

INTRODUCTION
EFFECT OF EXERCISE ON THE HPA AXIS
THE EFFECT OF EXERCISE TRAINING ON THE HPA AXIS
EXERCISE AND ABNORMALITIES OF THE HPA AXIS
REFERENCES

INTRODUCTION

In response to any external stimulus that is perceived as a threat to homeostasis (stress), activation of the autonomic nervous system occurs and plasma cortisol levels increase as a result of activation of the hypothalamo–pituitary–adrenal (HPA) axis. The hypothalamic hormones corticotropin-releasing hormone (CRH) and arginine vasopressin (AVP) are the major regulators of corticotropin (adrenocorticotrophic hormone; ACTH) secretion from the corticotropes of the anterior pituitary gland *(1)*. ACTH in turn stimulates the production and release of cortisol from the zona fasciculata of the adrenal cortex at a rate of about 12–15 mg/m^2/d in nonstressed adults. Approximately 90–93% of circulating cortisol is bound to a protein, cortisol binding globulin (CBG), and only the free fraction can readily diffuse through cell membranes and exert biological effects. Plasma cortisol levels peak at about the time of waking and have their nadir around midnight. Although light is the main entrainer of the cortisol rhythm, other influences, for example, physical activity, also have a significant effect on the human circadian pacemaker *(2)*.

Cortisol inhibits the activity of the HPA axis at the level of the pituitary and hypothalamus, as well as other regions of the brain, to influence their input into the hypothalamus *(3)*. Sensitivity to cortisol feedback is an important mechanism for regulation of the HPA axis. The nature and duration of the stress can alter the sensitivity to cortisol feedback in humans. For example, strenuous physical activity can induce alterations in the glucocorticoid sensitivity of peripheral blood lymphocytes *(4,5)*. There is

From: *Contemporary Endocrinology: Sports Endocrinology*
Edited by: M. P. Warren and N. W. Constantini © Humana Press Inc., Totowa, NJ

also evidence that differences in the response of the HPA axis to intense exercise between individuals may relate to differences in glucocorticoid sensitivity (6).

In addition to its effect on the HPA axis, CRH regulates the activity of the sympathetic nervous system as well as many of the behavioral changes that occur during stress (7,8). In the anterior pituitary, CRH originating from neurons in the parvicellular division of the paraventricular nucleus (PVN), stimulates the synthesis, as well as the secretion of ACTH by inducing transcription of the propiomelanocortin (POMC) gene. Many CRH-containing parvicellular neurons also contain AVP (9). AVP increases the release, but not the synthesis of ACTH. AVP originating from magnocellular neurons is principally involved in the regulation of water balance, but some of these neurons provide projections to the median eminence and are involved in the regulation of ACTH secretion (10). A synergistic effect of CRH and AVP on ACTH release has been shown in humans (1). Studies in animals have demonstrated a variation in the CRH:AVP ratio that is specific to the nature as well as the magnitude and duration of the stimulus (11,12). Furthermore, different populations of corticotropes have different sensitivities to CRH and AVP (13). Based on animal studies, it has been suggested that AVP may be important in maintaining pituitary adrenal responsiveness to acute stressors in chronic stress conditions (14,15). In humans, an increase in peripheral plasma AVP levels is a regular accompaniment to acute stress (1). At rest and during exercise, the endogenous opioid peptide, β-endorphin, inhibits the activity of the HPA axis (16).

Increasingly there is evidence for sexual dimorphism in the regulation of the HPA axis. The CRH gene has functional estrogen-response elements (17), and in the human female, the hypothalamus has higher CRH levels than in the male (18). Estradiol downregulates glucocorticoid receptor binding (19). There is evidence for increased tone of the central stress system in women (20), and generally female humans and animals have higher basal cortisol levels than males.

EFFECT OF EXERCISE ON THE HPA AXIS

Intense physical activity induces increases in the activity of the HPA axis. The mechanism by which physical exercise activates the HPA axis has not been fully elucidated. Physical exercise induces an effect on ACTH and cortisol secretion greater than that which can be accounted for by CRH alone (21). In humans, exercise is accompanied by increases in AVP release into the systemic circulation (22–24), which occur in proportion to the intensity of the exercise (22,23). Pulses of ACTH and AVP secretion are concordant during exercise in humans (24), and when pituitary venous effluent is sampled from galloping horses, synchronous pulses of ACTH and AVP occur (25).

Increases in plasma lactate have been implicated as one of the mechanisms responsible for activation of the HPA axis during exercise (26). Other humoral mediators, for example, angiotensin II (22) and interleukins (27), which increase during exercise, are also capable of activating the HPA axis. However, their role in humans in activating the HPA axis during exercise has not been defined. Impulses in afferent nerves from working muscles have been shown to be essential for the activation of the HPA axis during exercise (28,29). Furthermore, impulses generated from peripheral nerves originating in muscle tissue contribute to the increase in plasma AVP, which occurs during exercise (23). Changes in plasma volume and osmolality also occur during exercise accompanied by proportional changes in plasma AVP (23). Several factors have been identified to influence the cortisol response to exercise.

Intensity, Duration, and Timing of Exercise

Activation of the HPA axis was initially described to occur during aerobic physical activity that exceeded 60% of the maximum aerobic power *(30)*. However, in many studies, the response of plasma cortisol to exercise was determined relative to the usual pre-exercise baseline, rather than relative to the hormone's circadian baseline. This may result in a significant underestimation of the effect of exercise on plasma cortisol *(31)*. When evaluated relative to the circadian baseline, responses of plasma cortisol to 90 min of exercise at 55% and even 25% VO_2max, may be quite large *(32,33)*. Furthermore, in response to intense physical activity, the magnitude of the increase in free cortisol may be much greater that total cortisol *(34)*.

Activation of the HPA axis during aerobic exercise is proportional to the relative intensity of the exercise and is independent of the fitness level of the subject *(26,35)*. Prolonged submaximal physical activity *(36)* and very brief high-intensity exercise *(37)* result in activation of the HPA axis. However, brief high-intensity exercise produces an increase in plasma ACTH levels *(37)* that is greater than those found during prolonged submaximal exercise *(36)*, yet less than those seen following graded exercise to exhaustion *(36,38)*. In ultralong-distance races, an increase in plasma cortisol may be observed either prior to the onset of the race (reflecting prerace anxiety) *(39)* or after an initial delay, and thereafter remains elevated for the duration of the event *(39,40)*, overriding the usual circadian variation *(40,41)*. Duration of physical activity may be important in determining the response of plasma cortisol to exercise. For example, plasma cortisol increased more after a 42-km than a 19-km kayak race *(41)*. During a 6-d Nordic ski race, plasma ACTH levels increased and then remained similar throughout the race, whereas plasma cortisol was highest on the initial 2 d *(41)*. Wide interindividual differences are observed, and a number of psychological factors may modify the response of the HPA axis to physical stress *(42,43)*.

Type of Exercise

Plasma cortisol levels have been reported to increase in response to a 50-mile walking race in male volunteers *(44)* and in response to handball in women *(45)*. The response of the HPA axis to kayaking appears to induce a greater increase in plasma cortisol than marathon running *(46)*. In contrast to sustained aerobic activity, intermittent exercise of varying intensities, such as matchplay tennis, does not appear to induce activation of the HPA axis *(47)*. When associated with the stress of competition, cortisol levels may increase, but this is related more to psychological factors than the physical activity as such *(48)*.

Isometric (resistance) exercise induces activation of the HPA axis *(49–51)*, which is intensity-dependent *(50)*. The duration and number of repetitions in each set, and the interset rest period length are the primary determinants of the cortisol response *(52)*. Anaerobic exercise has been shown to induce a greater increase in plasma cortisol than aerobic exercise of the same total work output *(53)*.

Age

The response of the HPA axis to physical activity is independent of age. In male children, plasma cortisol increased in response to 30 min of exercise at VO_2max *(54)*. In adolescents, exercise to exhaustion on a cycle ergometer also resulted in activation of the HPA axis *(55)*. Plasma cortisol increases in response to weightlifting in adolescent males *(56)*.

In elderly males, the cortisol response to heavy-resistance exercise is diminished *(57)*, although this may reflect reduced effort. During submaximal aerobic exercise, elderly subjects have been observed to have an earlier activation of the HPA axis accompanied by a more pronounced increase in the activity of the sympathetic nervous system *(58)*. However, when exercised to the same relative intensity, the cortisol response to aerobic exercise is similar in both trained and untrained elderly subjects as compared to young controls *(59)*. Furthermore, the effect of endurance training on the activity of the HPA axis is similar in health elderly and younger subjects *(60)*.

Gender

Although there is a theoretical basis for a difference in the response of the HPA axis to physical activity between males and females, there are very few studies where this issue has been examined. Resting levels of plasma cortisol and responses to exercise appear to be independent of the menstrual phase in healthy women *(61,62)*. The response of plasma ACTH and cortisol to treadmill running for 30 min at 80% of VO_2max is similar in males and females *(63)*. However, the intensity of resistance exercise required to activate the HPA axis appears to be greater in females than males *(64)*. In one study, female marathon runners were shown to have lower baseline concentrations and larger increases in ACTH concentration in response to both incremental exercise and marathon running in comparison to men *(65)*. Another study has shown that the response of plasma cortisol to endurance exercise is not affected by the gender of the subject *(66)*. The delay before HPA axis activity returns to normal after a marathon is similar in males and females *(65)*.

Other Factors

A number of factors may modify the response of the HPA axis to physical activity. Cortisol responses to exercise are blunted when exercise is initiated at the peak of the cortisol response to a meal *(32)*. During exercise at low altitude, the response of plasma ACTH, but not cortisol, is increased compared to when exercise is undertaken at moderate level of altitude *(67)*. At high altitude, both ski-training *(68)* and marathon running *(69)* produce greater increases in plasma cortisol than training at moderate or low altitude. Mild dehydration does not affect the response of plasma cortisol to prolonged low-intensity exercise *(70)*. The response of plasma cortisol to short-duration, high-intensity exercise is not modified by an increase in environmental temperature *(71)*.

During prolonged, low-intensity exercise in humans, decreased blood glucose concentrations (<3.3 mmol/L) result in increased activation of the HPA axis, which can be prevented by maintaining the blood glucose constant *(72,73)*. During acute cycling exercise, the ingestion of carbohydrate attenuates the cortisol response *(74,75)*. By contrast carbohydrate ingestion during prolonged running exercise has been shown to result in either no change *(76)*, or an increased serum cortisol compared to placebo-treated controls *(77)*.

A number of other factors have been shown to affect the cortisol response to exercise. In dogs with moderate anemia (25% reduction in hematocrit), exercise results in greater increases in plasma cortisol than control animals *(78)*. In athletes, the environmental setting and focus of attention may affect the cortisol response to exercise, particularly if they alter the emotional experience associated with exercise *(79)*. Interestingly, although acute alcohol consumption may affect the HPA axis, alcohol consumption does not appear to affect the cortisol response to exercise *(80)*.

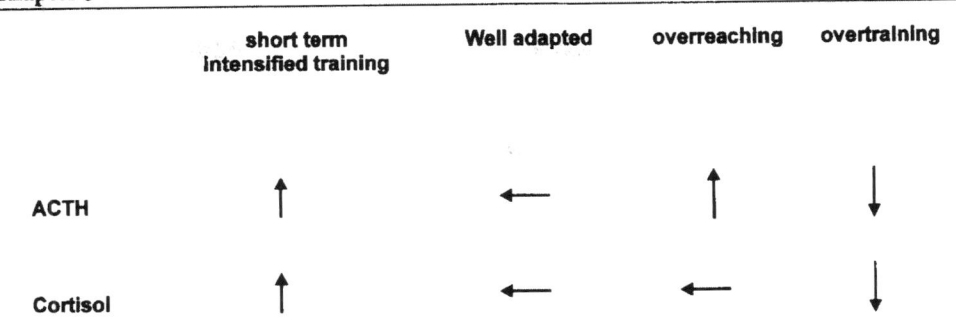

	short term intensified training	Well adapted	overreaching	overtraining
ACTH	↑	←	↑	↓
Cortisol	↑	←	←	↓

Fig. 1. Effect of exercise training on the HPA axis.

THE EFFECT OF EXERCISE TRAINING ON THE HPA AXIS

Training does not affect the cortisol response to exercise of the same relative intensity (81,82), but the response to the same absolute intensity may decrease (82–85). However, in response to supramaximal exercise, activation of the HPA axis in endurance-trained subjects is greater than in untrained subjects (86,87). The nature of the exercise training may to some extent determine the response of the HPA axis to subsequent acute exercise; when a substantial anaerobic component is present, the cortisol response to subsequent exercise may be increased (see Fig. 1) (88).

After prolonged endurance exercise, normalization of plasma cortisol levels may take up to 18–24 h (46,65). In trained athletes as compared to control subjects, recovery from intense, prolonged exercise is associated with greater plasma ACTH levels, but similar plasma cortisol levels (89). However, very intense physical training as such may result in adaptations characterized by increased ACTH, but not basal cortisol levels (90,91).

The nature of the effect of training on basal activity of the HPA axis remains unresolved. In prepubescent gymnasts, after five consecutive days of training (3 h each day at moderate intensity), plasma cortisol levels were similar to those of control subjects. A season of training did not affect basal plasma cortisol levels in either male or female joggers (92). Neither an increase in training intensity in middle- and long-distance runners nor 12 wk of intense training in competitive swimmers (93) affected basal plasma cortisol levels (94,95). There was no effect of up to 2 yr of intensive weight training on basal cortisol levels in adolescent males (56). However, 1 wk of overreaching stimulus induced an increase in early morning cortisol levels in this group of subjects (96). Intensive training for an endurance ultramarathon (91,97) or experimentally in recreational athletes (98) has been shown to increase pituitary ACTH secretion without affecting plasma cortisol levels. (Fig. 2) Another study has shown that intensive training on a treadmill increased resting plasma cortisol levels, but did not effect basal ACTH (88). In competitive swimmers, a short-term increase in training distance may increase basal plasma cortisol levels (without necessarily affecting performance) (99), and trained cyclists have been reported to have higher basal cortisol levels than untrained controls (59). There is no difference in the response of male and female athletes to a sudden increase in training (100).

The response of plasma cortisol may be determined by both the duration and the nature of the training program, because sprint interval (associated with a substantial anaerobic component to training), but not endurance training has been observed to increase basal plasma cortisol (88,91). An increase in training volume as opposed to intensity has

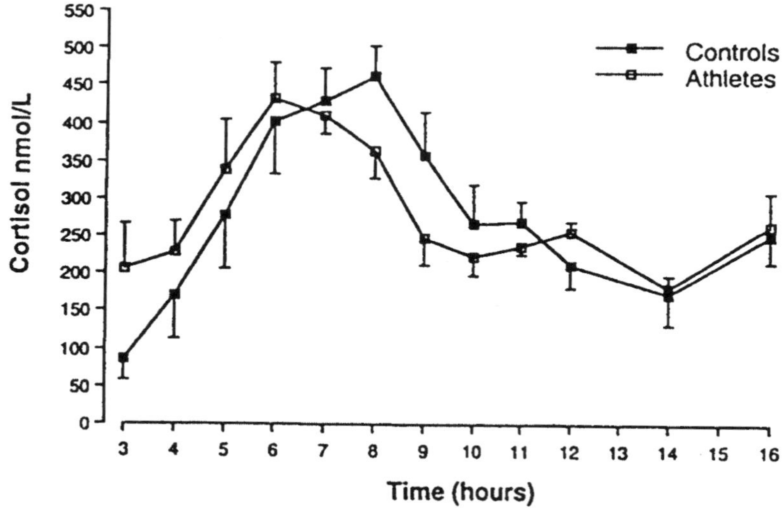
Controls
Athletes
Cortisol nmol/L
0
50
100
150
200
250
300
350
400
450
500
550
3
4
5
6
7
8
9
10
11
12
13
14
15
16
Time (hours)

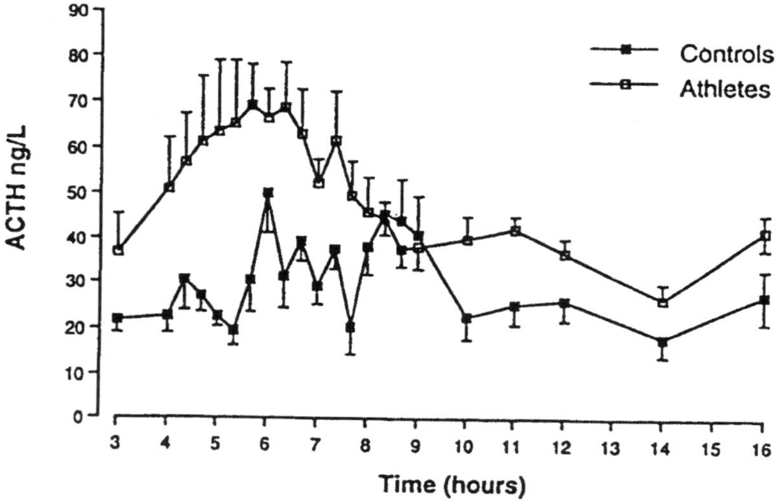
Controls
Athletes
ACTH ng/L
0
10
20
30
40
50
60
70
80
90
3
4
5
6
7
8
9
10
11
12
13
14
15
16
Time (hours)

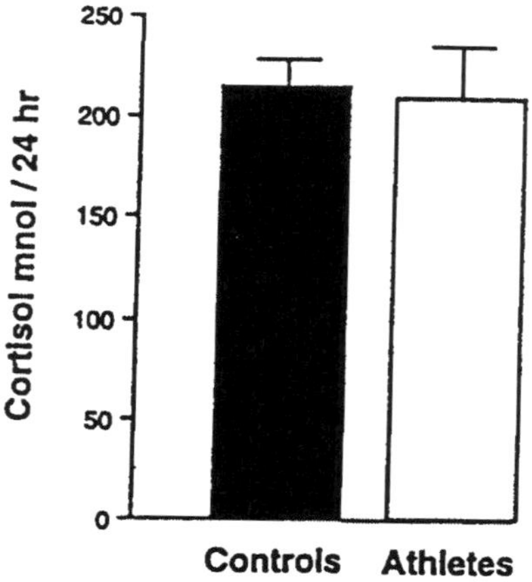
Cortisol mnol / 24 hr
0
50
100
150
200
250
Controls
Athletes

been observed to induce an overtraining syndrome, which is associated with a decrease in both resting and exercise-induced cortisol levels *(94)*. However, in another study, a twofold increase in training volume did not affect plasma cortisol levels, and there was no difference in the endocrine responses to an increase in training volume with crosstraining as compared to mode-specific training *(95)*. After 5 wk of training, the hormonal response to exercise is similar regardless of whether training was carried out under conditions to simulate increased altitude (2500 m) or at sea level *(101)*.

The effect of resistance exercise training on basal plasma cortisol levels is variable, and either no change *(96,102,103)* or a decrease has been reported *(104)*, the difference probably being related to lower training volumes. However, as with aerobic exercise, increasing resistance training volume or intensity increases resting cortisol levels, although a doubling of training volume has also been observed to result in a decrease in exercise-induced increases in cortisol levels when these are intensity-dependent *(105)*.

The objective of training is to optimize human performance. Training itself and short-term increases in training produce a number of neuroendocrine adaptations, which result in alterations of the activity of the HPA axis. This response is determined by the training volume, intensity, type of exercise, optimum periods of rest (regeneration), and poorly defined psychological factors. These various factors, in addition to the observation that responses of plasma cortisol and ACTH may not necessarily be concordant, may account for the discrepancies between the above studies.

In general, it appears that the response to short-term intensified training is an increased plasma cortisol level, particularly if an anaerobic element is involved. With overreaching, increased ACTH occurs, but the cortisol response is decreased, whereas with overtraining, HPA axis activity is decreased as a whole *(106)*.

EXERCISE AND ABNORMALITIES OF THE HPA AXIS

Overreaching and Overtraining

If adaptation to the increased training regimen does not occur, or if insufficient recovery time is included in training regimens, overreaching and subsequently overtraining may occur. Overreaching may be considered as short-term overtraining and may be a normal part of athletic training, or may be seen as a short-term consequence of ultraendurance events. By contrast, overtraining syndrome results in a state described as burnout or staleness, which is characterized by increased fatigue, altered mood state, increased infections, and suppressed reproductive function. Overtraining may be, at least in part, the consequence of inadequate periods of "regeneration" *(10–110)*.

From the HPA axis standpoint, it has been suggested that the earliest stage of overreaching (or very early overtraining) may be reflected by a reduced responsiveness to ACTH, which is initially compensated for by an increased pituitary ACTH response, but a decreased adrenal cortisol response *(91,110)*. When fully evolved, the overtraining syndrome is characterized by both a reduced ACTH and cortisol response *(94,106,111)*. In highly trained distance runners, who undertook a 38% increase in training intensity

---

Fig. 2. *(see opposite page)* Adaptation of the HPA axis to chorionic exercise stress is humans. Mean (± SEM) plasma concentrations of cortisol in ultramarathon (**top**) and ACTH (**middle**) athletes (⊟) and control subjects (■), and 24-h urinary free cortisol (**bottom**) excretion in ultramarathon athletes and control subjects.

over 3 wk, six of the subjects developed sustained fatigue and the increase of serum cortisol, normally induced by 30 min of submaximal exercise, was lost *(112)*.

Whether overtraining induced by high volume resistance exercise produces similar effects to highly aerobic activities is not entirely clear. Maximal-intensity, resistance exercise overtraining does not affect basal plasma cortisol or ACTH levels, and the response to exercise is decreased *(105)*.

Athletic Amenorrhea

Exercise-associated disorders of the reproductive axis in women are associated with abnormalities of the HPA axis. The response of plasma cortisol to both maximal and submaximal acute exercise is reduced in amenorrheic compared to eumenorrheic athletes *(62,113)*. Amenorrheic athletes have been found to have higher mean basal *(114,115)* early morning *(115)* or midafternoon *(62)* blood and 24-h urine *(115,116)* cortisol levels. There is also evidence that basal CRH stimulation is increased *(115,117)* and that adrenal sensitivity to ACTH is reduced *(62,118)*.

In conclusion, although a great deal has been learned about the effects of physical activity on the HPA axis, there is still much conflicting information and many areas of confusion. The response of the HPA axis to any stress is dependent not only on the nature of the stress, but also on the environment in which the stress is imposed as well the inherent characteristics of the individual concerned (genetic factors, gender, personality, prior experience), concomitant stressors, and nutritional state. In addition, the timing and manner in which samples are collected will also influence the results obtained.

The extent to which abnormalities of the HPA axis are simply consequences of, or are inherent to the pathophysiology of a variety of conditions related to exercise training, is not entirely clear. It is also not clear whether activity of the HPA axis can be used as a marker of training stress and adaptation, for example, by establishing the activity of and following longitudinally the HPA axis of individual athletes.

REFERENCES

1. Donald RA, Wittert GA. Stress and ACTH regulation. In: Kohler PO, ed. Current Opinion in Endocrinology and Diabetes. Current Science, Philadelphia, PA; 1994, pp. 93–99.
2. Van Reeth O, Sturis J, Byrne MM, Blackman JD, L'Hermite Baleriaux M, Leproult R, et al. Nocturnal exercise phase delays circadian rhythms of melatonin and thyrotropin secretion in normal men. Am J Physiol 1994;266:E964–E974.
3. Levin N, Shinsako J, Dallman M. Cortisocsterone acts on the brain to inhibit adrenalectomy-induced adrenocorticotropin secretion. Endocrinology 1988;122:694–701.
4. DeRijk RH, Petrides J, Deuster P, Gold PW, Sternberg EM. Changes in corticosteroid sensitivity of peripheral blood lymphocytes after strenuous exercise in humans. J Clin Endocrinol Metab 1996;81:228–235.
5. Grasso G, Lodi L, Lupo C, Muscettola M. Glucocorticoid receptors in human peripheral blood mononuclear cells in relation to age and to sport activity. Life Sci 1997;61:301–308.
6. Petrides JS, Mueller GP, Kalogeras KT, Chrousos GP, Gold PW, Deuster PA Exercise-induced activation of the hypothalamic-pituitary-adrenal axis: marked differences in the sensitivity to glucocorticoid suppression. J Clin Endocrinol Metab 1994;79:377–383.
7. Kalin NH. Behavioural effects of ovine corticotropin-releasing factor administered to rhesus monkeys. Fed Proc 1985;44:249–253.
8. Koob GF, Bloom FE. Corticotropin-releasing factor and behavior. Fed Proc 1991;44:259–263.
9. Whitnall MH. Stress selectively activates the vasopressin-containing subset of corticotropin-releasing hormone neurons. Neuroendocrinology 1989;50:702–707.

10. Holmes MC, Antoni FA, Aguilera G, Catt KJ. Magnocellular axons in passage through the median eminence release vasopressin. Nature 1986;319:326–329.
11. Plotsky PM Pathways to the secretion of adrenocorticotropin: a view from the portal. J Neuroendocrinol 1991;3:1–9.
12. Canny BJ, Funder JW, Clarke IJ. Glucocorticoids regulate ovine hypophysial portal levels of corticotropin-releasing factor and arginine vasopressin in a stress-specific manner. Endocrinology 1989;125:2532–2539.
13. Jia LG, Canny BJ, Orth DN, Leong DA. Distinct classes of corticotropes mediate corticotropin-releasing hormone- and arginine vasopressin-stimulated adrenocorticotropin release. Endocrinology 1991;128:197–203.
14. De Goeij DC, Dijksstra S, Tilders FJH. Chronic psychosocial stress enhances vasopressin, but not corticotropin-releasing factor, in the external zone of the median eminence of males rats. Endocrinology 1991;101:847–853.
15. De Goeij DC, Binnekade R, Tilders FJ. Chronic stress enhances vasopressin but not corticotropin-releasing factor secretion during hypoglycemia. Am J Physiol 1992;263:E394–99.
16. Staessen J, Fiocchi R, Bouillon R, Fagard R, Hespel P, Lijnen P, et al. Effects of opioid antagonism on the haemodynamic and hormonal responses to exercise. Clin Sci 1988;75:293–300.
17. Vamvakopoulos NC, Chrousos GP. Hormonal regulation of human corticotropin-releasing factor gene expression: implications for the stress response and immune/inflammatory reaction. Endocr Rev 1994;15:409–420.
18. Frederiksen SO, Ekman R, Gottfries CG, Widerlov E, Jonsson S. Reduced concentrations of galanin, arginine vasopressin, neuropeptide Y and peptide YY in the temporal cortex but not in the hypothalamus of brains from schizophrenics. Acta Psychiatr Scand 1991;83:273–277.
19. Turner BB. Sex difference in glucocorticoid binding in rat pituitary is estrogen dependent. Life Sci 1990;46:1399–1406.
20. Gallucci WT, Baum A, Laue L, Rabin DS, Chrousos GP, Gold PW, Kling MA. Sex differences in sensitivity of the hypothalamic–pituitary–adrenal axis. Health Psychol 1993;12:420–425.
21. Smoak B, Deuster P, Rabin D, Chrousos G. Corticotropin-releasing hormone is not the sole factor mediating exercise-induced adrenocorticotropin release in humans. J Clin Endocrinol Metab 1991;73:302–306.
22. Convertino VA, Keil LC, Bernauer EM, Greenleaf JE. Plasma volume, osmolality, vasopressin and renin activity during graded exercise in man. J Appl Physiol 1981;50:123–128 (Abstract).
23. Wade CE. Response, regulation and actions of vasopressin during exercise: a review. Med Sci Sports Exerc 1984;16:506–511 (Abstract).
24. Wittert GA, Stewart DE, Graves MP, Ellis MJ, Evans MJ, Wells JE, et al. Plasma corticotrophin releasing factor and vasopressin responses to exercise in normal man. Clin Endocrinol Oxford 1991;35:311–317.
25. Alexander SL, Irvine CH, Ellis MJ, Donald RA. The effect of acute exercise on the secretion of corticotropin-releasing factor, arginine vasopressin, and adrenocorticotropin as measured in pituitary venous blood from the horse. Endocrinology 1991;128:65–72.
26. Luger A, Deuster PA, Kyle SB, Gallucci WT, Montgomery LC, Gold PW, et al. Acute hypothalamic-pituitary-adrenal responses to the stress of treadmill exercise. Physiologic adaptations to physical training. N Engl J Med 1987;316:1309–1315.
27. Cannon JG, Kluger MJ. Endogenous pyrogen activity in human plasma after execise. Science 1983;220:617–619.
28. Kjaer M. Secher NH, Bach FW, Sheikh S, Galbo H. Hormonal and metabolic responses to exercise in humans: effect of sensory nervous blockade. Am J Physiol 1989;257:E95–101.
29. Kjaer M, Secher NH, Bangsbo J, Perko G, Horn A, Mohr T, et al. Hormonal and metabolic responses to electrically induced cycling during epidural anesthesia in humans. J Appl Physiol 1996;80:2156–2162.
30. Few JD. Effect of exercise on the secretion and metabolism of cortisol in man. J Endocrinol 1974;62:341–353.
31. Thuma JR, Gilders R, Verdun M, Loucks AB. Circadian rhythm of cortisol confounds cortisol responses to exercise: implications for future research. J Appl Physiol 1995;78:1657–1664.
32. Brandenberger G, Follenius M. Influence of timing and intensity of musclar exercise on temporal patterns of plasma cortisol levels. J Clin Endocrinol Metab 1975;40:845–849.

33. Brandenberger G, Follenius M, Hietter B. Feedback from meal-related peaks determines diurnal changes in cortisol response to exercise. J Clin Endocrinol Metab 1982;54:592–596.
34. Rowbottom DG, Keast D, Garcia Webb P, Morton AR. Serum free cortisol responses to a standard exercise test among elite triathletes. Aust J Sci Med Sport 1995;27:103–107.
35. Oleshansky MA, Zoltick JM, Herman RH, Mougey EH, Meyerhoff JL. The influence of fitness on neuroendocrine responses to exhaustive treadmill exercise. Eur J Appl Physiol 1990;59:405–410.
36. Farrell PA, Garthwaite TL, Gustafson AB. Plasma adrenocorticotropin and cortisol responses to submaximal and exhaustive exercise. J Appl Physiol 1983;55:1441–1444.
37. Buono MJ, Yeager JE, Hodgdon JA. Plasma adrenocorticotropin and cortisol responses to brief high-intensity exercise in humans. J Appl Physiol 1986;61:1337–1339.
38. Fraioli F, Moretti C, Paolucci D, Alicicco E, Crescenzi F, Fortunio G. Physical exercise stimulates marked concomitant release of beta-endorphin and adrenocorticotropic hormone (ACTH) in peripheral blood in man. Experientia 1980;36:987–989.
39. Fournier PE, Stalder J, Mermillod B, Chantraine A. Effects of a 110 kilometer ultra-marathon race on plasma hormone levels. Int J Sports Med 1997;18:252–256.
40. Nagel D, Seiler D, Franz H. Biochemical, hematological and endocrinological parameters during repeated intense short-term running in comparison to ultra-long-distance running. Int J Sports Med 1992;13:337–343.
41. Fellmann N, Bedu M, Boudet G, Mage M, Sagnol M, Pequignot JM, et al. Inter-relationships between pituitary-adrenal hormones and catecholamines during a 6-day Nordic ski race. Eur J Appl Physiol 1992;64:258–265.
42. Voigt K, Ziegler M, Grunert Fuchs M, Bickel U, Fehm Wolfsdorf G. Hormonal responses to exhausting physical exercise: the role of predictability and controllability of the situation. Psychoneuroendocrinology 1990;15:173–184.
43. Mason JW, Hartley LH, Kotchen TA, Mougey EH, Ricketts PT, Jones LG. Plasma cortisol and norepinephrine responses in anticipation of muscular exercise. Psychosom Med 1973;35:406–414.
44. Fukatsu A, Sato N, Shimizu H. 50-mile walking race suppresses neutrophil bactericidal function by inducing increases in cortisol and ketone bodies. Life Sci 1996;58:2337–2343.
45. Filaire E, Duche P, Lac G, Robert A. Saliva cortisol, physical exercise and training: influences of swimming and handball on cortisol concentrations in women. Eur J Appl Physiol 1996;74:274–278.
46. Lutoslawska G, Obminski Z, Krogulski A, Sendecki W. Plasma cortisol and testosterone following 19-km and 42-km kayak races. J Sports Med Phys Fitness 1991;31:538–542.
47. Bergeron MF, Maresh CM, Kraemer WJ, Abraham A, Conroy B, Gabaree C. Tennis: a physiological profile during match play. Int J Sports Med 1991;12:474–479.
48. Petraglia F, Barletta C, Facchinetti F, Spinazzola F, Monzani A, Scavo D, et al. Response of circulating adrenocorticotropin, beta-endorphin, beta-lipotropin and cortisol to athletic competition. Acta Endocrinol Copenh 1988;118:332–336.
49. Few JD, Imms FJ, Weiner JS. Pituitary-adrenal response to static exercise in man. Clin Sci Mol Med 1975;49:201–206.
50. Hakkinen K, Pakarinen A. Acute hormonal responses to two different fatiguing heavy-resistance protocols in male athletes. J Appl Physiol 1993;74:882–887.
51. Jurimae T, Karelson K, Smirnova T, Viru A. The effect of a single-circuit weight-training session on the blood biochemistry of untrained university students. Eur J Appl Physiol 1990;61:344–348.
52. Kraemer WJ, Dziados JE, Marchitelli LJ, Gordon SE, Harman EA, Mello R, et al. Effects of different heavy-resistance exercise protocols on plasma beta-endorphin concentrations. J Appl Physiol 1993;74:450–459.
53. Hackney AC, Premo MC, McMurray RG. Influence of aerobic versus anaerobic exercise on the relationship between reproductive hormones in men. J Sports Sci 1995;13:305–311.
54. del Corral P, Mahon AD, Duncan GE, Howe CA, Craig BW. The effect of exercise on serum and salivary cortisol in male children. Med Sci Sports Exerc 1994;26:1297–1301.
55. Winter JS. The metabolic response to exercise and exhaustion in normal and growth-hormone-deficient children. Can J Physiol Pharmacol 1974;52:575–582.
56. Kraemer WJ, Fry AC, Warren BJ, Stone MH, Fleck SJ, Kearney JT, et al. Acute hormonal responses in elite junior weightlifters. Int J Sports Med 1992;13:103–109.
57. Hakkinen K, Pakarinen A. Acute hormonal responses to heavy resistance exercise in men and women at different ages. Int J Sports Med 1995;16:507–513.

58. Korkushko OV, Frolkis MV, Shatilo VB, Yaroschenko Yu T. Hormonal and autonomic reactions to exercise in elderly healthy subjects and patients with ischemic heart disease. Acta Clin Belg 1990;45:164–175.
59. Silverman HG, Mazzeo RS. Hormonal responses to maximal and submaximal exercise in trained and untrained men of various ages. J Gerontol A Biol Sci Med Sci 1996;51:B30–7.
60. Carroll JF, Convertino VA, Wood CE, Graves JE, Lowenthal DT, Pollock ML. Effect of training on blood volume and plasma hormone concentrations in the elderly (see comments). Med Sci Sports Exerc 1995;27:79–84.
61. Kanaley JA, Boileau RA, Bahr JM, Misner JE, Nelson RA. Cortisol levels during prolonged exercise: the influence of menstrual phase and menstrual status. Int J Sports Med 1992;13:332–336.
62. De Souza MJ, Maguire MS, Maresh CM, Kraemer WJ, Rubin KR, Loucks AB. Adrenal activation and the prolactin response to exercise in eumenorrheic and amenorrheic runners. J Appl Physiol 1991;70:2378–2387.
63. Kraemer RR, Blair S, Kraemer GR, Castracane VD. Effects of treadmill running on plasma beta-endorphin, corticotropin, and cortisol levels in male and female 10K runners. Eur J Appl Physiol 1989;58:845–851.
64. Kraemer WJ, Fleck SJ, Dziados JE, Harman EA, Marchitelli LJ, et al. Changes in hormonal concentrations after different heavy-resistance exercise protocols in women. J Appl Physiol 1993;75: 594–604.
65. Heitkamp HC, Huber W, Scheib K. beta-Endorphin and adrenocorticotrophin after incremental exercise and marathon running—female responses. Eur J Appl Physiol 1996;72:417–424.
66. Friedmann B, Kindermann W. Energy metabolism and regulatory hormones in women and men during endurance exercise. Eur J Appl Physiol 1989;59:1–9.
67. Bashir N, el Migdadi F, Hasan Z, al Hader AA, Wezermes I, Gharaibeh M. Acute effects of exercise at low altitude (350 meters below sea level) on hormones of the anterior pituitary & cortisol in athletes. Endocr Res 1996;22:289–298.
68. Vasankari TJ, Rusko H, Kujala UM, Huhtaniemi IT. The effect of ski training at altitude and racing on pituitary, adrenal and testicular function in men. Eur J Appl Physiol 1993;66:221–225.
69. Marinelli M, Roi GS, Giacometti M, Bonini P, Banfi G. Cortisol, testosterone, and free testosterone in athletes performing a marathon at 4,000 m altitude. Horm Res 1994;41:225–229.
70. Hoffman JR. Maresh CM, Armstrong LE, Gabaree CL, Bergeron MF, Kenefick RW, et al. Effects of hydration state on plasma testosterone, cortisol and catecholamine concentrations before and during mild exercise at elevated temperature. Eur J Appl Physiol 1994;69:294–300.
71. Hoffman JR, Falk B, Radom Isaac S, Weinstein Y, Magazanik A, Wang Y, et al. The effect of environmental temperature on testosterone and cortisol responses to high intensity, intermittent exercise in humans. Eur J Appl Physiol 1997;75:83–87.
72. Tabata I, Ogita F, Miyachi M, Shibayama H. Effect of low blood glucose on plasma CRF, ACTH, and cortisol during prolonged physical exercise. J Appl Physiol 1991;71:1807–1812.
73. Tabata I, Atomi Y, Miyashita M. Blood glucose concentration dependent ACTH and cortisol responses to prolonged exercise. Clin Physiol 1984;4:299–307.
74. Lavoie JM, Helie R, Peronnet F, Cousineau D, Provencher PJ. Effects of muscle CHO-loading manipulations on hormonal responses during prolonged exercise. Int J Sports Med 1985;6:95–99.
75. Mitchell JB, Costill DL, Houmard JA, Flynn MG, Fink WJ, Beltz JD. Influence of carbohydrate ingestion on counterregulatory hormones during prolonged exercise. Int J Sports Med 1990;11:33–36.
76. Tsintzas OK, Williams C, Wilson W, Burrin J. Influence of carbohydrate supplementation early in exercise on endurance running capacity. Med Sci Sports Exerc 1996;28:1373–1379.
77. Vasankari TJ, Kujala UM, Viljanen,TT, Huhtaniemi IT. Carbohydrate ingestion during prolonged running exercise results in an increase of serum cortisol and decrease of gonadotrophins. Acta Physiol Scand 1991;141:373–377.
78. Wasserman DH, Lavina H, Lickley A, Vranic M. Effect of hematocrit reduction on hormonal and metabolic responses to exercise. J Appl Physiol 1985;58:1257–1262.
79. Harte JL, Eifert GH. The effects of running, environment, and attentional focus on athletes' catecholamine and cortisol levels and mood. Psychophysiology 1995;32:49–54.
80. Heikkonen E, Ylikahri R, Roine R, Valimaki M, Harkonen M, Salaspuro M. The combined effect of alcohol and physical exercise on serum testosterone, luteinizing hormone, and cortisol in males. Alcohol Clin Exp Res 1996;20:711–716.

81. Rolandi E, Reggiani E, Franceschini R, Bavastro G, Messina V, Odaglia G, et al. Comparison of pituitary responses to physical exercise in athletes and sedentary subjects. Horm Res 1985;21: 209–213.
82. Deuster,PA, Chrousos GP, Luger A, DeBolt JE, Bernier LL, Trostmann UH, et al. Hormonal and metabolic responses of untrained, moderately trained, and highly trained men to three exercise intensities. Metabolism 1989;38:141–148.
83. Hickson RC, Hidaka K, Foster C, Falduto MT, Chatterton RT Jr. Successive time courses of strength development and steroid hormone responses to heavy-resistance training. J Appl Physiol 1994;76:663–670.
84. Buono MJ, Yeager JE, Sucec AA. Effect of aerobic training on the plasma ACTH response to exercise. J Appl Physiol 1987;63:2499–2501.
85. Botticelli G, Bacchi Modena A, Bresciani D, Villa P, Aguzzoli L, Florio P, et al. Effect of naltrexone treatment on the treadmill exercise-induced hormone release in amenorrheic women. J Endocrinol Invest 1992;15:839–847.
86. Farrell PA, Kjaer M, Bach FW, Galbo H. Beta-endorphin and adrenocorticotropin response to supramaximal treadmill exercise in trained and untrained males. Acta Physiol Scand 1987;130: 619–625.
87. Snegovskaya,V, Viru A. Steroid and pituitary hormone responses to rowing: relative significance of exercise intensity and duration and performance level. Eur J Appl Physiol 1993;67:59–65.
88. Kraemer WJ, Fleck SJ, Callister R, Shealy M, Dudley GA, Maresh CM, et al. Training responses of plasma beta-endorphin, adrenocorticotropin, and cortisol. Med Sci Sports Exerc 1989;21:146–153.
89. Duclos M, Corcuff JB, Rashedi M, Fougere V, Manier G. Trained versus untrained men: different immediate post-exercise responses of pituitary adrenal axis. A preliminary study. Eur J Appl Physiol 1997;75:343–350.
90. Pestell RG, Hurley DM, Vandongen R. Biochemical and hormonal changes during a 1000 km ultramarathon. Clin Exp Pharmacol Physiol 1989;16:353–361.
91. Wittert GA, Livesey JH, Espiner EA, Donald RA. Adaptation of the hypothalamopituitary adrenal axis to chronic exercise stress in humans. Med Sci Sports Exerc 1996;28:1015–1019.
92. Ronkainen HR, Pakarinen AJ, Kauppila AJ. Adrenocortical function of female endurance runners and joggers. Med Sci Sports Exerc 1986;18:385–389.
93. Mujika I, Chatard JC, Padilla S, Guezennec CY, Geyssant A. Hormonal responses to training and its tapering off in competitive swimmers: relationships with performance. Eur J Appl Physiol 1996;74:361–366.
94. Lehmann M, Gastmann U, Petersen KG, Bachl N, Seidel A, Khalaf AN, et al. Training-overtraining: performance, and hormone levels, after a defined increase in training volume versus intensity in experienced middle- and long-distance runners. Br J Sports Med 1992;26:233–242.
95. Flynn MG, Pizza FX, Brolinson PG. Hormonal responses to excessive training: influence of cross training. Int J Sports Med 1997;18:191–196.
96. Fry AC, Kraemer WJ, Stone MH, Warren BJ, Fleck SJ, Kearney JT, et al. Endocrine responses to overreaching before and after 1 year of weightlifting. Can J Appl Physiol 1994;19:400–410.
97. Tharp GD, Buuck RJ. Adrenal adaptation to chronic exercise. J Appl Physiol 1974;37:720–722.
98. Lehmann M, Knizia K, Gastmann U, Petersen KG, Khalaf AN, Bauer S, et al. Influence of 6-week, 6 days per week, training on pituitary function in recreational athletes. Br J Sports Med 1993;27: 186–192.
99. Kirwan JP, Costill DL, Flynn MG, Mitchell JB, Fink WJ, Neufer PD, et al. Physiological responses to successive days of intense training in competitive swimmers. Med Sci Sports Exerc 1988;20: 255–259.
100. O'Connor PJ, Morgan WP, Raglin JS. Psychobiologic effects of 3 d of increased training in female and male swimmers. Med Sci Sports Exerc 1991;23:1055–1061.
101. Engfred K, Kjaer M, Secher NH, Friedman DB, Hanel B, Nielsen OJ, et al. Hypoxia and training-induced adaptation of hormonal responses to exercise in humans. Eur J Appl Physiol 1994;68: 303–309.
102. Hakkinen K, Pakarinen A, Alen M, Kauhanen H, Komi PV. Neuromuscular and hormonal responses in elite athletes to two successive strength training sessions in one day. Eur J Appl Physiol 1988; 57:133–139.
103. Hakkinen K, Pakarinen A, Alen M, Kauhanen H, Komi PV. Neuromuscular and hormonal adaptations in athletes to strength training in two years. J Appl Physiol 1988;65:2406–2412.

104. Alen M, Pakarinen A, Hakkinen K, Komi PV. Responses of serum androgenic-anabolic and catabolic hormones to prolonged strength training. Int J Sports Med 1988;9:229–233.
105. Fry AC, Kraemer WJ. Resistance exercise overtraining and overreaching. Neuroendocrine responses. Sports Med 1997;23:106–129.
106. Barron JL, Noakes TD, Levy W, Smith C, Millar RP. Hypothalamic dysfunction in overtrained athletes. J Clin Endocrinol Metab 1985;60:803–806.
107. Budgett R. Overtraining syndrome. Br J Sports Med 1990;24:231–236.
108. Fry RW, Morton AR, Keast D. Overtraining in athletes. An update. Sports Med 1991;12:32–65.
109. Fry RW, Morton AR, Garcia Webb P, Crawford GP, Keast D. Biological responses to overload training in endurance sports. Eur J Appl Physiol 1992;64:335–344.
110. Lehmann MJ, Lormes W, Opitzgress A, Steinacker JM, Netzer N, Foster C, et al. Training and overtraining—an overview and experimental results in endurance sports. J Sports Med Phys Fitness 1997;37:7–17.
111. Urhausen A, Gabriel H, Kindermann W. Blood hormones as markers of training stress and overtraining. Sports Med 1995;20:251–276.
112. Verde T, Thomas S, Shephard RJ. Potential markers of heavy training in highly trained distance runners. Br J Sports Med 1992;26:167–175.
113. Loucks AB, Horvath SM. Exercise-induced stress responses of amenorrheic and eumenorrheic runners. J Clin Endocrinol Metab 1984;59:1109–1120.
114. Ding JH, Sheckter CB, Drinkwater BL, Soules MR, Bremner WJ. High serum cortisol levels in exercise-associated amenorrhea. Ann Intern Med 1988;108:530–534.
115. Loucks AB, Mortola JF. Girton L, Yen SS. Alterations in the hypothalamic–pituitary–ovarian and the hypothalamic–pituitary–adrenal axes in athletic women. J Clin Endocrinol Metab 1989;68:402–411.
116. Villanueva AL, Schlosser C, Hopper B, Liu JH, Hoffman DI, Rebar RW. Increased cortisol production in women runners. J Clin Endocrinol Metab 1986;63:133–136.
117. Hohtari H, Salminen Lappalainen K, Laatikainen T. Response of plasma endorphins, corticotropin, cortisol, and luteinizing hormone in the corticotropin-releasing hormone stimulation test in eumenorrheic and amenorrheic athletes. Fertil Steril 1991;55:276–280.
118. De Souza MJ, Luciano AA, Arce JC, Demers LM, Loucks AB. Clinical tests explain blunted cortisol responsiveness but not mild hypercortisolism in amenorrheic runners. J Appl Physiol 1994;76:1302–1309.

4 Impact of Chronic Training on Pituitary Hormone Secretion in the Human

Johannes D. Veldhuis, MD and Kohji Yoshida, MD

CONTENTS

INTRODUCTION
MULTIPLE DETERMINANTS OF PITUITARY RESPONSES
  TO EXERCISE TRAINING
OTHER CONFOUNDING ISSUES
NEUROENDOCRINE AXES AS FEEDBACK AND FEEDFORWARD
  CONTROL SYSTEMS
INTERACTIONS AMONG NEUROENDOCRINE AXES
METABOLIC MECHANISMS
IMPLICATIONS
SUMMARY
ACKNOWLEDGMENTS
REFERENCES

INTRODUCTION

The impact of chronic training on pituitary function is best understood by a basic appraisal of the neuroendocrine physiology of any given individual axis and the more complex interactive pathophysiology among axes *(1–12)*. Interaxes interactions have received relatively little attention. Even evaluating a single neuroendocrine axis in its dynamic state is a complicated challenge, given combined feedforward and feedback activities among the key control loci within any given axis *(13,14)*. For example, in the case of the growth hormone (GH) and insulin-like growth factor 1 (IGF-1) axis, hypothalamic GH-releasing hormone (GHRH) secreted by arcuate nuclei stimulates pituitary GH secretion acutely, whereas the somatostatinergic system originating in the paraventricular nuclei opposes GHRH action *(15)*. These two neuronal inputs are reciprocally interconnected by intrahypothalamic synapses and common impinging neuromodulator pathways *(14)*. In addition, secreted GH feeds back on brain GH receptors, stimulating somatostatin secretion and possibly inhibiting GHRH release. Available GH secreted into the bloodstream triggers IGF-1 production in various target tissues,

From: *Contemporary Endocrinology: Sports Endocrinology*
Edited by: M. P. Warren and N. W. Constantini © Humana Press Inc., Totowa, NJ

and circulating IGF-1 is capable of inhibiting pituitary GH secretion indirectly and directly (*see* Fig. 1). Such feedforward (GHRH's driving GH secretion) and feedback (GH's inhibiting its own secretion, IGF-1's inhibiting GH secretion, and so forth) dynamic control mechanisms in principle can be modified by the effects of exercise at one or more levels within the axis. Moreover, multiple determinants modulate neuroendocrine responses to training, such as the body composition of the individual, concurrent stress and/or weight loss, gender, diet and energy balance, concomitant drug or hormone use, age, puberty, pregnancy, and/or lactational status *(16–18)*.

Here, we will examine the neuroendocrine determinants of pituitary responses to exercise training, explore some of the confounding issues (e.g., species differences, varying modes of neurohormone secretion, within- and between-axis regualtion, and so on), and explore the overall notion of neuroendocrine axes as feedback and feedforward control systems capable of within-axis as well as between-axes interactions. Finally, metabolic mechanisms, although likely multifactorial, will be examined briefly, and their clinical implications underscored.

MULTIPLE DETERMINANTS OF PITUITARY RESPONSES TO EXERCISE TRAINING

Among other determinants of neuroendocrine responses to exercise training is the acuteness vs chronicity of the training or exercise stimulus *(2,5,11,12,19–22)*. In particular, numerous studies demonstrate that acute exercise induces a variety of short-term changes in multiple hypothalamo–pituitary axes, including the nearly immediate secretion of GH and adrenocorticotrophic hormone (ACTH), β-endorphin and cortisol, whereas the results of chronic training are not necessarily identical *(20,21,23–30)*. Moreover, stress or acute exercise imposed in an untrained individual will elicit endocrine responses potentially distinct from those observed in a highly physically trained subject *(3,8,9,11, 31–40)*. Thus, many studies are confounded in part by the nature of the prior or concomitant training regimen, its duration, and its intensity. Finally, extreme physical exertion, "overreaching," often evokes neuroendocrine disturbances that are not typical of either short-term submaximal exertion or chronic training *(5,9,41–43)*.

Neuroendocrine axes are exquisitely sensitive to nutrient intake, body composition, and total (and percentage) body fat *(44–51)*. Recent studies of the GH axis document unequivocally that percentage body fat, and in particular visceral (intra-abdominal) fat accumulation *(52)*, negatively influences pulsatile GH secretion by suppressing the mass of GH secreted per burst and shortening the half-life of GH in the circulation *(44,45, 53–56)*. The reciprocal relationship between visceral fat mass and GH secretion is illustrated in Fig. 2. Impaired GH secretion and more rapid GH removal jointly serve to reduce 24-h pulsatile serum GH concentrations in otherwise healthy but relatively more (viscerally) obese individuals. In contrast, acute weight loss or nutrient deprivation potently stimulates GH secretion in the human (while suppressing it in the rat) by 3- to 10-fold, with augmentation in both men and women of GH secretory pulse amplitude and mass and, to a lesser degree, burst frequency *(47,57,58)*. Consequently, nutrition, body weight, and body composition are prime determinants of pituitary (GH) secretory activity, which likely condition responses to exercise *(59)*. In addition, in men, as well as more recently recognized in women, body mass index (relative obesity) is a negative

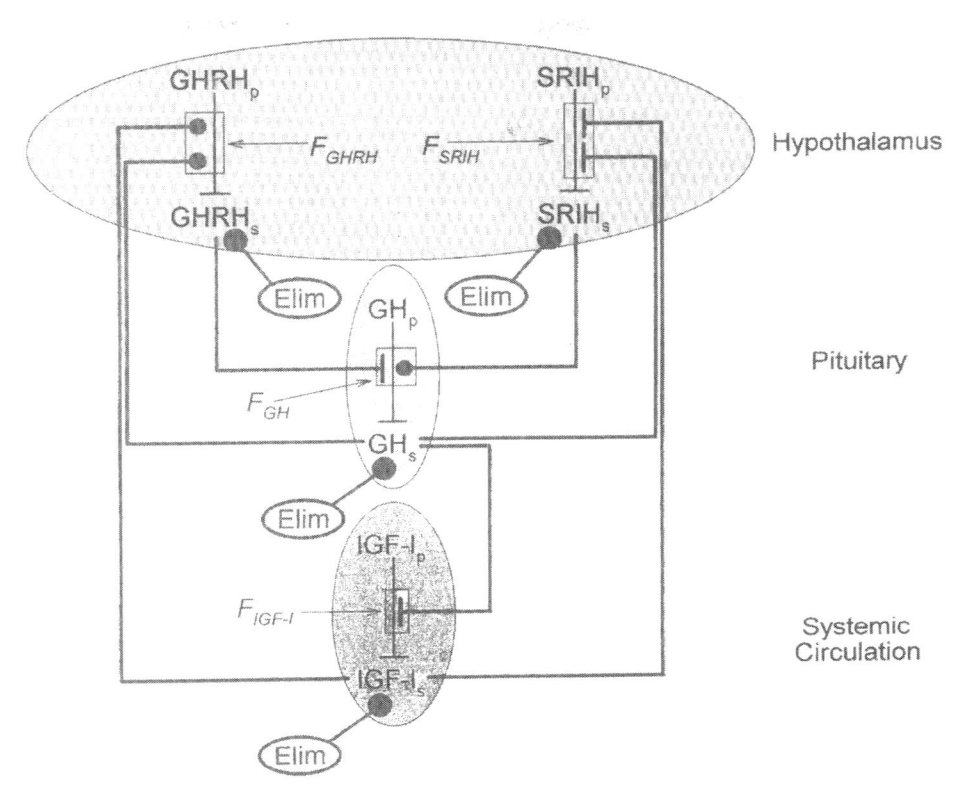

Fig. 1. Network feedback and feedforward linkages within the basic GHRH–somatostatin/GH–IGF-1 axis. Somatostatin is abbreviated here as SRIH. "Elim" denotes metabolic elimination; "F" defines selective input functions, e.g., F_{GHRH} indicates relevant input into GHRH neurons via SRIH and other neuromodulators; F_{SRIH} defines input into SRIH neurons by GHRH and other neurotransmitters; and subscripts "p" and "s" represent particular (tissue or secretory-granule contained) and secreted hormone or peptide, respectively. Some lines denote negative feedback (or feedforward) onto the target node marked by a dot, whereas other lines mark a positive effector pathway terminating with a bar. The interconnected dynamic system shown is simplified from a larger family of interrelated parameters anticipated within the full GH–IGF-1 axis. Additional possible secretagogue input via a putative GHRP-like ligand family is not illustrated, although GHRP receptors (*see text*) are expressed in the hypothalamus and pituitary gland. No endogenous GHRP-receptor ligand(s) has (have) been isolated definitively. Adapted with permission from Straume et al. *(14)*.

correlate of LH pulse amplitude *(49,60)* and of the serum testosterone concentration in middle-aged men *(49)*.

Gender distinctions also strongly influence the secretory output of several neuroendocrine axes. Foremost, the gonadotropin-releasing hormone–luteinizing hormone (GnRH–LH) follicle-stimulating hormone (FSH)–sex steroid axes in men and women exhibit clarion differences, particularly at the level of so-called positive feedback, which is mechanistically required to achieve a preovulatory LH surge in women *(61)*. The GH–IGF-1 axis is also strongly sexually dimorphic in the human (as well as in the rat, as reviewed earlier *[15]*). For example, in healthy premenopausal men and women,

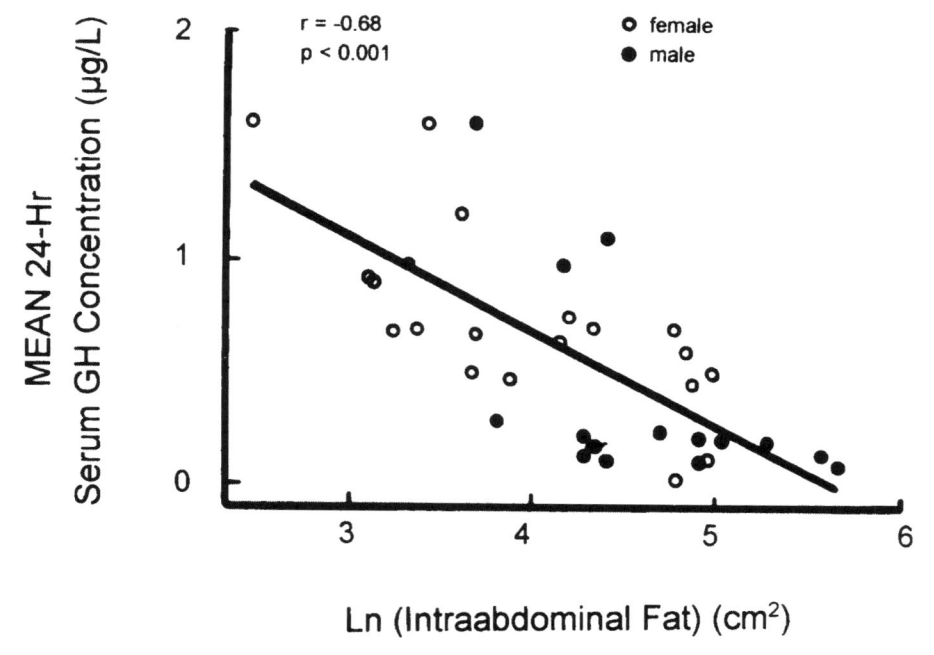

Fig. 2. Negative relationship between 24-h mean serum GH concentration and intra-abdominal (visceral) fat mass, as determined by computerized axial tomographic scanning of the abdomen, in a cohort of healthy middle-aged men and women. GH concentrations were determined by 20-min blood sampling for 24 h and subsequent assay by immunofluorometry. The solid circles denote male subjects, and the open circles females. The regression line shows a strongly negative relationship between the natural logarithm of intra-abdominal adiposity and daily GH secretory activity in both men and women. In multiple linear regression analyses, intra-abdominal fat mass accounted for the majority of the variability in integrated serum GH concentrations, exceeding that owing to age and gender in this population. Redrawn with permission from Vahl et al. *(56)*.

GH secretion differs quantitatively by way of a nearly twofold greater mean (24-h) serum GH concentration, higher plasma IGF-1 level, greater mass of GH secreted per burst, and a more disorderly pattern of GH release in women compared to men *(62)*. In addition, the individual negative impact of age, body mass index, or percentage body fat on GH secretion is 1.5- to 2-fold more evident in men than women (48); the positive effect of physical conditioning (increased VO_2max) on GH release is also more prominent in the male *(48)* (Fig. 3). The tissue responses to GH also may be sex-specific in part, since estrogen can antagonize GH-driven IGF-1 production by the liver *(15)*. Consequently, gender must be identified as a major determinant of neuroendocrine responses in the GH–IGF-1 axis. Exercise-stimulated GH secretion may be less gender-dependent *(63)*.

A lesser gender difference is observed for the corticotropin-releasing hormone (CRH)–arginine vasopressin (AVP)/ACTH–cortisol axis, where in the female, relatively increased expression of the CRH gene and increased adrenal responsiveness to ACTH are proposed *(64)*. However, the orderliness of individual 24-h ACTH and cortisol release (approximate entropy) or their relative synchrony (crossentropy) in men and women is similar *(65)*.

Another significant confounding influence on neuroendocrine axes is age. For example, in the case of the LH–testosterone axis in men, there is progressive deterioration of LH or testosterone's individual orderliness of release over 24 h and of LH–testosterone

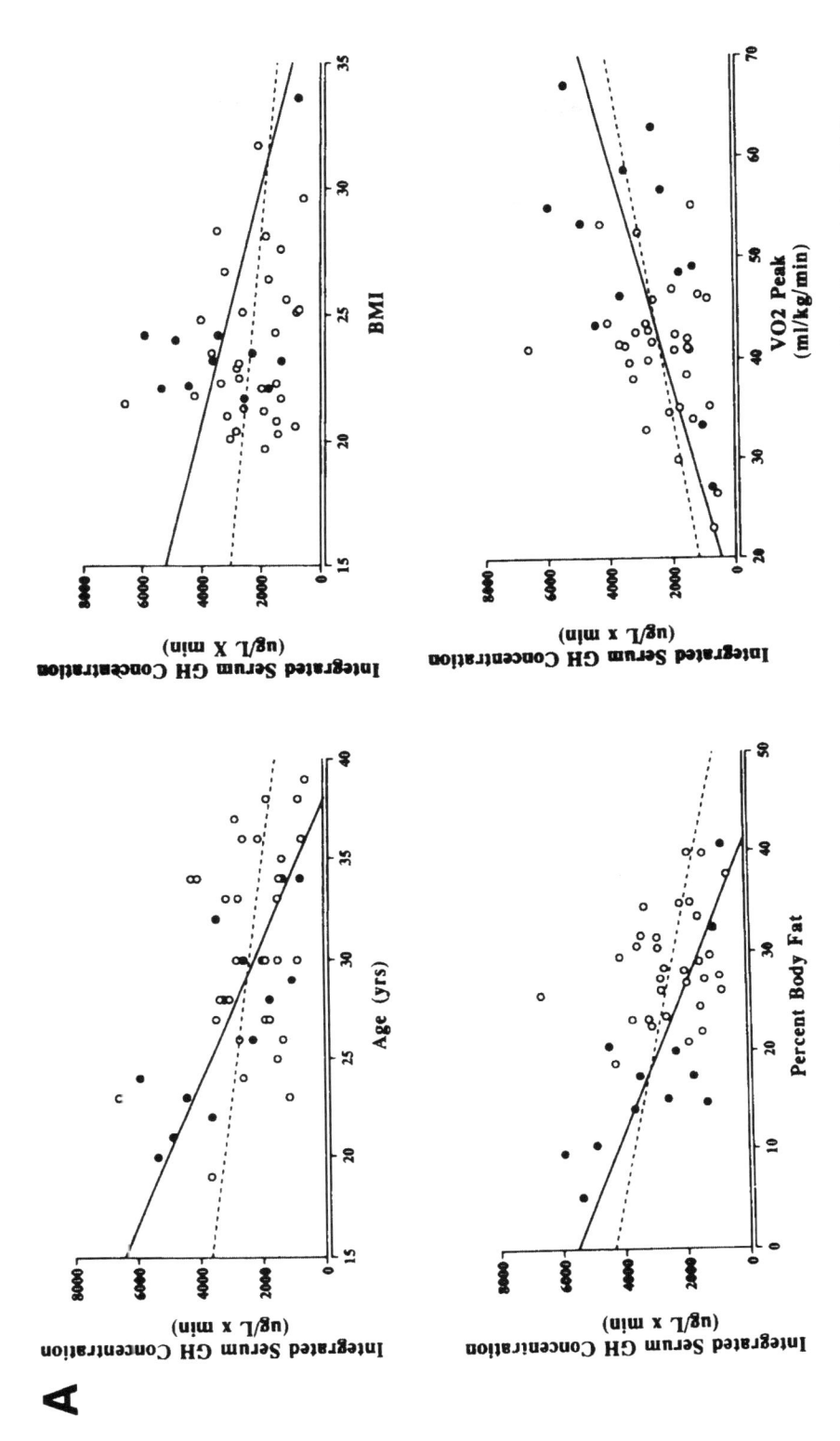

Fig. 3. (A) Impact of gender on the effects of age, adiposity as measured by body mass index (BMI) or percentage body fat, and physical fitness as quantitated by maximal oxygen consumption (VO_2 max peak or max) on integrated (24-h) serum GH concentrations in normal men (●, $N = 12$) and women (○, $N = 32$). Linear regression plots are given for each sex. The solid lines denote regression in men, and the interrupted lines depict women's data.

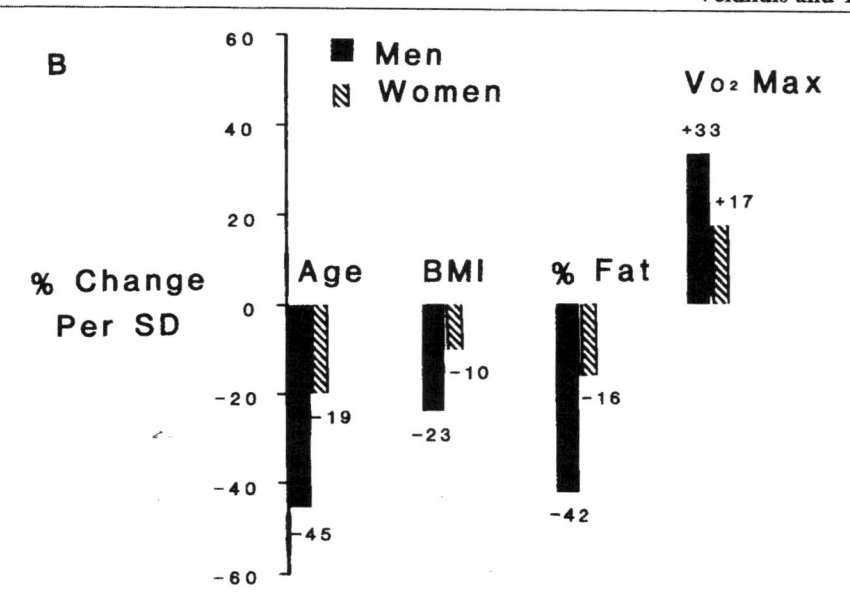

Fig. 3. (B) Approximately twofold greater impact of age, BMI, percentage body fat, and VO₂max on 240-h mean serum GH concentrations in men than women. Data are means ± SEM expressed as standardized regression coefficients for the regression lines in (A). The gender-specific standardized regression coefficient is the slope of the linear relationship (given as a percentage) adjusted per unit standard deviation (SD) of the male or female group as pertinent. Redrawn with permission from Weltman et al. *(48)*.

coupling or synchrony, when assessed by either crosscorrelation analysis (indicating diminished feedforward control) *(66)* or crossapproximate entropy (indicating decreased pattern synchrony within the reproductive axis' feedback system) *(67)*. The regularity of GH or ACTH/cortisol release also deteriorates with age in men and women *(65,68)*. In addition, in both men and women, there are marked quantitative decreases in overall GH axis secretory activity, with a progressive fall in plasma IGF-1 and daily GH secretion rates with aging, especially in men compared to women of premenopausal age *(44,45,48,54)*.

Concurrent drug and/or hormone use can also markedly modify several pituitary-target tissue axes. For example, prescribed or self-use of anabolic steroids will profoundly suppress LH and FSH release and reduce levels of endogenous sex steroids, while potentially stimulating the GH–IGF-1 axis (if aromatizable androgens are employed) *(13,63,69–71)*. Likewise, the use of birth control pills in young women stimulates GH secretion significantly, and may produce some alterations in body composition *(72)*. At puberty, when sex-steroid hormone secretion changes more dramatically *(73,74)*, the individual's GH–IGF-1 and/or GnRH–LH axis may be uniquely susceptible to the impact of exercise training (at least prior to pubertal onset), resulting in a significant delay in sexual maturation and adolescence and possibly reduced predicted adult height *(75)* (*see* Chapter 17).

We infer that an array of important factors, such as exercise intensity and duration, its acuteness vs chronicity, associated weight loss and/or stress (discussed further below), diet and energy balance, body composition, gender, age, and maturational status (e.g., prepubertal vs pubertal) may all codetermine the neuroendocrine and pituitary responses to a stress pertubation, such as exercise.

OTHER CONFOUNDING ISSUES

One confounding issue experimentally in evaluating the impact of acute or chronic physical training on pituitary function is species differences. For example, in the rat, physical exertion reduces GH secretion *(15)*, whereas in the human acute and chronic exercise both increase GH secretion significantly, the former within 15–30 min and the latter following sustained exercise at an intensity above the individual lactate threshold *(15,20,21,24,76,77)*. Indeed, chronic physical training in women results in a doubling of the 24-h mean serum GH level even on days when exercise is not undertaken *(21)* (*see* Fig. 4 *[20]*). Consequently, many experiments carried out in the rodent do not find applicability, especially for the GH–IGF-1 axis, to human studies. Moreover, the gender differences in the GH axis in the rat and human are readily distinguishable mechanistically in the two species, with a greater mean amplitude (and mass) of GH secretory bursts in women than men (but the converse occurs in the rat) *(62)*. A similarity in the two species is a more disorderly pattern of GH release in the female *(78)*.

Further complicating interpretation and analysis of pituitary secretion are the multifold temporal modes of physiological pituitary-hormone release:

1. Pulsatile.
2. Nyctohemeral or circadian.
3. Entropic, or moment-to-moment variations in the orderliness of secretion *(67,79–81)*.

Pulsatile hormone secretion typically mirrors episodic neural input that acts via intermittent secretagog delivery to a responsive pituitary cell population in the absence of significant inhibitory input concurrently. Indeed, a pulse of pituitary hormone secretion can be viewed as a collection of secretory rates, centered about some moment in time. This concept is illustrated in Fig. 5.

In contrast to the foregoing episodic (pulsatile) secretory mode are less rapid, 24-h variations in serum hormone concentrations, which are well established for ACTH, LH, GH, thyroid-stimulating hormone (TSH), prolactin, cortisol, and so forth *(82)*. These nyctohemeral (night–day) variations constitute only a small part of the total variation in daily neurohormone release. True circadian rhythms are so-called free-running with a periodicity of 24 h, temperature-compensated, and susceptible to Zeitgebers or specific phase-entraining cues *(83)*. Not all human 24-h neuroendocrine rhythms conform to this definition, which would denote true (suprachiasmatic nucleus-driven) circadian activity. Based on sleep-reversal studies, and so forth, circadian rhythmicity clearly does exist for ACTH/cortisol release in the human and GH secretion (approx 50% of the 24-h GH rhythm is sleep- and activity-entrained, and 50% is circadian) *(15,84)*.

Neurohormone release also exhibits features of minute-to-minute patterning, serial orderliness, or relative regularity, which can be quantified by an approximate entropy statistic *(67,78)*. Higher values of approximate entropy denote greater disorderliness of hormone release, and are a feature of female GH secretory patterns (compared to male), healthy aging of the human insulin, GH, LH, and ACTH/cortisol axes *(54,65,67,78,85,86)*, as well as aldosteronomas *(87)*, tumoral pituitary hormone secretion (acromegaly, Cushing's disease, and prolactinomas *[65,88]*), and insulin release in type II diabetes

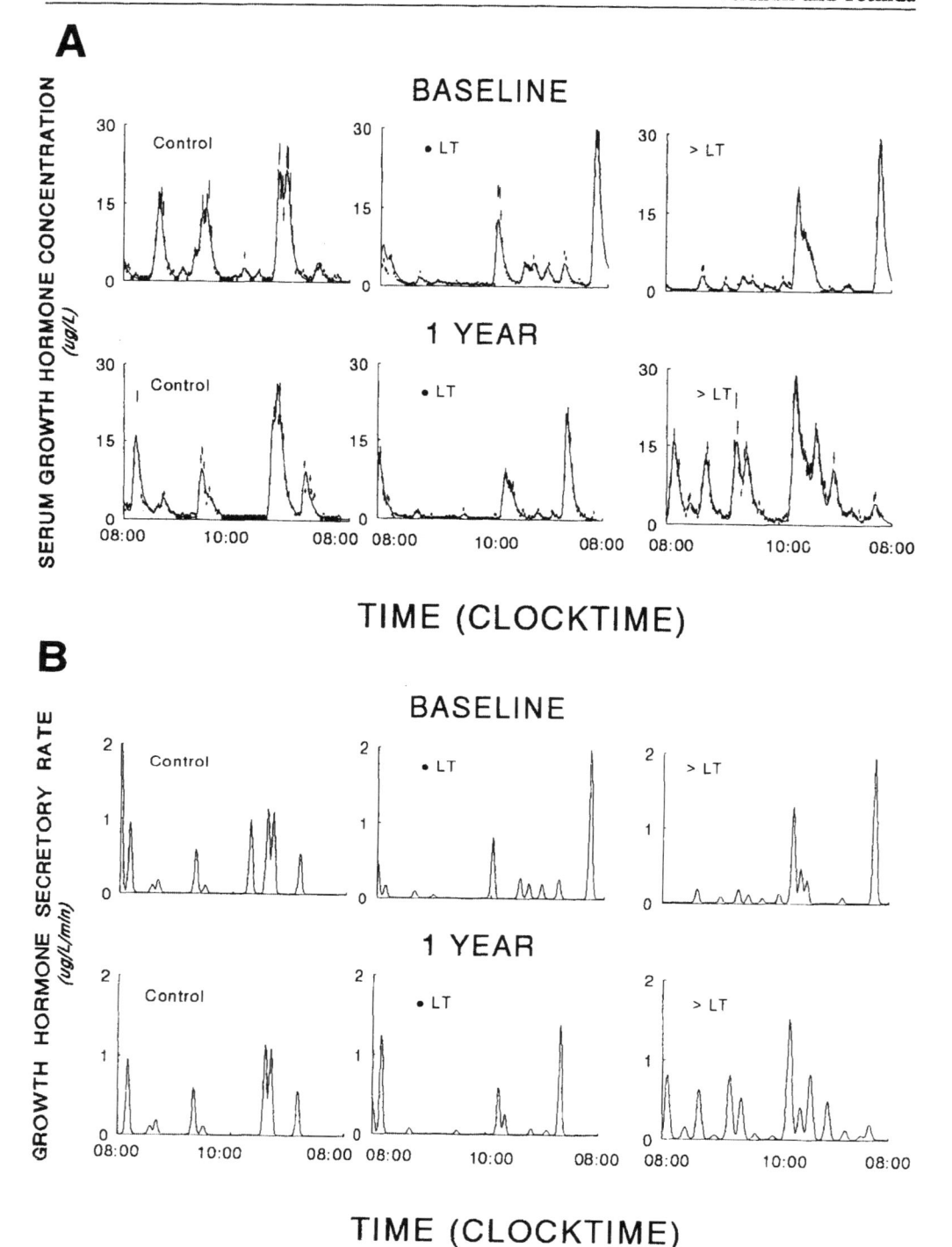

Fig. 4. Twenty-four hour serum GH concentration or secretion profiles in three different premenopasual women each studied twice: control (left; no exercise training, sedentary volunteer); before (baseline) and after 1 yr of exercise training below (middle-panel), or at or above (right panel) the individually determined lactate threshold (LT). Adapted with permission from ref. (20).

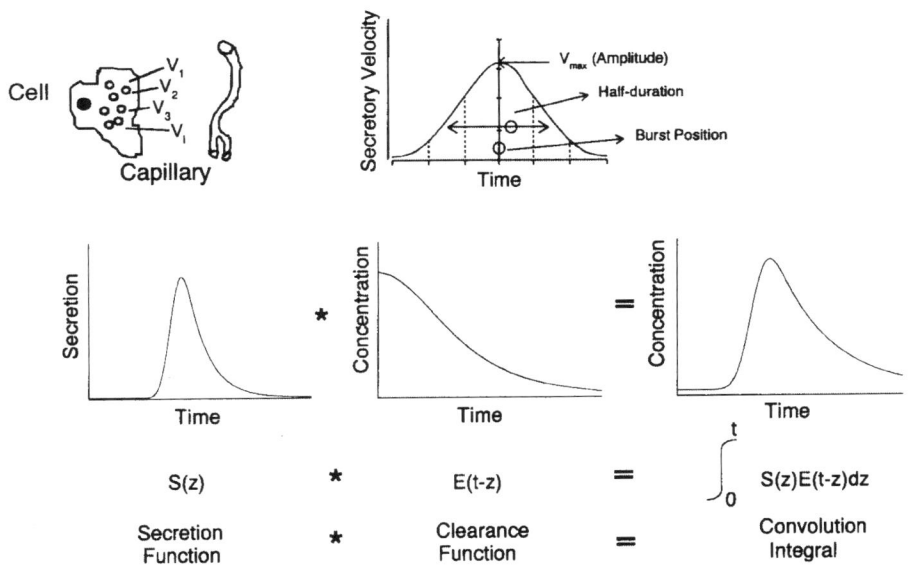

Fig. 5. Schematized illustration of a model-specific deconvolution concept implemented to quantitate (GH) secretion. The upper landscape depicts an intuitive formulation of a hormone secretory burst, as arising from (multi-)cellular discharge of individual hormone molecules more or less in concert temporally, each at its own particular secretory rate (velocity). A secretory burst (or pulse) is visualized as an array of such molecular secretory velocities centered about some moment in time, and dispersed around this center with a finite standard duration (SD) or half-width. The burst event may or may not be symmetric over time. The lower landscape with the algebraic subheads shows the mathematical notion, whereby a plasma hormone concentration peak (far right) is viewed as developing from a burst-like secretory process (far left) and a finite hormone-specific removal rate (half-life of elimination). The so-called convolution (intertwining or interaction) of the simultaneous secretory and elimination functions creates a resultant (skewed) plasma concentration pulse. Deconvolution analysis consists of mathematically estimating the constituent underlying secretory features (and/or associated half-life), given (a series of) blood hormone concentration peaks as the starting point. A variety of model-independent (waveform-invariant) deconvolution strategies can also be applied, if *a priori* knowledge of the pertinent (biexponential) hormone elimination rate process is available. Adapted with permission from ref. *(15)*.

mellitus *(89,90)*. Thus, entropy measures can identify secretory disturbances complementary to pulsatile or circadian variations.

The complex mode of pituitary hormone secretion imposes the need for appropriately rigorous sampling intensity and duration to capture the pulsatile, circadian, and entropic features, followed by application of relevant analytical tools appropriately validated under those conditions of study. Such technical issues have been reviewed recently *(80,91–93)*.

Further confounding in the literature arises because biochemically measurable endocrine changes do not always imply definite biological or clinical sequelae. For example, studies of the thyrotropin-releasing factor (TRH)–TSH–thyroidal axis have revealed numerous biochemically measurable changes during acute or chronic exercise, but their clinical sequelae are not known *(94)*. Similarly, in relation to the male reproductive axis, a variety of pituitary–gonadal changes are well established in response to chronic exercise, such as diminished LH pulse frequency at least in a subset of men, and relatively decreased spermatogenesis (e.g. a 30–50% decline in sperm number). However, clinical signs and symptoms of androgen deficiency rarely, if ever, occur, and male infertility is not known to be associated with chronic physical training *(5,32–35,43,95–100)*. Finally, multiple hormones are produced by the anterior pituitary gland, and, as discussed further below, the corresponding individual axes may evince significant interactions.

NEUROENDOCRINE AXES AS FEEDBACK AND FEEDFORWARD CONTROL SYSTEMS

As intimated in the Introduction, neuroendocrine axes should be viewed as dynamic feedforward and feedback control systems. The term feedforward defines the ability of a secreted agonist to act on a remote or proximal tissue and evoke a typically sigmoidal (e.g., log-logistic) dose–response curve, e.g., as anticipated for GHRH's acting on somatotrope cells in the anterior pituitary gland, GnRH's acting on gonadotrope cells, and so forth *(15,101)*. Conversely, feedback denotes the ability of a secreted product from a target tissue to inhibit the production of the agonistic signal, e.g., testosterone feeds back on hypothalamic GnRH secretion in the male, IGF-1 feeds back on pituitary somatotrope secretion of GH, L-thyroxine feeds back on TSH secretion at the pituitary and hypothalamic levels, and so forth. As highlighted in Figs. 1 and 6, both the GHRH–somatostatin/GH–IGF-1 axis *(14)*, and the GnRH–LH/FSH/sex steroid *(101)* axes should be viewed as complex feedback and feedforward control systems *(13,14,79,101–103)*. This concept is physiologically critical, since most pathophysiological stimuli impinge on several points within the feedback control system, thus impacting on the overall dynamics. Such system-level responses cannot be observed readily when separated components are studied individually. Similarly, the stress-responsive ACTH–adrenal axis comprises CRH–AVP/ACTH–cortisol, with corresponding feedforward and interactive feedback mechanisms inherent *(3,40,104)*.

An important notion in future studies of chronic exercise effects on the pituitary will be to limit isolation of individual components of the axis, and rather study the overall axis dynamics. Technology, such as approximate entropy *(67,105)* and network analysis *(14,101)*, for accomplishing the latter is just beginning to emerge. To date, the vast majority of published literature (as discussed throughout this volume) has enunciated changes at individual control points, which unfortunately subdivides the feedback system artificially, and limits insights into its interactive properties, which function from minute to minute and day to day.

INTERACTIONS AMONG NEUROENDOCRINE AXES

Foremost among the challenges to be addressed in investigative and clinical neuroendocrine pathophysiology are the nature and mechanisms of interaction between two, or among three or more, neuroendocrine axes. For example, in relation to chronic exercise or other stressors in experimental animals, alterations occur not only in hypothalamic GHRH and somatostatin gene expression, but also in the GnRH neuronal ensemble and neuropeptide Y (NPY)- and CRH-secreting neurons *(104,106)*. In conjunction with concurrent changes in dietary intake, activity of TRH neurons in the hypothalamus may also be suppressed (reviewed in ref. *107*). Relevantly, these multiple neuronal pathways are directed by corresponding families of neurotransmitters (e.g., norepinephrine, serotonin, acetylcholine, and so forth), as well as various potent neuromodulators (e.g.,

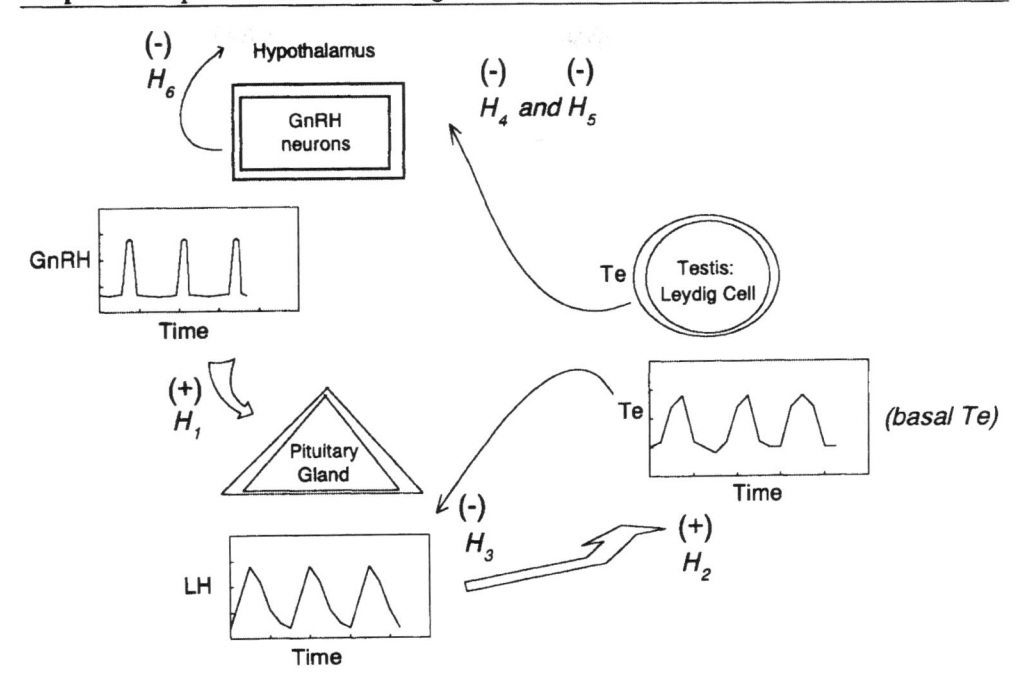

Fig. 6. Schematic illustration of the time-delayed negative feedback (–) and positive feedforward (+) within the human male GnRH–LH–testosterone (Te) axis. The broad arrows indicate feedforward (+) stimulus-secretion linkages, and the narrow arrows denote feedback (–) inhibition. The "H" functions are developed further in ref. *(101)*, and serve to define the dose–response relationships at each feedback interface within the axis. Adapted with permission from ref. *(101)*.

neuropeptide Y, galanin, and so on). Thus, a major focus in understanding the whole-body neuroendocrine responses of an intact organism to chronic exercise training must eventually include the articulation of not only individual neuronal pathway changes, but also their collective and interconnected alterations owing to common neuromodulatory inputs. For example, infusion of leptin, the product of the *ob* gene in adipocytes, is capable of: rescuing suppressed hypothalamic TRH secretion in fasting; relieving inhibited GnRH gene expression in certain stress models; and stimulating GH secretion in the fasted male rat (presumptively by reducing hypothalamic somatostatin gene expression). Thereby, leptin may integrate a complex response pattern via concerted hypothalamic actions that supervise diverse pituitary hormone secretory activities *(107–109)*. However, in the human, leptin levels correlate inversely (rather than directly, as in the rat) with GH axis secretory activity, as illustrated in Fig. 7 *(55)*.

METABOLIC MECHANISMS

The exact metabolic mechanisms that subserve hypothalamo–pituitary responses to exercise training are not known. Among those extensively considered are free fatty acids, which clearly can inhibit GH secretion *(15)*. On the other hand, any direct role of free fatty acids in modifying the GnRH–LH–gonadal axis is not evident. Similarly, both insulin and free IGF-1 can inhibit GH secretion directly at the anterior pituitary level, and indirectly via hypothalamic effects under several conditions in certain species *(15)*.

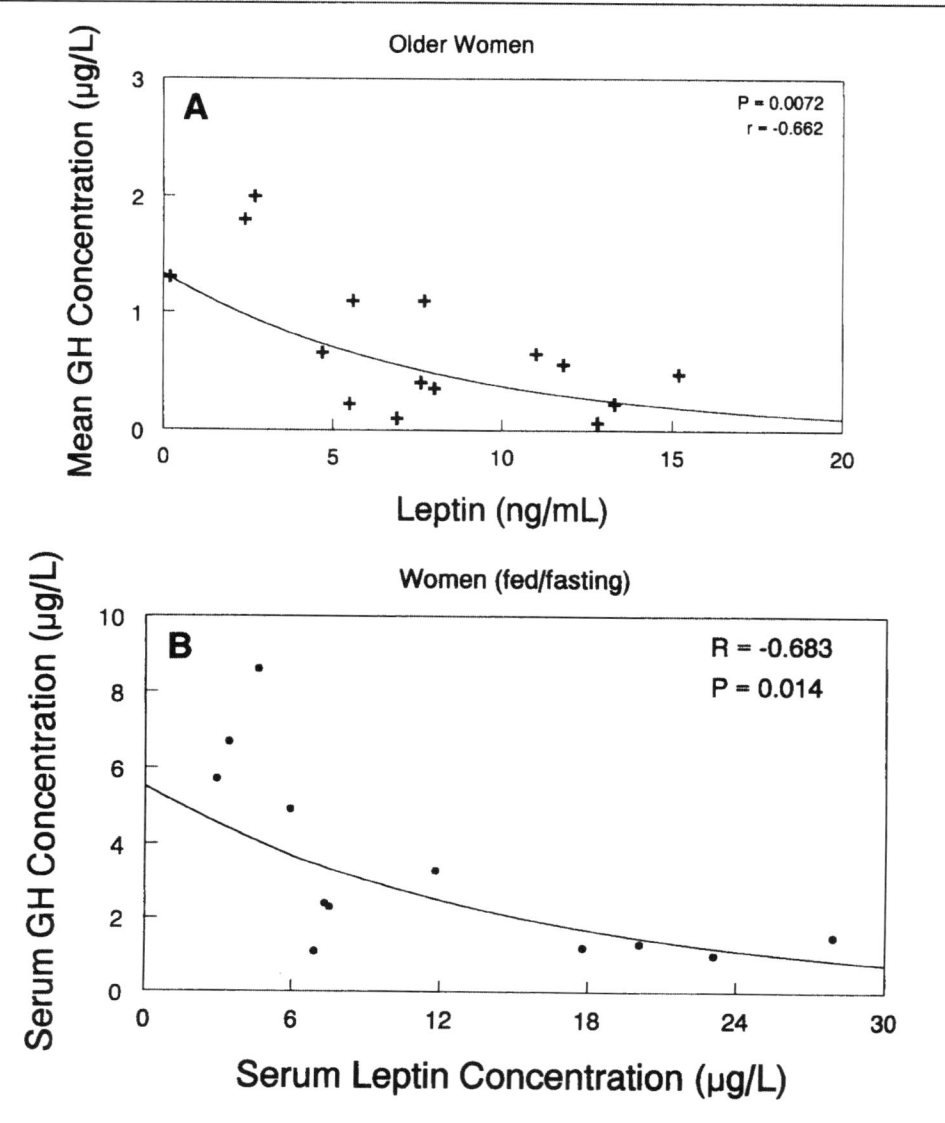

Fig. 7. (A) Inverse log-linear relationship between fasting serum leptin concentrations and integrated 24-h serum GH concentrations in 15 healthy postmenopausal women *(55)*. **(B)** Similar inverse (exponential) regression between serum leptin and GH output in young women fed or fasted *(58)*. *P* and *r* values for the linear regressions are shown. Adapted with permission.

Moreover, prolonged nutrient and/or glucose deprivation can arrest puberty in the immature sheep, and modify hypothalamic peptide secretion (e.g., stimulate CRH and/ or AVP, while inhibiting GnRH, secretion) *(104)*. In contrast, carbohydrate ingestion during exercise in one study in the human seemed to increase cortisol and decrease gonadotropin release *(110)*, whereas maintenance of euglycemia in another study abolished exercise-induced ACTH–cortisol release in nearly exhaustively exercised volunteers *(111)*. Finally, as intimated above, the peptide leptin can modify somatostatin, GnRH, TRH, and NPY gene expression, among other hypothalamic responses to the stress of fasting *(55,58)*. Overall, we postulate that such multifactorial metabolic cues and the sex steroid milieu significantly codetermine neuroendocrine responses to exercise training *(112–114)*. In addition, under the most severe exercise stimulus, overall "final-common-pathway" stressor responses may prevail, such as secretion of reproductively inhibitory CRH and endogenous opioids, with consequent suppression of GnRH–LH secretion and conversely (in a species-specific manner) stress-driven alterations in the GH–IGF-1 axis *(10,15,38,115–123)*.

IMPLICATIONS

Among other implications of chronic training are favorable nonendocrine adaptations of hemodynamic and cardiovascular function. These changes are likely to be important in long-term health risk. Moreover, body compositional changes, motivated in part by the above neuroendocrine alterations, would be predicted to have a propitious impact on population-wide morbidity and mortality *(12,117)*. In contrast, alterations in bone density accompanying chronic exercise have bipotential implications, e.g., with putatively increased fracture risk owing to sex steroid deprivation (amenorrhea) and possibly reduced total (height) growth potential *(75)*, and, conversely, variably decreased fracture risk owing to increased bone density associated with the stress-strain mechanism of enhanced bone apposition accompanying sustained physical training *(22,124–126)*. However, other confounding factors, such as concurrent estrogen status, activity of the GH–IGF-1 axis, ethnicity, and gender, can also modify bone density and fracture risk. For example, we recently observed that black men and women show increased bone mass over their Caucasian counterparts, but that only in men is the higher bone density in blacks associated with correspondingly increased GH secretion *(127)*. The mechanisms underlying such ethnic differences are also not yet understood, nor are possible ethnic differences in endocrine responsiveness to exercise stress well investigated.

SUMMARY

The impact of chronic exercise training on the neuroendocrine control of the anterior pituitary gland, and its feedback and feedforward inputs, is complex. Multiple determinants influence adaptive hypothalamo–pituitary secretory responses to physical stress, namely, training intensity and duration, including overreaching exercise, concurrent weight loss, diet and energy balance, other associated stressors (both psychological and physical), body composition, gender, age, the sex steroid milieu, and developmental/maturational status. Confounding variables include interspecies differences, the complexity of neurohormone secretion (pulsatile, circadian, and entropic rhythms), the difficulty in interpreting earlier cross-sectional studies (with possible ascertainment bias) compared to longitudinal data, and the distinction between biochemical changes in and clinically significant sequelae of neurohormonal alterations with exercise. We emphasize that measurable pituitary responses to exercise should be viewed as part of a feedforward and feedback control system, as exemplified for the GH–IGF-1, GnRH–LH, CRH–AVP–ACTH, and other axes, with yet additional between-axes interactions. Although the final metabolic mechanisms that direct neuroendocrine changes in chronic training are not known definitively (e.g., free fatty acids, insulin, IGF-1, glucose, sex hormones, leptin, and/or others), their nature is likely multifactorial. In response to extremely strenuous exercise, stress-like neuroendocrine reactivity may predominate, whereas with appropriately modulated exercise intensity and volume, favorable clinical benefits, such as augmented GH secretion, cardiovascular conditioning, improved sense of well-being, and preserved reproductive function and bone density, likely ensue.

ACKNOWLEDGMENTS

We thank Patsy Craig for her skillful preparation of the manuscript and Paula P. Azimi for the data analysis, management, and graphics. This work was supported in part by NIH Grant MO1 RR00847 (to the General Clinical Research Center of the University of Virginia Health Sciences Center), Research Career Development Award 1-KO4-HD-00634 (to J. D. V.), the Baxter Healthcare Corporation (Round Lake, IL to J. D. V.), the NIH-supported Clinfo Data Reduction Systems, the University of Virginia Pratt Foundation and Academic Enhancement Program, the National Science Foundation Center for Biological Timing (Grant DIR89-20162), and the NIH NICHD U54 Center for Reproduction Research (HD96008).

REFERENCES

1. Veldhuis JD, Yoshida K, Iranmanesh A. The effect of mental and metabolic stress on the female reproductive system and female reproductive hormones. In: Hubbard J, Workman EA, eds. Handbook of Stress Medicine: an Organ System Approach. CRC, Boca Raton, FL, 1997, pp. 115–140.
2. Veldhuis JD, Evans WS, Weltman AL, Weltman JY, Rogol AD. Impact of exercise, as a paradigm of a physical stressor, on the female hypothalamo-pituitary-gonadal axis. In: Genazzani AR, Pertraglia F, eds. Hormones in Gynecological Endocrinology. Parthenon Publishing, UK, 1992, pp. 337–349.
3. Luger A, Deuster PA, Gold PW, Loriaux DL, Chrousos GP. Hormonal responses to the stress of exercise. Adv Exp Med Biol 1988;245:273–280.
4. Bullen BA, Skrinar GS, Beitins IZ, Carr DB, Reppert SM, Dotson CO, et al. Endurance training effects of plasma hormonal responsiveness and sex hormone excretion. J Appl Physiol Respir Environ Exerc Physiol 1984;56:1453–1463.
5. Roberts AC, McClure RD, Weiner RI, Brooks GA. Overtraining affects male reproductive status. Fertil Steril 1993;60:686–692.
6. Crist DM, Hill JM. Diet and insulin-like growth factor I in relation to body composition in women with exercise-induced hypothalamic amenorrhea. J Am Coll Nutr 1990;9:200–204.
7. Loucks AB. Effects of exercise training on the menstrual cycle: existence and mechanisms. Med Sci Sports Exerc 1990;22:275–280.
8. Wittet GA, Livesey JH, Espiner EA, Donald RA. Adaptation of the hypothalamopituitary adrenal axis to chronic exercise stress in humans. Med Sci Sports Exerc 1996;28:1015–1019.
9. Viru A, Karelson K, Smirnova T. Stability and variability in hormonal responses to prolonged exercise. Int J Sports Med 1992;13:230–235.
10. Dishman RK. Brain monoamines, exercise, and behavioral stress: animal models. Med Sci Sports Exerc 1997;29:63–74.
11. Deuste PA, Chrousos GP, Luger A, DeBolt JE, Bernier LL, Trostmann UH, et al. Hormonal and metabolic responses of untrained, moderately trained, and highly trained men to three exercise intensities. Metab Clin Exp 1989;38:141–148.
12. Rogol AD, Weltman JY, Evans WS, Veldhuis JD, Weltman AL. Long-term endurance training alters the hypothalamic-pituitary axes for gonadotropins and growth hormone. In: Veldhuis JD, ed. Endocrinology and Metablism Clinics of North America. WB Saunders, Philadelphia, PA, 1992, pp. 817–832.
13. Veldhuis JD. Male hypothalamic-pituitary-gonadal axis. In: Yen SC, Jaffe RB, Barbieri RL, eds. Reproductive Endocrinology. WB Saunders, Philadelphia, PA, 1999; pp. 622–631.
14. Straume M, Chen L, Johnson ML, Veldhuis JD. Systems-level analysis of physiological regulation interactions controlling complex secretory dynamics of growth hormone axis: a connectionist network model. Methods Neurosci 1995;28:270–310.

15. Giustina A, Veldhuis JD. Pathophysiology of the neuroregulation of GH secretion in experimetnal animals and the human. Endocr Rev 1998;19:717–797.
16. Clapp JF. The effects of maternal exercise on early pregnancy outcome. Am J Obstet Gynecol 1989;161:1453–1457.
17. Altemus M, Deuster PA, Galliven E, Carter CS, Gold PW. Suppression of hypothalamic–pituitary–adrenal axis responses to stress in lactating women. J Clin Endocrinol Metab 1995;80:2954–2959.
18. Bonen A, Campagna P, Gilchrist L, Young DC, Beresford P. Substrate and endocrine responses during exercise at selected stages of pregnancy. J Appl Physiol 1992;73:134–142.
19. Veldhuis JD, Evans WS, Demers LM, Thorner MO, Wakat D, Rogol AD. Altered neuroendocrine regulation of gonadotropin secretion in women distance runners. J Clin Endocrinol Metab 1985;61:557–563.
20. Weltman A, Weltman JY, Schurrer R, Evans WS, Veldhuis JD, Rogol AD. Endurance training amplifies the pulsatile release of growth hormone: effects of training intensity. J Appl Physiol 1992;76(6):2188–2196.
21. Rogol AD, Weltman A, Weltman JY, Seip RL, Snead DB, Levine S, et al. Durability of the reproductive axis in eumenorrheic women during one year of endurance training. J Appl Physiol 1992;72(4):1571–1580.
22. Snead DB, Weltman JY, Weltman A, Evans WS, Veldhuis JD, Varma MM, et al. Reproductive hormones and bone mineral density in women runners. J Appl Physiol 1992;72(6):2149–2156.
23. Alexander SL, Irvine CH, Ellis MJ, Donald RA. The effect of acute exercise on the secretion of corticotropin-releasing factor, arginine vasopressin, and adrenocorticotropin as measured in pituitary venous blood from the horse. Endocrinology 1991;128:65–72.
24. Thompson DL. Weltman JY, Rogol AD, Metzger D, Veldhuis JD, Weltman A. Cholinergic and opioid involvement in release of growth hormone during exercise and recovery. J Appl Physiol 1993;75:870–878.
25. Fryburg DA, Weltman A, Jahn LA, Weltman JY, Samolijik E, Veldhuis JD. Short-term modulation of the androgen milieu alters pulsatile but not exercise or GHRH-stimulated GH secretion in healthy men. J Clin Endocrinol Metab 1997;82:3710–3719.
26. Wideman L, Weltman JY, Shah N, Story S, Veldhuis JD, Weltman A. The effects of gender on exercise-induced growth hormone (GH) release. J Applied Physiol 1999; in press.
27. Kanaley JA, Weltman JY, Veldhuis JD, Rogol AD, Harman ML, Weltman A. Human growth hormone response to repeated bouts of aerobic exercise. J Appl Physiol 1997;83:1756–1761.
28. Weltman JY, Seip RL, Weltman AL, Snead D, Veldhuis JD, Rogol AD. Release of luteinizing hormone and growth hormone after recovery from maximal exercise. J Appl Physiol 1990;69(1):196–200.
29. Pritzlaff CJ, Wideman L, Weltman JY, Gutgesell ME, Hartman ML, Veldhuis JD, et al. Impact of acute exercise intensity on pulsatile growth hormone (GH) release in men. J Appl Physiol 1999, in press.
30. Weltman A, Pritzlaff CJ, Wideman L, Considine RV, Fryburg DA, Gutgesell ME, et al. Acute exercise of varying intensity does not affect serum leptin levels. J Appl Physiol 1998, submitted.
31. Lehmann M, Knizia K, Gastmann U, Petersen KG, Khalaf AN, Bauer S, et al. Influence of 6-week, 6 days per week, training on pituitary function in recreational athletes. Br J Sports Med 1993;27: 186–192.
32. Elias AN, Wilson AF. Exercise and gonadal function. Hum Reprod 1993;8:1747–1761.
33. Cumming DC, Wheeler GD, MCColl EM. The effects of exercise on reproductive function in men. Sports Med 1989;7:1–17.
34. McColl EM, Wheeler GD, Gomes P, Bhambhani Y, Cumming DC. The effects of acute exercise on pulsatile LH release in high-mileage male runners. Clin Endocrinol 1989;31:617–621.
35. Hackney AC. Endurance training and testosterone levels. Sports Med 1989;8:117–127.
36. Caston AL, Farrell PA, Deaver DR. Exercise training-induced changes in anterior pituitary gonadotrope of the female rat. J Appl Physiol 1995;79:194–201.
37. Blaney J, Sothmann M, Raff H, Hart B, Horn T. Impact of exercise training on plasma adrenocorticotropin response to a well-learned vigilance task. Psychoneuoendocrinology 1990;15:453–462.
38. Watanabe T, Morimoto A, Sakata Y, Wada M, Murakami N. The effect of chronic exercise on the pituitary-adrenocortical response in conscious rats. J Physiol 1991;439:691–699.
39. Fellmann N, Bedu M, Boudet G, Mage M, Sagnol M, Pequignot JM, et al. Inter-relationships between pituitary-adrenal hormones and catecholamines during a 6-day Nordic ski race. Eur J Appl Physiol Occup Physiol 1992;64:258–265.
40. Laatikainen TJ. Corticotropin-releasing hormone and opioid peptides in reproduction and stress. Ann Med 1991;23:489–496.

41. Bonen A, Keizer HA. Pituitary, ovarian, and adrenal hormone responses to marathon running. Int J Sports Med 1987;3:161–167.
42. Pestell RG, Hurley DM, Vandongen R. Biochemical and hormonal changes during a 1000 km ultramarathon. Clin Exp Pharmacol Physiol 1989;16:353–361.
43. Friedl KE, Plymate SR, Bernhard WN, Mohr LC. Elevation of plasma estradiol in healthy men during a mountaineering expedition. Horm Metab Res 1988;20:239–242.
44. Iranmanesh A, Lizarralde G, Veldhuis JD. Age and relative adiposity are specific negative determinants of the frequency and amplitude of growth hormone (GH) secretory bursts and the half-life of endogenous GH in healthy men. J Clin Endocrinol Metab 1991;73:1081–1088.
45. Veldhuis JD, Iranmanesh A, Ho KKY, Lizarralde G, Waters MJ, Johnson ML. Dual defects in pulsatile growth hormone secretion and clearance subserve the hyposomatotropism of obesity in man. J Clin Endocrinol Metab 1991;72:51–59.
46. Veldhuis JD, Iranmanesh A, Evans WS, Lizarralde G, Thorner MO, Vance ML. Amplitude suppression of the pulsatile mode of immunoradiometric LH release in fasting-induced hypoandrogenemia in normal men. J Clin Endocrinol Metab 1993;76:587–593.
47. Hartman ML, Veldhuis JD, Johnson ML, Lee MM, Alberti KG, Samojlik E, et al. Augmented growth hormone (GH) secretory burst frequency and amplitude mediate enhanced GH secretion during a two-day fast in normal men. J Clin Endocrinol Metabol 1992;74:757–765.
48. Weltman A, Weltman JY, Hartman ML, Abbott RA, Rogol AD, Evans WS, et al. Relationship between age, percentage body fat, fitness and 24 hour growth hormone release in healthy young adults: effects of gender. J Clin Endocrinol Metab 1994;78:543–548.
49. Veldhuis JD, Urban RJ, Lizarralde G, Johnson ML, Iranmanesh A. Attenuation of luteinizing hormone secretory burst amplitude is a proximate basis for the hypoandrogenism of healthy aging in men. J Clin Endocrinol Metab 1992;75:52–58.
50. Bergendahl M, Vance ML, Iranmanesh A, Thorner MO, Veldhuis JD. Fasting as a metabolic stress paradigm selectively amplifies cortisol secretory burst mass and delays the time of maximal nyctohemeral cortisol concentrations in healthy men. J Clin Endocrinol Metab 1996;81:692–699.
51. Aloi JA, Bergendahl M, Iranmanesh A, Veldhuis JD. Pulsatile intravenous gonadotropin-releasing hormone administration averts fasting-induced hypogonadotropism and hypoandrogenemia in healthy, normal-weight men. J Clin Endocrinol Metab 1997;82:1543–1548.
52. Veldhuis JD, Kulin HE, Warner BA, Santner SJ. Responsiveness of gonadotropin secretion to infusion of an opiate-receptor antagonist in hypogonadotropic individuals. J Clin Endocrinol Metab 1982;55:649–653.
53. Iranmanesh A, Grisso B, Veldhuis JD. Low basal and persistent pulsatile growth hormone secretion are revealed in normal and hyposomatotropic men studied with a new ultrasensitive chemiluminescence assay. J Clin Endocrinol Metab 1994;78:526–535.
54. Veldhuis JD, Liem AY, South S, Weltman A, Weltman J, Clemmons DA, et al. Differential impact of age, sex-steroid hormones, and obesity on basal versus pulsatile growth hormone secretion in men as assessed in an ultrasensitive chemiluminescence assay. J Clin Endocrinol Metab 1995;80:3209–3222.
55. Roubenoff R, Rall LC, Veldhuis JD, Kehayias JJ, Rosen C, Nicolson M, et al. The relationship between growth hormone kinetics and sarcopenia in postmenopausal women: the role of fat mass and leptin. J Clin Endocrinol Metab 1998;83:1502–1506.
56. Vahl N, Jorgensen JOL, Skjaerback C, Veldhuis JD, Orskov HJ, Christiansen J. Abdominal adiposity rather than age and sex predicts the mass and patterned regularity of growth hormone secretion in mid-life healthy adults. Am J Physiol 1997;272:E1108–E1116.
57. Ho KY, Veldhuis JD, Johnson ML, Furlanetto R, Evans WS, Alberti KG, et al. Fasting enhances growth hormone secretion and amplifies the complex rhythms of growth hormone secretion in man. J Clin Invest 1988;81:968–975.
58. Bergendahl M, Iranmanesh A, Evans WS, Veldhuis JD. Short-term fasting selectively suppresses leptin pulse mass and 24-hour rhythmic leptin release in healthy mid-luteal phase women without disturbing leptin pulse frequency or its entropy control (pattern orderliness). J Clin Endocrinol Metab 1999;83:883–894.
59. Walberg-Rankin J, Gwazdauskas FC. Response of beta-endorphin and estradiol to resistance exercise in female during energy balance and energy restriction. Int J Sports Med 1992;13:542–547.
60. Garcia-Rudaz MC, Ropelato, MG, Escobar ME, Veldhuis JD, Barontini M. Augmented frequency and mass of LH discharged per burst are accompanied by marked disorderliness of LH secretion in adolescents with polycystic ovary syndrome. Eur J Endo 1998;139:621–630.

61. Veldhuis JD, Johnson ML, Bolton WK. Analyzing pulsatile endocrine data in patients with chronic renal failure: a brief review of deconvolution techniques. Pediatr Nephrol 1991;5:522–528.
62. Van den Berg G, Veldhuis JD, Frolich M, Roelfsema F. An amplitude-specific divergence in the pulsatile mode of GH secretion underlies the gender difference in mean GH concentrations in men and premenopausal women. J Clin Endocrinol Metab 1996;81:2460–2466.
63. Veldhuis JD, Metzger DL, Martha PM Jr, Mauras N, Kerrigan JR, Keenan B, et al. Estrogen and testosterone, but not a non-aromatizable androgen, direct network integration of the hypothalamo-somatotrope (growth hormone)-insulin-like growth factor I axis in the human: evidence from pubertal pathophysiology and sex-steroid hormone replacement. J Clin Endocrinol Metab 1997;82:3414–3420.
64. Roelfsema F, Van den Berg G, Frolich M, Veldhuis JD, van Eijk A, Buurman MM, et al. Sex-dependent alteration in cortisol response to endogenous adrenocorticotropin. J Clin Endocrinol Metab 1993;77:234–240.
65. Van den Berg G, Pincus SM, Veldhuis JD, Frolich M, Roelfsema F. Greater disorderliness of ACTH and cortisol release accompanies pituitary-dependent Cushing's Disease. Eur J Endocrinol 1997;136:394–400.
66. Mulligan T, Iranmanesh A, Johnson ML, Straume M, Veldhuis JD. Aging alters feedforward and feedback linkages between LH and testosterone in healthy men. Am J Physiol 1997;42:R1407–R1413.
67. Pincus SM, Mulligan T, Iranmanesh A, Gheorghiu S, Godschalk M, Veldhuis JD. Older males secrete luteinizing hormone and testosterone more irregularly, and jointly more asynchronously, than younger males: dual novel facets. Proc Natl Acad Sci USA 1996;93:14,100–14,105.
68. Keenan DM, Yang R, Veldhuis JD. Statistical estimation of the parameters of pulsatile hormone concentration data. Siam J Appl Methods 1999; in press.
69. Rogol AD, Martha PM Jr, Johnson ML, Veldhuis JD, Blizzard RM. Growth hormone secretory dynamics during puberty. In: Adashi EY, Thorner MO, eds., The Somatotrophic Axis and the Reproductive Process in Health and Disease. Springer-Verlag, New York, 1996, pp. 69–82.
70. Veldhuis JD. Male hypothalamic–pituitary–gonadal axis. In: Lipshultz LI, Howards SS, eds., Infertility in the Male. Mosby-Year Book, Philadelphia, PA, 1996, pp. 23–58.
71. Veldhuis JD, Iranmanesh A, Rogol AD, Urban RJ. Regulatory actions of testosterone on pulsatile growth hormone secretion in the human: studies using deconvolution analysis. In: Adashi EY, Thorner MO, eds., Somatotropic Axis and the Reproductive Process in Health and Disease. Springer-Verlag, New York, 1995, pp. 40–57.
72. Veldhuis JD. Gender differences in secretory activity of the human somatotropic (GH) axis. Eur J Endocrinol 1997;134:287–295.
73. Veldhuis JD. Neuroendocrine mechanisms mediating awakening of the gonadotropic axis in puberty. Pediatr Nephrol 1996;10:304–317.
74. Mauras N, Rogol AD, Haymond MW, Veldhuis JD. Sex steroids, growth hormone, IGF-I: neuroendocrine and metabolic regulation in puberty. Horm Res 1996;45:74–80.
75. Theintz GE, Howald H, Weiss U, Sizonenko PC. Evidence for a reduction of growth potential in adolescent female gymnasts. J Pediatr 1993;122:306–313.
76. Dawson-Hughes B, Stern D, Goldman J, Reichlin S. Regulation of growth hormone and somatomedin-C secretion in postmenopausal women: effect of physiological estrogen replacement therapy. J Clin Endocrinol Metab 1986;63:424–432.
77. Weltman A, Seip RL, Snead D, Weltman JY, Evans WS, Veldhuis JD, et al. Exercise training at and above the lactate threshold in previously untrained women. Int J Sports Med 1992;13(3):257–263.
78. Pincus SM, Gevers E, Robinson ICA, Roelfsema F, Hartman ML, Veldhuis JD. Females secrete growth hormone with more process irregularity than males in both human and rat. Am J Physiol 1996;270:E107–E115.
79. Veldhuis JD. Pulsatile hormone release as a window into the brain's control of the anterior pituitary gland in health and disease: implications and consequences of pulsatile luteinizing hormone secretion. The Endocrinologist 1995;5:454–469.
80. Veldhuis JD. Issues in quantifying pulsatile neurohormone release. In: Van de Kar LD, ed. Methods in Neuroendocrinology: The Cellular and Molecular Neuropharmacology Series. CRC, Boca Raton, FL, 1998; pp. 181–203.
81. Veldhuis JD. New modalities for understanding dynamic regulation of the somatotropic (GH) axis: explication of gender differences in GH neuroregulation in the human. J Pediatr Endocrinol 1996;9:237–253.

82. Veldhuis JD, Iranmanesh A, Johnson ML, Lizarralde G. Twenty-four hour rhythms in plasma concentrations of adenohypophyseal hormones are generated by distinct amplitude and/or frequency modulation of underlying pituitary secretory bursts. J Clin Endocrinol Metab 1990;71:1616–1623.
83. Veldhuis JD. A parismonious model of amplitude and frequency modulation of episodic hormone secretory bursts as a mechanism for ultradian signaling by endocrine glands. In: Wever R, Kleitman N, eds. Ultradian Rhythms in Life Processes: an Inquiry into Fundamental Principles. Springer-Verlag, London, 1992, pp. 139–172.
84. Veldhuis JD, Iranmanesh A, Johnson ML, Lizarralde G. Amplitude, but not frequency, modulation of ACTH secretory bursts gives rise to the nyctohemeral rhythm of the corticotropic axis in man. J Clin Endocrinol Metab 1990;71:452–463.
85. Hartman ML, Pincus SM, Johnson ML, Matthews DH, Faunt LM, Vance ML, et al. Enhanced basal and disorderly growth hormone (GH) secretion distinguish acromegalic from normal pulsatile GH release. J Clin Invest 1994;94:1277–1288.
86. Pincus SM, Veldhuis JD, Mulligan T, Iranmanesh A, Evans WS. Effects of age on the irregularity of LH and FSH serum concentrations in women and men. Am J Physiol 1997;273:E989–E995.
87. Siragy HM, Vieweg WVR, Pincus SM, Veldhuis JD. Increased disorderliness and amplified basal and pulsatile aldosterone secretion in patients with primary aldosteronism. J Clin Endocrinol Metab 1995;80:28–33.
88. Van den Berg G, Pincus SM, Frolich M, Veldhuis JD, Roelfsema F. Reduced disorderliness of growth hormone release in biochemically inactive acromegaly after pituitary surgery. Eur J Endocrinol 1998;138:164–169.
89. Schmitz O, Porksen N, Nyholm B, Skjaerback C, Butler PC, Veldhuis JD, et al. Disorderly and nonstationary insulin secretion in glucose-tolerant relatives of patients with NIDDM. Am J Physiol 1997;35:E218–E226.
90. Meneilly GS, Ryan AS, Veldhuis JD, Elahi D. Increased disorderliness of basal insulin release, attenuated insulin secretory burst mass, and reduced ultradian rhythmicity of insulin secretion in older individuals. J Clin Endocrinol Metab 1997;82:4088–4093.
91. Johnson ML, Veldhuis JD. Evolution of deconvolution analysis as a hormone pulse detection method. Methods Neurosci 1995;28:1–24.
92. Veldhuis JD, Johnson ML. Specific methodological approaches to selected contemporary issues in deconvolution analysis of pulsatile neuroendocrine data. Methods Neurosci 1995;28:25–92.
93. Veldhuis JD, Evans WS, Johnson ML. Complicating effects of highly correlated model variables on nonlinear least-squares estimates of unique parameter values and their statistical confidence intervals: estimating basal secretion and neurohormone half-life by deconvolution analysis. Methods Neurosci 1995;28:130–138.
94. Loucks AB, Laughlin GA, Mortola JF, Girton L, Nelson JC, Yen SS. Hypothalamic–pituitary–thyroidal fucntion in eumenorrheic and amenorrheic athletes. J Clin Endocrinol Metab 1992;75:514–518.
95. Rogol AD, Veldhuis JD, Williams FT, Johnson ML. Pulsatile secretion of gonadotropins and prolactin in male marathon runners: relation to the endogenous opiate system. J Androl 1983;5:21–27.
96. Bagatell CJ, Bremner WJ. Sperm counts and reproductive hormones in male marathoners and lean controls. Fertil Steril 1990;53:688–692.
97. Arce JC, De Souza MJ. Exercise and male factor infertility. Sports Med 1993;15:146–149.
98. Lucia A, Chicharro JL, Perez M, Serratosa L, Bandres EF, Legido JC. Reproductive function in male endurance athletes: sperm analysis and hormonal profiles. J Appl Physiol 1996;81:2627–2636.
99. Celani MF, Grandi M. The pituitary-testicular axis in non-professional soccer players. Exp Clin Endocrinol 1989;94:244–252.
100. Vasankari TJ, Kujala UM, Taimela S, Huhtaniemi IT. Pituitary-gonadal response to gonadotropin-releasing hormone stimulation is enhanced in men after strenuous physical exercise. Acta Endocrinol 1993;129:9–14.
101. Keenan DM, Veldhuis JD. A biomathematical model of time-delayed feedback in the human male hypothalamic–pituitary–Leydig cell axis. Am J Physiol 1998;275:E157–E176.
102. Veldhuis JD, Johnson ML. Analytical methods for evaluating episodic secretory activity within neuroendocrine axes. Neurosci Biobehav Rev 1994;18:605–612.

103. Keenan D, Veldhuis JD. A stochastic model of admixed basal and pulsatile hormone secretion as modulated by a deterministic oscillator. Am J Physiol: Regul Integrative Comp Physiol 1997;273:R1182–R1192.
104. Bergendahl M, Veldhuis JD. Altered pulsatile gonadotropin signaling in nutritional deficiency in the male. Trends Endocrinol Metab 1995;6:145–159.
105. Frager MS, Pieper DR, Tonetta SA, Duncan JA, Marshall JC. Pituitary gonadotropin-releasing hormone receptors: effects of castration, steroid replacement, and the role of gonadotropin-releasing hormone in modulating receptors in the rat. J Clin Invest 1991;615–623.
106. Bergendahl M, Evans WS, Veldhuis JD. Current concepts on ultradian rhythms of luteinizing hormone secretion in the human. Hum Reprod Update 1996;2:507–518.
107. Licinio J, Negrao AB, Mantzoros C, Kaklamani V, Wong M-L, Bongiorno PB, et al. Synchronicity of frequently-sampled 24-hour concentrations of circulating leptin, luteinizing hormone, and estradiol in healthy women. Proc Natl Acad Sci USA 1998;95:2541–2546.
108. Schwartz MW, Seeley RJ, Campfield LA, Burn P, Baskin DG. Identification of targets on leptin action in rat hypothalamus. J Clin Invest 1996;98:1101–1106.
109. Ahima RS, Dushay J, Flier SN, Prabakaran D, Flier JS. Leptin accelerates the onset of puberty in normal female mice. J Clin Invest 1997;99:391–395.
110. Vasankari TJ, Kujala UM, Viljanen TT, Huhtaniemi IT. Carbohydrate ingestion during prolonged running exercise results in an increase of serum cortisol and decrease of gonadotrophins. Acta Physiol Scand 1991;141:373–377.
111. Tabata I, Ogita F, Miyachi M, Shibayama H. Effect of low blood glucose on plasma CRF, ACTH, and cortisol during prolonged physical exercise. J Appl Physiol 1991;71:1807–1812.
112. Matkovic V, Ilich JZ, Skugor M, Badenhop NE, Goel P, Clairmont A, et al. Leptin is inversely related to age at menarche in human females. J Clin Endocrinol Metab 1997;82:3239–3245.
113. Wade GN, Schneider JE, Li HY. Control of fertility by metabolic cues. Am J Physiol 1996;270: E1–E19.
114. Mastrogiacomo I, Toderini D, Bonanni G, Bordin D. Gonadotropin decrease induced by prolonged exercise at about 55% of the VO_{2max} in different phases of the menstrual cycle. Int J Sports Med 1990:11:198–203.
115. Botticelli G, Bacchi Modena A, Bresciani D, Villa P, Aguzzoli L, Florio P, et al. Effect of naltrexone treatment on the treadmill exercise-induced hormone release in amenorrheic women. J Endocrinol Invest 1992;15:839–847.
116. Kanaley JA, Boileau RA, Bahr JM, Misner JE, Nelson RA. Cortisol levels during prolonged exercise: the influence of menstrual phase and menstrual status. Int J Sports Med 1992;13:332–336.
117. Hohtari H, Elovainio R, Salminen K, Laatikainen T. Plasma corticotropin-releasing hormone, corticotropin, and endorphins at rest and during exercise in eumenorrheic and amenorrheic athletes. Fertil Steril 1988;50:233–238.
118. Samuels MH, Sanborn CF, Hofeldt F, Robbins R. The role of endogenous opiates in athletic amenorrhea. Fertil Steril 1991;565:507–512.
119. Harber VJ, Sutton JR, MacDougall JD, Woolever CA, Bhavnani BR. Plasma concentrations of beta-endorphin in trained eumenorrheic and amenorrheic women. Fertil Steril 1997;67:648–653.
120. Hohtari H, Salminen-Lappalainen K, Laatikainen T. Response of plasma endorphins, corticotropin, cortisol, and luteinizing hormone in the corticotropin-releasing hormone stimulation test in eumenorrheic and amenorrheic athletes. Fertil Steril 1991;55:276–280.
121. Armeanu MC, Lambalk CB, Berkhout GM, Schoemaker J. Effects of opioid antagonism with naltrexone on pulsatile luteinizing hormone secretion in women with hypothalamic amenorrhea in basal conditions and after discontinuation of treatment with pulsatile LHRH. Gynecol Endocrinol 1992;6:3–12.
122. Loucks AB, Mortola JF, Girton L, Yen SS. Alterations in the hypothalamic–pituitary–ovarian and the hypothalamic–pituitary–adrenal axes in athletic women. J Clin Endocrinol Metab 1989;68:402–411.
123. De Cree C, Van Kranenburg G, Geurten P, Fujimori Y, Keizer HA. 4-Hydroxycatecholestrogen metabolism responses to exercise and training: possible implications for menstrual cycle irregularities and breast cancer. Fertil Steril 1997;67:505–516.
124. Dugowson CE, Drinkwater BL, Clark JM. Nontraumatic femur fracture in an oligomenorrheic athlete. Med Sci Sports Exerc 1991;23:1323–1325.
125. Baker E, Demers L. Menstrual status in female athletes: correlations with reproductive hormones and bone density. Obstet Gynecol 1988;72:683–687.

126. Marcus R, Cann C, Madvig P, Minkoff J, Goddard M, Bayer M, et al. Menstrual function and bone mass in elite women distance runners: endocrine and metabolic features. Ann Intern Med 1985;102:158–163.
127. Wright NM, Renault J, Willi S, Veldhuis JD, Gordon L, Key LL, et al. Greater secretion of growth hormone in black than in white males: possible factor in greater bone mineral density. J Clin Endocrinol Metab 1995;80:2291–2297.

5 Exercise and the Growth Hormone–Insulin-Like Growth Factor-1 Axis

Alon Eliakim, MD, Jo Anne Brasel, MD, and Dan M. Cooper, MD

CONTENTS

INTRODUCTION
THE GH–IGF-1 AXIS
ACUTE EXERCISE AND THE GH–IGF-1 AXIS GROWTH HORMONE
INSULIN-LIKE GROWTH FACTORS (IGFs)
INSULIN-LIKE GROWTH FACTOR BINDING PROTEINS (IGFBPs)
EXERCISE TRAINING AND THE GH–IGF-1 AXIS
REFERENCES

INTRODUCTION

Naturally occurring physical activity in humans plays a profound role in tissue anabolism, growth, and development, yet little is known about the mechanisms that link patterns of exercise with tissue anabolism. Anabolic effects of exercise are not limited to individuals engaged in competitive sports who are particularly focused on improvements in strength or cardiovascular functions. For example, limb immobilization, neural injury, and prolonged bed rest cause reduction of muscle mass and bone density even in individuals who live a sedentary lifestyle (1). These observations imply that a sizeble anabolic stimulus arises from a relatively modest physical activity of daily living. Conversely, excessive exercise may have adverse effects. For example, Theintz et al. (2) recently reported a reduction in the growth potential of female adolescent gymnasts engaging in intense training.

The magnitude and tissue specificity of anabolic effects of exercise likely change with maturation and aging. It is striking that naturally occurring levels of physical activity, energy expenditure, and muscle strength exhibit some of their most rapid increases during childhood and adolescence. This particular combination of rapid growth and development, high levels of naturally occurring physical activity, and spontaneous, puberty-related increases in anabolic hormones (growth hormone [GH], insulin-like

From: *Contemporary Endocrinology: Sports Endocrinology*
Edited by: M. P. Warren and N. W. Constantini © Humana Press Inc., Totowa, NJ

growth factor-1 [IGF-1], and sex steroids) suggests the possibility of integrated mechanisms linking exercise with a variety of anabolic responses. This chapter will focus on the relationship between fitness and components of the GH–IGF-1 axis, and the effect of exercise and exercise training on circulating and local (i.e., muscle) component of this system.

THE GH–IGF-1 AXIS

The GH–IGF-1 axis regulates many essential life processes, including growth, development, metabolic, and reparative processes, and may affect several other physiologic activities (e.g., aging). During the past several decades, the understanding of this axis has increased markedly as various components of the axis have been identified and characterized and their molecular and clinical regulation have been clarified.

The axis is composed of hormones, growth factors, binding proteins, and receptors. The understanding of the axis must, therefore, consider each individual component and the interaction between them under both normal physiologic and pathological conditions. The axis starts in the central nervous system (CNS), which secretes a series of neurotransmitters (catecholamines, serotonin and cholinergic agents) that cause the hypothalamus to synthesize growth hormone-releasing hormone (GHRH) and somatostatin (SMS). GHRH stimulates the anterior pituitary to synthesize and secrete GH. In contrast, SMS directly inhibits GH secretion. However, SMS is produced in many other tissues as well, and exerts many different biologic activities, most of which are not related to the GH–IGF-1 axis.

GH is the major secretory product of the somatotroph axis. One of GH's most important actions is the stimulation of IGF-1 synthesis. However, other effects of GH on metabolism, body composition, and tissue differentiation are independent of IGF-1. GH exerts direct feedback effect on the two hypothalamic hormones that control its secretion. Tissue GH effects are mediated by the interaction between GH and the GH receptor. The GH receptor contains an intracellular and extracellular transmembrane domains. The extracellular domain is identical in structure to GH binding protein (GHBP) *(3)*. Therefore, a unique feature of this axis is that the measurable circulating GHBP levels likely reflect GH receptor number and overall tissue responsiveness to GH.

IGF-1 is part of the insulin-related peptides. As noted earlier, the endocrine form, secreted mainly by the liver, is GH-dependent. However, the paracrine and autocrine forms are only partially regulated by GH. Although IGF-1 can act in an endocrine manner, its action probably occurs primarily as a result of paracrine or autocrine secretion and regulation. IGF-1 actions are numerous and reproduce most, but not all, of the anabolic and growth-promoting effects of GH. IGF-1 stimulates SMS secretion and inhibits GH by a negative feedback mechanism *(4)*, but it is not clear whether circulating or central IGF-1 is responsible for this feedback mechanism.

The majority of circulating IGF-1 is bound to one of six IGFBPs. The most abundant circulating BP during adult life is IGFBP-3, which is synthesized mainly in the liver, and is GH-dependent. When bound to IGF-1, it complexes with an acid-labile subunit to form the circulating complex that carries most of the IGF-1 in the serum. As noted earlier, some of these binding proteins are GH-dependent (e.g., IGFBP-3), but others, such as IGFBP-1 and 2, are insulin-, rather than GH-, dependent (being high when insulin levels are low). The interaction between IGF-1 and its binding proteins is even more complicated, since some binding proteins were found to inhibit (e.g., IGFBP-4), but others to stimulate (e.g., IGFBP-5) IGF-1 anabolic effects *(5)*.

IGF-1 binds to two different receptors: type I and II. Type I receptor exhibit similarities to the insulin receptor, has tyrosine-kinase activity, and mediates most of IGF-1's effects. The type II receptor is identical to the mannose-6-phosphate receptor, and binds IGF-2 as well.

Pulsatility is characteristic of the hormones in the GH–IGF axis (i.e., GHRH, SMS, and GH). It has been shown in many experimental models that the pulsatile pattern of GH secretion is significantly important for accelerated growth rate *(6)*. In contrast, circulating levels of IGF-1 and IGFBP's level are relatively stable during the day.

Several components of the axis are age-dependent. Both GHRH, GH, GHBP, IGF-1, and IGFBP-3 reach their peak circulating levels during puberty *(7,8)*, and decrease with aging *(9)*. These changes are partially sex-hormone-dependent. Nutritional state has a remarkable influence on the GH–IGF-1 axis as well. For example, fasting and malnutrition increase GH secretion, but reduce IGF-1 levels *(10)*, probably owing to a decrease in GH receptors. This chapter will focus on exercise, another environmental regulator of the hormonal cascade of the GH–IGF-1 axis.

ACUTE EXERCISE AND THE GH–IGF-1 AXIS
GROWTH HORMONE (GH)

It is important to distinguish the acute effects of a single bout of exercise on components of the GH–IGF axis from what appear to be more profound neuroendocrinological adaptations that occur in physically active people or in response to long-term programs of endurance training.

It was first shown by Roth et al. *(11)* that physical exercise increases circulating GH levels. However, GH response to exercise is dependent on the duration and intensity of the exercise bout, the fitness level of the exercising subject, the timing of blood sampling, refractoriness of pituitary GH secretion to the exercise stimuli, and other environmental factors. Therefore, standardized exercise protocols should be used to evaluate the GH response to acute exercise.

Several previous studies reported that the GH response to exercise is greater in less fit subjects *(12)*. However, in those earlier studies, subjects were asked to perform exercise tests at the same absolute, rather than relative power. Since fitness varies so greatly in any population, the use of an absolute rather than relative work intensity can lead to the potentially confounding circumstance in which some subjects exercise below, whereas others exercise above their lactic/anaerobic threshold (LAT). This is an important distinction, since hormonal and metabolic responses to exercise are not related to exercise in a simple linear manner *(13,14)*. For example, several investigators *(15)* have demonstrated that circulating GH levels increased only in response to above, but not below LAT. This is consistent with other reports *(12,16,17)*, which demonstrated that loads of 75–90% of maximal aerobic power yielded a greater GH rise than milder loads. Therefore, results of studies in which the GH response to exercise was tested at an absolute work rate would superficially lead to the conclusion that fitter subjects have smaller rather than larger GH responses. In fact, these studies demonstrate simply that as individuals become fitter, the stress associated with exercise at an absolute work rate diminishes.

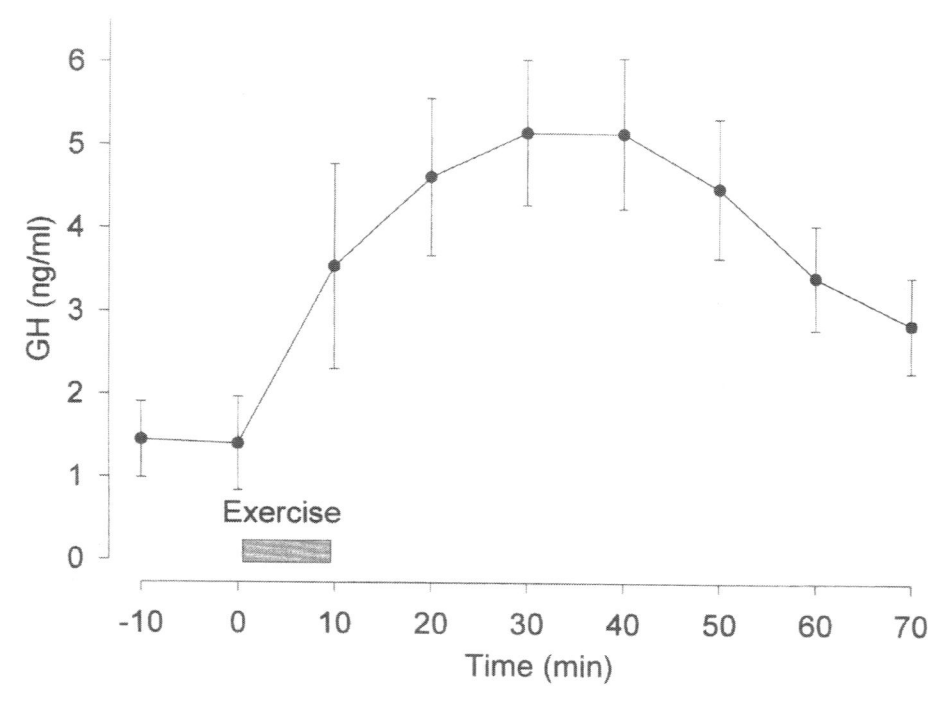

Fig. 1. The effect of a 10-min high-intensity exercise bout on GH secretion. Peak GH was observed at about 30 min after the onset of exercise.

The exercise duration should be at least 10 min *(18)*, since exercise of shorter duration (e.g., 5 min at 50% between LAT and VO_2max *[15]*) was not accompanied by increases in circulating GH levels. Moreover, exercise-induced GH peak occurs 25–30 min after the start of the exercise (Fig. 1), irrespective of the exercise duration *(12,15,19–21)*. Thus, when the task is brief (e.g., 10 min) a peak may be reached after its cessation, but when the task is long (e.g., 45 min), the peak may be reached while the individual is still exercising. Blood sampling, however, should be targeted to obtain the exercise-induced GH peak.

Another confounding factor in the GH response to exercise is the possibility of a "refractory period" in which the normal pituitary gland will not respond sufficiently to a stimulus for GH release. We previously studied *(20)* the GH response to exercise immediately following multiple (every 20 min), overnight GH sampling. The GH response to exercise appeared to be inhibited if a spontaneous, early morning GH pulse had occurred within 1 h prior to the exercise test. Cappon et al. *(22)* previously demonstrated a refractory period of at least 1 h following exercise-induced GH secretion (i.e., the subsequent GH response to exercise was attenuated: Fig. 2), and postulated that exercise-specific factors, like elevated free fatty acids or alterations in parasympathetic-sympathetic tone, might have been responsible *(23–26)*. However, these mechanisms were probably not operant in the refractory period that followed a spontaneous early morning GH pulse, since the subjects were sleeping when the pulse occurred. A more likely possibility is the phenomenon of GH autoinhibition *(27)* in which the elevated circulating GH from the previous spontaneous pulse played a role in inhibiting the subsequent pituitary response to exercise.

Chapter 5 / Exercise and the GH–IGF-1 Axis

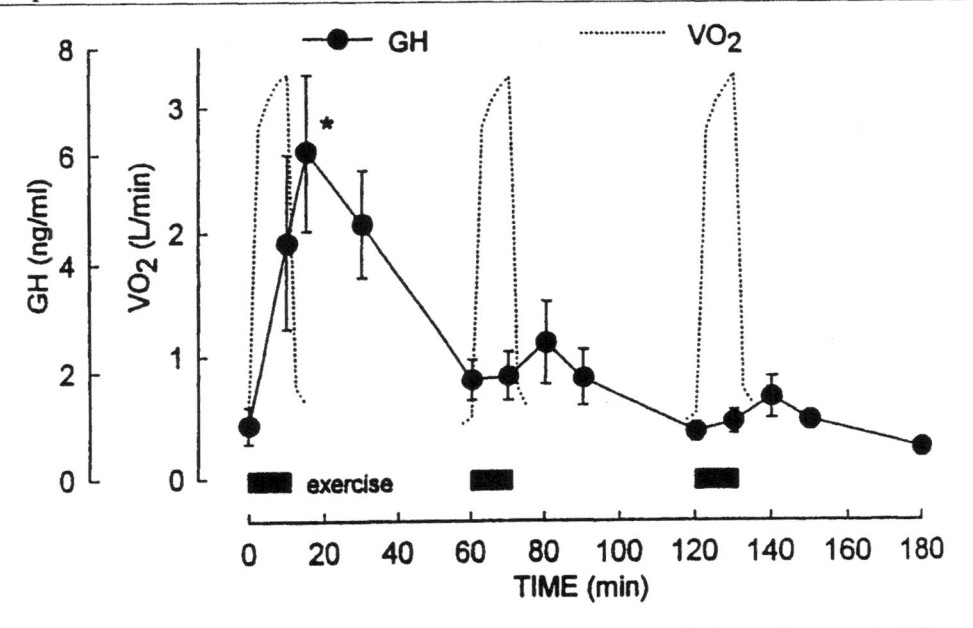

Fig. 2. GH and maximal oxygen uptake (VO_2max) of three 10-min exercise bouts. Increases in VO_2max were the same for all three exercise tests, and demonstrated slopes typical to above lactate threshold work intensities. GH increased significantly only after the first exercise bout (with courtesy by Cappon et al. [22]).

Environmental and nutritional factors as well as some pathological states may interfere with GH response to exercise. Cappon et al. (28) postulated that a high-fat meal (known to stimulate somatostatin from gastrointestinal tissues [29]) would inhibit the magnitude of GH response to exercise, and indeed, the GH response to exercise in their study was attenuated 45 min after administration of high-fat meal. The inhibition of the exercise-induced GH response was correlated with circulating levels of somatostatin. (Fig. 3).

High ambient temperature may in itself increase circulating GH levels (30), whereas low temperature attenuates GH release (31). Obesity and/or polycystic ovarian syndrome (32) are characterized by attenuated GH response to exercise.

There are some clinical, practical implications for the increase in circulating GH levels following exercise. The first is as a physiological "provocation" for GH secretion in the diagnosis of GH deficiency. As noted earlier, GH is secreted in pulses. Therefore, a single random blood sample cannot differentiate between a healthy and GH-deficient child. To overcome this, a number of provocation procedures to stimulate pituitary GH release have been developed (33). Most of the GH stimulation tests currently in use involve the use of pharmacological agents (34). These tests are uncomfortable for the patient and present some risk (e.g., hypoglycemia). Moreover, even a "positive" stimulus test can be questioned because information about physiological GH secretory patterns is lacking. These confounding factors have led a number of investigators to emphasize the role of physiological stimulation tests or, on the other hand, to focus on less variable circulating substances, like IGF-1 and/or its binding proteins, in the diagnosis of GH deficiency in children (35). Second, if indeed GH plays a key role in the anabolic effects of exercise and exercise training (i.e., muscle hypertrophy), attention

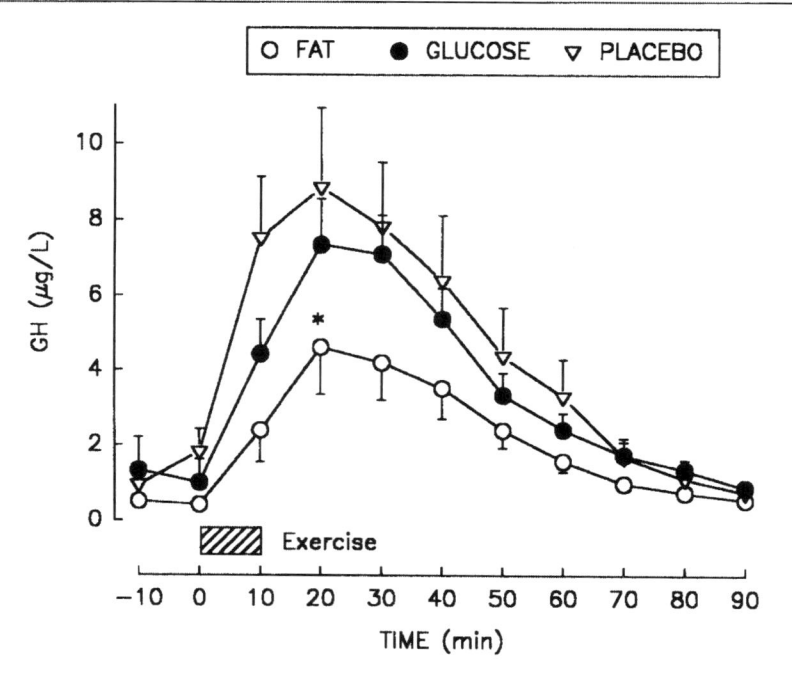

Fig. 3. The effect of high-fat and high-carbohydrate meals on exercise-induced GH secretion. High-fat meal (but not carbohydrate meal) significantly attenuated the exercise-associated GH increase (with courtesy by Cappon et al. *[28]*).

should be paid by athletes and trainers to factors that may inhibit the GH response to exercise and, therefore, attenuate the training effect (i.e., exercise intensity, short intervals between exercise sessions, exercise training in cold climate, following high-fat meal, and so forth).

INSULIN-LIKE GROWTH FACTORS (IGFS)

The effect of exercise on circulating IGF-1 has been examined by several investigators with differing results. For example, Wilson and Horowitz *(36)* reported no increase in serum IGF-1 in children after 15 min of an unspecified cycle ergometer exercise protocol, nor did Hagberg and coworkers *(37)* find an increase in IGF-1 after 60 min of treadmill exercise comparable to 70% of the subject's VO_2max in young and old adults. In addition, the effect of exercise on IGF-1 appears to depend on the type of the exercise performed. For example, increases in circulating IGF-1 are not observed in training programs that consist primarily of resistance exercise (i.e., weight lifting) *(38)*. More recently Bang and coworkers *(39)* reported a 26% increase in IGF-1 at the 10-min point of a 30-min exercise protocol in six healthy subjects (three women). Consistent with these results, Schwarz et al. *(21)* demonstrated increases in serum IGF-1 following 10 min of exercise of both below and above LAT. The mechanism of these different IGF responses to the type of exercise is not known.

The determinants of the transient increase in circulating IGF-1 in response to exercise are not readily apparent. One possibility would be the "classic" mechanism of increased hepatic IGF release owing to exercise-induced secretion of GH. However, data from

Bang et al. *(39)* and Schwarz et al. *(21)* suggest that the increase in IGF-1 accompanying exercise is, in fact, not related to GH. As noted earlier, GH increases significantly only in response to high-intensity exercise, yet IGF-1 increases for both low- and high-intensity exercise. Moreover, circulating IGF-1 reaches its peak before the GH peak (i.e., 10 min compared to 30 min), whereas increases in serum IGF-1, owing to *de novo* IGF-1 synthesis in the liver and transport to the circulation, occur several hours after the administration of endogenous GH *(40)*. In addition, Bang et al. *(39)* showed that exercise led to increases in IGF even in subjects with pituitary insufficiency.

The observed changes in circulating IGFs must reflect rapid changes in the balance among one or all of:

1. IGF input into the circulation from the liver and/or other sources.
2. Distribution within the circulating blood.
3. Removal from the circulation.

The transient nature of the increases suggests that hemodynamic or metabolic effects of exercise *per se* might play a role. Exercise in humans is accompanied by the rapid "autotransfusion" of hemoconcentrated blood from the spleen into the cellular circulation *(41)* by increased blood flow to the exercising muscle and by loss of plasma water *(42)*. Each of these phenomena might explain, in part, an increased IGF concentration by changes in IGF flux and/or volume of distribution, but measurements of circulating IGF concentration alone are not sufficient to determine which of these mechanisms is most important.

There have been far fewer investigations in humans of the physiological responses of IGF-2 compared with IGF-1. In part, this lack of attention to IGF-2 may have resulted because in the rat (the most commonly used animal model for IGF-1 molecular biology and physiology), IGF-2 appears to exert its most important effects prenatally, and circulating levels are quite low during all of postnatal life *(43)*. In contrast, IGF-2 levels remain high throughout life in humans *(44)*, and may play a particularly important role in bone growth and development *(45)*. Studies by Bang et al. *(39)* and Schwarz et al. *(21)* showed an acute, endurance exercise-associated rise in IGF-2; however, the biological importance of this finding has yet to be determined.

INSULIN-LIKE GROWTH FACTOR BINDING PROTEINS (IGFBPs)

There have been few studies of IGFBPs in response to brief exercise. Most have concentrated on IGFBP-1, even though IGFBP-1 exists in the circulation in much smaller quantities than IGFBP-3 and appears to play a lesser role in circulating IGF-1 bioavailability than does IGFBP-3 *(46)*. Suikkari et al. *(47)* noted an increase in IGFBP-1 following 3 h of cycle ergometer exercise at a work rate comparable to 45–50% of the subjects' VO_2max. Similarly, Hopkins et al. *(48)* reported an increase in IGFBP-1 following prolonged exercise to exhaustion.

Schwarz and coworkers *(21)* have demonstrated that IGFBP-3 levels measured by radioimmunoassay (RIA) increased with both low- and high-intensity exercise, and were greater during the above-LAT protocols. In contrast to their RIA measurements, IGFBP-3 measured by Western ligand blotting (WLB) did not change. As a potential explanation for the discrepancy between RIA and WLB data, they suggested that the antibody used in the RIA recognizes both intact and fragment forms of IGFBP-3, but the WLB method measures only the intact form of IGFBP-3. They, therefore, measured the rate of IGFBP-3 proteolysis as a function of exercise, and were intrigued to find that proteolysis did occur consequent to high-intensity exercise, and that this increased proteolysis was associated with the peak increase in IGF-1 and IGF-2 serum concentrations. It is important, however, to note that increases in IGFBP-3 proteolytic activity occurred in this study only for high-intensity exercise, but increases in IGFBP-3, IGF-1, and IGF-2 occurred for both low- and high-intensity exercise.

The mechanism for the increased IGFBP-3 proteolysis following high-intensity exercise is not clearly understood. However, IGFBP-3 protease activity has been shown to be calcium-dependent *(49)*, and brief periods of heavy exercise can lead to increases in total and free-ionized serum calcium concentrations with a time-course similar to the observed changes in IGFBP-3 proteolysis *(50)*. Interestingly, Belcastro *(51)* demonstrated in the rat that exercise increases nonlysosomal calcium-specific protease activity of calpain, a protease that in vitro causes morphological changes in striated muscle similar to exercise. Although all IGFBP-3 proteases that have been observed clinically are not identical *(52)*, the original pregnancy-associated IGFBP-3 protease(s) was characterized as a calcium-dependent serine protease *(49)*. The cleavage patterns of the exercise-induced IGFBP-3 protease seems similar to the pregnancy-associated patterns supporting, indirectly, the possibility that calcium may play a role in exercise-induced IGFBP-3 proteolysis.

The modest proteolytic activity observed in the circulating blood may actually reflect more substantial proteolytic activity in the local milieu of the exercising muscle. Along these lines, Lalou and Binoux *(53)* suggested that IGFBP-3 protease activity is more marked in the tissues than in the circulation. Schwarz et al. *(21)* showed that marked acid-base changes had occurred during high-intensity exercise protocols (10 min cycling at 50% between LAT and VO_2max), and serum changes of this magnitude are known to be associated with even more profound changes in the exercising muscle *(54)*. In vitro studies demonstrate that IGFBP-3 undergoes limited proteolysis at acid pH *(55)*. Whether or not the magnitude of these local changes in pH somehow stimulate IGFBP-3 proteolysis and the local release of bioactive IGFs into the exercising muscle has yet to be determined.

EXERCISE TRAINING AND THE GH–IGF-1 AXIS

Several independent studies of healthy human beings have demonstrated significant correlation between physical fitness and circulating components of the GH–IGF-1 axis. Weltman et al. *(58)* demonstrated a significant positive correlation between 24-h integrated GH concentrations and peak VO_2 in young healthy male, but not female adults. They also demonstrated an inverse correlation between 24-h integrated GH concentrations and body fat in both males and females. They concluded that a gender effect exists with respect to the influence of physical fitness on the neuroendocrine control of the somatotrophic axis. They suggested that hyperinsulinemia associated with excess body fat and decreased levels of physical activity may reduce GH release *(61)*, and since men, in general, have more central fat than women *(62)*, this may account for the greater influence of adiposity on GH secretion in men. They further speculated that the higher estradiol levels in adult females, which stimulate GH release *(63)*, may oppose the inhibitory effect of insulin and therefore explain the gender-related differences in the correlation between fitness and GH concentration.

The positive correlation between fitness and GH levels is consistent with animal experiments of Borer et al. *(64)*, who noted an increased GH pulse amplitude in physically active, rapidly growing hamsters compared with less rapidly growing, sedentary controls. They suggested that the fit state was associated with increased circulating endorphins and/or increased tissue sensitivity to endorphins. Endorphins inhibit somatostatin (known to attenuate pituitary GH secretion), and this leads to increased pituitary GH secretion.

Kelley and coworkers *(57)* found a significant positive correlation between VO_2max and both circulating GH and IGF-1 levels in healthy pre- and postmenopausal females. They found that both VO_2max and IGF-1 concentrations decline with age. However, when the influence of both age and fitness was analyzed using multiple regression, VO_2max remained the only independent predictor of IGF-1 concentrations. Therefore, they concluded that the decrease in serum IGF-1 with age is not related to aging *per se*, but probably to age-related decline in physical activity and fitness. Along with these observations, Poehlman and Copeland *(56)* reported a significant positive correlation between VO_2max and circulating IGF-1 levels in young (18–36 yr old) and old (59–76 yr old) adults.

We recently described *(59)* that both functional (i.e., VO_2max) and structural (i.e. thigh muscle volume determined by serial magnetic resonance images) indices of fitness were correlated with mean overnight GH levels, GHBP, and serum IGF-1 levels in late pubertal adolescent girls (Fig. 4). Moreover, thigh muscle volume was inversely correlated with IGFBP-2 and IGFBP-4. These cross-sectional data suggest that fitness in healthy, adolescent females is associated with adaptations of the GH–IGF-1 system consistent with an hormonally expressed, anabolic state.

Similar to the findings of Weltman et al. *(58)* and Borer et al. *(64)*, the significant correlation between fitness and mean overnight GH levels resulted probably from an increase in peak GH amplitude, since only peak amplitude (and not peak frequency or width) was significantly correlated with mean GH.

The positive correlation between GHBP and fitness is unique. GHBP is the extracellular domain of the GH receptor *(65)*, and is believed to reflect tissue GH receptor capacity. Ligand-mediated receptor regulation appears to exist for GH and GHBP in a number of situations. GHBP decreases when exogenous recombinant human growth hormone (rhGH) is administered to humans *(66)*, is low in acromegaly *(67)*, and is high in obesity despite low GH *(68)*. However, ligand-mediated receptor downregulation does not appear to operate during normal growth when both GH and GHBP increase in the prepubertal years *(69)*. Our data suggest that the relatively trained or "fit" state in adolescent females is another example of simultaneous increases in both GH and GHBP. The mechanism of these responses is not known, but suggests anabolic adaptations of both the ligand and receptor.

The simultaneous higher levels of GH, GHBP, and IGF-1 in fitter adolescent females suggest that the increased circulating IGF-1 resulted from the "traditional" pathway of GH- mediated increases in hepatic IGF-1 production. Our data also suggest that the generally increased circulating IGF-1 in fitter adolescent females might be related to IGFBPs. IGFBP-2 and IGFBP-4 were inversely correlated with thigh muscle volume. The role of these binding proteins in the circulation is yet not known; however, it is intriguing that an inverse correlation between IGF-1 and IGFBP-2 has been noted in several pathological conditions *(70,71)*, and during states of protein restriction *(72)*. In

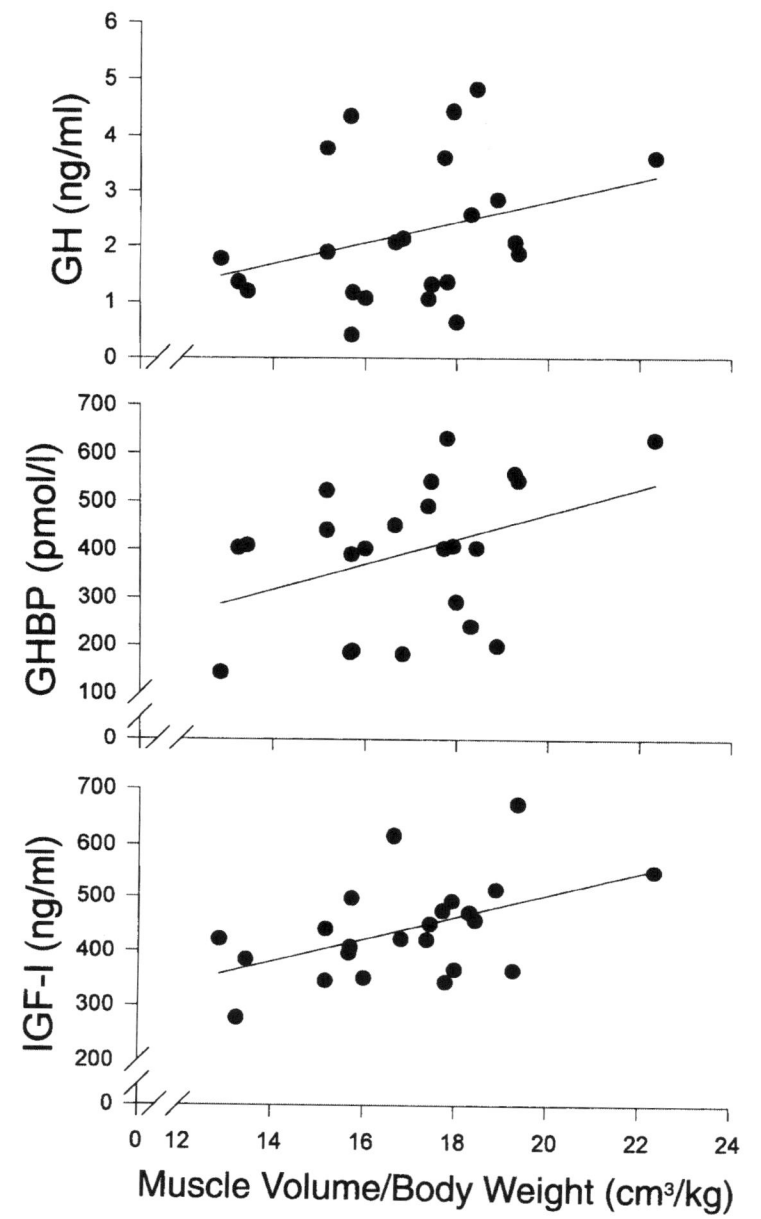

Fig. 4. Cross-sectional relationships between thigh muscle volume and mean overnight GH concentrations ($r = 0.35$, $p < 0.05$) **(top)**; GHBP ($r = 0.39$, $p < 0.04$) **(middle)**; and circulating IGF-1 ($r = 0.5$, $p < 0.008$) **(bottom)** in late pubertal females.

addition, cell-culture experiments indicate that IGFBP-4 inhibits the anabolic functions of IGF-1 *(73)*. Thus, IGFBP-2 and IGFBP-4 might attenuate IGF-1 anabolic effects, and, therefore, the lower level of these binding proteins in fitter subjects may increase IGF-1 bioactivity.

More recently, we studied *(60)* cross-sectionally the relationship between fitness and circulating components of the GH–IGF-1 axis in a group of late pubertal adolescent males. Mean GH was positively correlated with fitness. However, in contrast to adolescent females, GHBP was negatively correlated, and IGF-1 was not correlated with fitness in adolescent males. Interestingly, consistent with the findings in adolescent females, the strongest relationship observed was the inverse correlation between fitness and IGFBP-4.

The increased mean GH resulted from an increase in peak width and amplitude, since both were significantly correlated with fitness, whereas GH peak frequency was not. There are several possible explanations for the inverse relationship between GH and GHBP in fit subjects. Ligand-mediated receptor downregulation is, of course, a possibility in which higher circulating GH levels lead to lower tissue GH receptor. In this paradigm, GH secretion is enhanced in fit subjects, and the increased secretion eventually downregulates the GH receptor. A different explanation is that fitness-associated downregulation of GH receptors may be the primary adaptation. The lower levels of circulating GHBP (as noted, reflecting lower tissue GH receptor number) in fit subjects may represent widespread tissue insensitivity to GH. Circulating GH itself is known to inhibit pituitary GH secretion *(27)*. Thus, in the fit, relatively GH-insensitive state, higher levels of GH would be required to limit pituitary secretion of GH, once initiated. A similar mechanism has been demonstrated in the clinical syndrome of "thyroid resistance" in which reduced tissue sensitivity to thyroid hormone results in generally greater pituitary thyroid-stimulating hormone (TSH) secretion *(74)*.

As a result of the low GHBP levels in fitter adolescent boys, IGF-1 was not correlated with fitness. As noted earlier, these observations contradict our findings in adolescent girls *(59)*. These differences, however, are at least internally consistent: both mean GH and GH sensitivity (i.e., increased tissue GH receptor) were enhanced in the fitter females, likely leading to increased hepatic production of IGF-1 and, consequently, greater circulating IGF-1.

However, the mechanism for the different gender-related relationships among fitness, GHBP, and IGF-1 is not readily apparent. Recently discovered effects of estrogen and testosterone on GHBP could play a role: testosterone appears to decrease GHBP *(75)*, whereas estrogen increases GHBP *(76,77)*. Perhaps these large, sex-steroid-related effects masked more subtle fitness-associated effects on GHBP.

There was a substantial inverse correlation between IGFBP-4 and both muscle mass and peak VO_2. As noted, IGFBP-4 appears to inhibit mitogenic effects of IGF-1 in bone-culture studies *(73)*. Interestingly, IGF-1 itself leads to proteolysis of IGFBP-4, suggesting a possible mechanism whereby IGF-1 acts to enhance its own bioactivity *(78,79)*. These observations suggest a novel mechanism in which the fit state is anabolic not by acting on GH or IGF-1, but by altering their binding proteins.

Most of the male and female adolescents who participated in the cross-sectional study participated in a brief (5-wk), randomized, prospective endurance-type training intervention. Based on the cross-sectional data, we hypothesized that training would lead to increases in circulating GH and IGF-1 levels. Training was accompanied by a 15% higher total energy expenditure (by the doubly labeled water technique), and resulted in significant increases in VO_2max and thigh muscle volume in the trained, but not the control subjects (both females and males) *(80)*. In contrast to our hypotheses, there was a significant decrease in IGF-1 and IGFBP-5 in the trained, but not the control females *(59)*, as well as a significant decrease in GHBP and IGF-1, and a significant increase in IGFBP-2 in the trained, but not control males (Fig. 5) *(81)*.

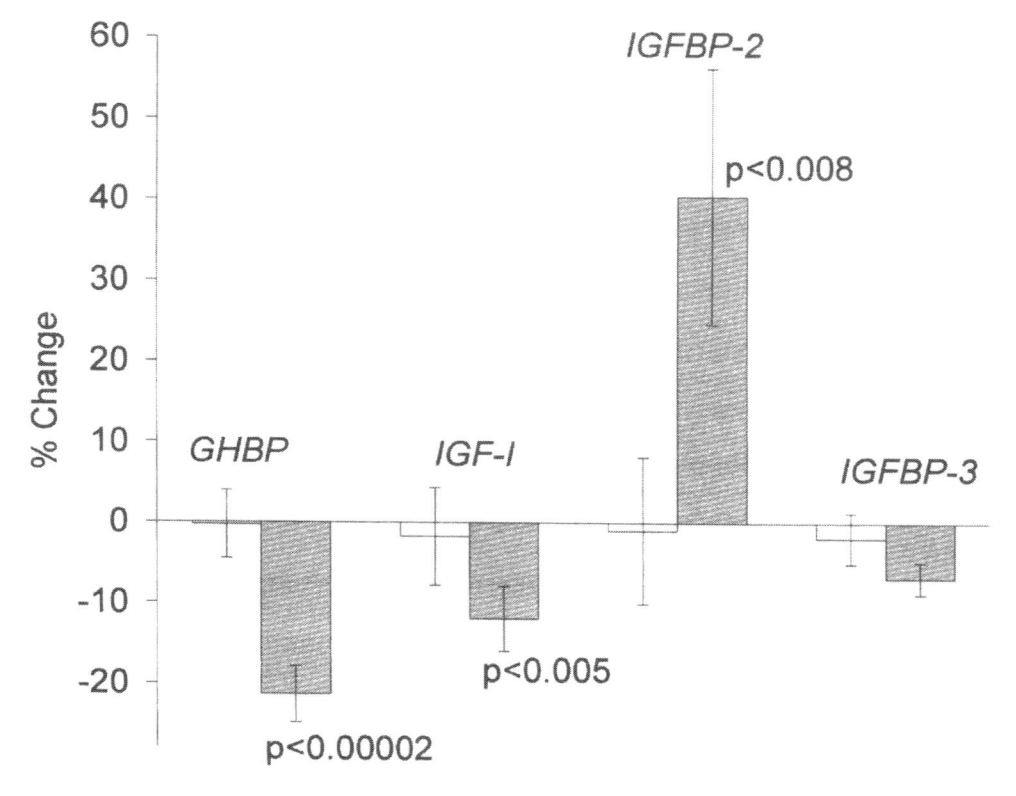

Fig. 5. Changes in GHBP, IGF-1, IGFBP-2, and IGFBP-3 following 5 wk of endurance-type training protocol in control (open bars) and trained (hatched bars) subjects. GHBP and IGF-1 were significantly decreased, and IGFBP-2 significantly increased in the training, but not control group subjects. These changes are typically found in catabolic states.

These effects are commonly observed in energy-deficient states, like food deprivation or disease-associated malnutrition *(70–72)*, but "catabolic" neuroendocrine adjustments occurred in the present study, even though training increased thigh muscle volume. Moreover, although energy expenditure was significantly greater in the training group, it was not accompanied by weight loss.

A potential mechanism for this seemingly paradoxical "catabolic" adaptation was the substantial reduction in circulating GHBP in the trained male subjects. As noted earlier, the lower GHBP circulating levels may reflect fewer tissue receptors and reduced tissue responsiveness to GH *(65)*. This is consistent with the lower levels of IGF-1 that we found in the training group, since as previously noted, circulating IGF-1 depends on its GH-induced, hepatic production *(82)*.

The exercise training effect on GHBP observed here appears to be unique. In several pathological states (malnutrition *[83]*, obesity *[68]*), the relationship between GH and GHBP suggest the well-described phenomenon of ligand-induced receptor regulation. In this study, training did lead to a reduction in GHBP, but without any change in mean GH or GH pulsatility. Thus, the possibility exists that lower GH receptor is the initiating mechanism in the neuroendocrine response to training. The mechanism for such a direct training effect on GH receptors or GHBPs is not known.

Interestingly, we found a training-associated reduction in IGFBP-5 in adolescent females. IGFBP-5 is one of the binding proteins that seems to enhance some of the IGF-1 mitogenic effects (i.e., in bones *[84]*). These observations emphasize again that the exercise training-induced decrease in IGF-1 bioavailability is mediated not only by acting on IGF-1 itself, but also by altering its binding proteins.

What emerges from our observations is the hypothesis that the sudden imposition of an endurance training program first leads to hormonal adaptations suggestive of a catabolic state, but at some point, presumably after 5 wk, an anabolic "rebound" occurs (similar perhaps to the phenomenon of catch-up growth following a period of nutritional deprivation). Exactly how and when this switch takes place, and whether the initial catabolic-type stage is necessary for the ultimate anabolic adaptation remain unknown.

Along with this hypothesis, Weltman et al. *(85)* noted a significant increase in the amplitude of spontaneously occurring GH pulses in women following a longer training program (1 yr of training at above LAT work intensities). They suggested that it is possible that the women who trained at above LAT were habitually exposed to increased circulating levels of both endorphins and catecholamines *(86–88)* and, as a consequence, decreased somatostatin tone and increased GH secretion. However, the mechanism for training-induced increases in GH secretion is not clearly understood.

There is increasing awareness that the effect of stimuli like exercise on growth factors may be different in local tissues than in the circulation *(89)*. Very few studies have examined the effect of brief exercise or training on muscle IGF-1 levels. Yan et al. *(90)* demonstrated that an acute bout of eccentric exercise led to an increase in IGF-1 immunoreactivity in rat type II muscle 4 d postexercise. Consistent with Yan's observation, we found *(91)* that 5 d of treadmill training in young female rats resulted in a significant increase in muscle IGF-1 protein, without changes in IGF-1 gene expression (i.e., mRNA), and without changes in circulating IGF-1 (Fig. 6). These results suggest that the early mechanisms of the training adaptation involve translational or posttranslational increases in muscle tissue IGF-1, and that local IGF-1 regulation (e.g., muscle tissue) may be dissociated from central neuroendocrine control mechanisms. Along these lines, Phillip et al. *(92)* examined the mechanisms responsible for the rapid (24–48 h) accumulation of IGF-1 in the experimental nephropathic kidney. They concluded that the increase in IGF-1 was not owing to an increase in local synthesis of IGF-1, but rather to an increase in IGF-1 uptake from the circulation resulting from nonmembrane-associated IGFBP. This observation emphasized again the role of IGFBPs (which may possess a cell-membrane integrin binding domain allowing them to associate strongly with the surface of the cells) in the regulation of the early adaptation of local IGF-1 to exercise training.

Moreover, there is evidence that early changes in other, non-IGF, components of the local adaptation to exercise training are mediated largely by translational and posttranslational events *(93)*. Town and Essig *(94)*, for example, examined the effect of endurance training on mitochondrial enzymes and related proteins in the rat. They demonstrated increased aminolevulinate synthase activity after 3 d of training, and elevated cytochrome oxidase activity following 7 d of training, but the investigators found no changes in the gene expression of these enzymes.

In contrast, DeVol et al. *(95)* showed that a significant increase in IGF-1 mRNA accompanied compensatory hypertrophy of the plantaris and soleus muscle only 2 d after unilateral excision of the gastrocnemius tendon (levels of IGF-1 protein were not

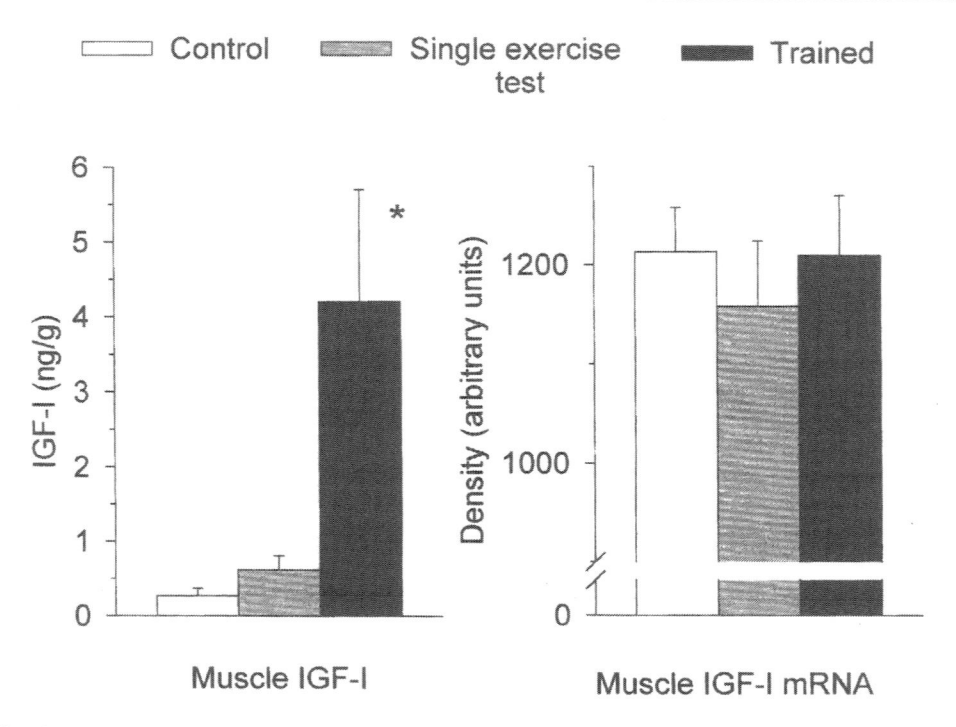

Fig. 6. Effect of a single maximal exercise test and 5 d of endurance-type treadmill training on muscle IGF-1 levels and IGF-1 gene expression. Training led to a significant increase in muscle IGF-1 protein, but not IGF-1 mRNA.

measured in these studies). The apparent discrepancy between the results of DeVol et al. and other studies suggests that different types and amounts of muscular work could lead to a different time-course and pattern of IGF-1 increase.

Longer periods of exercise training, however, do lead to stimulation of IGF-1 gene expression both in the central neuroendocrine and local tissue components of the GH–IGF-1 system. Zanconato et al. *(89)*, for example, found that by 4 wk of endurance training in young rats, hepatic IGF-1 gene expression was increased. Yeh et al. *(96)* observed an increase in circulating IGF-1 in rats after 9 wk of training. Finally, Zanconato et al. *(89)* showed that 4 wk of endurance-type training in the rat led to increases in exercising muscle IGF-1 gene expression and protein. Interestingly, however, inhibition of GH (by hypophysectomy *[95]* and by GH-releasing hormone antibody *[89]*) actually enhanced the local IGF-1 response to increased muscular work. It is clear from these observations that experimental inhibition of GH alone cannot succeed in blocking possible autocrine and paracrine effects of IGF-1 in the anabolic adaptations to physical activity. These data emphasize the GH independence of the "local" vs the GH-dependent "central" IGF-1 responses to exercise and training.

What is the advantage of the organism of simultaneous central "catabolism" and local anabolism early in the adaptation to increased physical activity? In this we can only speculate that this adaptive mechanism might reduce global anabolic function, thereby conserving energy sources, but still allow for local tissue growth in response to environmental stresses like exercise training.

Supporting this idea is the state of "marginal malnutrition" seen in highly trained, nutritionally self-deprived athletes (e.g., female gymnasts *[2]*) or impoverished, poorly nourished children whose daily lives include strenuous physical work *(97)*. In these populations, adaptation to hard physical activity does occur, but somatic growth is reduced, and circulating IGF-1 is low. We also recently demonstrated in the rat a dissociation between target tissue and central neuroendocrine GH-IGF-1 responses using a very different environmental condition *(98)*. Rats exposed to hypoxia were found to have a reduction in body growth rate and circulating IGF-1. However, surprisingly, the relative size of the heart and lung was increased along with IGF-1 gene expression. An important anabolic anatomic/structural adjustment to reduced oxygen-carrying capacity had occurred locally, but the central response was catabolic, and overall growth was reduced.

In summary, we speculate that there are at least two phases in the GH-IGF-1 response to a training program: the first is an acute catabolic-type response. During this initial phase, local muscle IGF-1 might actually increase *(89,95)* as circulating IGF-1 falls, reflecting an important mechanistic role for autocrine/paracrine effects of IGF-1 in the response to training. At some later point (presumably after 5 wk), and dependent on the nutritional and energy balance of the individual, a chronic anabolic adjustment of the GH-IGF-1 axis occurs. Understanding that the neuroendocrine response to exercise training is bi- or perhaps multiphasic is important. First, from a methodological perspective, what is observed after 5 wk of training, roughly the duration of training used in many studies focused on the metabolic effects of exercise (e.g., *99*), might not reflect the ultimate, steady-state responses of the GH-IGF-1 axis or other neuroendocrine systems.

Second, our data also are relevant to current attempts to define a possible therapeutic role for GH and other growth factors in a variety of clinical situations. Indeed, if some "downregulation" of these circulating factors is a necessary component of the complete adaptation to increased physical activity, then the timing of exogenous administration is critical. Moreover, the optimization of using exercise with (or without) exogenous growth factors must ultimately rest on greater understanding of the interaction between local tissue growth responses to exercise and the seemingly paradoxical catabolic-type, neuroendocrine responses observed in the present study.

REFERENCES

1. Leblanc AD, Schneider VS, Evans HJ, Engelbretson DA, Krebs JM. Bone mineral loss and recovery after 17 weeks of bed rest. J Bone Miner Res 1990;5:843–850.
2. Theintz GE, Howald H, Weiss U, Sizonenko PC. Evidence for a reduction of growth potential in adolescent female gymnasts. J Pediatr 1993;122:306–313.
3. Leung DW, Spencer SA, Cachianes G, Hammonds RG, Collins C, Henzel WJ, et al. Growth hormone receptor and serum binding protein: purification, cloning, and expression. Nature 1987;330:537–540.
4. Berelowitz M, Szabo M, Frohman LA, Firestone S, Chu L, Hintz RL. Somatomedin-C mediates growth hormone negative feedback by effects on both the hypothalamus and the pituitary. Science 1981;212:1281–1297.
5. Rajaram S, Baylink DJ, Mohan S. Insulin-like growth factor binding proteins in serum and other biological fluids: regulation and functions. Endocr Rev 1997;18:801–831.
6. Clark RG, Jansson J-O, Isaksson O, Robinson IC. Intravenous growth hormone: growth responses to patterned infusions in hypophysectomized rats. J Endocrinol 1985;104:53–61.
7. Mauras N, Blizzard RM, Link K, Johnson ML, Rogol AD, Veldhuis JD. Augmentation of growth hormone secretion during puberty: evidence for a pulse amplitude-modulated phenomenon. J Clin Endocrinol Metb 1987;64:596–601.

8. Silbergeld A, Litwin A, Bruchis S, Versano I, Laron Z. Insulin-like growth factor-I in healthy children adolescents and adults as determined by radioimmunoassay specific for the synthetic 53-70 peptide region. Clin Endocrinol 1986;25:67–74.
9. Corpas E, Harman SM, Blackman MR. Human growth hormone and human aging. Endocr Rev 1993;14:20–39.
10. Marimme TJ, Zapf J, Froesch ER. Insulin-like growth factors in the fed and fasted states. J Clin Endocrinol Metab 1982;55:999–1002.
11. Roth J, Glick SM, Yalow RS. Hypoglycemia: A potent stimulus to the secretion of growth hormone. Science 1963;140:987,988.
12. Buckler JMH. Exercise as a screening test for growth hormone release. Acta Endocrinol 1972;69:219–229.
13. Cooper DM, Barstow TJ, Bergner A, Lee W-NP. Blood glucose turnover during high- and low-intensity exercise. Am J Physiol 1989;257:405–412.
14. Coggan AR, Kohrt WM, Spina RJ, Kirwan JP, Bier DM, Holloszy JO. Plasma glucose kinetics during exercise in subjects with high and low lactate thresholds. J Appl Physiol 1992;73:1873–1880.
15. Felsing NE, Brasel J, Cooper DM. Effect of low- and high-intensity exercise on circulating growth hormone in men. J Clin Endocrinol Metab 1992;75:157–162.
16. Sutton JR, Lazarus L. Growth hormone and exercise comparison of physiological and pharmacological stimuli. J Appl Physiol 1976;41:523–527.
17. Hartley LH, Mason JW, Hogan RP, et al. Multiple hormonal responses to graded exercise in relation to physical training. J Appl Physiol 1972;33:602–606.
18. Bar-Or O. Growth hormone deficiency-using exercise in the diagnosis. In: Bar-Or O, ed. Pediatric Sports Medicine for the Practitioner. Springer-Verlag, New York, 1983, pp. 182–191.
19. Winter JSD. The metabolic response to exercise and exhaustion in normal and growth hormone deficient children. Can J Physiol Pharmacol 1974;52:575–582.
20. Eliakim A, Brasel JA, Cooper DM. GH response to exercise: assessment of the pituitary refractory period, and relationship with circulating components of the GH–IGF-1 axis in adolescent females. J Pediatr Endocrinol Metab 1999;12:47–55.
21. Schwarz AJ, Brasel JA, Hintz RL, Mohan S, Cooper DM. Acute effect of brief low- and high-intensity exercise on circulating IGF-1, II, and IGF binding protein-3 and its proteolysis in young healthy men. J Clin Endocrinol Metab 1996;81:3492–3497.
22. Cappon J, Brasel JA, Mohan S, Cooper DM. Effect of brief exercise on circulating insulin-like growth factor-I. J Appl Physiol 1994;76:1418–1422.
23. Hicks AL, MacDougall JD, Muckle TJ. Acute changes in high-density lipoprotein cholesterol with exercise of different intensities. J Appl Physiol 1987;63:1956–1960.
24. Casanueva FF, Villanueva L, Cabezas J, Fernandez-Cruz A. Cholinergic mediation of growth hormone secretion elicited by arginine clonidine and physical exercise in man. J Clin Endocrinol Metab 1984;59:526–532.
25. Casanueva FF, Villanueva L, Dieguez C, Diaz Y, Cabranes JA, Szoke B, et al. Free fatty acids block growth hormone (GH) releasing hormone-stimulated GH secretion in man directly at the pituitary. J Clin Endocrinol Metab 1987;65:634–642.
26. Kelijman M, Frohman LA. Beta-adrenergic modulation of growth hormone (GH) autofeedback on sleep-associated and pharmacologically induced GH secretion. J Clin Endocrinol Metab 1989;69:1187–1194.
27. Pontiroli AE, Lanzi R, Monti LD, Sandoli E, Pozza G. Growth hormone (GH) autofeedback on GH response to GH-releasing hormone. Role of free fatty acids and somatostatin. J Clin Endocrinol Metab 1991;72:492–495.
28. Cappon JP, Ipp E, Brasel JA, Cooper DM. Acute effects of high-fat and high-glucose meals on the growth hormone response to exercise. J Clin Endocrinol Metab 1993;76:1418–1422.
29. Penman E, Wass JAH, Medbak S, Morgan L, Lewis JM, Besser GM, et al. Response of circulating immunoreactive somatostatin to nutritional stimuli in normal subjects. Gastroenterology 1981;81: 692–699.
30. Okada Y, Hikita T, Ishitobi K, et al. Human growth hormone secretion during exposure to hot air in normal adult male subjects. J Clin Endocrinol Metab 1972;34:759–763.
31. Buckler JM. The relationship between changes in plasma growth hormone levels and body temperature occurring with exercise in man. Biomedicine 1973;19:193–197.
32. Wilkinson PW, Parkin JM. Growth hormone response to exercise in obese children. Lancet 1974;2:55.
33. Frasier SD. A review of growth hormone stimulation tests in children. Pediatrics 1974;53:929–937.

34. Cowell CT. Short stature. In: Brook CGD, ed. Clinical Paediatric Endocrinology. Blackwell Science, Oxford, 1995, pp. 136–172.
35. Rosenfeld RG, Albertsson-Wikland K, Cassorla F, Frasier SD, Hasegawa Y, Hintz RL. Diagnostic controversy: The diagnosis of childhood growth hormone deficiency revisited. J Clin Endocrinol Metab 1995;80:1532–1540.
36. Wilson DP, Horowitz JL. Exercise-induced changes in growth hormone and somatomedine-C. Am J Med Sci 1987;293:216–217.
37. Hagberg JM, Seals DR, Yerg JE, et al. Metabolic responses to exercise in young and older athletes and sedentary men. J Appl Physiol 1988;65:900–908.
38. Kraemer WJ, Marchitelli L, Gordon SE, et al. Hormonal and growth factor responses to heavy resistance exercise protocols. J Appl Physiol 1990;69:1442–1450.
39. Bang P, Brandt J, Degerblad M, Enberg G, Kaijser L, Thoren M, et al. Exercise-induced changes in insulin-like growth factors and their low molecular weight binding protein in healthy subjects and patients with growth hormone deficiency. Eur J Clin Invest 1990;20:285–292.
40. Marcus RG, Butterfield G, Holloway L, et al. Effects of short term administration of recombinant human growth hormone to elderly people. J Clin Endocrinol Metab 1990;70:519–527.
41. Flamm SD, Taki J, Moore R, Lewis SF, Keech F, Maltais F, et al. Redistribution of regional and organ blood volume and effect on cardiac function in relation to upright exercise intensity in healthy human subjects. Circulation 1990;81:1550–1559.
42. Convertino VA, Keil LC, Bernauer EM, Greenleaf JE. Plasma volume, osmolality, vasopressin, and renin activity during graded exercise in man. J Appl Physiol 1981;50:123–128.
43. Moses AC, Nissley SP, Short PA, Rechler MM, White RM, Knight AB, et al. Increased levels of multiplication stimulating activity, an insulin like growth factor, in fetal rat serum. Proc Natl Acad Sci USA 1980;77:3649.
44. Argente J, Barrios V, Pozo J, Munoz MT, Hervas F, Stene M, et al. Normative data for insulin-like growth factors (IGFs), IGF- binding proteins, and growth hormone-binding protein in a healthy Spanish pediatric population: age- and sex-related changes. J Clin Endocrinol Metab 1993;77:1522–1528.
45. Mohan S, Baylink DJ. The role of insulin-like growth factor-II in the coupling of bone formation to resorption. In: Spencer EM, ed. Modern Concepts of Insulin-like Growth Factors. New York, Elsevier, 1991, pp. 169–184.
46. Baxter RC. Physiological roles of IGF binding proteins. In: Spencer EM, ed. Modern Concepts of Insulin-Like Growth Factors. Elsevier Science Publishing, New York, 1991, pp. 371–380.
47. Suikkari AM, Sane T, Seppala M, Yki Jarvinen H, Karonen SL, Koivisto VA. Prolonged exercise increases serum insulin-like growth factor-binding protein concentrations. J Clin Endocrinol Metab 1989;68:141–144.
48. Hopkins NJ, Jakeman PM, Cwyfan Hughes SC, Holly JMP. Changes in circulating insulin-like growth factor-binding protein-I (IGFBP-1) during prolonged exercise: effect of carbohydrate feeding. J Clin Endocrinol Metab 1994;79:1887–1890.
49. Lamson G, Giudice LC, Cohen P, Liu F, Gargosky S, Muller HL, et al. Proteolysis of IGFBP-3 may be a common regulatory mechanism of IGF action in vivo. Growth Regul 1993;3:91–95.
50. Vora NM, Kukreja SC, York PAJ, Bowser N, Hargis GK, Williams GA. Effect of exercise on serum calcium and parathyroid hormone. J Clin Endocrinol Metab 1983;57:1067–1069.
51. Belcastro AN. Skeletal muscle-activated neutral protease (calpain) with exercise. J Appl Physiol 1993;74:1381–1386.
52. Davenport ML, Isley WL, Pucilowska JB, Pemberton LB, Lyman B, Underwood LE, et al. Insulin-like growth factor-binding protein-3 proteolysis is induced after elective surgery. J Clin Endocrinol Metab 1992;75:590–595.
53. Lalou C, Binoux M. Evidence that limited proteolysis of insulin-like growth factor binding protein-3 (IGFBP-3) occurs in the normal state outside of the bloodstream. Regul Pept 1993;48:179–188.
54. Barstow TJ, Buchthal C, Zanconato S, Cooper DM. Changes in potential controllers of human skeletal muscle respiration during incremental calf exercise. J Appl Physiol 1994;77:2169–2176.
55. Martin JL, Baxter RC. Insulin-like growth factor binding protein from human plasma J Biol Chem 1986;261:8754–8760.
56. Poehlman ET, Copeland KC. Influence of physical activity on insulin-like growth factor-I in healthy younger and older men. J Clin Endocrinol Metab 1990;71:1468–1473.
57. Kelley PJ, Eisman JA, Stuart MC, Pocock NA, Sambrook PN, Gwinn TH. Somatomedin-c, physical fitness, and bone density. J Clin Endocrinol Metab 1990;70:718–723.

58. Weltman A, Weltman JY, Hartman ML, Abbot RD, Rogol AD, Evan WS, et al. Relationship between age, percentage body fat, fitness, and 24-hour growth hormone release in healthy young adults: effects of gender. J Clin Endocrinol Metab 1994;78:543–548.
59. Eliakim A, Brasel JA, Mohan S, Barstow TJ, Berman N, Cooper DM. Physical fitness, endurance training, and the GH-IGF-1 system in adolescent females. J Clin Endocrinol Metab 1996;81:3986–3992.
60. Eliakim A, Brasel JA, Barstow TJ, Mohan, S, Cooper DM. Fitness and the growth hormone-insulin-like growth factor-I axis in adolescent males. Med Sci Sports Exerc 1998;30:512–517.
61. Yamashita S, Melmed S. Effects of insulin on rat anterior pituitary cells: inhibition of growth hormone secretion and mRNA levels. Diabetes 1986;35:440–447.
62. Bouchard C, Despres JP. Variation in fat distribution with age and health implications. In: Spirduso WW, Eckert HM, eds. Physical Activity and Aging. Human Kinetics Champain, IL, 1989; pp. 78–106.
63. Ho KY, Evans WS, Blizzard RM. Effects of sex and age on the 24H profile of growth hormone secretion in man: Importance of endogenous estradiol concentration. J Clin Endocrinol Metab 1987;64:51–58.
64. Borer KT, Nicoski DR, Owens V. Alteration of pulsatile growth hormone secretion by growth-inducing exercise: involvement of endogenous opiates and somatostatin. Endocrinology 1986;118:844–850.
65. Rosenfeld RG. Circulating growth hormone binding proteins. Horm Res 1994;42:129–132.
66. Leger J, Noel M, Czernichow P, Postel-Vinay MC. Progressive normalization of growth hormone binding protein and IGF-1 levels in treated growth hormone deficient children. Pediatr Res 1995;37:731–735.
67. Kratzsch J, Blum WF, Ventz M, Selisko T, Birkenmeyer G, Keller E. Growth hormone binding protein related immunoreactivity in the serum of patients with acromegaly is regulated inversely by growth hormone concentration. Eur J Endocrinol 1995;132:306–312.
68. Jorgensen JO, Pedersen SB, Borglum J, Frystyk J, Ho KK, Christiansen JS, Orskov H, Blum WF, Richelsen B. Serum concentration of insulin-like growth factors, IGF binding proteins 1 and 3, and growth hormone binding proteins in obese women and the effect of growth hormone administration: a double blind, placebo-controlled study. Eur J Endocrinol 1995;133:65–70.
69. Baumann G, Shaw MA, Amburn K. Regulation of plasma growth hormone binding proteins in health and disease. Metabolism 1989;38:683–689.
70. Mohnike K, Kluba U, Blum WF, Aumann V, Vorwerk P, Mittler U. Serum concentrations of insulin-like growth factors (IGF)-I and IGF-II and IGF binding proteins (IGFBP)-2 and GFBP-3 in 49 children with ALL, NHL or solid tumors. Klin Padiat 1995;207:225–229.
71. Tonshoff B, Blum WF, Wingen AM, Mehls O. Serum insulin-like growth factors (IGFs) and IGF binding proteins 1, 2, and 3 in children with chronic renal failure: relationship to height and glomerular filtration rate. The European Study Group for Nutritional Treatment of Chronic Renal Failure in Childhood. J Clin Endocrinol Metab 1995;80:2684–2691.
72. Smith WJ, Underwood LE, Clemmons DR. Effects of caloric or protein restriction on insulin-like growth factor-I (IGF-1) and IGF-binding proteins in children and adults. J Clin Endocrinol Metab 1995;80:443–449.
73. Mohan S, Bautista CM, Wergedal J, Baylink DJ. Isolation of an inhibitory insulin-like growth factor (IGF) binding protein from bone cell-conditioned medium: a potential local regulator of IGF action. Proc Natl Acad Sci USA 1989;86:8338–8342.
74. McDermott MT, Ridgway EC. Thyroid hormone resistance syndromes. Am J Med 1993;94:424–432.
75. Ip T-P, Hoffman DM, O'Sullivan AJ, Leung K-C, Ho KKY. Do androgen regulate growth hormone binding protein in adult men? J Clin Endocrinol Metab 1995;80:1278–1282.
76. Jospe N, Orlowski CC, Furlanetto RW. Comparison of transdermal and oral estrogen therapy in girls with Turner syndrome. J Pediatr Endocrinol Metab 1995;8:111–116.
77. Rajkovic IA, Valiontis E, Ho KK. Direct quantitation of growth hormone binding protein in human serum by ligand-immunofunctional assay: comparison with immunoprecipitation and chromatographic methods. J Clin Endocrinol Metab 1994;78:772–777.
78. Donnelly MJ, Holly JM. The role of IGFBP-3 in the regulation of IGFBP-4 proteolysis. J Endocrinol 1996;149:R1–R7.
79. Noll K, Wegmann BR, Havemann K, Jaques G. Insulin like growth factors stimulate the release of insulin like binding protein-3 and degradation of IGFBP-4 in non-small cell lung cancer cell lines. J Clin Endocrinol Metab 1996;81:2653–2662.

80. Eliakim A, Barstow TJ, Brasel JA, Ajie H, Lee WN, Renslo R, et al. The effect of exercise training on energy expenditure, muscle volume and maximal oxygen uptake in adolescent females. J Pediatr 1996;129:347–353.
81. Eliakim A, Brasel JA, Mohan S, Wong WLT, Cooper DM. Increased physical activity and the growth hormone-insulin like growth factor-I axis in adolescent males. Am J Physiol, 1998;44:12,308–12,314.
82. Lowe WL Jr. Biological actions of the insulin-like growth factors. In: LeRoith D, ed. Insulin-Like Growth Factors: Molecular and Cellular Aspects. CRC, Boca Raton, 1991, pp. 49–86.
83. Postel-Vinay MC, Saab C, Gourmelen M. Nutritional status and growth hormone binding protein. Horm Res 1995;44:177–181.
84. Mohan S, Nakao Y, Honda Y, Landale E, Leser U, Dony C, et al. Studies on the mechanisms by which insulin-like growth factor (IGF) binding protein-4 (IGFBP-4) and IGFBP-5 modulate IGF actions in bone cells. J Biol Chem 1995;270:20,424–20,431.
85. Weltman A, Weltman JY, Schurrer R, Evans WS, Veldhuis JD, Rogol AD. Endurance training amplifies the pulsatile release of growth hormone: effects of training intensity. J Appl Physiol 1992;72:2188–2196.
86. Borer KT. Exercise-induced facilitation of pulsatile growth hormone secretion and somatic growth. In: Laron Z, Rogol AD, eds. Hormones and Sports. Raven, New York, 1989, pp. 21–35.
87. Coplan NL, Gleim GW, Nicholas JA. Exercise related changes in serum catecholamines and potassium: effect of sustained exercise above and below lactate threshold. Am Heart J 1989;117:1070–1075.
88. Goldfarb AH, Hatfield BD, Armstrong D, Potts J. Plasma beta-endorphin concentration: response to intensity and duration of exercise. Med Sci Sports Exerc 1990;22:241–244.
89. Zanconato S, Moromisato DY, Moromisato MY, Woods J, Brasel JA, LeRoith D, et al. Effect of training and growth hormone suppression on insulin-like growth factor-I mRNA in young rats. J Appl Physiol 1994;76:2204–2209.
90. Yan Z, Biggs RB, Booth FW. Insulin-like growth factor immunoreactivity increases in muscle after acute eccentric contractions. J Appl Physiol 1993;74:410–414.
91. Eliakim A, Moromisato MY, Moromisato DY, Brasel JA, Roberts C Jr, Cooper DM. Increase in muscle IGF-1 protein but not IGF-1 mRNA after 5 days of endurance training in young rats. Am J Physiol 1997;273:R1557–R1561.
92. Phillip M, Werner H, Palese T, Kowarski AA, Stannard B, Bach LA, et al. Differential accumulation of insulin-like growth factor-I in kidneys of pre- and postpubertal streptozotocin-diabetic rats. J Mol Endocrin 1994;12:215–224.
93. Booth FW, Kirby CR. Changes in skeletal muscle gene expression consequent to altered weight bearing. Am J Physiol 1992;262:R329–R332.
94. Town GP, Essig DA. Cytochrome oxidase in muscle of endurance-trained rats: subunit mRNA contents and heme synthesis. J Appl Physiol 1993;74:192–196.
95. DeVol DL, Rotwein P, Sadow JL, Novakofski J, Bechtel PJ. Activation of insulin-like growth factor gene expression during work-induced skeletal muscle growth. Am J Physiol 1990;259:E89–E95.
96. Yeh JK, Aloia JF, Chen M, Ling N, Koo HC, Millard WJ. Effect of growth hormone administration and treadmill exercise on serum and skeletal IGF-1 in rats. Am J Physiol 1994;266:E129–E135.
97. Spurr GB, Reina JC. Marginal malnutrition in school-aged Colombian girls: dietary intervention and daily energy expenditure. Hum Nutr Clin Nutr 1987;41:93–104.
98. Moromisato DY, Moromisato MY, Zanconato S, Roberts CT Jr, Cooper DM. Effect of hypoxia on lung, heart, and liver insulin-like growth factor-I gene and receptor expression in the newborn rat. Crit Care Med 1996;24:919–924.
99. Perseghin G, Price TB, Petersen KE, Roden M, Cline CW, Gerow K, et al. Increased glucose transport phosphorylation and muscle glycogen synthesis after exercise training in insulin resistant subjects. N Engl J Med 1996;335:1357–1362.

6 Thyroid Function and Exercise*

Victor J. Bernet, MD and Leonard Wartofsky, MD

CONTENTS

INTRODUCTION
THYROID PHYSIOLOGY
THYROID HORMONE AND PULMONARY FUNCTION
EXERCISE AND THYROID AXIS RESPONSE
REFERENCES

INTRODUCTION

Thyroid hormone receptors are present in virtually every tissue in the body, thereby permitting an important physiologic role for the two thyroid hormones, thyroxine (T4) and triiodothyronine (T3). Skeletal and cardiac muscle function, pulmonary performance, metabolism, and the neurophysiologic axis are only a few of the important areas that are affected by thyroid hormone levels (1). Any abnormality in thyroid function causing either an excess or deficiency in circulating thyroid hormone levels can lead to changes in body function at rest and during exercise. The presence of thyroid disease can have a major impact on exercise tolerance resulting in reduced performance of strenuous activities. On the other hand, exercise itself may have direct or indirect effects on thyroid function, either secondary to acute alterations in the integrity of the pituitary–thyroid axis or to the more long-lasting changes noted in well-trained athletes to be discussed below. Alterations in thyroid function in well-trained athletes might be viewed as an adaptive mechanism associated with enhanced performance possibly serving to provide a better balance between energy consumption and expenditure. Underlying energy balance does appear to play an important role in the effects exercise may have on the pituitary and thyroid axis. Reports in the literature indicate that athletes with excessive weight loss may exhibit a "low T3 syndrome" accompanied by amenorrhea (in women) as well as other alterations in pituitary function (2). Fortunately, thyroid diseases usually can be treated effectively, and most individuals with thyroid disorders should expect to

---

*The opinions or assertions contained herein are the private views of the authors and are not to be construed as official or reflecting the views of the Department of the Army or the Department of Defense.

From: *Contemporary Endocrinology: Sports Endocrinology*
Edited by: M. P. Warren and N. W. Constantini © Humana Press Inc., Totowa, NJ

obtain resolution of their thyroid-related symptoms, including those associated with a negative impact on their exercise tolerance. Gail Devers, who has been very public about her experience with Graves' disease, is a well-known sprinter who went on to win Olympic fame following treatment for her Graves' disease and may act as a case in point.

After a brief overview of normal thyroid physiology, this chapter will provide a survey of the literature describing effects of abnormal thyroid hormone levels on exercise tolerance, with a special focus on alterations in cardiac, muscle, and respiratory function. The chapter will conclude with a review of existing data on the response of the pituitary–thyroid axis to varying levels and types of exercise.

THYROID PHYSIOLOGY

All steps in thyroid hormone (TH) biosynthesis are driven by thyrotropin (TSH) and are intimately linked to iodine metabolism. Dietary iodine (I) is reduced to iodide, absorbed by the small intestine, and then enters the circulation. Tissues that extract iodide from plasma include the thyroid, kidneys, salivary glands, choroid plexus, gastric glands, and lactating breast tissue. However, iodide clearance is predominately a function of either the thyroid gland or the kidneys. Iodide "trapped" by the thyroid gland subsequently undergoes oxidation by thyroid peroxidase (TPO), iodinating tyrosyl residues in the storage protein, thyroglobulin, to form the iodothyronines, monoiodotyrosine (MIT) and diiodotyrosine (DIT). MIT and DIT molecules can then couple to form either tetraiodothyronine (thyroxine or T4) and/or triiodothyronine (T3), which are the two major thyroid hormones *(3)*. T4 and T3 are bound within peptide linkage within thyroglobulin and stored within the thyroid follicles. Under control of TSH, thyroglobulin undergoes endocytosis and proteolytic digestion, releasing T4 and T3 into the circulation. The feedback loop is completed at the hypothalamic level where declining levels of circulating T4 or T3 will prompt secretion of thyrotropin-releasing hormone (TRH), which stimulates synthesis and secretion of TSH. After binding to its specific receptor on the thyroid cell membrane, TSH leads to stimulation of T4 and T3 production and secretion mediated by cyclic AMP. Only 20% of circulating T3 is derived from thyroid secretion, whereas 80% is derived from the monodeiodination of T4 by 5′-deiodinase (type I) in the periphery (*see* Fig. 1) *(4)*. Since T3 is some 10–15 times more biologically potent than T4 is, this latter conversion has been termed the "activating" pathway of thyroid hormone metabolism. Alternatively and in certain physiologic and pathologic states, the deiodination of T4 proceeds via a 5-deiodinase (type II), which leads instead to reverse T3 (rT3) or 3,3′,5′- triiodothyronine production. Since rT3 is a biologically inactive thyroid compound *(4)*, this route of metabolism has been termed the "inactivating" pathway. A precise metabolic role for rT3 has not been described, but diversion of T4 metabolism from the activating to the inactivating pathway serves a nitrogen-sparing and protective effect for the body during times of stress and has been viewed as a homeostatic mechanism.

After binding to a cellular receptor, the thyroid hormones have both genomic *(5)* and nongenomic *(6)* effects, the former leading to increased expression of nuclear actions, whereas the latter appears to involve plasma membrane/mitochondrial responses *(7)*. Genomic effects, such as induction of gene expression, require some time for response, such as the effect of T3 on α-myosin heavy-chain regulation in the heart. The T3 nuclear

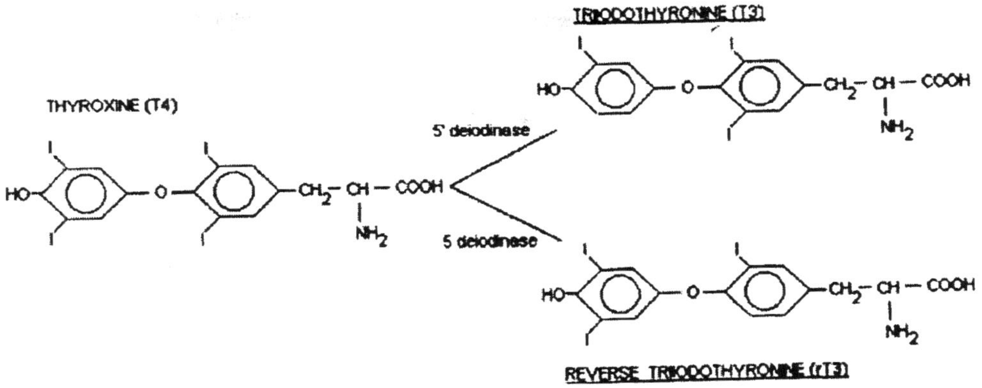

Fig. 1. Thyroxine, triiodothyronine, and reverse triiodothyronine.

receptor is encoded by c-erb A genes, which have several T3 binding protein isoforms *(8)*. Nongenomic effects utilize messenger pathways, such as cyclic AMP, to control cellular respiration, sarcoplasmic reticulum Ca-ATPase activity (SERCA), or actin polymerization and ion homeostasis, and hence have a more rapid response time *(9)*.

Thyroid Hormone Effects

Exercise capacity, the maximal capacity for oxygen consumption (VO_2max), and endurance, the ability to perform prolonged exercise at 75% VO_2max, are the two main components of exercise tolerance *(10)*. Hyper- and hypothyroidism, associated with either excess or deficiency of thyroid hormone (TH), respectively, may have a negative impact on exercise performance. Hypothyroidism is marked by a decrease in skeletal muscle blood flow with a concomitant reduction in O_2 delivery. Free fatty acid (FFA) mobilization is also reduced and with it delivery of fatty acids to the muscles. Blood flow alterations explain part of the muscle dysfunction in hypothyroidism, since muscle contractility has been shown to recover with return of normal blood flow in rat studies *(11)*. However, studies do not reveal a global hypoperfusion of muscle, but instead, a reduction in flow to the fast twitch type II fibers of high-oxidative type muscles *(12)*. Hypothyroidism has not been found to alter the metabolic cost of exercise *(13)*. Hyperthyroid subjects also have an impairment in cellular respiration and reduced exercise endurance *(14)*. In distinction to hypothyroid individuals, muscle blood flow is enhanced in hyperthyroid subjects including fast twitch sections of muscle *(15)*. Excess heat generation from the elevated metabolic activity associated with thyrotoxicosis and secondary hyperthermia may adversely impact heat dissipation during exercise and exercise tolerance. However, despite a baseline temperature increase of 0.5°C in thyrotoxic subjects, exercise-induced temperature rise has been observed not to differ from that in controls *(16)*. Although the thyroid hormones have pervasive effects on virtually all functions of the body, the following discussion emphasizes thyroid-related influences on exercise tolerance as mediated via involvement with cellular metabolism and the function of skeletal muscle and the cardiac, vascular, and pulmonary systems.

Cardiac

Cardiac performance/output is dependent on the contractility of the heart as well as systemic vascular resistance. Resting tachycardia is very common in hyperthyroidism, and many patients complain of having a "racing" or "pounding" heart. The heart, being itself a muscle, is affected by thyroid hormone levels as is skeletal muscle. TH has specific effects on protein synthesis in muscle and on synthesis of the various forms of myosin isoenzymes in many animals [17]. Although β-myosin is the primary muscle fiber, unlike α-myosin, its expression is unaffected by TH levels in the human adult heart [18]. Instead, the enhanced contractility associated with TH may be owing to increases in sarcoplasmic reticulum Ca^{2+} ATPase. LT4 therapy has been reported to improve exercise tolerance even in euthyroid patients, as seen in subjects with idiopathic dilated cardiomyopathy [19]. In these studies, LT4 administration was associated with an increase in cardiac output (CO), reduction in systemic vascular resistance (SVR), and an improved left ventricular ejection fraction (LVEF).

Hypothyroidism has been associated with a decrease in intravascular volume, stroke volume, diastolic hypertension, and cardiac index, and an increase in SVR (see Table 1) [20]. Vascular control mechanisms may be abnormal in hypothyroidism with blunted vasodilatation secondary to reduced endothelium-dependent vasodilatation [21,22]. In patients with transient hypothyroidism owing to thyroidectomy, radionuclide ventriculography and right heart catheterization revealed lower cardiac output, stroke volume, and end-diastolic volume at rest, but increased systemic peripheral resistance [23]. Pulmonary capillary wedge pressure (PCWP), right atrial pressure, heart rate, and LVEF were unchanged. In comparison to the euthyroid state in the same individuals, heart rate, cardiac output, end diastolic volume and stroke volume were lower during exercise with hypothyroidism. These results lead to the hypothesis that hypothyroidism impacts on cardiac function through alterations in load parameters and not through an effect on contractility.

LVEF at rest and with exercise appears to be altered with TH deficiency. The baseline LVEF and peak LVEF were shown to be lower in hypothyroid subjects (average age 52 yr) in comparison with results when the same individuals were euthyroid, although the rise of LVEF in the two states was similar [24]. As assessed by radionuclide gated-pool ventriculography in a younger group (average age 24 yr), there was no noticeable change in LVEF with hypothyroidism, although exercise tolerance did improve after LT4 replacement [25]. Even hypothyroidism of a brief duration of only 10 d was associated with an impaired (i.e., <5% increase) LVEF response to exercise; LVEF response returned to normal with restoration of the euthyroid state [26]. Of interest, the patients still achieved the same workload in either state.

Hypothyroid individuals may have a form of reversible coronary dysfunction as found in a study of six patients undergoing stress testing before and after LT4 replacement therapy. Prior to replacement therapy, SPECT (thallium-201) scanning revealed notable regional perfusion defects in four of six patients, which resolved within 8 wk of LT4 therapy [27]. In another study, LVEF dropped with exercise in hypothyroid individuals and the calcium channel blocker, verapamil, attenuated this drop [28]. Replacement LT4 was associated with normalization of LVEF response, and verapamil did not affect LVEF during euthyroidism. That verapamil attenuated the fall of LVEF with exercise during the hypothyroid phase, and the increase of LVEF was appropriate with euthyroidism, could be consistent with reversible ischemia from TH deficiency.

Table 1
Cardiovascular Changes in Thyroid Disease

	Hyperthyroidism	Hypothyroidism
Heart rate	↑ NC	↓/NC
Vascular volume	↑	↓
Stroke volume	↑	↓
Cardiac output	↑	↓
SVR	↓	↑
LVEF		
Rest	↑↓ NC	↓ NC
Exercise	↓	↓
Diastolic blood pressure	↓	↑
Systolic blood pressure	↑	↓
LV pre-ejection period	↓ Time	↑ Time
LV ejection time	↓ Time	↑ Time

"Subclinical" hypothyroidism is a term that has been applied to patients with mild elevations of serum TSH (usually in the range of 5–15 mU/L), but with normal levels of total and free thyroxine or triiodothyronine. It has been a matter of investigative interest whether the mild hypofunction associated with subclinical hypothyroidism affected any measureable cardiac parameters (29). Patients with TSH levels of 14.8 ± 9.4 mIU/L were studied during rest and exercise, pre- and post-LT4 therapy. Overall cardiac structure and function were not significantly altered, except for LV diastolic dimension, which was slightly larger with the euthyroid state, and shortening of the pre-ejection period at stage III exercise from 51 to 39 s was noted. However, this study was somewhat limited by a small sample size. Resting LVEF may be lower in hypothyroid subjects than in controls (30), although in one study, treatment of individuals with subclinical hypothyroidism revealed a similar resting LVEF in comparison to untreated subjects. A small increase in LVEF was seen with submaximal exercise with LT4 therapy, but no difference was noted with moderate exercise (31). Additionally, the LV pressure–volume relationship at end systole during exercise showed a steeper pressure–volume slope in the euthyroid compared with subclinically hypothyroid subjects.

Conflicting data exist on whether or not asymmetric septal hypertrophy (ASH) is present in many hypothyroid patients. Bernstein assessed intraventricular septum thickness by echocardiography in 13 hypothyroid patients with TSH levels between 47 and 324 mIU/L (32). Contrary to older reports, septal thickness was normal in all the subjects (33).

The effects of hyperthyroidism on cardiac function both during rest and exercise are numerous (see Table 1) (34). In thyrotoxicosis, the extent of the various cardiac responses to excess TH is somewhat dependent on the duration and severity of the disorder. Resting tachycardia, a slow decline in postexercise heart rate, atrial fibrillation, decreased exercise tolerance, and rarely, congestive heart failure (CHF) are seen in thyrotoxic patients. Cardiac complications from hyperthyroidism tend to occur in patients with a history of prior ischemia, hypertension, and valvular heart disease (35). Augmented blood volume and blood flow to the skin, muscles, and kidneys are seen and may be owing to vasodilators released secondary to increased cellular respiration (36). A rise in cellular oxygen consumption leads to a higher demand for O_2 and the need to get fuel to the peripheral tissues *(36)*. An increase in the velocity of cardiac muscle contraction is present, as well as a rise in myosin ATPase activity *(37)*. Evaluation of systolic time intervals in thyrotoxic subjects reveals a shortening of the LV pre-ejection period along with quicker LV ejection time and isovolumic contraction *(38,39)*.

"Subclinical" hyperthyroidism is a term that has been applied to patients with undetectable levels of serum TSH in a highly sensitive assay, but with normal levels of total and free thyroxine or triiodothyronine. In one study, there was no difference in LVEF at rest and exercise between subclinical hyperthyroidism and controls, whereas overt hyperthyroid subjects had a reduction in LVEF with exercise, increased heart rate, and cardiac output at both rest and exercise *(40)*. Another study found an inverse correlation between serum T4 levels and LVEF during thyrotoxicosis *(41)*. LVEF may be greater at rest in hyperthyroidism, but the lack of an increase or even a drop in LVEF with exercise seems to be a reproducible finding *(42)*. β-adrenergic blockade did not alter the drop in LVEF with exercise, yet the LVEF response normalized with a return to the euthyroid state. These results would implicate a direct effect of thyroid hormones on LVEF not mediated by β-adrenergic receptors *(42)*. However, β-blockers can decrease tachycardia at rest and exercise. Studies using β-adrenergic blocking agents in hyperthyroid human subjects reveal a decrease in tachycardia, pulse pressure, and an increased circulation time with β-blocker therapy. However, the enhanced ventricular function appeared to be independent of β-adrenergic status as assessed by such contractility indexes as pre-ejection period (PEP), left ventricular ejection time (LVET), PEP/LVET ratio, and the isovolemic contraction period (ICP). Cyclic AMP levels have been found to be mildly elevated in hyperthyroid individuals and infusion of the β-blocker, propranolol, has reduced the levels back into the normal range, thereby indirectly suggesting an enhanced β-adrenergic receptor *(43)*.

The significance of the role of β-adrenergic receptors in hyperthyroidism is somewhat controversial *(44)*. Initially, it was believed that catecholamines, directly or indirectly through enhanced catecholamine receptor sensitivity, mediated the effect of excess TH levels on the heart *(45)*. Animal studies have revealed that the effect of hyper- and hypothyroidism on α- and β-adrenergic receptor number, and responsiveness appears to vary from tissue to tissue, and may either increase, decrease, or remain unchanged *(46)*. One study supporting the concept that β-receptor stimulation influences cardiac function during hyperthyroidism revealed a faster heart rate and a 36% steeper incline in hormonal response (HR) along with a faster LV fiber circumferential shortening to isoproterenol infusion than during euthyroidism *(47)*. This result would indicate that hyperthyroidism of even a brief duration can sensitize the heart to β-adrenergic stimulation affecting HR and LV shortening without any changes in LV mass or loading conditions. However, several other studies have revealed no apparent enhancement of β-adrenergic stimulation with thyrotoxicosis *(42,48–50)*. A recent study by Hoit et al. of thyrotoxic baboons tends to refute a role of $β_1$- or $β_2$-adrenergic receptors in any cardiac response to hyperthyroidism *(51)*. TH excess was not associated with enhanced LV sensitivity to catecholamines.

The effect of triiodothyronine-induced thyrotoxicosis on exercise tolerance has been studied, with increases noted in resting oxygen uptake, heart rate, and cardiac output *(52)*. Lactic acid levels rose with submaximal exercise to a 25% higher peak in hyperthyroid subjects. Additionally, skeletal muscle oxidative and glycolytic activities were reduced by 21–37%. Even after only 2 wk of elevated T3 levels, type IIA muscle fibers were reduced by 15% in size. Protein breakdown and loss of lean body mass were also seen in these subjects. The fact that exercise ability was also found to be diminished despite an increase in HR and CO indicates that cardiac dysfunction is not the primary etiology of the reduction in exercise capacity. Much data point to the decrease in SVR (50%) seen in h yperthyroidism as the cause for the rise in cardiac output. In this regard, phenylephrine administration was associated with an increase in SVR and a decrease in CO not seen in euthyroid subjects *(53)*. Another study in young hyperthyroid adults revealed normal response on LVEF to exercise in 11 of 15 subjects *(25)*. The four subjects with a subnormal rise in LVEF tended to have higher T4 levels, resting HR, and reduced peak workload. Conceivably, an inability to lower SVR during exercise in the hyperthyroid state might lead to impaired exercise tolerance *(54)*. Of note, hyperthyroid patients with CHF tended to have higher SVR values and/or a disproportionate rise with strenuous activity *(55)*. The reduced SVR causes a cascade of physiologic responses. The low SVR leads to a decrease in renal perfusion followed by a rise in angiotensin causing increased sodium reabsorption and a concomitant rise in total body sodium and then plasma volume *(44)*. An exogenously administered excess of T4 can lead to growth in LV mass that usually reverts with resolution of the hyperthyroidism *(56)*. In additon, β-blockers may be able to prevent the increase in LV mass during thyrotoxicosis *(57)*.

Thyroid hormone has been shown to increase number and size of mitochondria and play an important role in oxidative metabolism *(58,59)*. With cardiac and muscular function being adversely affected by excess TH, one would postulate that work capacity must be reduced in hyperthyroid individuals. A study of maximum power output in hyperthyroid individuals with measurements of work capacity both while thyrotoxic and then euthyroid on propylthiouracil (PTU) therapy revealed a 19% increase from a low maximum power output during the thyrotoxic phase at 1.65 ± 0.15 W/kg^{-1} to 1.84 ± 0.15 W/kg^{-1} in a euthyroid state 3 mo later. A subset of patients were retested 12 mo later, and maximum power output in comparison to controls was in the low-normal range at 2.75 ± 0.15 W/kg^{-1}, representing a +13% rise from the 3-mo test *(60)*. Oxygen uptake at maximal effort was low during thyrotoxicosis and did not increase at 3 and 12 mo. Net mechanical efficiency was also low at baseline and at 3 mo, but returned back up to normal at 25.2% by 12 mo. Of interest, blood lactate levels during maximal effort only rose to 50% of the normal response at all three time-points.

Muscle

Muscle weakness is a common complaint in patients with either thyroid excess or deficiency, and a variety of investigations have addressed muscle changes secondary to thyroid disease. Hypothyroidism may underlie up to 5% of acquired myopathies *(61)*. At least mild elevations in creatine kinase levels are seen in about 90% of hypothyroid patients *(62)*. Exertional rhabdomyolysis has been reported with hypothyroidism (four cases) and may be secondary to an acquired, reversible defect in muscle glycogenolysis *(63)*. One case of exercise-induced rhabdomyolysis was associated with significant hypothyroidism (TSH > 100) after the patient had walked just a 4-km distance. Type II fiber atrophy has been reported in muscle biopsies in hypothyroid subjects, and a subsequent muscle biopsy of the latter patient's quadriceps revealed marked type II group atrophy *(64,65)*. In hypothyroid subjects, the alterations in lipid, protein, and carbohydrate metabolism in muscle may have pronounced effects on muscle function. Thus, exercise may exacerbate this situation and be associated with rhabdomyolysis. In

Hoffmann's syndrome, another muscle disorder related to hypothyroidism, abnormalities include increased muscle mass, muscle stiffness and weakness, creatine kinase of as much as >10 times normal levels, and repetitive positive waves on electromyograph (EMG) *(66)*. Resolution of symptoms is expected with thyroid hormone replacement. Electromyographic testing in hypothyroidism may reveal normal patterns or possibly myopathic characteristics *(67)*. EMG patterns that can be seen with hypothyroidism include: fibrillations, increased polyphasic waves, unusual high-frequency discharges, and reduced motor unit recruitment *(66)*. Reduced duration of action potentials and increased polyphasic potentials can be seen with thyrotoxicosis *(68)*.

An abnormal increase in lactate during exercise has been described in "subclinical" hypothyroidism. In one study, baseline lactate and pyruvate levels were similar between euthyroid and normal subjects *(69)*. However, during exercise, lactate was significantly higher in subclinical hypothyroidism in comparison to controls, whereas pyruvate response was similar between the groups. It was also noted that the increments in lactate were positively correlated with the duration of subclinical hypothyroidism, but not with the levels of TSH, FT4, or FT3. It was hypothesized that mitochondrial oxidative dysfunction was present and that this dysfunction worsens with length of disease; glycolysis may exceed pyruvate oxidation explaining the lactate buildup. T3 receptors on the mitochondrial membranes of skeletal muscle point to a possible direct effect of thyroid hormones on oxidative metabolism.

Muscle function is based on the interaction of myosin and actin filaments powered by ATP hydrolysis, which is regulated by Ca^{2+} from the sarcoplasmic reticulum *(17)*. Hyperthyroidism seems to cause an increase, and hypothyroidism a decrease in Ca^{2+} uptake and ATP hydrolysis by SERCA (*see* Table 2) *(70)*. Phosphorous nuclear magnetic resonance spectroscopy has been utilized to measure muscle phosphate metabolites, such as phosphocreatine (PCr), ATP, inorganic phosphate (Pi), phosphodiesterase (PDE), and intracellular pH (pHi). The PCr/Pi ratio and PCr recovery rate following exercise are reliable indicators for assessment of oxidative phosphorylation *(71)*. In addition, intracellular changes in pH are related to lactate production *(72)*. Kaminisky assessed these parameters in hypothyroid women subdivided into either moderate hypothyroidism (normal FT4 with elevated TSH), subacute thyroid deficiency (s/p I-131 or thyroidectomy with low FT4 and high TSH > 50), and severe/chronic hypothyroidism (of which one had overt myopathy). In comparison to controls, the hypothyroid group had a significant increase in the Pi/ATP ratio at rest and a decrease in the PCr/Pi ratio during exercise, although the latter ratio change is not specific and can be seen in other disease states. Chronic hypothyroidism was associated with an increased PDE/ATP ratio.

The pHi decreased during exercise to a lower nadir in the hypothyroid patients, and more so in the subacute or moderately hypothyroid groups. Finally, PCr recovery rate was much slower in hypothyroid than control subjects *(73)*. This study demonstrated a dysfunction of muscle bioenergetics with even mild TH deficiencies. The increased PCR/Pi ratio at rest and PCr recovery rate following exercise indicate an impairment of oxidative phosphorylation. Several postulates exist for the aforementioned metabolic muscle changes: 1) transition of white type II to red type I fibers, which could change PCR/Pi ratio and/or an increased PDE/ATP ratio in severe hypothyroidism consistent with fiber change and 2) PCr resynthesis and PCr/Pi have been shown to be lower in conditions with mitochondrial myopathies *(74)*. It was postulated that PCr decline was most likely owing to altered ATP synthesis, either by impaired oxidative phosphorylation or slower

Table 2
Muscle Changes in Thyroid Disease

	Hyperthyroidism	Hypothyroidism
Muscle strength	↓	↓
Creatinine kinase	↓	↑
Type II fibers	↑	↓
Lactate: exercise response	↑	↑
Sarcoplasmic reticulum Ca^{2+} uptake	↑	↓
PCr/Pi ratio—exercise	↑	↓
PCr recovery rate	↑	↓

rate of oxidative substrate availability. Argov also reported results using ^{31}P-nuclear magnetic resonance (NMR) to see the response of PCr/Pi in two hypothyroid patients. PCr/Pi was lower at rest in these subjects (4.8 and 5.5) in comparison to controls (8.5). There was a depletion of PCr during exercise and a delayed recovery of PCr/Pi that was also noted in parallel studies on thyroidectomized rats. L-Thyroxine reversed the abnormalities in both groups (rats and humans) after about 1 mo of therapy. Also, the slope of work rate improved from 14 J/min to 48 J/min. Studies in five hyperthyroid patients demonstrated no difference from controls, except for a very rapid recovery time for PCr/Pi (4.2–5.8 U/min). The exercise and recovery response in the hypothyroid group point to an in vivo mitochondrial impairment in hypothyroid muscle (75). Animal studies of hypothyroidism reveal that glycogen levels in muscle appear to be normal to increased at rest, whereas during exercise, muscle utilization of glycogen rises as may lactate production (76,77).

Hyperthyroidism is associated with an increase in fast and a decrease in slow twitch muscle fibers (14). Thyrotoxicosis appears to induce an oxidative muscular injury secondary to an increase in mitochondrial metabolism and a decrease in glutathione peroxidase, which may be protective against such injury (78). Glycogen is lower at baseline in thyrotoxicosis and is utilized at a faster rate with an associated increase of serum lactate (79). The increase in glycogen use may be secondary to augmented β-adrenergic receptors in the muscle facilitating glycogen degradation by elevating glycolytic enzymes as well as modulators of such enzymes (10).

Thyrotoxic periodic paralysis (TPP) is an unusual complication of hyperthyroidism more typically seen in thyrotoxic Asian subjects, although not exclusively so. Patients with TPP suffer from attacks of para- or quadriplegia incited by exercise, high carbohydrate meals, or high salt intake. We have seen patients present with flaccid, paralytic attacks several hours following their military physical fitness test as the presenting manifestation of hyperthyroidism. The muscular function of these patients may appear grossly normal before and between episodes, although some patients have a prodrome of muscle stiffness and aching. Other patients may have a chronic myopathy and tremor from the hyperthyroidism. The proximal muscles of the lower extremities are usually first involved, and episodes usually resolve over a time period of several hours to a day. The pathophysiology revolves around an imbalance in Na/K pump. Nerve conduction and EMG studies reveal that the muscle has reduced excitability during TPP episodes, and low-amplitude muscle action potentials are seen following a paralytic episode (80).

Decreased compound motor action potential amplitudes are found postexercise in TPP *(81)* and improve following treatment *(82)*. Of note, muscle fiber conduction velocity measured in two patients with TPP was within normal limits (4.0 and 3.6 m/s, respectively) before and during paralysis episodes, although muscle strength was reduced by 40% during an attack *(83)*. The attacks usually resolve once the patient's TH levels are lowered into the euthyroid range.

THYROID HORMONE AND PULMONARY FUNCTION

Performance of any strenuous activity especially of endurance training requires the ability of the respiratory system to augment oxygen utilization, and this ability can be affected by altered thyroid structure or function. Large goiters, especially firm, nodular substernal goiters can cause an extrathoracic tracheal obstruction, which can limit air flow to the lungs. Altered TH levels can lead to impairment in optimal pulmonary function. Myxedema or profound hypothyroidism is associated with alveolar hypoventilation related to a reversible reduction in hypoxic ventilatory drive *(84)*. Reductions in lung volumes are seen and include: vital capacity, total lung capacity, functional residual capacity, and expiratory reserve volume, as well as a decrease in diffusing capacity for carbon monoxide (DLCO) *(85)*. Thyroxine replacement therapy is associated with resolution of the aforementioned changes, but a concomitant reduction in patient weight may also be an important factor in pulmonary function improvement *(86)*. Frank respiratory failure is unusual.

In hyperthyroidism, oxygen demand is increased, and the respiratory systems adjust to the increase in demand by increasing respiratory rate and minute ventilation *(87)*. Alveolar ventilation remains normal, but a rise in dead space ventilation is seen. Pulmonary function is dependent on not just intrinsic lung function, but also the accessory muscles for respiration. Pulmonary compliance and airway resistance tend to remain unchanged, whereas vital capacity and expiratory reserve volume are reduced, implicating respiratory muscle weakness *(88)*. Other supporting evidence for respiratory muscle dysfunction in thyrotoxic patients is the reduction of maximal static inspiratory and expiratory efforts, which are seen to resolve on restoration of euthyroidism *(89)*. It appears that ventilation is increased beyond the oxygen uptake and is related to dead space ventilation *(90)*. These changes also appear to resolve with appropriate therapeutic intervention *(90)*. Studies have shown changes in TH levels modify diaphragmatic function as well as muscle fiber type. Hyperthyroid patients tend to have increased fast-twitch fibers and improved diaphragm energy transduction, whereas hypothyroidism is associated with poor energy transduction and slow-twitch fibers. DLCO may be reduced during periods of strenuous exercise during thyrotoxicosis *(91)*. Another finding has been that TH excess does not appear to alter the airway hyperesponsiveness seen in asthma, although exercise-induced asthma was not specifically studied *(92)*.

EXERCISE AND THYROID AXIS RESPONSE

When evaluating TH responses to exercise, one must look for potential changes in thyroid hormone levels and in the response of the pituitary–thyroid axis to both acute and chronic exercise patterns. Other variables to consider would include: baseline individual physical status, duration and intensity of training, type, duration, and intensity of exercise being evaluated, as well as the parameters that were measured during testing. In at least one study, TSH was noted to rise from 3.1 to 4.0, µU/mL just in anticipation of strenuous exercise, although the response dissipated with repetitive testing, which might implicate a psychologic influence on the TSH rise *(93)*. In one study, healthy men undergoing bicycle ergometry for 20 min were noted to have a drop in T4 and T3 levels at 20 and 40 min postexercise, respectively *(94)*. TRH stimulation yielded a normal TSH response. A free T4 increase of 25% has been seen postexercise *(95)*, although an associated rise in FFAs was seen in that study, and interference by the FFAs in the assay results is possible. TSH also rose by 41%, but could not be correlated with T4/T3 levels. Another ergometry study examining the response to 30 min of submaximal exercise revealed no change in TSH and a 35% rise in free T4 above controls *(96)*. The response of thyroid function to short-duration, graded exercise at 47, 77, and 100% maximal oxygen uptake and prolonged exercise at 76% oxygen uptake has been assessed. TSH was noted to rise progressively with increasing workload to a peak TSH of 107% of baseline serum level. A rise in TSH was also seen with prolonged exercise, but with a peak 33% lower than graded exercise *(97)*. Another study compared the effect of submaximal and maximal exercise effect on TH levels *(98)*. Maximal exercise was associated with a decrease in TSH, FT4, stable rT3, and rise in T3 during activity, whereas submaximal exercise was associated with an increase in TSH, but T3, rT3, and FT4 were unchanged. Another test in subjects swimming either 0.9 or 1.8 km or exercising with bicycle ergometry for 60–90 min demonstrated no significant change in FT4 and a small increase (partially from hemoconcentration) in serum T3 and rT3 *(99)*.

TH changes in ultradistance and long-distance runners have also been investigated *(100)*. Hesse et al. studied the effect of three distances of 75 km, 45 km, and marathon (42.2 km) with the subjects performing the 45-km run being slightly older (36 yr) than the other two groups. T4 levels increased in the 75-km and marathon group, but decreased in the 45-km group postrace. T3 also dropped only in the 45-km group. Reverse T3, measured only in the marathon and 75-km groups, rose in both groups. Other correlations revealed that TSH, T4, and T3 were lower in the older-age runners, whereas faster runners with better conditioning had higher T4 and TSH levels in comparison to slower runners. The authors speculated whether the increase in rT3 might be protective against excess glucose metabolism, especially if intracellular glucose deficiency were present *(100)*. Dessypris et al. investigated TH responses in tri-athletes grouped as either young (mean age 23 yr) or older (mean age 60 yr) subjects *(101)*. Both groups had a rise in TSH, which returned to normal over 18 h postevent *(102)*. Semple et al.'s report on marathon runners revealed no change in TSH, T4, T3, or rT3 levels before and after the marathon *(103)*. However, another study revealed an increase in TSH and free T4 postmarathon, with a decrease in FT3 and rise in T4 to free rT3 conversion, which was still detectable 22 h following race completion *(104)*. The level of training of athletes has been shown to affect the TH response to acute exercise. In one investigation, untrained athletes had a rise in T3, a decrease in rT3, and no change in T4, whereas the well-trained athletes were found to have a rise in rT3, no change in T3, and a decrease in T4 levels. It was hypothesized that the rT3 elevation in well-trained athletes might be adaptive in that there is a more efficient cellular oxidation process *(105)*. Of note, Rone et al. found an increase in T3 production and turnover in well-trained male athletes in comparison to sedentary men *(106)*. Following a treadmill stem test (TMST), TH levels and TRH simulation revealed responses similar in nature among sedentary subjects (VO_2max 38.5 mL/kg · min), regular joggers (VO_2max 45.0 mL/kg · min), and marathon runners (VO_2max 60.3 mL/kg · min) *(107)*.

Variation in ambient temperature appears to alter the body's TH response to exercise. One study looked at proficient swimmers exercising in three water temperatures, 20, 26, and 32°C, for approx 30 min at a moderate speed; TSH and free T4 rose in the colder water, were unchanged at 26°C, and fell at the warmer temperature, but T3 levels were not affected *(108)*. Cold receptors appear to regulate a rise in TRH and TSH level in cold water, and exposure duration may affect the peak TSH with higher levels owing to longer times in the water *(109,110)*.

The chronic effects on thyroid hormone parameters have also been studied in endurance athletes. The results of the studies conflict with regard to whether or not baseline TH levels are shifted in well-trained athletes. Baseline TH levels have been found to be unchanged, increased, or decreased *(107,111)*. Identical twins that were studied during an observed 93-d endurance training period with stable energy intake had an average 5-kg weight loss (primarily fat), and lower baseline FT3, TT3, and TT4 with a nonsignificant drop in FT4 by the end of the 93-d exercise period *(112)*. A shorter study in recreational athletes over 6 wk revealed no change in TSH or TSH response to TRH stimulation with regular bicycle ergometry training (although the exercise endurance improved) *(113)*. Also, a 1-mo aerobic conditioning program in six healthy women revealed no change in either TSH, T4, T3, or rT3, and Rone et al. reported no difference in baseline values for T4, T3, TSH, or T3U between endurance athletes and sedentary controls over time *(114)*. In the latter study, oral liothyronine sodium (50 µg) was administered, and its metabolism assessed. The endurance group exhibited an increase in the following parameters: T3 metabolic clearance rate, T3 total volume of distribution, T3 disposal rate, and total body T3 pool even when normalized for total body weight, lean body mass, and body surface area.

There is evidence that T3 production and utilization correlate strongly with the amount of lean body mass in physically trained males *(106)*. Radioactive iodine uptake may be altered secondary to chronic exercise. T3 metabolism may be altered in endurance athletes as compared with sedentary controls. A lower thyroid uptake of I-123 has been found in regular exercising rats and humans (RAIU 8%) in comparison to sedentary subjects (RAIU 14%) *(111)*.

Energy balance plays a role in the body's TH response to exercise. Energy balance amounts to the difference between daily caloric intake minus the energy used by the body in the form of metabolism, muscle work, and baseline functional needs of various organs. Much data exist on the response of TH to fasting or malnutrition *(115,116)*. T3 tends to decrease, whereas rT3 tends to increase with fasting, which appears to be a regulatory mechanism to regulate catabolism and energy expenditure. The TH levels return to normal with refeeding. Loucks et al. *(117)* found a decrease in TT3 (−15%) and FT3 (−18%) along with an increase in rT3 (+24%) in healthy women undergoing aerobic exercise testing with low caloric intake of 8 kcal · kg body wt^{-1}/d. This "low T3 syndrome" was not seen in individuals receiving a diet of 30 kcal/kg body wt/·d, a level more in balance with energy expenditure. Low-caloric diets high in carbohydrate appear to blunt the drop in T3 in comparison to low-carbohydrate intake *(118)*. Even a mild energy deficiency may have an effect on TH levels. Female gymnasts with borderline energy deficit had a decrease in T3 and increase in T4 during 3 d of heavy workouts *(119)*. Glucose infusion has been found to diminish the increase in rT3 and T4 along

Chapter 6 / Thyroid and Exercise

with decrease in T3 from a 30-min ergometry test *(120)*. Participants in a 90-km crosscountry ski race exhibited an increase in T4 and FT4, which resolved by 1 d postrace. Skiers were exposed to cold temperatures over a period of 5.4–8.1 h. With an approximate 7000-kcal exercise demand noted, an acute negative energy balance was believed to be evident, and a factor in TH changes *(121)*.

A study of military troop exercises in the Arctic lasting 3 d revealed a TSH decline throughout the time period, which took >48 h for return to baseline. Serum TT4/FT4 and TT3 initially increased, then declined below baseline, and then reverted toward normal by 48 h posttests *(122)*. Cold, sleep deprivation, and varying physical activity were all mitigating factors. A negative energy balance may have been present secondary to the cold and significant physical activity. In another military study, rangers were assessed over 4 d of grueling training in conjunction with sleep and caloric deprivation. The physical strain associated with this training was associated with an initial increase of T4, FT4, T3, rT3, and thyroxine-binding globulin (TBG) during the first 24 h. After 4 d of training, there was a gradual decrease in T4, FT4, T3 (65%), and TBG, whereas rT3 continued to rise. The group that received a higher caloric intake, and therefore less energy deficiency, had a continued increase in T3 instead. Also, T4 increased in the energy-sufficient group and TBG remained elevated, too. TSH decreased during the first day and remained low throughout the training period in energy-deficient groups. An acute exercise challenge (bicycle erometry) during this training period was associated with a small, but significant increase in T4, T3, rT3, and TBG, but TSH and FT4 remained unchanged. Subsequently, T4, T3, rT3, and TBG also decreased significantly following the exercise challenge. The response of TSH to TRH was reduced in all groups, but much less so in the energy-sufficient group. Energy deficiency correlates with a decrease in T3 and increase in rT3 *(123)*. Higher altitudes have been shown to be associated with an increase in T4 and FT4 *(124)*. Stock et al. reported that exercise at elevated altitudes is also notable for a significant increase in T4 and FT4 with even mild activity *(125)*.

Energy balance in women runners has also been investigated. Subjects with negative energy balance had a decrease in T3 (−15%) and FT3 (−18%), but a +24% increase in rT3 was noted *(117)*. This "low T3 syndrome" was prevented by dietary adjustment, but not by reduction in exercise intensity. Rat studies indicate that serum T4 and T3 remain stable with exercise-induced weight loss, whereas TH changes are noted in underfed, sedentary rats *(126)*. A study of subjects on bicycle ergometry revealed a rise in rT3 from 29 to 40 ng/gL with a decrease in T3 from 154 to 147 ng/dL. Glucose infusion during a repeat test reduced the rT3 and T3 changes. A positive correlation during exercise between rT3 and FFAs was found ($r = 0.95$). The glucose infusion reduced this correlation to $r = 0.81$ for FFA. Of note, exercise stress was minimal in this study with heart rate of 120 beats/min and working at 40% of maximal oxygen consumption *(127)*. As mentioned above, restriction of dietary carbohydrate has been associated with lower serum T3 level. Thyroidal responses to exercise were measured in groups with either a fat-enriched or carbohydrate-enriched diet. The T3 level tended to be lower at any point in exercise with the fat diet in comparison to the carbohydrate diet *(128)*. Similarly, patients with anorexia nervosa have been found to have lower T4 and T3 levels. When muscle metabolism was investigated in anorexia nervosa with ^{31}Phosphorous magnetic resonance spectroscopy (^{31}P-MRS), there was little difference between anorexics with low-normal T3 and below-normal T4 levels than in controls. The Pi/PCr ratio was slightly higher in anorexics at 20–30% exercise capacity, but not at higher workloads, and the Pi/PCr recovery rate was not different from controls *(129)*.

TH changes secondary to exercise have been assessed in patients with known or suspected coronary artery disease. Tests results are conflicting with at least one exercise study revealing no changes in TSH, T4, T3, or rT3, but another bicycle ergometry stress test yielded a TSH decline and increase in TT4 and FT4, which all resolved within 1 h posttest *(130,131)*. Of note, combined oral L-T4/L-T3 overdosage has been reported to cause ST wave depressions with TMST that resolve with the euthyroid state *(132)*. In general, diagnostic treadmill testing is best delayed until patients are euthyroid.

Amenorrhea is commonly seen in well-trained female athletes. Studies have compared the TH differences between women athletes with normal menses and amenorrhea. One study found TT4/FT4, TT3/FT3, and rT3 were all lower in the amenorrheic group in comparison to sedentary women, whereas the athletes with regular menses had only a slightly lower FT4 level. TSH circadian rhythm was unaltered *(133)*. Caloric balance was similar in the two groups. Thyroid hormone levels in eumenorrheic nonathletes and eumenorrheic endurance-trained athletes were compared with amenorrheic endurance-trained athletes. The amenorrheic subjects had lower T4 and T3 levels then the eumenorrehic groups, but the trained eumenorrehic females had slightly lower T4 and T3 levels than the eumenorrheic nonathletes as well. Of interest, the amenorrheic athletes tended to eat less fat and eat more carbohydrates with a similar caloric intake in comparison to the two other groups. Also, the amenorrheic group tended to train more hours and more strenuously then the other two groups. VO_2 was similar in the trained groups, who also weighed less and had lower body fat. As measured by ^{31}P-MRS, Pi/Cr was not different at rest or at exercise, and pH did not differ at any activity level. However, PCr recovery was substantially faster in the eumenorrehic endurance-trained group (26.3 ± 3.3 s) than in the eumenorrheic nonathletes (42.6 ± 4.6 s) and amenorrheic athletes (41.2 ± 6.6 s); however, the Pi/PCr recovery was only different between the eumenorrheic trained athletes and nonathletes *(134)*. It is of interest that T3 was lower in the trained athletes vs in the nonathletes. Also, one must wonder that even if the caloric intake in the amenorrheic athletes was equal, the T3/T4 changes may have been secondary to an energy deficiency, since their activity level was higher. However, even the trained eumenorrheic athletes had lower levels of TH, yet many trained athletes have been found to have higher levels of T3 at rest. PCr recovery is related to oxidative metabolism, and the fast recovery in trained eumenorrheic athletes indicates a potentially more efficient metabolism, yet amenorrheic individuals did not appear to obtain this advantage. The other parameters for exercise metabolism were similar. In another study, levels of TSH, T3, and T4 were not found to be different in oligomenorrheic heavily trained adolescents vs adolescent athletes without "strenuous" exercise (defined as >5 h/d) with regular menses *(135)*.

In summary, the thyroid function changes secondary to exercise represent a complex physiologic response, which is difficult to characterize fully. Mitigating factors in the TH response to exercise include: age, baseline fitness, nutrition status, ambient temperature, altitude, as well as time, intensity, and type of exercise performed. Another important factor in interpretation of the extant literature is that not all TH blood tests were assessed in every study. Moreover, older studies employed less sensitive assay techniques, for example, first-generation TSH immunoassay, whereas our various assays

Table 3
Reported Changes of Thyroid Hormones in Association with Exercise

Reference	Exercise type	Caloric status	TSH	TT4	FT4	TT3	FT3	rT3	Comments
93	Pre-exercise	NA[l]	↑[n]						Anticipation of exercise[i]
94	Ergometry	NA	NC[m]	↓		↓			
95	Ergometry	NA	↑	↑		↑			Normal TRH stim
97	Treadmill	NA	↑	NC		NC			Graded exercise
128	Treadmill	NA	NC	NC		NC			
98	Running	NA	↓[o]		↓	↑		NC	Maximal exericse
99	Swimming	NA			NC	↑		↑	
100	Ultradistance	NA		↑		NC		↑	75 km (age 2? yr)[f]
100	Ultradistance	NA		↓		↓		∅	45 km (age 36 yr)[f]
100	Ultradistance	NA	NC	↑		↓		↑	42.2 km (marathon)[f]
101	Marathon	NA	NC	NC		NC		NC	
102	Triathalon	NA	↑	↑					Groups age 23 and age 60
103	Marathon	NA	NC	NC		NC		NC	
104	Marathon	NA	↑	↑	↑		↓	↑	Rise T4 to rT3 conversion
121	Crosscountry Skiing	Deficient		↑	↑				Cold exposure
122	Military training	Deficient	↓	↑↓[a]	↑↓[a]	↑↓[a]	↓		Arctic weather[a] Sleep deprivation
123	Military training	Deficient	↓	↑↓[b]	↑↓[b]	↑↓[b]		↑↑	Sleep deprivation
123	Military training	Sufficient	↓	↑	↑↓↑[b]	↑		↑	
123	Ergometry[c]	Deficient and Sufficient	NC	↑	NC	↑		↑	TSH response to TRH reduced[d]
105	Ergometry	NA		NC		↑		↓	Untrained athletes
105	Ergometry	NA		↓		NC		↑	Well-trained athletes
107	TMST	NA		NC	NC	NC		NC	Sedentary, joggers, and well-trained athletes[j]
131	Ergometry	NA		NC	NC	NC		NC	Suspected CAD patients
130	Ergometry	NA	↓	↑	↑	NC		NC	
108	Swimming	NA	↑		↑	NC			20°C[g]
108	Swimming	NA	NC		NC	NC			26°C
108	Swimming	NA	↓		↓	NC			32°C
112	Chronic endurance exercise	NA		↓	NC	↓	↓		Identical twins
113	Chronic Ergometry	NA	NC						Recreational athletes NC TSH response to TRH
133	Chronic endurance exercise	NA	NC[i]	↓	↓	↓	↓	↓	Amenorrheic[e]
114	Aerobic exercise 4 wk	NA	NC	NC		NC		NC	Healthy women

(continued)

Table 3 (continued)
Reported Changes of Thyroid Hormones in Association with Exercise

Reference	Exercise type	Caloric status	TSH	TT4	FT4	TT3	FT3	rT3	Comments
106	Running		NC	NC		NC			Endurance athletes[h] vs. controls: baseline
2	Aerobic exercise	Deficient		↑		↓	↓	↑	Not seen in energy balanced group
119	Gymnastic exercise	Deficient		↓		↓			
117	Runners	Deficient	NC	↑		↓			Prevented by caloric increase
120	Ergometry	NA		↑		↓		↑	Glucose infusion[k]
96	Ergometry	NA	NC	↑	↑				Submaximal exercise
98	Running	NA	↑		NC	NC		NC	Submaximal exercise
124	High-altitude exercise	NA	NC	↑	↑	↑			TT4/FT4 increase with higher altitude alone pre-exercise
134	Ergometry	Anorexia		↓		↓			Amenorrheic vs eumenorrheic controls and athletes[i]
127	Ergometry	NA				↑		↑	Hypothyroidism
135	Ballet	NA	NC	NC		NC			

[a]Initial increase of TT4/FT4 and TT3 first 24 h, then decrease, then resolve 48 h posttraining.
[b]Initial increase of TT4/FT4 and TT3 first 24 h, then decrease. However, T3 continued to rise in the energy-sufficient group, whereas T4 initially rose, then fell, and finally rose again.
[c]Acute exercise challenge during military training.
[d]TSH response to TRH reduced more in energy-deficient than energy-sufficient group.
[e]TT4/FT4, TT3/FT3, and rT3 were lower in exercise amenorrheic group vs sedentary women. The eumenorrheic exercise group only a slightly lower FT4 level, but T4 and T3 were slightly lower than the eumenorrheic sedentary group.
[f]TSH, T4, and T3 lower in older runners, whereas faster runners had higher T4 and TSH in relation to slower runners.
[g]High TSH with longer cold water exposure.
[h]Endurance athletes had balanced increase in T3 production and disposal rates in comparison to active and sedentary men.
[i]TSH response to TRH stimulation was blunted in amenorrheic vs eumenorrheic athletes.
[j]TSH response to TRH stimulation was unchanged by exercise in all three groups.
[k]A glucose infusion blunted the exercise-induced changes of rT3, T3, and T4.
[l]NA = not assessed in study.
[m]NC = no change.
[n]↑ = increase.
[o]↓ = decrease.

have improved over the collective time span of these many studies. The detection of increased FFAs in several studies, which may interfere with some FT4 assays, also cannot be overlooked. However, despite these issues, review of the literature does reveal certain trends, and some are more evident then others (*see* Table 3). One of the more consistent findings is that rT3 tends to increase with exercise especially with associated caloric energy deficiency or ultradistance exercise. TSH appears to be unaffected by exercise in about 50% of studies with an increase in TSH secondary to cold exposure being a noted exception. TT4 was found to increase in 46%, decrease in 26%, and be unchanged in 28% of investigations, although an increase was more typically found with caloric energy deficiency, cold exposure, or ultradistance exercise. Free T4 follows a similar pattern to TT4. TT3 was found to be decreased or be unchanged in 73% of study subjects, and usually is low with caloric energy deficiency (as in low T3 syndrome or euthyroid sick states). FT3 was infrequently assessed in the protocols, but when measured, tended to rise with exercise. The response of thyroid hormones to swimming exercise is altered by water temperature, and changes seen with altitude include a rise in TT4/FT4. Many of the TH changes seen especially in athletes with negative energy balance can be reversed with either a high-carbohydrate intake or even glucose infusion. Although well-trained athletes may exhibit an increased production and turnover of T4 and/or T3, baseline TH levels do not appear to be affected by chronic endurance exercise.

REFERENCES

1. Wartofsky L. The approach to the patient with thyroid disease. In: Becker KL, ed. Principles and Practice of Endocrinology and Metabolism, 2nd ed. J.B. Lippincott, Philadelphia, 1995, pp. 278–280.
2. Loucks AB, Callister R. Induction and prevention of low-T3 syndrome in exercising women. Am J Physiol 1993;264(5Pt2):R924–R930.
3. Reed L, Pangaro LN. Physiology of the thyroid gland I: synthesis and release, iodine metabolism, and binding and transport. In: Becker KL, ed. Principles and Practice of Endocrinology and Metabolism, 2nd ed. J.B. Lippincott, Philadelphia,1995, pp. 285–291.
4. Leonard JL, Koehrle J. Intracellular pathways of iodothyronine metabolism. In: Braverman LE, Utiger RD, eds. Werner and Ingbar's The Thyroid, 7th ed. Lippincott-Raven, Philadelphia, 1996, pp. 125–160.
5. Brent GA. The molecular basis of thyroid hormone action. N Engl J Med, 1994;331:847–853.
6. Davis PJ, Davis FB. Nongenomic actions of thyroid hormone. Thyroid 1996;6:497–504.
7. Motomura K, Brent GA. Mechanisms of thyroid hormone action: Implications for the clinical manifestation of thyrotoxicosis. Endocrinol Metab Clin North Am 1998;27(1):1–19.
8. Dillmann WH. Biochemical basis of thyroid hormone action in the heart. Am J Med 1990;V88:626–629.
9. Davis PJ, Davis FB. Acute cellular actions of thyroid hormone and myocardial function. Ann Thorac Surg 1993;56:S16–S23.
10. McAllister RM, Delp MD, Laughlin MH. Thyroid status and exercise tolerance: Cardiovascular and metabolic considerations. Sports Med 1995;20(3):189–198.
11. McAllister RM, Ogilvie RW, Terjung RL. Functional and metabolic consequences of skeletal muscle remodeling in hypothyroidism. Am J Physiol 1991;260:E272–E279.
12. McAllister RM, Delp MD, Laughlin MH. Muscle blood flow during exercse in sedentary and trained hypothyroid rats. Am J Physiol 1995;269:H1949–H1954.
13. Burack R, Edwards RHT, Grun M, et al. The response to exercise before and after treatment of myxedema with thyroxine. J Pharm Exp Ther 1970;176:212–218.
14. Martin WH, Spina RJ, Korte E, et al. Mechanisms of impaired exercise capacity in short duration experimental hyperthyroidism. J Clin Invest 1991;88:2047–2053.
15. McAllister RM, Sansone JC, Laughlin MH. Effects of hyperthyroidism on muscle blood flow during exercise in the rat. Am J Physiol 1995;268:H330–335.

16. Nazar K, Chwalbinska-Moneta J, Machalla J, Kaciuba-Uscilko H. Metabolic and body temperature changes during exercise in hyperthyroid patients. Clin Sci Mol Med 1978;54:323–327.
17. Morkin E, Flink IL, Goldman S. Biochemical and physiologic effects of thyroid hormones on cardiac performance. Prog Cardiovasc Dis 1983;25(5):435–459.
18. Klein I, Ojamaa K. Cardiovascular manifestations of endocrine disease. J Clin Endocrinol Metab 1992;75:339.
19. Moruzzi P, Doria E, Agostoni PG, Capacchione V, Sganzrela P. Usefulness of L-thyroxine to improve cardiac and exercise performance in idiopathic dilated cardiomyopathy. Am J Cardiol 1994;73(5):374–378.
20. Amidi M, Leon DF, DeGroot WJ, Kroetz FW, Leonard JJ. Effect of the thyroid state on myocardial contractility and ventricular ejection rate in man. Circulation 1968;38:229–239.
21. McAllister RM, Delp MD, Laughlin MH. A review of effects of hypothyroidism on vascular transport in skeletal muscle during exercise. Can J Appl Physiol 1997;22(1):1–10.
22. Delp MD, McAllister RM, Laughlin MH. Exercise training alters aortic vascular reactivity in hypothyroid rats. Am J Physiol 1995;268:H1428–H1435.
23. Wieshammer S, Keck FS, Waitzinger J, Kohler J, Adam W, Stauch M, et al. Left ventricular function at rest and during exercise in acute hypothyroidism. Br Heart J 1988;60:204–211.
24. Forfar JC, Muir AL, Toft AD. Left ventricular function in hypothyroidism: Responses to exercise and beta adrenoceptor blockade. Br Heart J 1982;48:278–284.
25. Smallridge RC, Goldman MH, Raines K, Jones S, Van Nostrand D. Rest and exercise left ventricular ejection fraction before and after therapy in young adults with hyperthyroidism and hypothyroism. Am J Cardiol 1987;60:929–930.
26. Donaghue K, Hales I, Allwright S, et al. Cardiac function in acute hypothyroidism. Eur J Nuclear Med 1985;11:147–149.
27. Bernstein R, Muller C, Midtbo K, Smith G, Huag E, Hertzenberg L. Silent myocardial ischemia in hypothyroidism. Thyroid 1995; V5(6):443–446.
28. Bernstein R, Muller C, Midtbo K, Haug E, Nakken KF, Hertzenberg L et al. Cardiac left ventricualr function before and during early thyroxine treatment in severe hypothyroidism. J Intern Med 1991;230:493–500.
29. Arem R, Rokey R, Kiefe C, Escalante DA, Rodriguez A. Cardiac systolic and diastolic function at rest and exercise in subclinical hypothyroidism: effect of thyroid hormone therapy. Thyroid 1996; 6(5):397–401.
30. Forfar JC, Wathen CG, Todd TA, Bell GW, Hannan WJ, Muir AL, et al. Left ventricular performance in subclinical hypothyroidism. Q J Med 1995;57:857–865.
31. Bell GM, Todd TA, Forfar JC, et al. End-organ responses to thyroxine therapy in subclinical hypothyroidism. Clin Endocr 1985;22:83–89.
32. Bernstein R, Midtbo K, Smith G, Muller C, Haug E, Holme I, et al. Incidence of hypertrophic cardiomyopathy in hypothyroidism. Thyroid, 1995;5(4):277–281.
33. Santos AD, Miller RP, Puthepurakal KM. Echocardiographic characterization of the reversible cardiomyopathy of hypothyroidism. Am J Med 1980;86:675.
34. Amidi M, Leon DF, DeGroot WJ, Kroetz FW, Leonard JJ. Effect of the thyroid state on myocardial contractility and ventricular ejection rate in man. Circulation 1968;38:229–239.
35. Sandler G, Wilson GM. The nature and prognosis of heart disease in thyrotoxicosis. Q J Med 1959;28:247–269.
36. Klein I. Thyroid hormone and the cardiovascular system. Am J Med 1988;88(6):631–637.
37. Schwartz K, Lecarpenter Y, Martin JL, et al. Myosin isoenzyme distribution correlates with speed of myocardial contraction. J Mol Cell Cardiol 1981;13:1071–1075.
38. Parisi AF, Hamilton BP, Thomas CN, et al. The short cardiac pre-ejection period, an index of thyrotoxicosis. Circulation 1974;49:900–904.
39. Amidi M, Leon DF, DeGroot WJ, et al. Effect of the thyroid state on myocardial contractility and venrticular ejection rate in man. Circulation 1968;38:229–239.
40. Foldes J, Istvanffy M, Halmagyi M, Varadi A, Lakatos P, Partos O. Hyperthyroidism and the heart: Study of the left ventricular function in preclinical hyperthyroidism. Acta Med Hungar 1986;43(1):23–29.
41. Shafer RB, Bianco JA. Assessment of cardiac reserve in patients with hyperthyroidism. Chest 1980;78:269–273.
42. Forfar JC, Muir AL, Sawers SA, Toft AD. Abnormal left ventricular function in hyperthyroidism. New Engl J Med 1982;V307(19):1165–1170.

43. Karlberg BE, Henriksson KG, Anderson GG. Cyclic adenosine 3',5'- monophosphate concentration in plsama, adipose tissue and skeletal muscle in normal subjects and in patients with hyper- and hypothyroidism. J Clin Endocrinol Metab 1974;39(1):96–101.
44. Klein I, Ojamaa K. Thyrotoxicosis and the heart. Endocrinol Metab Clin North Am 1998;27(1):51–62.
45. Levy GS, Klein I. Catecholamine-thyroid hormone interactions and the cardiovascular manifestatuions of hyperthyroidism. Am J Med 1990;88:947.
46. Bilezikian JP, Loeb JN. The influence of hyperthyroidism and hypothyroidism on α- and β-adrenergic receptor systems and adrenergic responsivesness. Endocr Rev 1983;4(4)378–388.
47. Martin WH, Spina RJ, Korte E. Effect of hyperthyroidism of short duration on cardiac sensitivity to beta-adrenergic stimulation. J Am Cardiol 1992;19:1185–1191.
48. Liggett SB, Shah SD, Cryer PE. Increased fat and skeletal muscle B-adrenergic receptors but unaltered metabolic and hemodynamic sensitivity to epinephrine in vivo experimental human thyrotoxicosis. J Clin Invest 1989;83:830–839.
49. Merillon JP, Passa PH, Chastre J, et al. Left ventricular function and hyperthyroidism. Br Heart J 1981;46:137–143.
50. Aoki VS, Wilson WR, Theilen EO, et al. The effects of triiodothyronine on hemodynamic responses to epinephrine and norepinephrine in man. J Pharmacol Exp Ther 1967;157:62–68.
51. Hoit BD, Khoury SF, Shao Y. Effects of thyroid hormone on cardiac beta-adrenergic responsiveness in conscious baboons. Circulation 1997;96:592.
52. Martin WH, Spina RJ, Korte E, Yarasheski KE, et al. Mechanisms of impaired exercise capacity in short duration experimental hyperthyroidism. J Clin Invest 1991;88:2047–2053.
53. Theilen EO, Wilson WR. Hemodynamic effects of peripheral vasoconstriction in normal and thyrotoxic patients. J Appl Physiol 1967;22:207–210.
54. Graettinger JS, Muenster JJ, Selverstone LA, Campbell JA. A correlation of clinical and hemodynamic studies in patients with hyperthyroidism with and without congestive heart failure. J Clin Invest 1959;1316–1327.
55. Forfar JC, Caldwell GC. Hyperthyroid heart disease. Clin Endocrinol Metab 1985;14:491–509.
56. Nixon JV, Anderson RJ, Cohen ML. Alterations in left ventricular mass and performance in patients treated effectively for thyrotoxicosis. Am J Med 1979;67:268–276.
57. Klein I. Thyroxine-induced cardiac hypertrophy:time course of development and inhibition by propranolol. Endocrinology 1988;123:203–210.
58. Frey H, Skjorsten F. Peripheral circulatory and metabolic consequences of thyrotoxciosis. Scand J Clin Lan Invest 1967;19:351–362.
59. Winder WW, Baldwin KM, Terjung RL, Hollozsy JO. Effects of thyroid hormone administration on skeletal muscle mitochondria. Am J Physiol 1975;228:1341–1345.
60. Sestoft L, Saltin B. The low physical working capacity of thyrotoxic patients is not normalized by oral antithyroid treatment. Clin Physiol 1988;8:9–15.
61. Fessel WJ. Myopathy of hypothyroidism. Ann Rheum Dis 1968;14:574.
62. Graig FA, Smith JC. Serum creatinine phosphokinase activity in altered thyroid states. J Clin Endocrinol and Metab 1965;25:723–731.
63. Riggs JE. Acute exertional rhabdomyolysis in hypothyroidism: The result of a reversible defect in glycogenolysis. Military Med 1990;155(4):171,172.
64. Emser W, Schimrigk K. Myxedema myopathy: A case report. Eur Neurol 1977;16:286.
65. Sekine N, Yamamoto M, Michikawa M, et al. Rhabdomyolsis and acute renal failure in a patient with hypothyroidism. Intern Med 1993;32(3):269–271.
66. Klein I, Parker M, Shebert R. Hypothyroidism presenting as muscle stiffness and pseudohypertrophy: Hoffmann's syndrome. Am J Med 1981;70:891–894.
67. Astrom KE, Kugelberg E, Muller R. Hypothyroid myopathy. Arch Neurol, 1961;5:472.
68. Ramsay ID. Electromyography in thyrotoxicosis. Q J Med 1965;34:255.
69. Monzani F, Caraccio N, Siciliano G, et al. Clinical and biochemical features of muscle dysfunction in subclinical hypothyroidism. J Clin Endocrinol Metab 1997;82(10):3315–3318.
70. Sukp J. Alterations of Ca^{2+} uptake and Ca^{2+}-activated ATPase of cardiac sarcoplasmic reticulum in hyper- and hypothyroidism. Biochim Biophys Acta 1971;252:324–337.
71. Arnold DL, Matthews PM, Radda GK. Metabolic recovery after exercise and the assessment of mitochondrial function in vivo in human skeletal muscle by means of 31-P NMR study. Magnet Res Med 1994;1:307–315.

72. Chance B, Eleff S, Leigh JS, Sokolov D, Sapega A. Mitochondrial regulation of phosphocreatinine/inorganic phosphate ratios in exercising human muscle: a gated 31-P NMR study. Proc Natl Acad Sci USA 1981:78:6714–6718.
73. Kaminsky P, Robin-Lherbier B, Brunotte F, et al. Energetic metabolism in hypothyroid skeletal muscle, as studied by phosphorous magnetic resonance spectroscopy. J Clin Endocrinol Metab 1992;74(1):124–129.
74. Argov Z, Bank WJ, Maris J, Peterson P, Chance B. Bioenergetic heterogeneity of human mitochondrial myopathies as demonstarted by in vivo phosphorous magnetic resonance spectroscopy. Neurology1987;37:257–262.
75. Argov ZJ, Renshaw PF, Boden B, Winokur A, Bank W. Effects of thyroid hormones on skeletal muscle bioenergetics: In vivo phosphorous-31 magnetic resonance spectroscopy study of humans and rats. J Clin Invest 1988;81:1695–1701.
76. Kaciuba-Uscilko H, Brzezinska Z, Kruk B, et al. Thyroid hormone deficiency and muscle metabolism during light and heavy exercise in dogs. Pflugers Arch 1988;412:366,367.
77. Ramsay ID. Muscle dysfunction in hyperthyroidism. Lancet 1966;2:931–934.
78. Asayama K, Kato K. Oxidative muscular injury and its relevance to hyperthyroidism. Free Radical Biol Med 1990;8:293–303.
79. Fitts RH, Brimmer CJ, Troup JP, et al. Contractile and fatigue properties of thyrotoxic rat skeletal muscle. Muscle Nerve 1984;7:470–477.
80. Kelley DE, Garhib H, Kennedy FP, Duda RJ, McManis PG. Thyrotoxic Periodic Paralysis: Report of 10 cases and review of the electromyographic findings. Arch Intern Med 1989;149(11):2597–2600.
81. McManis PG, Lambert EH, Daube JR. The exercise test in periodic paralysis. Muscle Nerve 1986;9:704–710.
82. Jackson CE, Barohn RJ. Improvement of the exercise test after therapy in thyrotoxic periodic paralysis. Muscle Nerve 1992;15:1069–1071.
83. Links TP, van der Hoeven JH. Improvement of the exercise test after therapy in thyrotoxic periodic paralysis. Muscle Nerve 1993;16(10):1132–1133.
84. Zwillich CW, Pierson DJ, Hofeldt FD, Lufkin EG, Weh JV. Ventilatory control in myxedema and hypothyroidism. N Eng J Med 1975;292(13):662–665.
85. Ingbar DH. The respiratory system in hypothyroidism. In: Braverman LE, Utiger RD, eds. Werner and Ingbar's The Thyroid, 7th ed. Philadelphia, Lippincott-Raven Publishers 1996, pp. 805–810.
86. Wilson WR, Bedell GN. The pulmonary abnormalities in myxedema. J Clin Invest 1960;39:42.
87. Kahaly G, Hellerman J, Mohr-Kahaly S, Treese N. Impaired cardiopulmonary exercise capacity in patients with hyperthyroidism. Chest 1996;109(1):57–61.
88. Massey DG, Becklake MR, McKenzie JM, Bates DV. Circulatory and ventilatory response to exercise in thyrotoxicosis. N Eng J Med 1967;276(20):1104–1112.
89. Siafakas NM, Milona I, Salesiotou V, et al. Respiratory muscle strength in hyperthyroidism before and after treatment. Am Rev Respir Dis 1992;146(4):1025–1029.
90. Stein M, Kimbel P, Johnson RL. Pulomonary function in hyperthyroidism. J Clin Invest 1960;40:348–363.
91. Ayers J, Clark TH, Maisey MN. Thyrotoxicosis and dyspnea. Clin Endocrinol (Oxf) 1982;164:645.
92. Hollinsworth HM, Pratter MR, Dubois JM, Braverman LE, Irwin RS. Effect of triiodothyronine-induced thyrotoxicosis on airway hyperresponsiveness. J Appl Physiol 1991;71(2):438–444.
93. Mason JW, Hartley LH, Kotchen TA, et al. Plasma thyroid-stimulating hormone response in anticipation of muscular exercise in the human. J Clin Endo Metab 1973;37(3):403–406.
94. Sawhney RC, Malhotra AS, Gupta RB, Rai RM. A study of pituitary-thyroid function during exercise in man. Indian J Physiol Pharm 1984;28(2):153–158.
95. Liewendahl K, Helenius T, Näveri H, Tikkanen H. Fatty acid-induced increase in serum dialyzable free thyroxine after physiocal exercise: implication for nonthyroidal illness. J Clin Endocrinol Metab 1992;74(6):1361–1365.
96. Terjung RL, Tipton CM. Plasma thyroxine and thyroid-stimulating hormone levels during submaximal exercise in humans. Am J Physiol 1971;220(6):1840–1845.
97. Galbo H, Hummer L, Petersen IB, Christensen NJ, Bie N. Thyroid and testicular hormone responses to graded and prolonged exercise in man. Eur J Appl Physiol 1977;36:101–106.
98. Schmid P, Wolf W, Pilger E, et al. TSH, T3, rT3 and FT4 in maximal and submaximal physical exercise. Eur J Appl Physiol 1982;48:31–39.

99. Premachandra BN, Winder WW, Hickson R, Lang S, Hollozy JO. Circulating reverese triiodothronine in humans during exercise. Eur J Appl Physiol 1981;47:281–288.
100. Hesse V, Vilser C, Scheibe J, Jahreis G, Foley T. Thyroid hormone metabolism under extreme body exercise. Exp Clin Endocrinol 1989;94(1/2):82–88.
101. Dessypris A, Wager G, Fyhrquist F, Makinen T, Welin MG, Lamberg BA. Marathon run: effects on blood cortisol-ACTH, iodothyronines- TSH and vasopressin. Acta Endocrinol 1980;95:151–157.
102. Malarkey WB, Hall JC, Rice RR, et al. The influence of age on endocrine responses to ultraendurance stress. J Gerontol 1993;48(4):M134–39.
103. Semple CG, Thomson JA, Beastall GH. Endocrine responses to marathon running. Br J Sports Med 1985;19(3):148–151.
104. Sander M, Röcker L. Influence of marathon running on thyroid hormones. Int J Sports Med 1988;9:123–126.
105. Limanova Z, Sonka J, Kratochvil O, Sonka K, Kanka J, Sprynarova S. Effects of exercise on serum cortisol and thyroid hormones. Exp Clin Endocrinol 1983;81(3):308–314.
106. Rone JK, Dons RF, Reed HL. The effect of endurance training on serum triiodothyronine kinetics in man: physical conditioning marked by enhanced thyroid hormone metabolism. Clin Endocrinol 1992;37:325–330.
107. Smallridge RC, Whorton NE, Burman KD, Ferguson EW. Effects of exercise and physical fitness on the pituitary-thyroid axis and on prolactin secretion in male runners. Metabolism 1985;34(10): 949–954.
108. Deligiannis A, Karamouzis M, Kouidi E, Mougios V, Kallaras C. Plasma TSH, T3, T4 and cortisol responses to swimming at varying water temperatures. Br J Sp Med 1993;27(4):247–250.
109. Dulac S, Quirion A, DeCarufel D, et al. Metabolic and hormonal responses to long-distance swimming in cold water. Int J Sports Med 1987;8:352–356.
110. Reichlin S, Martin JB, Jackson JM. Regulation of thyroid stimulating hormone (TSH) secretion. In: Jeffcoate SL, Hutchinson JSM, eds. The Endocrine Hypothalamus. London, UK: Academic, 1978, pp. 237–243.
111. Rhodes BA, Conway MJ. Exercise lowers thyroid radioiodine uptake: Concise communication. J Nuclear Med 1980; 21(9):835–837.
112. Tremblay A, Poehlman ET, Despres JP, Theriault G, Danforth E, Bouchard C. Endurance training with constant energy intake in identical twins: Changes over time in energy expenditure and related hormones. Metabolism 1997;46(5):499–503.
113. Lehmann M, Knizia K, Gastmann U, et al. Influence of 6-week, 6 days per week, training on pituitary function in recreational athletes. Br J Sp Med 1993;27(3):186–192.
114. Caron PJ, Sopko G, Stolk JM, Jacobs DR, Nisula BC. Effect of physical conditioning measures on thyroid hormone action. Horm Metab Res 1986;18:206–208.
115. Vagenakis AG, Burger A, Portnay GI, et al. Diversion of peripheral thyroxine metabolism from activating to inactivating pathways during complete fasting. J Clin Endocrinol Metab 1975;41:191–194.
116. Burman KD, Diamond RC, Harvey GS, O'Brien JT, Georges LP, Bruton J, et al. Glucose modulation of alterations in serum iodothyronine concentrations induced by fasting. Metabolism 1979;28(4):291–299.
117. Loucks AB, Heath EM. Induction of Low-T3 syndrome in exercising women occurs at a threshold of energy availability. Am J Physiol 1994;264(3Pt2):R817–823.
118. Mathieson RA, Walberg JT, Gwazdauskas FC, Hinkle DE, Gregg JM. The effect of varying carbohydrate content of a very-low-caloric-diet on resting metabolic rate and thyroid hormones. Metabolism 1986;35(5):394–398.
119. Jahreis G, Kauf E, Frohner G, Schmidt HE. Influence of intensive exercise on insulin-like growth factor I, thyroid and steroid hormones in female gymnasts. Growth Regul 1991;1:95–99.
120. O'Connell M, Robbins DC, Horton ES, Sims EAH. Changes in serum concentrations of 3,3',5'-triiodothyronine and 3,5,3'-triiodothyronine during prolonged moderate exercise. J Clin Endocrinol Metab 1979;49(2):242–246.
121. Kirkeby K, Strömme SB, et al. Effects of prolonged, strenuous exercise on lipids and thyroxine in serum. Acta Med Scand 1977;202:463–467.
122. Hackney AC, Hodgdon JA, Hesslink R, Trygg K. Thyroid hormone responses to military winter exercises in the Arctic region. Arctic Med Res 1995;54:82–90.
123. Opstad PK, Falch D, Oktedalen O, Fonnum F, Wergeland R. The thyroid function in young men during prolonged exercise and the effect of energy and sleep deprivation. Clin Endocrinol 1984;20:657–669.

124. Sawhney RC, Malhotra AS. Thyroid function in sojourners and acclimatized low landers at high altitude in man. Horm Metab Res 1991;23:81.
125. Stock MJ, Chapman C, Stirling JL, Campbell IT. Effects of exercise, altitude, and food on blood hormone and metabolic levels. J Appl Physiol 1978;45(3):350–354.
126. Katzeff HL, Selgrad C. Maintenance of thyroid hormone production during exercise-induced weight loss. Am J Physiol 1991:261(3Pt1):E382–388.
127. Burack R, Edwards RHT, Grun M, et al. The response to exercise before and after treatment of myxedema with thyroxine. J Pharm Exp Ther 1970;176:212–218.
128. Johannessen A, Hagen C, Galbo H. Prolactin, growth hormone, thyrtropin,3,5,3'-triiodothyronine, and thyroxine responses to exercise after fat- and carbohydrate-enriched diet. J Clin Endocrinol Metab 1981;52:56–61.
129. Harber VJ, Petersen SR, Chilbeck PD. Thyroid hormone concentrations and skeletal muscle metabolism during exercise in anorexic females. Can J Appl Physiol Pharm1997;75(10–11):1197–1202.
130. Licata G, Scaglione R, Novo S, Dichiara MA, Di Vincenzio D. Behavior of serum T3, rT3,TT4, FT4 and TSH levels after exercise on a bicycle ergometer in healthy euthyroid male young subjects. Boll Soc Ital Biol Sper 1984;30–60(4):753–759.
131. Siddiqui AR, Hinnefeld RB, Dillon T, Judson WE. Immediate effects of heavy exercise on the circulating thyroid hormones. Br J Sports Med 1983;17(3):180–183.
132. Peterson CR, Jones RC. Abnormal post-exercise electrocardiogram due to iatrogenic hyperthyroidism. Military Med 134(9):694–697.
133. Loucks AB, Laughlin GA, Mortola JF, Girton L, Nelson JC, Yen SSC. Hypothalamic–pituitary–thyroidal function in eumenorrheic and amenorrheic athletes. J Clin Endocrinol Metab 1992;75: 514–518.
134. Harber VJ, Petersen SR, Chilibeck PD. Thyroid hormone concentrations and muscle metabolism in amenorrheic and eumenorrheic athletes. Can J Appl Physiol 1998;23(3):293–306.
135. Creatsas G, Salakos N, Averkiou M, Miras K, Aravantinos D. Endocrinological profile of oligomenorrheic strenuously exercising adolescents. Int J Gynecol Obstet 1992;38:215–221.

7 The Male Reproductive System, Exercise, and Training

David C. Cumming, MBChB, FRCSC

CONTENTS

    INTRODUCTION
    MALE REPRODUCTIVE PHYSIOLOGY
    ACUTE EXERCISE AND THE HYPOTHALAMIC-PITUITARY GONADOTROPHIN
        (HPG) AXIS IN MEN
    THE EFFECTS OF PROLONGED EXERCISE ON THE HPG AXIS IN MEN
    EFFECT OF ENDURANCE TRAINING ON THE HPG AXIS IN MEN
    MECHANISMS OF EXERCISE-ASSOCIATED REDUCTIONS
        IN SERUM TESTOSTERONE LEVELS
    REFERENCES

INTRODUCTION

The hormonal rhythms that regulate reproduction are generally robust in both men and women, but they are subject to changes with short- or longer-term physiological and psychological stresses. Such changes may be clinically significant or more commonly clinically insignificant. The effects of physical activity on the male reproductive axis vary with the intensity and duration of the activity, the fitness of the individual, and and probably his nutritional-metabolic status. Relatively short, intense exercise usually increases and more prolonged exercise usually decreases serum testosterone levels. Endurance and other forms of training can induce subclinical inhibition of normal reproductive function, but clinical expression of reproductive dysfunction with exercise is uncommon in men. Long-term, exercise-associated suppression of hormone and sperm production by the testis is rarely of clinical significance, or at least few athletes are prepared to admit publicly that they have problems. The goal of this chapter is to examine the effects of physical activity on the male reproductive system and the mechanisms through which such changes could occur.

From: *Contemporary Endocrinology: Sports Endocrinology*
Edited by: M. P. Warren and N. W. Constantini © Humana Press Inc., Totowa, NJ

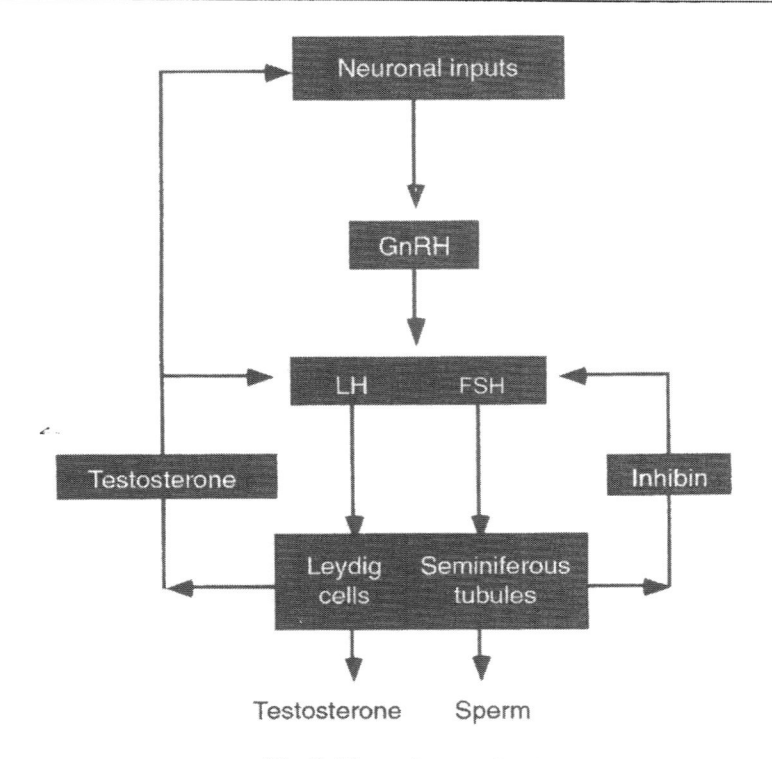

Fig. 1. The male reproductive axis.

MALE REPRODUCTIVE PHYSIOLOGY

As shown in Fig. 1, the male reproductive system consists of the testes and the hypothalamic–pituitary unit which controls their function. Recent detailed reviews of male reproductive physiology are available (1). The testes mature spermatozoa, and manufacture testosterone and other androgenic steroids, together with some nonsteroidal substances, notably inhibin. Peripheral conversion of precursor steroids results in production of other steroids, such as dihydrotestosterone and estradiol; 20% of these two hormones is secreted directly and 80% is made in the periphery from precursors. Maturation of spermatozoa, which transmit the genetic material from the male takes over 2 mo, a feature that is essential to remember when planning studies that examine the response of spermatogenesis to training. There is also substantial temporal and perhaps seasonal variation in sperm counts in the same individual (2,3).

Androgens are responsible for the development and maintenance of male secondary sex characteristics, but may also influence such diverse functions as muscle growth and repair, hepatic enzyme function, red blood cell manufacture, sex drive, and some nonsexual aspects of behavior, including perhaps aggressive behavior.

Testicular function is controlled by gonadotropins, luteinizing hormone (LH), and follicle-stimulating hormone (FSH); prolactin also has a biphasic effect on testicular steroid synthesis. LH regulates androgenesis; FSH, together with locally produced testosterone, is responsible for spermatogenesis. Gonadotropin-releasing hormone (GnRH) is secreted from the hypothalamus in 90- to 120-min, pulses and controls LH and FSH

Table 1
Factors Determining Exercise and/or Training-Associated Changes
in Levels of Testosterone in Circulation

Synthesis/secretion	Gonadotropin mediated (LH and FSH)
	Other (prolactin, catecholamines)
Testicular blood flow	Catecholaminergic and other controls
Protein binding in blood	Specific, high affinity (SHBG, CBG[a])
	Nonspecific, low affinity (albumin)
Metabolic clearance	Target tissue uptake and metabolism
	Hepatic metabolism

[a]CBG = cortisol-binding globulin.

release interactively with testosterone and inhibin and perhaps other steroidal and nonsteroidal substances produced by the testis. Inhibin exerts inhibitory feedback on FSH levels, whereas testosterone exerts a simple inhibitory "servo" effect on LH. Pulsatile GnRH also responds to inputs to the hypothalamus from elsewhere in the brain and from local nerve cell systems, including those producing corticotropin-releasing hormone (CRH), prolactin, dopamine, norepinephrine, GABA, and β-endorphin. Dopamine, CRH, prolactin, and β-endorphin are usually considered to be inhibitory, but noradrenaline and GABA stimulate LH release. Testicular interstitial fluid contains many secretory products, defined and undefined. The role of many substances in local and systemic function and their importance in exercise are unclear. Assumptions are frequently made that are difficult to prove.

Serum testosterone and LH levels change according to certain natural rhythms. Testosterone levels show a small diurnal variation, but pulsatile testosterone release is difficult to demonstrate, despite the pulsatile nature of LH release. Response to an LH pulse does not occur in <20–30 min (4). This is important in examining testosterone responses to short-term, strenuous physical activity. It is also important to recognize that modifications of binding or clearance can be as significant as changes in synthesis and secretion in determining the effects of physical activity on circulating testosterone levels. Exercise and training can change several factors that modulate the circulating testosterone levels (see Table 1).

ACUTE EXERCISE AND THE HYPOTHALAMIC-PITUITARY GONADAL (HPG) AXIS IN MEN

Increased serum testosterone levels have been reported during relatively strenuous free and treadmill running, weight training, and ergometer cycling, and have ranged from 13 to 185% (5–17). The response appears to be modified by intensity of activity and other variables. Short-term immersion in maximal swimming exercise appears to decrease circulating testosterone levels (18). The testosterone response has been reported to increase with increased exercise load (19,20). Similar workloads produce similar responses, regardless of whether the load is aerobic or anaerobic (21); in this situation, the response seems to differ from that of cortisol, in which the increase begins at the anaerobic threshold. Dietary intake may modify basal levels of testosterone, but not the exercise response to high-intensity, resistance exercise (22). Increased and decreased ambient temperature, altitude and dehydration similarly have no effect on testosterone responses to intense exercise *(23–25)*. Acute exercise-induced testosterone increments are also seen in older men, despite their very different hormonal milieu (higher estradiol, higher sex hormone binding globulin [SHBG], and lower free testosterone) *(26–28)*.

There is conflicting evidence about gonadotropin response, since LH and FSH levels have been reported as unchanged, increased, or rarely, decreased by short-term strenuous exercise *(5,7,12,13,17,29,30)*. Since the LH response to exercise is inconsistent and since testosterone levels increase in response to exercise more quickly than their response to LH (with a few minutes of strenuous exercise vs 20–30 min following LH), it is usually accepted that the exercise-associated increment in circulating testosterone levels is not mediated by LH. Possible mechanisms could be nonspecific (i.e., influence all steroid hormones in the same way) or specific involving only an increase in production of testosterone.

Possible nonspecific mechanisms associated with short-term exercise-induced serum testosterone increases include decreased metabolic clearance rate (MCR) and hemoconcentration through decreased plasma volume. Testosterone is cleared via the liver and extrahepatic mechanisms. The metabolic clearance rate of testosterone through the liver has been described as reduced during moderate physical activity *(31,32)*. The change in clearance, however, seems to be later than that of testosterone increments reported elsewhere. Suitable markers for extrahepatic clearance have not been described. Measurement of 3 α-androstanediol glucuronide may provide a marker for clearance through tissues that convert testosterone to dihydrotestosterone prior to use. Although this excludes the liver, it also excludes muscle, which uses testosterone directly.

Changes in hemoconcentration were considered important in some *(7,11,17,30)*, but by no means all studies *(5,12,13,16,29,33–36)*. Testosterone in circulation is bound to SHBG (60%) and albumin (38%) with a small amount free (2%). Because the binding affinity of testosterone to SHBG is 5000-fold greater than binding to albumin, substantial changes can occur in serum albumin without significant effect on total testosterone levels *(37)*. Although variable hemoconcentration has been reported with different forms of exercise, circulating SHBG, unlike serum protein, changes little with short- or longer-term running, and increases in the testosterone/SHBG ratio suggest that hemoconcentration played no significant role *(13)*.

For nonspecific mechanisms to be responsible for the acute exercise-induced serum testosterone increase, we would expect all circulating steroids to be affected in the same manner given that MCR and hemoconcentration do not differentiate among hormones. The timing of the testosterone increase was distinct from those of androstenedione and dehydroepiandrosterone (DHEA), predominantly adrenal androgens whose increments were simultaneous with that of cortisol *(5)*. The clear difference in responses among hormones suggests that specific testicular mechanisms are involved.

What mechanism could exist independent from gonadotropin stimulation of testosterone? The involvement of the sympathetic system in testicular testosterone production suggested that a direct neural pathway may stimulate testosterone production during exercise in some species *(38)*. Circulating catecholamine levels also increase substantially during exercise. β-Adrenergic blockade inhibits testosterone responses to exercise, whereas *l*-dopa, phentolamine, and clonidine had no effect *(39,40)*. β-Adrenergic blockade reduces hepatic perfusion and should increase rather than decrease testosterone responses if impaired hepatic blood flow were the mechanism. Investigation was undertaken in individuals with paraplegia; in contrast, the normal testosterone increment that accompanies short-term strenuous exercise in paraplegic subjects was eliminated during exercise under conditions of autonomic dysreflexia, characterized by elevated norepinephrine levels *(41)*. In a subsequent study, functional electrical stimulation- (FES) assisted resistance training induced an increase in serum testosterone levels without change in sex hormone binding globulin levels or hematocrit *(42)*. This increment was accompanied by an equally large increase in norepinephrine—which in this instance failed to suppress the testosterone increase. These studies suggest that norepinephrine at least is unrelated to exercise-induced changes in testosterone.

An anticipatory increase in circulating testosterone levels has been described and is presumably independent of hepatic perfusion or hemoconcentration *(5,17)*. It remains unclear exactly what mechanisms may be operative in increasing serum testosterone levels in any particular exercise protocol, and it is possible that the mechanisms responsible early in exercise may differ from those observed subsequently—for example, direct secretion by an unknown mechanism could be augmented later by changes in clearance and/or hemoconcentration. The definitive work remains to be designed

THE EFFECTS OF PROLONGED EXERCISE ON THE HPG AXIS IN MEN

A further difficulty is that in contrast to the short-term testosterone increment, which varies with intensity, prolonged submaximal exercise (exceeding 2 h) is generally associated with a complex series of changes in circulating androgen. Responses have been examined under laboratory conditions and during free activity, such as marathon and ultramarathon races, as well as crosscountry skiing. Several studies have reported an initial testosterone increase followed by a decline to or below baseline values *(14,43–56)*. The decrease appears proportional to the preceding workload *(43)*. Serum testosterone levels may also transiently decline following short-term, strenuous physical activity *(7,13)*. Physical and psychological stresses, such as surgery, myocardial infarction, and simulated warfare training, also result in decreased testosterone levels *(5)*.

Several mechanisms could potentially be important in decreased circulating testosterone levels during and following prolonged exercise, including suppressed gonadotropin release, or by elevated prolactin, cortisol, CRH, or catecholamine levels directly on the testis or indirectly via suppression of gonadotropins. Alterations in circulating β-endorphin levels have been considered responsible for short-term and chronic exercise-associated suppression of the HPG axis in both men and women. This has been difficult to prove, since opiate antagonism does not prevent the exercise-induced decrease in LH observed by some, but by no means all investigators *(14,49,52,53,57,58)*. Gonadotropin response to GnRH has been reported as reduced and increased following prolonged, exhaustive exercise *(53,59)*. Pulsatile LH release did not decrease following 60 and 120 min of treadmill running in men, although the area under the multiple sample curve was decreased after exercise *(49,58)*. The testosterone response to human chorionic gonadotropin (HCG) stimulation is reduced *(59)*.

How do we account for the decreased serum testosterone levels following prolonged exercise, which cannot be invariably explained by inhibition through changes in central control? The mild, transient prolactin increase with intense or prolonged exertion is unlikely to suppress postexercise testosterone levels. Short-term hypercortisolemia induced by insulin or injection of hydrocortisone hemisuccinate suppresses testosterone levels; since both centrally induced and peripherally injected cortisol increases influence testosterone levels, it is likely that the effect is mediated directly on the testis without intervening effects on the hypothalamic–pituitary axis *(60)*. The testosterone decrease that occurs with increasing cortisol levels during short-term, symptom-limited physical activity supports this contention *(5,45)*. Since CRH mediates its effect centrally, it is unlikely to be involved. As indicated earlier, there is an exercise-induced increment in catecholamines; the persistence of the increment beyond the end of exercise has been considered as a possible mechanism through which there could be testicular resistance to circulating gonadotropins *(53)*. The cause for the decrease in serum testosterone levels which occurs with prolonged exercise remains unclear. It is possible that the decline could result from a subtle interference at either hypothalamic or gonadal levels or because of increased androgen utilization following strenuous exercise for repair of structural and metabolic injury to the tissues.

EFFECT OF ENDURANCE TRAINING ON THE HPG AXIS IN MEN

The consistent testosterone decline following prolonged submaximal exercise suggested that there may be a physiological suppression of circulating testosterone associated with chronic involvement in endurance training *(61)*. Several cross-sectional and prospective studies have now supported this idea. Subjects include runners, strength-trained individuals, rowers, wrestlers, and cyclists *(62–77)*. Military training including a heavy physical exercise component resulted in an increase in mean plasma testosterone, androstenedione, and LH without change in SHBG levels *(78)*. Prospective studies using relatively light training regimes also produced increased testosterone levels *(79–81)*. Some cross-sectional and prospective studies have reported no change in serum testosterone even with heavy training *(82,83)*.

Symptomatic changes in testicular androgenesis and spermatogenesis are less clearly defined than equivalent changes in the reproductive system of women in whom the endocrine control of reproduction is both interactive and cyclic. Although measures of sperm function are generally normal in runners with very strenuous training regimens even with low physiological androgen levels *(62,82)*, there is some evidence that males with a high level of physical activity may have some abnormalities of semenanalysis *(77,83)*. In an artificial insemination program, donors with a high physical activity profile and low semen volume had significantly lower pregnancy rates than those with "normal" activity and low semen volume *(84,85)*. When semen volume was normal, there was no reduction in fertility. Anecdotal data have also suggested that libido may be impaired in some runners during periods of intense endurance training *(4,62,86–87)*. Reduced testosterone levels may play a role in this, but chronic fatigue may also be significant. A large-scale study of sexuality in runners was published in *The Runner* *(87)*. Although the scientific validity may be questioned, it is surprising that almost one-quarter of the male respondents to the questionnaire would be prepared to give up sex before running and almost half have admitted that they sometimes felt too tired from running to engage in sex. The positive replies to this question increased with increasing mileage. In contrast, fitness training in middle-aged men has been reported to increase sexual drive and sexual activity in a group of previously sedentary men (mean age 44 yr) *(88)*. There is some evidence that sex of offspring may also be affected by endurance training *(89)*; the observed increase in female sex of offspring is very difficult to explain.

So little is known of short- or long-term problems with exercise-induced symptomatic reproductive change in men that it is impossible at present to provide advice on the management of problems other than to review with the athlete having problems the possibility of decreasing the exercise load.

Androgen-dependent skeletal muscle hypertrophy and androgen synergism with growth hormone are well accepted. A consequence of severe training regimes with relatively low circulating testosterone levels could be to reduce repair of muscle damage. A decline in circulating testosterone levels in rats undergoing endurance training was accompanied by increased excretion of products of muscle catabolism *(90)*. Increased utilization of testosterone may be needed to maintain muscle in chronic exercisers so that basal testosterone or testosterone/cortisol ratios may be important. Concomitant catabolic effects of high cortisol levels (for example, in "overtraining syndrome") and inability of testosterone to prevent muscle breakdown could be contributory in this regard. Testosterone and growth hormone also interact in stimulating cardiac muscle hypertrophy: it is possible that significant lowering of testosterone levels could influence repair of cardiac muscle *(91)*.

The number of lower-limb injuries, particularly "shin splints" and stress fractures, has increased dramatically in the high-mileage runner *(92)*. Shin splints represent the effects of chronic mechanical stress on the bone with possible associated impairment of bone repair mechanisms. Maintenance of bone mass in men is at least in part dependent on circulating testosterone levels *(93)*. The declining testosterone levels associated with high-mileage runners particularly in the fourth and fifth decade of their lives raises the question of implications of the early development of osteoporosis in these men. Exercise in the well-nourished male runners may prevent age-related decreases in bone mineral content, but a case report has described osteoporotic fractures in a hypogonadal marathoner with anorexia nervosa *(94)*. Clearly, the anorexia is more significant, but the report raised the question of how much exercise-associated hypogonadism could produce a similar, if less dramatic, effect *(95)*.

It has been postulated that the physiological reduction in circulating testosterone levels could also be involved in lowered red blood cell manufacturing because of lowered erythropoietin and improvement in lipid profiles, reducing the risk of atherosclerotic heart disease *(96–99)*. Androgens may also be important in hepatic and renal function, in the brain, including effects on aggression, and in the immune system. Although there have been concerns over the normal functioning of the immune system in endurance-trained athletes, any effect of lowered, but still physiological serum testosterone levels on the immune system and hepatic and renal function remains speculative. Social and other pressures influence aggression, so that any short-term increases or longer-term reduction in serum testosterone levels would be likely to have little influence on mood and behavior. It is, therefore, unlikely that the reductions in circulating testosterone levels within the physiological range could play a significant role in any of these systems.

MECHANISMS OF EXERCISE-ASSOCIATED REDUCTIONS IN SERUM TESTOSTERONE LEVELS

The fall in serum testosterone levels must result from decreased production rates, decreased binding, or increased clearance. There is little evidence of decreased binding

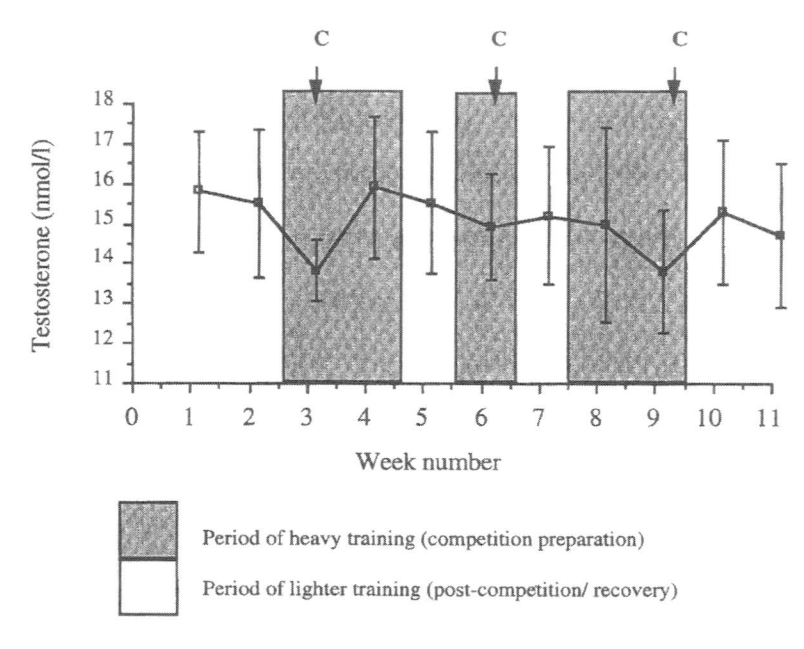

Fig. 2. Serum testosterone levels during periods of heavy and lighter training in teenage wrestlers.

(61). No studies have shown long-term increases in hepatic or extrahepatic clearance of testosterone in endurance-trained or other athletes, although basal estradiol clearance is increased in women athletes, presumably through increased hepatic metabolism *(100)*. Testicular tissue stimulated by HCG responds normally with an appropriate increase in testosterone *(49)*. Serum testosterone levels also increase in response to an acute exercise load in men with chronically low levels *(101)*. If testosterone levels fell because of increased hormone utilization by muscle, one might expect a compensatory gonadotropin increase to restore normal testicular androgenesis. Evidence has suggested a reduction in LH activity that could be responsible for the reductions in total and free testosterone associated with chronic involvement in running, but this has not been consistent in all studies. Evidence of altered LH pulsatile release in male runners is conflicting *(49,58,66,102,103)*. LH pulse frequency is not significantly altered in runners with exercise. GnRH-induced LH response appears to be impaired *(58)*. No evidence has supported increased opioidergic tone as being important in the generation of GnRH-LH suppression in athletes, but the effects of catecholamines have received little attention *(57,102)*. Chronic elevation of serum cortisol levels has been associated with overtraining, but cortisol levels are usually normal in male endurance-trained runners *(104)*. In contrast, both cyclists and wrestlers have increased serum levels and increased production rates, respectively *(75,76)*. The lack of elevation of cortisol would also suggest that CRH is not responsible for inhibition of serum testosterone levels. Serum prolactin levels are chronically depressed rather than elevated and, therefore, not likely involved in the change in testosterone in highly trained male runners *(61)*.

Suppression of the HPG axis in men is associated with starvation, vegetarian diet, and low-fat, high-fiber diet *(96,105,106)*. An anorectic subgroup with reduced total and free testosterone and a preoccupation with caloric intake and lean body mass was described among a group of 20 high-mileage runners *(62)*. The significant reductions in total and free testosterone in wrestlers during the season were associated with their practices in trying to "make weight." Within the season, as shown in Fig. 2, times of dietary and fluid restriction around competition were responsible for further loss of weight in wrestlers *(75)*. Although there were significant correlations among total and free testosterone and body weight and body fat in young male wrestlers, no correlation was observed between physiological reductions in serum testosterone levels and body fat in cross-sectional studies of runners and controls or in young wrestlers followed longitudinally *(61,75)*. A longitudinal study of sedentary individuals undergoing a 6-mo training schedule found that with running the initial dietary surplus was converted to a deficit as the running increased, but sedentary controls over the same time actually increased their surplus. Serum testosterone levels fell by some 30% over the 6 mo, and a regression analysis indicated that caloric deficit per kg of body weight was the most significant predictor of posttraining testosterone levels ($p < 0.05$) *(4)*. Other evidence in men has been published both supporting *(107)* and contradicting *(108)* this suggestion. Studies have generally been small, and well-designed studies remain to be completed.

It seems likely that chronic effects of endurance training on the HPG axis in men result from a mechanism of inhibition that is central and analogous to that described in women, perhaps involving a nutritional-metabolic influence. The possibility of peripheral effects of increased steroids utilization is worthy of further investigation. It is unlikely that clinical expression of reproductive suppression with training is common in men.

REFERENCES

1. Millette CF. Reproductive physiology in men. In: Seibel MM, ed. Infertility. A Comprehensive Text, 2nd ed. Appleton & Lange, Stamford, CT, 1997, pp. 221–251.
2. World Health Organisation. Collection and examination of human semen. In: WHO Laboratory Manual for the Examination of Human Semen and Semen-Cervical Mucus Interaction. 2nd ed. Cambridge University Press for the WHO, Cambridge, UK; 1987, pp. 3–15.
3. Leven RJ. Male factors contributing to the seasonality of human reproduction. In: Campbell KL, Wood JW, eds. Human Reproductive Ecology. Interaction of environment, fertility and behavior. Ann NY Acad Sci 1994;709:29–45.
4. Cumming DC, Wheeler GD. Exercise, training, and the male reproductive system. In: Bouchard C, Shephard RJ, Stephens T, eds. Physical Activity, Fitness, and Health. Human Kinetics Publishers, Champaign, IL, 1994, pp. 980–992.
5. Cumming DC, Brunsting LA III, Strich G, Greenberg L, Ries AL, Rebar RW. Reproductive hormone increases in response to acute exercise in men. Med Sci Sports Exerc 1986;18:369–373.
6. Fahey TD, Rolph R, Moongee P, Nagel J, Mortara S. Serum testosterone, body composition, and strength of young adults. Med Sci Sports Exerc 1976;1:31–34.
7. Galbo H, Hummer L, Petersen IB, Christensen NJ, Bie N. Thyroid and testicular hormone responses to graded and prolonged exercise in man. Eur J Appl Physiol 1977;36:101–106.
8. Gawel MJ, Park DM, Alaghband-Zadeh, J, Rose FC. Exercise and hormonal secretion. Postgrad Med J 1979;55:373–376.
9. Jezova D, Vigas M. Testosterone response to exercise during blockade and stimulation of adrenergic receptors in man. Horm Res 1981;15:141–147.
10. Karvonen J, Peltola E, Saarela J, Nieminen MM. Changes in running speed, blood lactic acid concentration and hormone balance during sprint training performed at an altitude of 1860 metres. J Sports Med Phys Fit 1990;30:122–126.
11. Kindermann W, Schnabel A, Schmitt WM, Biro G, Cassens J, Weber F. Catecholamines, growth hormone, cortisol, insulin and sex hormones in aerobic and anaerobic exercise. Eur J Appl Physiol 1982;49:389–399.

12. Kuoppasalmi K, Naveri H, Rehunen S, Harkonen M, Adlercreutz H. Effect of strenuous anaerobic running on plasma growth hormone, cortisol, luteinizing hormone, testosterone, androstenedione and estrone and estradiol. J Steroid Biochem 1976;7:823–829.
13. Kuopposalmi K. Plasma testosterone and sex-hormone-binding capacity in physical exercise. Scand J Clin Lab Invest 1980;40:411–418.
14. Schmid P, Pusch PP, Wolf WW, Pilger E, Pessenhofer H, Schwaberger G, et al. Serum FSH, LH and testosterone in humans after physical exercise. Int J Sports Med 1982;3:84–89.
15. Sutton JR, Coleman MJ, Casey J, Lazarus L. Androgen responses during physical exercise. Br Med J 1973:i:520–522.
16. Vogel RB, Books CA, Ketchum C, Zauner CW, Murray FT. Increase of free and total testosterone during submaximal exercise in normal males. Med Sci Sports Exerc 1984;17:119–123.
17. Wilkerson JE, Horvath SM, Gutin B. Plasma testosterone during treadmill exercise. J Appl Physiol 1980;49:249–253.
18. Cumming DC, Wall SR, Quinney HA, Belcastro AN. Decrease in serum testosterone levels with maximal intensity swimming exercise in trained male and female swimmers. Endocr Res 1987; 13:31–41.
19. Gotshalk LA, Loebel CC, Nindl BC, Putukian M, Sebastianelli WJ, Newton RU, et al. Hormonal responses of multiset versus single-set heavy-resistance exercise protocols. Can J Appl Physiol 1997;22:244–255.
20. Duclos M, Corcuff JB, Rashedi M, Fougere V, Manier G. Does functional alteration of the gonadotropic axis occur in endurance trained athletes during and after exercise? A preliminary study. Eur J Appl Physiol Occup Physiol 1996;73:427–433.
21. Hackney AC, Premo MC, McMurray RG. Influence of aerobic versus anaerobic exercise on the relationship between reproductive hormones in men. J Sports Sci 1995;13:305–311.
22. Volek JS, Kraemer WJ, Bush JA, Incledon T, Boetes M. Testosterone and cortisol in relationship to dietary nutrients and resistance exercise. J Appl Physiol 1997;82:49–54.
23. Hoffman JR, Falk B, Radom-Isaac S, Weinstein Y, Magazanik A, Wang Y. The effect of environmental temperature on testosterone and cortisol responses to high intensity, intermittent exercise in humans. Eur J Appl Physiol Occup Physiol 1997;75:83–87.
24. Sakamoto K, Wakabayashi I, Yoshimoto S, Masui H, Katsuno S. Effects of physical exercise and cold stimulation on serum testosterone level in men. Nipp Eiseigaku Zasshi—Jpn J Hyg 1991;46:635–638.
25. Hoffman JR, Maresh CM, Armstrong LE, Gabaree CL, Bergeron MF, Kenefick RW, et al. Effects of hydration state on plasma testosterone, cortisol and catecholamine concentrations before and during mild exercise at elevated temperature. Eur J Appl Physiol Occup Physiol 1994;69:294–300.
26. Zmuda JM, Thompson PD, Winters SJ. Exercise increases serum testosterone and sex hormone-binding globulin levels in older men. Metab Clin Exp 1996;45:935–939.
27. Hakkinen K, Pakarinen A. Acute hormonal responses to heavy resistance exercise in men and women at different ages. Int J Sports Med 1995;16:507–513.
28. Nicklas BJ, Ryan AJ, Treuth MM, Harman SM, Blackman MR, Hurley BF. Testosterone, growth hormone and IGF-I responses to acute and chronic resistive exercise in men aged 55–70 years. Int J Sports Med 1995;16:445–450.
29. Schmid P, Pusch PP, Wolf WW, Pilger E, Pessenhofer H, Schwaberger G, et al. Serum FSH, LH and testosterone in humans after physical exercise. Int J Sports Med 1982;3:84–89.
30. Metivier G, Gauthier R, de la Chevotriere J, Grymala D. The effect of acute exercise on the serum levels of testosterone and luteinizing (LH) hormone in human male athletes. J Sports Med Phys Fit 1980;20:235–237.
31. Cadoux-Hudson TA, Few JD, Imms FJ. The effect of exercise on the production and clearance of testosterone in well trained young men. Eur J Appl Physiol 1985;54:321–325.
32. Sutton JR, Coleman MJ, Casey JH. Testosterone production rate during exercise. In: Landry F, Orban WAR, eds. 3rd International Symposium on Biochemistry of Exercise. Symposium Specialists, Miami, FL, 1978, pp. 227–234.
33. Kuopposalmi K, Naveri H, Harkonen N, Adlerkreutz H. Plasma cortisol, a'dione, testosterone and luteinizing hormone in running exercise of various intensities. Scand J Clin Lab Invest 1980;40: 403–409.
34. Mathur DN, Toriola, AL, Dada OA. Serum cortisol and testosterone levels in conditioned male distance runners and non-athletes after maximal exercise. J Sports Med Phys Fit 1986;26:245–250.

35. McConnell TR, Sinning WE. Exercise and temperature effects on human sperm production and testosterone levels. Med Sci Sports Exerc 1984;16:51–55.
36. Urhausen A, Kinderman W. Behaviour of testosterone, sex hormone binding globulin (SHBG) and cortisol before and after a triathlon. Int J Sports Med 1987;8:305–308.
37. Burke CW, Anderson DC. Sex hormone binding globulin is an estrogen amplifier. Nature 1972;240: 38–40.
38. Levin J, Lloyd CW, Lobotsky J, Friedrich EH. The effect of epinephrine on testosterone production. Acta Endocrinol 1967;55:184–192.
39. Jezova D, Vigas M. Testosterone response to exercise during blockade and stimulation of adrenergic receptors in man. Horm Res 1981;15:141–147.
40. Kindermann W, Schnabel A, Schmitt WM, Biro G, Hippchen M. Catecholamine, STH, cortisol, glucagon, insulin und sexualhormone bei korperlicher belastung und beta1-blockade. Klin Wohenschr 1982;60:505–512, 525.
41. Wheeler G, Cumming D, Burnham R, Maclean I, Slolely BD, Bhambhani Y, et al. Testosterone, cortisol and catecholamine responses to exercise stress and autonomic dysreflexia in elite quadriplegic athletes. Paraplegia 1994;32:292–299.
42. Wheeler GD, Ashley EA, Harber V, Laskin JJ, Olenik LM, Sloley D, et al. Hormonal responses to graded-resistance, FES-assisted strength training in spinal cord-injured. Spinal Cord 1996;34:264–267.
43. Berchtold P, Berger M, Cuppers HJ, Herrmann J, Nieschlag E, Rudorff K, et al. Non-glucoregulatory hormones (T4, T3, rT3, TSH, testosterone) during physical exercise in juvenile-type diabetics. Horm Metab Res 1978:10:269–273.
44. de Lignieres B, Plas J-N, Commandre F, Morville R, Viani J-L, Plas F. Secretion testiculaire d'androgenes apres effort physique prolongue chez l'homme. La Nouv Presse Med 1976;5: 2060–2064.
45. Dessypris K, Adlercreutz H. Plasma cortisol, testosterone, androstenedione and luteinizing hormone (LH) in a non-competitive marathon run. J Steroid Biochem 1976;7:33–37.
46. Hakkinen K, Pakarinen A, Alen M, Kauhanen H, Komi PV. Neuromuscular and hormonal responses in elite athletes to two successive strength training sessions in one day. Eur J Appl Physiol 1988;57: 133–139.
47. Johansson C, Tsai L, Hultman E, Tegelman R, Pousette A. Restoration of anabolic deficit and muscle glycogen consumption in competitive orienteering. Int J Sports Med 1990;11:204–207.
48. Keizer H, Janssen GM, Menheere P, Kranenburg G. Changes in basal plasma testosterone, cortisol, and dehydroepiandrosterone sulfate in previously untrained males and females preparing for a marathon. Int J Sports Med 1989;10(Suppl. 3):S139–S145.
49. MacConnie SE, Barkan A, Lampman RM, Schork MA, Beitins IZ. Decreased hypothalamic gonadotropin releasing hormone secretion in male marathon runners. N Engl J Med 1986;315:411–417.
50. Mateev G, Djarova T, Ilkov A, Sachanska T, Klissurov L. Hormonal and cardiorespiratory changes following simulated saturation dives to 4 and 11 ATA. Undersea Biomed Res 1990;17:1–11.
51. Morville R, Pesquies PC, Guezzenec CY, Serrurier BD, Guignard M. Plasma variations in testicular and adrenal androgens during prolonged physical exercise in man. Ann d'Endocrinol 1979;40:501–510.
52. Schurmeyer T, Jung K, Nieschlag E. The effects of an 1100 kilometer run on testicular adrenal and thyroid hormones. Int J Androl 1984:7:276–282.
53. Tanaka H, Cleroux J, de Champlain J, Ducharme JR, Collu RJ. Persistent effects of a marathon run on the pituitary–testicular axis. Endocrinol Invest 1986;9:97–101.
54. Tegelman R, Carlstrom K, Pousette A. Hormone levels in male ice hockey players during the night after a 26-hour cup tournament. Andrologia 1990;22:261–268.
55. Urhausen A, Kinderman W. Behaviour of testosterone, sex hormone binding globulin (SHBG) and cortisol before and after a triathlon. Int J Sports Med 1987;8:305–308.
56. Webb ML, Wallace JP, Hamill C, Hodgson JL, Mashaly MM. Serum testosterone concentration during two hours of moderate intensity treadmill running in trained men and women Endocr Res 1984;10:27–38.
57. Elias AN, Fairshter R, Pandian MR, Domurat E, Kayaleh R. Beta-endorphin/beta-lipotropin release and gonadotropin secretion after acute exercise in physically conditioned males. Eur J Appl Physiol 1989;58:522–527.
58. McColl EM, Wheeler GD, Gomes P, Bhambhani Y, Cumming DC. The effects of acute exercise on LH pulsatile release in high mileage male runners. Clin Endocrinol 1989;31:617–629.

59. Kujala UM, Alen M, Huhtaniemi IT. Gonadotrophin-releasing hormone and human chorionic gonadotrophin tests reveal that both hypothalamic and testicular endocrine functions are suppressed during acute prolonged physical exercise. Clin Endocrinol 1990;33:219–225.
60. Cumming DC, Quigley ME, Yen SSC. Acute suppression of circulating testosterone levels by cortisol in man. J Clin Endocrinol Metab 1983;57:671–673.
61. Wheeler GD, Wall SR, Belcastro AN, Cumming DC. Reduced serum testosterone and prolactin levels in male distance runners. JAMA 1984;252:514–516.
62. Ayers JWT, Komesu Y, Romain T, Ansbacher RA. Anthropometric, hormonal and psychologic correlates of semen quality in endurance trained male athletes. Fertil Steril 1985;43:917–921.
63. Frey MAB, Doerr BM, Srivastava LM, Glueck CJ. Exercise training, sex hormones and lipoprotein relationships in men. J Appl Physiol 1983;54:757–762.
64. Hackney AC, Sinning WE, Bruot BC. Reproductive hormonal profiles of endurance-trained and untrained males. Med Sci Sports Exerc 1988;2:60–65.
65. Hackney AC, Sinning WE, Bruot BC. Hypothalamic-pituitary-testicular axis function in endurance-trained males. Int J Sports Med 1990;11:98–103.
66. Wheeler GD, Singh M, Pierce WD, Epling WF, Cumming DC. Endurance training decreases serum testosterone levels in men without change in LH pulsatile release. J Clin Endocrinol Metab 1991;72:422–425.
67. Wheeler GD, Wall SR, Belcastro AN, Conger P, Cumming DC. (1986) Are anorexic tendencies prevalent in the habitual runner? Brit J Sportsmed 1986;20:77–81.
68. Morville R, Pesquies PC, Guezzenec CY, Serrurier BD, Guignard M. Plasma variations in testicular and adrenal androgens during prolonged physical exercise in man. Ann d'Endocrinol 1979;40:501–510.
69. Hakkinen K, Keskinen KL, Alen M, Komi PV, Kauhanen H. Serum hormone concentrations during prolonged training in elite endurance-trained and strength-trained athletes. Eur J Appl Physiol 1989;59:233–238.
70. Craig BW, Brown R, Everhart J. Effects of progressive resistance training on growth hormone and testosterone levels in young and elderly subjects. Mech Aging Dev 1989;49:159–169.
71. Hakkinen K, Pakarinen A, Alen M, Kauhanen H, Komi PV. Relationships between training volume, physical performance capacity and serum hormone concentrations during prolonged weight training in elite weight lifters. Int J Sports Med 1987;8(Suppl.):61–65.
72. Hakkinen K, Pakarinen A. Serum hormones in male strength athletes during intensive short term strength training. Eur J Appl Physiol 1991;63:194–199.
73. Urhausen A, Kullmer T, Kindermann W. A 7-week follow-up study of the behaviour of testosterone and cortisol during the competition period in rowers. Eur J Appl Physiol 1987;56:528–533.
74. Strauss RH, Lanese RR, Malarkey WB. Weight loss in amateur wrestlers and its effect on testosterone levels. JAMA 1985;254:3337,3338.
75. Wheeler GD, McFadyen SG, Symbaluk D, Pierce WD, Cumming DC. The Effects of training on serum testosterone and cortisol levels in wrestlers. Clin J Sports Med 1992;2:257–260.
76. Neary JP, Wheeler GD, McLean I, Cumming DC, Quinney HA. Urinary free cortisol as an indicator of exercise training stress. Clin J Sports Med 1994;4:160–165.
77. Arce JC, De Sousa MJ, Pescatello LS, Luciano AA. Subclinical alterations in hormone and semen orifile in athletes. Fertil Steril 1993;59:398–404.
78. Remes K, Kuopposalmi K, Adlercreutz H. Effects of longterm physical training on plasma testosterone, androstenedione, luteinizing hormone, sex hormone binding globulin capacity. Scand J Clin Lab Invest 1979;39:743–749.
79. Johnson CC, Stone MH, Byrd RJ, Lopez SA. The response of serum lipids and plasma androgens to weight training exercise in sedentary males. J Sports Med Phys Fit 1983;23:39–44.
80. Mendoza SG, Carrasco H, Zerpa A, Briceno Y, Rodriguez F, Speirs J, et al. Effect of physical training on lipids, lipoproteins, apolipoproteins, lipases, and endogenous sex hormones in men with premature myocardial infarction. Metabolism 1991;40:368–377.
81. Peltonen P, Marniemi J, Hietanen E, Vuori I, Enholm C. Changes in serum lipids, lipoproteins and heparin releasable lipolytic enzymes during moderate physical training in man, a longitudinal study. Metabolism 1981;30:518–526.
82. Bagatell CJ, Bremner WJ. Sperm counts and reproductive hormones in male marathoners and lean controls. Fertil Steril 1990;53:688–692.
83. Roberts AC, McClure RD, Weiner RL, Brooks GA. Overtraining affects males reproductive status. Fertil Steril 1993;60:686–692.

84. Baker ER, Leuker R, Stumpf PG. Relationship of exercise to semen parameters and fertility success of artificial insemination donors. Fertil Steril 1984;41:107S(abstract).
85. Baker ER, Stevens C, Leuker R. Relationship of exercise to semen parameters and fertility success of artificial insemination donors. JSC Med Assoc 1988;84:580–582.
86. Cumming DC, Wheeler GD, McColl EM. The effects of exercise on reproductive function in men. Sports Med 1989;7:1–17.
87. Editorial. Special survey. Running and Sex. The Runner. 1982;May:26–35.
88. White JR, Case DA, McWhirter D, Mattison AM. Enhanced sexual behavior in exercising men. Arch Sex Behav 1990;19:193–209.
89. Crawford EG, Gilmore D, James WH. Running in the family. Nature 1992;357:272.
90. Dohm GL, Louis TM. Changes in androstenedione, testosterone and protein metabolism as a result of exercise. Proc Soc Exp Biol Med 1978;158:622–625.
91. Mooradian AD, Morley JE, Korenman SG. Biological actions of androgens. Endocr Rev 1987; 8:1–28.
92. Stanish W. Overuse injuries in athletes, a perspective. Med Sci Sports Exerc 1984;16:1–7.
93. Foresta C, Ruzza G, Mioni R, Guarneri G, Gribaldo R, Meneghello A, et al. Osteoporosis and decline of gonadal function in the elderly man. Horm Res 1984;19:18–22.
94. Rigotti NA, Neer RM, Jameson L. Osteopenia and bone fractures in a man with anorexia nervosa and hypogonadism. JAMA 1986;256:385–388.
95. Riggs BL. Exercise, hypogonadism and osteopenia. JAMA 1986;256:392,393.
96. Enger S, Herbjornsen K, Erikssen P, Fretland A. High density lipoproteins and physical activity, the influence of physical exercise, age and smoking on HDL-cholesterol and the HDL/total cholesterol ratio. Scand J Clin Lab Invest 1977;37:251–255.
97. Hartung GH, Foreyt JP, Mitchell RE, Vlasek I, Gotto AM. Relation of diet to high-density-lioprotein cholesterol in middle aged marathon runners, joggers and inactive men. N Engl J Med 1980;302: 357–361.
98. Kantor MA, Cullinane EM, Herbert PN, Thompson PD. Acute increase in lipoprotein lipase following prolonged exercise. Metabolism 1984;33:454–457.
99. Schriewer H, Jung K, Gunnewiig V, Assmann G. Serum lipids and lipoproteins during a twenty day run of 1,100 kilometers. Ann Sports Med 1983;1:71–74.
100. Keizer HA, Doorfman J, Bunnik GSJ. Influence of physical exercise on sex hormone metabolism. Med Sci Sports Exerc 1980;48:765–769.
101. Hackney AC, Fahrner CL, Stupnicki R. Exp Clin Endocrinol Diabetes 1997;105:291–295.
102. Rogol AD, Veldhuis JD, Williams FA, Johnson ML. Pulsatile secretion of gonadotropins and prolactin in male marathon runners. Relation to the endogenous opiate system. J Androl 1984;5:21–27.
103. Jensen CE, Wiswedel K, McLoughlin J, van dey Spuy Z. Prospective study of of hormonal and semen profiles of marathon runners. Fertil Steril 1995;64:1189–1196.
104. Adlercreutz H, Harkonen M, Kuopposalmi K, Naveri H, Huhtaniemi H, Tikkanen H, et al. Effect of training on plasma anabolic and catabolic steroid hormones and their responses during physical exercise. Int J Sports Med 1986;7(Suppl.):27,28.
105. Hamalainen EK, Adlercreutz H, Puska P, Pietinen P. Decrease of serum total and free testosterone during a low-fat high fibre diet. J Steroid Biochem 1983;18:369,370.
106. Zubiran S, Gomez-Mont F. Endocrine disturbance in chronic human malnutrition. Vitam Horm 1952;11:97–102.
107. Thompson JL, Manore MM, Skinner JS, Revussin, Spraul M. Daily energy expenditure in male endurance athletes with differing energy intakes. Med Sci Sports Exerc 1995;27:347–354.
108. Sjodin AM, Andersson AB, Hogberg JM, Westerterp KR. Energy balance in cross country skiers: a study using doubly labelled water. Med Sci Sports Exerc 1994;26:720–724.

8 Exercise and the Hypothalamus
Ovulatory Adaptations

Moira A. Petit, BA, MS, PhD, and Jerilynn C. Prior, BA, MD, FRCPC

CONTENTS
INTRODUCTION
THE OVULATORY CYCLE
HYPOTHALAMIC ADAPTATION AND OVULATORY FUNCTION
ADAPTATIONS TO EXERCISE TRAINING
CLINICAL APPLICATIONS/TREATMENT
CONCLUSIONS
REFERENCES

INTRODUCTION

As early as 1939, Hans Selye, who later received the Nobel prize for work on the endocrinology of the adaptation response, reported that muscular exercise was often a cause for "menstrual irregularities" in women *(1)*. Selye performed controlled animal experiments showing that whether or not exercise suppresses reproduction depends on the abruptness of exercise onset *(1)*. Forty years later, Shangold et al. *(2)* published the first prospective observational study documenting gradual shortening of the luteal-phase length with increased running activity in one woman with regular menstrual cycles. Despite these early observations indicating that subtle alterations of ovulatory function occur within cycles of normal length, the exercise science literature has since focused on the absence (amenorrhea) or presence (eumenorrhea) of menstrual flow in women athletes. The purpose of this chapter is to review the subtle (and clinically important) ovulatory changes in response to exercise.

Hundreds of cross-sectional studies report "athletic amenorrhea," and inappropriately imply causal relationships between loss of flow and exercise. However, better-designed prospective studies observing normally ovulatory women and closely examining ovulatory function during progressively increasing exercise (subsequently termed "exercise training") show only subclinical changes and no amenorrhea when exercise training is the only stressor *(3–5)*. Prevalent but subtle changes in ovulatory function are the first

From: *Contemporary Endocrinology: Sports Endocrinology*
Edited by: M. P. Warren and N. W. Constantini © Humana Press Inc., Totowa, NJ

and most subtle hypothalamic adaptation to exercise training *(2,6)*. Failure of hypothalamic adaptation in response to intense stressors such as starvation, psychological distress, illness, or rapidly increasing exercise, results in significant disability. Overwhelming stress associated with excessive exercise training (Chapter 20) and extreme nutritional imbalance (Chapter 9) are discussed elsewhere in this volume.

In this chapter, we describe the subtle alterations in ovulatory function that occur as a result of hypothalamic adaptation (rather than failure to adapt) to exercise training and other "stressors." We will also discuss the consequences of ovulatory disturbances, including infertility and a negative bone balance. Before beginning that discussion, however, it is necessary to define both the language and the physiological processes of ovulation.

THE OVULATORY CYCLE

The words used to describe the release of an egg and the hormonal characteristics of a cycle in which that occurs need to be defined and described because both are usually obscured by the persuasive, yet unfounded expectation that regular cycles are normally ovulatory. We will start by defining the language of reproduction.

Terminology

In the exercise science literature, women are commonly classified as eumenorrheic if their menstrual flow occurs monthly, or oligo/amenorrheic if flow is sporadic or has been absent for three or more months *(7)*. However, cycles of normal length can also be described by their luteal phase or ovulatory characteristics. Ovulatory and cycle interval characteristics form a complex continuum (Fig. 1). This starts with the most normal cycle type, which is ovulatory with a normal luteal-phase length of 10–16 d and a normal cycle length of 21–36 d *(8)*. This spectrum ends with the most disturbed ovarian function, which is amenorrhea, the absence of flow for six or more months. Between these extremes, cycles that are normal in length may have a short (<10 d) or insufficient (normal length, but low progesterone) luteal phase, or be anovulatory. Anovulatory cycles are ones in which cycle intervals may be short, normal, or long, but no egg is released and progesterone levels never exceed 16 nmol/L (5 ng/mL).

DEFINITIONS

Given the importance of clarity in science, it is useful to define the terms meant to describe cycle types when ovulatory status is not known. Eumenorrhea implies menstrual cycles that are normal in length, with flow occurring each 21–36 d *(9)*. When a woman's flow occurs between 36 and 180 d, the term oligomenorrhea is appropriate. For cycle lengths longer than 180 d, women are classified as experiencing amenorrhea. Cycles of varying and abnormal lengths are called "cycle disturbances."

The words used to describe the ovulatory characteristics of a cycle are nearly independent of cycle intervals. Cycles are defined as having short luteal-phase lengths if ovulation occurs but the time from ovulation to the day before the start of flow (luteal phase) is < 10 d by quantitative basal temperature analysis *(8,10)*, or <12 d using the midcycle luteinizing hormone (LH) peak as the indicator of luteal-phase onset. An inadequate or insufficient luteal phase means ovulation occurs and luteal-phase length is normal, but progesterone levels during the luteal phase are lower than the usual midluteal peak progesterone level of 45 nmol/L. If ovulation and subsequent corpus luteal forma-

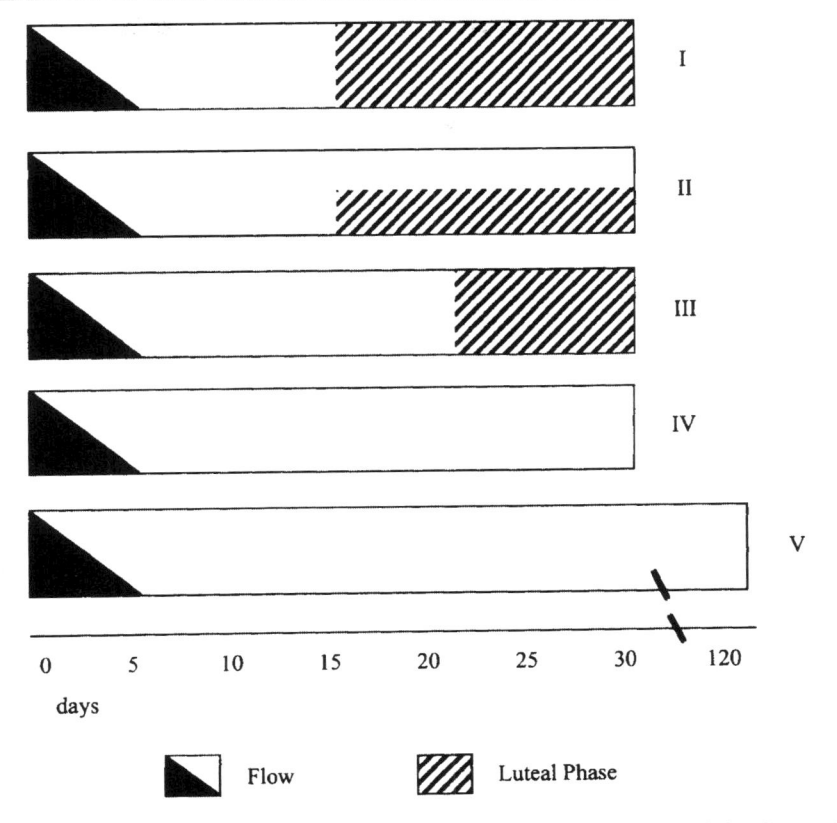

Fig. 1. A spectrum of cycle types starting at the top with the most normal, which is of normal length and ovulatory with a normal luteal-phase length. The next cycle is also of normal length and ovulatory, but has an insufficient but normal-length luteal phase. The third cycle, also of normal length, illustrates a short luteal-phase cycle. The fourth cycle is an anovulatory cycle of normal length, and the final cycle is a anovulatory cycle that is longer than normal in cycle length (oligomenorrhea).

tion do not occur, the cycle is anovulatory. Therefore, anovulation refers to cycles in which no eggs are formed (and released). "Subtle disturbances of ovulation" refers to cycles that are normal in length, but have either a short or inadequate luteal phase or are anovulatory. "Ovulatory disturbance" is a general term that includes the range of abnormal ovulatory characteristics, including short and inadequate luteal phase and anovulatory cycles, and generally implies that the cycle length is normal. Cycles that are irregular or abnormal in length and about which ovulatory characteristics are unknown should be termed "cycle disturbances," and include polymenorrhea (cycles shorter in interval than 21 d) as well as oligomenorrhea and amenorrhea.

IMPRECISE LANGUAGE ABOUT REPRODUCTION

There are several problems with classifying women as eumenorrheic. The term has recently been applied to women who "experienced at least 10 menstrual periods per year" *(11)*, even though this would give average cycle lengths of 36.5 d (which are abnormally long) and should be described as "oligomenorrhea." Another difficulty with the term eumenorrheic is that it presumes that all cycles of normal length display the same ovulatory and hormonal characteristics. Data from our 1-yr prospective study in ovulatory women of varying exercise habits *(4)* show that normal-length cycles can as easily be anovulatory as ovulatory. In that study, all of the anovulatory cycles were normal in length. Therefore, a further erroneous assumption often made in the literature is that only long or short cycles are hormonally abnormal.

The term "ovulatory" menstrual cycle is also often misused. Researchers often assume a woman is ovulatory if she reports that her cycles are normal in length and regular. Likewise, the term "anovulation" is commonly used as a synonym for amenorrhea, because women whose periods have stopped (unless they have become pregnant or have had a hysterectomy) are not ovulating.

Classifying women only by their cycle intervals implies that the reproductive system works in an on–off manner, rather than displaying the broad spectrum of potential responses described above. Classification of women's cycles needs to include the entire range of cycle types, because a distinctly different hormonal profile is present in each case. The variability and hormonal physiology of cycles, even those of normal length, are important to understand.

Physiology

Just as cycles vary in interval and ovulatory characteristics, so does the cascade of signals from the hypothalamic gonadotrophin-releasing hormone (GnRH) nucleus to the pituitary gonadotrophin-producing cells. Pituitary messages to the ovarian follicle also change, as do hormones from the ovary that give feedback to the pituitary and the hypothalamus. What follows is an effort to clarify the cycle manifestations of the hypothalamic changes described in earlier chapters.

OVARIAN HORMONE LEVELS DURING THE NORMAL CYCLE

An ovulatory menstrual cycle is characterized by systematic and major changes in the levels of estrogen prior to ovulation (follicular phase) and variations of both estrogen and progesterone postovulation (luteal phase). Follicular-phase estradiol levels during and just after flow average 60–200 pmol/L (levels that are similar to those in children and men). Estradiol levels subsequently rise over the next 7–18 d to a peak just prior to ovulation that is, on average, 220% above the follicular phase baseline *(12)*. There is then a decrease to about 100% above baseline for most of the luteal phase before estradiol levels again return to baseline just prior to menstruation *(12)*. In contrast, progesterone levels, which remain low during the follicular phase (approx 0.5 nmol/L, similar to levels in children and men) increase after ovulation to over 1400% of follicular-phase baseline values. Progesterone levels remain elevated over 1000% above baseline during the 10–16 d of active hormonal production by one corpus luteum *(12)*.

The production of estradiol and progesterone is coordinated by, and ultimately dependent on, the timing and magnitude of GnRH pulsatility in the hypothalamus. GnRH stimulates the gonadotrophins, LH and follicle-stimulating hormone (FSH), to be released from the pituitary. LH peaks at midcycle, and directly triggers follicle rupture and egg release. FSH plays an important role in recruiting intermediate-sized follicles and stimulating the dominant follicle that eventually ovulates. In addition, FSH increases LH receptors on ovarian granulosa cells. GnRH, LH, and FSH are all in feedback regulation by ovarian estradiol and progesterone levels. Also, FSH production is actively suppressed by inhibin, a polypeptide hormone whose probably important role in reproductive physiology is still poorly understood *(13)*.

HORMONAL PROFILE CHANGES DURING DISTURBED CYCLES

Hormonal characteristics of cycles that are abnormal in length will be briefly discussed followed by the hormonal characteristics of cycles that are abnormal in ovulatory characteristics. Although few studies have systematically measured estradiol levels in cycles that are short or long, the generalization that shorter cycles have higher estradiol levels is supported by a study in which hormone levels were measured daily during 68 cycles *(14)*. That study documents that shorter follicular-phase lengths are associated with statistically higher estradiol levels. The logic of this observation is that the more estradiol stimulation of the endometrium, the more likely it is to shed causing bleeding. The opposite is true of long cycles—less estradiol stimulation of the endometrium leads to delayed shedding and flow.

The hormonal characteristics of cycles with disturbed ovulation are less clear. The common feature of all disturbed cycles is the lower amount and/or duration of progesterone production. Estrogen and androgen productions are highly variable in individuals with ovulatory disturbances. Evidence for high estrogen levels with anovulatory cycles is most clearly found in studies of women shortly after puberty *(15)* and in perimenopausal women before menopause *(16)*. In both instances, estrogen levels exceed the midcycle peak equivalent levels for prolonged periods of time. Androgen excess, which is associated with anovulation, is also associated with high estradiol levels *(17)*, obesity, insulin resistance, and varying hirsutism.

Evidence that estradiol levels may be normal in anovulatory cycles comes from our observational prospective study *(4)*. In that group of initially ovulatory women (in whom perimenopause and androgen excess were excluded), the cycles without ovulation were normal in length, and the women who had entirely normal ovulation did not differ in mean estradiol level (measured twice in two cycles a year apart) from the women who experienced anovulation. This flies in the face of the expectation that cycles with disturbed ovulation will have low estradiol levels as had been observed in four women studied by Sherman and Korenman *(18)*. Sowers et al. also have reported low midfollicular estradiol levels in premenopausal women with disturbed ovulation *(19)*. However, several other authors in addition to ourselves have not observed consistently low estradiol levels associated with anovulation *(20,21)*.

In summary, disturbances of cycle interval are often associated with abnormally low or high estradiol levels (inversely related to cycle length), but ovulatory disturbances may have high, normal, or low estradiol levels and rates of production.

Documentation of Ovulatory Function

This section describes the currently available methods for documenting ovulatory function and the advantages and disadvantages of each. Our primary focus will be to describe the use of quantitative basal temperature (QBT), which we have found to be the best available method for continuous, longitudinal monitoring of ovulatory function.

CURRENTLY USED INDIRECT METHODS

All of the currently available methods for assessing ovulation are indirect, except actual visualization of extrusion of a secondary oocyte from the ovary. Because ovulation requires an LH surge and progesterone levels do not rise if ovulation does not occur, serum or urinary measures of the midcycle LH peak and/or progesterone levels are often used as indicators of ovulation. One method is to perform serial samples of serum or urine daily during the midcycle to detect the LH peak. Alternatively, in the week prior to menses, serum (or plasma) samples showing levels of progesterone above 16 nmol/L (5 ng/mL) are indicative of ovulation. The postovulatory increase in progesterone can also be measured in spots of whole blood *(22)*, urine *(23)*, or saliva *(24)*, or by its effect to increase the basal temperature or to inhibit the elasticity of cervical mucus (although this latter effect has not been scientifically evaluated to date).

An estradiol peak is necessary to trigger the midcycle LH peak. Therefore, another indirect assessment of ovulation involves collecting estradiol levels daily with serum samples. Samples must be taken until an estradiol level double the preceding level and over 750 pmol/L is documented. However, midcycle peak estradiol levels may occur and not be followed by an LH peak or by ovulation in premenopausal (as in perimenopausal) women *(21,25,26)*. Therefore, an estradiol peak level is not a specific test of ovulation. To a lesser degree, the same lack of specificity is also true of an LH peak *(26)*.

LIMITATIONS OF AVAILABLE METHODS FOR DIAGNOSIS OF OVULATION DISTURBANCES

Serial sampling of blood, saliva, or urine is required to document adequately all of the important ovulatory characteristics (including whether ovulation occurred, as well as luteal-phase adequacy and length) of a single cycle. Using these methods to document several consecutive cycles is very labor-intensive, invasive, expensive, and imposes a high degree of burden on the participating woman. Continuous longitudinal documentation of hormone levels in large numbers of women is, therefore, virtually impossible to obtain using these sampling techniques *(3,5,26)*. Similarly, although formerly endometrial biopsy analysis to show the histological changes related to progesterone was considered to be a gold standard for luteal-phase adequacy and length, it has a ± 2-d SD and is not useful *(27)*. In addition, although gynecologists commonly describe endometrial biopsies as a minor procedure, they are invasive and uncomfortable (and women who have had one often attempt to avoid a second!). Finally, vaginal or abdominal serial ultrasound assessments (to show a growing follicular cyst that enlarges to over 18 mm and then disappears) are considered reasonably accurate indicators of the occurrence of ovulation *(28)*, but they are impractical because they are uncomfortable for women, require expensive equipment and complex scheduling, and are expensive for long-term prospective research.

The logical question is: why not measure ovulatory characteristics during one cycle and then just monitor cycle intervals over the necessary period of time? Could you not infer that the subsequent cycles, if they are regular and normal in length, are similar in ovulatory status? That would be an accurate strategy if women's cycles were as stable in ovulatory characteristics as they are in cycle interval. However, ovulatory characteristics are highly variable over time within women *(4,8,29,30)*. For example, Hinney et al. *(29)* documented "corpus luteum insufficiency" by a late-luteal-phase progesterone level below 25 nmol/L in 109 women of whom only 55, when tested in the following cycle, continued to show corpus luteum insufficiency. Likewise, 5 yr after our intensive monitoring of continuous cycles for 1 yr in 66 women, cycle lengths (in 3 cycles) correlated well with previous ones ($r = 0.68$, $p < 0.05$), but luteal-phase lengths correlated considerably less well ($r = 0.39$, $p = < 0.05$) *(30)*.

Furthermore, as this chapter will subsequently document, ovulatory disturbances caused by hypothalamic adaptation occur rapidly and as quickly revert to normal ovulation. Thus, studies that measure ovulatory characteristics in only a few cycles or monitor cycles discontinuously (such as every other or every fourth cycle) are not likely to detect ovulatory disturbances (in general) and particularly not likely to document those related to hypothalamic adaptation to exercise. That is especially true if cycle characteristics are documented only in the cycle before exercise intensity is again increased, as has been done in two important prospective studies *(3,5)*.

At least 6 mo of continuous sampling, in which both ovulation and luteal-phase length are assessed, are necessary to characterize adequately a sedentary, weight-stable woman's menstrual and ovulatory characteristics *(31)*. In exercising women, it is even more critical to provide a robust baseline from which to examine potential changes associated with exercise training. For all of these reasons, a noninvasive, inexpensive, and habit-forming method for documenting ovulatory characteristics is necessary.

QUANTITATIVE BASAL TEMPERATURE (QBT)

Daily basal (meaning first thing after wakening in the morning, fasting, and when metabolism is stable) oral temperatures (often referred to as BBT) potentially allow continuous, longitudinal research into ovulatory characteristics to be conducted in large populations. High levels of progesterone during the luteal phase increase the basal temperature. This increase begins to be significant approx 24–48 h after the LH peak *(10)*. A monophasic set of basal temperatures during one cycle in which our least-squares program (Maximina®) detects no significant shift characterizes an anovulatory cycle with progesterone levels that do not rise sufficiently to alter temperatures. A biphasic cycle is indicative of ovulation, and the day of the significant temperature shift can be used to define the onset of the luteal phase *(10)*. In ovulatory cycles, the increased progesterone levels raise the basal temperature during the luteal phase by approx 0.3°C.

However, BBT was a clinical tool before it was a research method. Therefore, the early studies utilizing BBT as a method of detecting ovulation had a number of problems, including that women might take their temperature at different times of day, women had difficulties reading or shaking down the older mercury thermometers, women were expected to plot their own temperatures as a graph (which caused common inaccuracies of graphing), and the temperature patterns were evaluated for the presence or absence of ovulation using nonquantitative methods and often "eyeball" or equally nonreproducible methods *(32)*. Finally, even when more systematic methods of assessing changes in temperatures were described *(33)*, insufficient data relating the temperature shift to hormonal data were available.

In our laboratory, these problems have been solved by better instruction of women about what, in addition to fever, alters the basal temperature (such as wakening earlier or later than usual, or being up in the night) and providing a form on which to record these factors. In addition, we asked them to take their temperature with a digital thermometer reading to two decimal places and to record temperatures in a list, rather than plotting them on a graph. We then devised and applied a computer program (Maximina®) of least-square analysis to each cycle of temperature data and showed it to be valid against the independently assessed serum LH peak ($r = 0.88$) *(10)*. This more scientific method we term QBT to differentiate it from the crude and unscientific BBT methods used in the past.

Thus, we believe we have transformed the previously inaccurate and unreliable BBT method into a scientific tool for documentation of ovulatory characteristics. Furthermore, it is a method that can be easily taught, requires only a relatively inexpensive and durable digital thermometer, and is one that interested women can and will consistently use *(4,34)* for lengths of time exceeding a year. Taking of basal oral temperature quickly becomes a habit. However, for this to happen, it does require the interest and commitment of women and of those teaching them.

The major difficulty with widespread use of the QBT method is its lack of accuracy in those whose time of waking and sleeping is variable (e.g., those on shift work, with small children, or students). Ideally, a simpler method, not dependent on a stable life pattern, and requiring less commitment from women would be developed for documentation of ovulatory characteristics in longitudinal studies and for epidemiology.

HYPOTHALAMIC ADAPTATION AND OVULATORY FUNCTION

The neuroendocrine physiology of adaptation to exercise and other stressors is complex and not yet well understood. However, it was reviewed over 10 years ago and much remains the same *(35)*. It has also been covered by earlier chapters, and therefore, it will be reviewed only briefly here. The hypothalamus functions to maintain internal homeostasis in response to internal and external factors. Numerous influences, such as ambient and core temperature changes, energy balance changes, illness (which alters eating and sleeping patterns and may cause elevated temperature levels), and psychological stress, can directly or indirectly alter the pulsatile secretion of GnRH and thus change subsequent reproductive function *(36)*.

The thesis of this chapter is that the first and most subtle adaptive response to exercise training is a shortened luteal phase length in which estradiol levels are commonly normal, but total exposure to progesterone is decreased. As discussed, studies that examine hypothalamic control and the subtle changes that lead to shortening of luteal-phase length with exercise training require long-term, continuous monitoring of ovulatory function.

Ovulatory disturbances in response to exercise training can be viewed as a functional adaptation to the increased physiological stress of the exercise, rather than as part of a disease process (Table 1). The adaptation model suggests:

1. Ovulatory disturbances are caused by a hypothalamic process that is conservative, e.g., protects or saves energy for the individual.
2. They are induced by a variety of physical and psychological "stressors," which act through a common mechanism and manifest similar changes.
3. There are gradients of change in response to the severity or intensity of the threat.
4. The adaptive changes reverse to the normal baseline steady state when the threat is lessened or eliminated, or the individual has had sufficient time and is able to adapt.

Evidence for these points will be described in the following sections. The specific ovulatory adaptations to exercise training, including the gradients of change and reversibility will be described in the Adaptations to Exercise Training section.

Hypothalamic Adaptive Processes

Evidence that the subtle alterations that lead to shortening of luteal-phase length are controlled by the hypothalamus is largely circumstantial, because altering hypothalamic function biochemically or with direct nerve cell stimulation is impossible in humans. The strongest evidence that the hypothalamus controls changes in ovulatory function comes from the similar pattern of responses during exposures to a whole range of psychological and physiological stressors.

Table 1
Model Choices[a]

	Disease	Adaptation
Cause	A single agent or presumed etiology	An integrated interaction of personal and environmental factors
Time-course	Continuous or worsening	Labile and reversible
Disability	A present detriment in function/pain/discomfort	A present positive effect, rare discomfort/concern
Prognosis	Risk for chronic disease, harm/discomfort	Excellent, no permanent impairment (if reversed)
Therapy	Specific (external agent)	Modulation of attitude/environment/lifestyle
	Effective	Do nothing to interfere with the adaptation
	Without major side effects	Cause no harm
Therapeutic relationship (patient:physician)	Passive: authoritarian	Active: consultative, supportive

[a]Prior. Reprinted with permission of Human Kinetics Publisher (36b).

Corticotropin-releasing hormone (CRH) release increases when any internal or external environmental signal is perceived as stressful (as shown schematically in Fig. 2). The increased CRH may either directly or indirectly (via the β-endorphin system) slow the hypothalamic pulsatile release of GnRH (37,38) and, therefore, decrease pulsatile LH release. Because the pulses of LH stimulate progesterone and estradiol secretion, they provide an important modulator of ovulatory function, although the exact effector mechanisms are as yet unknown.

Reproductive and primarily ovulatory changes are "conservative" for the individual, because through multiple pathways, they effectively prevent pregnancy when the individual woman is under duress. They are also conservative of energy because less progesterone production, which decreases the otherwise increased core temperature by approx 0.3°C, would mean about 300 fewer dietary calories were needed to ensure energy balance (39).

STRESS MECHANISM

Selye (1) observed nearly 50 years ago that the adrenal glands were hypertrophied when various kind of stressors interrupted estrus in rats. He also observed similar patterns of response of the ovaries and the adrenals to excessive exercise, to interference with normal diet, and to emotional stressors. More recently a strong relationship was also documented between social stress and nonovulation in nonhuman primates. Subordinate primates experienced 16.5% of their cycles as nonovulatory, whereas dominant female primates had only 3.5% anovulatory cycles (40). Cortisol excess that was similar to levels seen in women under stress significantly increased the metabolic clearance of progesterone as well as increasing LH pulse amplitude in experimental studies by Kowalski, Chatterton, and colleagues. This research showed that monkeys who were

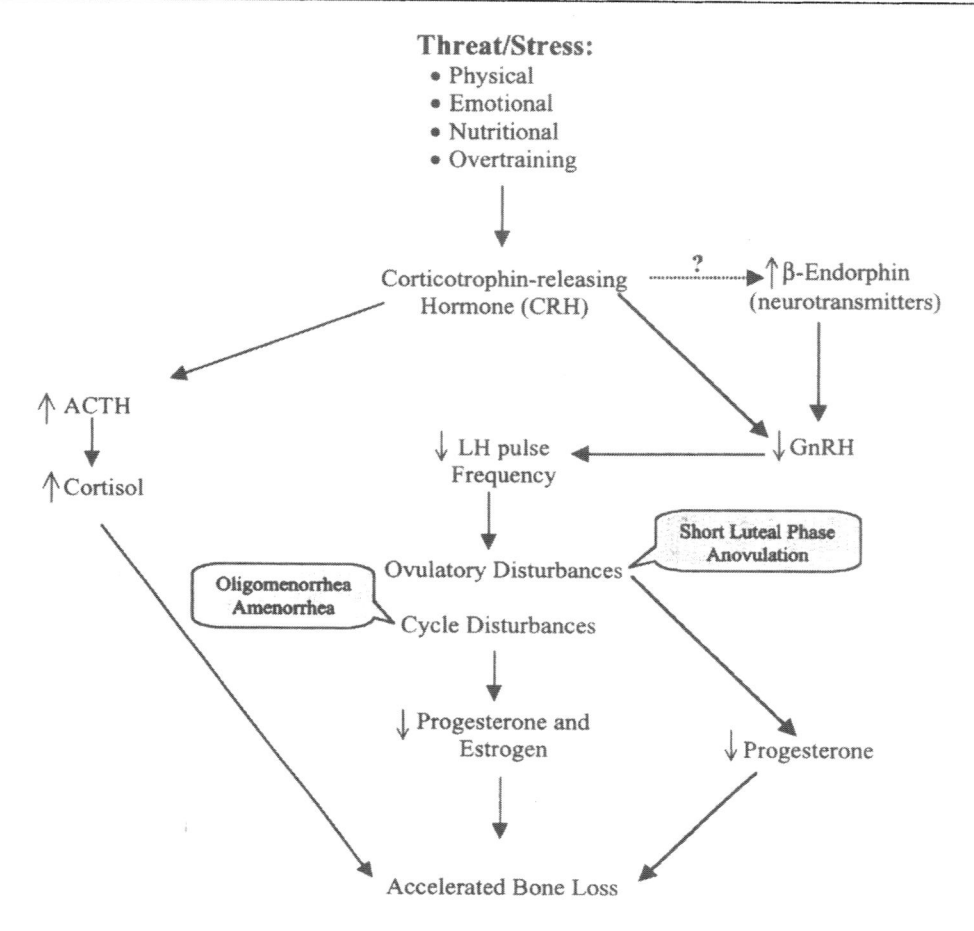

Fig. 2. Process through which physical, emotional, or nutritional challenges cause increased release of CRH from the hypothalamus. These factors suppress the reproductive system and stimulate the adrenal axis. Abbreviations: ACTH = corticotrophin; LH = luteinizing hormone (Adapted from Prior *[36a]*).

exposed to induced hypercortisolism had lower luteal-phase serum progesterone levels and ovulatory disturbances *(41,42)*.

In humans, downward modulation of reproduction during illness was documented by lower than normal LH levels in very ill postmenopausal women *(43)*. Evidence for an adaptive ovarian response to emotional or psychological stress is best illustrated by a prospective study in Japanese nursing students whose regular and apparently ovulatory cycles more commonly showed ovulatory disturbances during the stressful school year than in the summer break *(44)*. Weight loss is known to be one of the most powerful physiological hypothalamic stressors *(45,46)*. An experimental protocol involving fasting for 3 d in the late follicular phase appears to be more disruptive of follicle development and more likely to alter LH pulsatility in women who are initially very lean than in those who have normal body weights and fat *(47)*. There continues to be debate about what proportion of exercise-related effects on the reproductive system are causally related to relative energy imbalance or are caused by a separate exercise stressor *per se (48)*. Long-term prospective monitoring of ovulatory characteristics and cycle hormone levels, rather than cross-sectional data, are needed to answer this question.

Active women with amenorrhea, like overtrained male athletes *(49)*, have increased basal levels of cortisol *(50)* and blunted cortisol responses to exercise *(51,52)*. Berga et al. *(51)* reported high 24-h cortisol levels in those with hypothalamic forms of "anovulation" compared with normally menstruating women. This hypercortisolemia was not observed in women with other reasons for disturbed cycles, such as hyperandrogenism or hyperprolactemia. A few women initially deemed to have hypothalamic amenorrhea subsequently ovulated during the study and were shown to have concomitantly reduced levels of cortisol *(51)*. Ding and colleagues *(50)* could similarly predict women whose cycle intervals would subsequently become normal because their cortisol excretion was decreased. Active women with normal cycle intervals may also have decreased LH and increased cortisol compared to sedentary controls *(53)*. Because cycle lengths are normal, but LH and cortisol levels were altered, it is likely that these women were experiencing subtle ovulatory disturbances associated with exercise training (although ovulatory function was not assessed) *(53)*.

High cortisol secretion or urinary excretion has become a useful marker of hypothalamic adaptive responses to stressors including exercise, because all stressors apparently act through the hypothalamic CRH pathway. Therefore, studies in both humans and non-human primates demonstrate increased cortisol levels simultaneously with decreased LH pulsatility and/or disturbed ovulatory function during reproductive disturbances coinciding with a variety of stressful situations.

It should be noted that although hypothalamic disturbances of ovulation characterized by lower pulsatile release of LH are probably the most common cause for the menstrual cycle disturbances reported in athletes, short luteal-phase cycles or anovulation associated with androgen excess (and with high, rather than low, LH levels) *(54,55)* can also be documented. High androgen and LH levels were recently described as a cause of amenorrhea in swimmers *(54)*. In addition, defects of the large corpus luteum cells have been postulated to cause lower luteal-phase progesterone levels, although LH pulsatility and estradiol levels are both normal *(29)*.

ENERGY CONSERVATION

Cycle disturbances are termed "functional," because they do not represent disease processes. When discussing ovulatory disturbances as protective against excess energy expenditure, the severity of the disturbance is proportional to the amount of energy conserved. Basal metabolic rate (BMR) is 32% lower in severe cases of an energy deficit, such as with anorexia nervosa and amenorrhea, as well as anovulation *(56)*. Amenorrhea in women without an extreme eating disorder may be relatively less threatening, because compared with menstruating women, it appears to lower BMR only 17% *(57)*. Anovulatory cycles, which are normal in length, are also less metabolically costly to maintain than ovulatory cycles and prevent the risk for the high energy demands of pregnancy. The basal temperature rise during the luteal phase increases metabolic rate as evidenced by reported increases in energy intake after ovulation. Barr et al. *(39)* documented that women's dietary intake is increased approx 300 kcals/d during the luteal phase of cycles which were confirmed to be ovulatory compared with anovulatory cycles in the same women who had no exercise or weight changes during the six-cycle study.

A shortened luteal-phase length (in contrast to anovulation) occurs in response to the least threatening intensity or kind of stressor. Energy is relatively less conserved when the luteal-phase length is shortened than in anovulatory cycles, because there may be as many as 9 d of progesterone elevation. We believe that shortening of luteal-phase length is the most common adaptive response to stressors, such as weight loss, emotional stress, illness, or exercise training. It is of importance that despite the minimal alteration of ovarian physiology, fertilization and implantation of the egg are still prevented by corpus luteum insufficiency and short luteal-phase cycles.

Synergism or Interactions Among Factors Influencing Ovulatory Function

The concept of adaptation with a common hypothalamic change caused by many different stressors implies that the response to one, such as exercise, would depend on the current state of other factors, such as energy balance or emotional stress. Therefore, it is important to consider those factors that are known to influence ovulatory function and to acknowledge that individuals may respond differently to any given stress depending on the presence of many personal variables *(58)*. Such factors as the individual's current energy balance, underlying characteristics of the individual (i.e., the levels of reproductive maturation, weight, and emotional well-being), intensity of the threat, and the rapidity with which it is introduced all influence the adaptive response. Multiple emotional and psychological stressors, weight loss or restrictive eating, and the need to feel "in control" all are often perceived as stressful by the hypothalamus and influence reproductive function (Fig. 3). These stressors all appear to act through the common hypothalamic CRH pathway.

ENERGY BALANCE

It is likely that exercise and other stressors affect LH pulsatility through their influence on energy balance *(48)*. This is discussed in detail elsewhere in this volume (Chapter 9). It was postulated in 1982 that hypothalamic insulin receptors might provide a common signal *(6)*. Those who are ill or overexercising would have decreases in their insulin levels as a consequence of negative caloric balance. It is well accepted that severe weight loss or an extreme energy deficit, such as with anorexia nervosa, suppresses reproductive function. In such extreme cases, CRH levels are high *(59)*, and amenorrhea will likely result. More subtle reproductive disturbances often occur when the relative threat is less severe, but conditions that facilitate pregnancy are not optimal. For example, ovulatory disturbances may occur with healthy weight loss or dieting *(60)*, as well as when recreational exercise or emotional stress increase. In each case, the greater the need for energy conservation, the more severe the cycle disturbance *(46,61)*.

EATING RESTRAINT

Subtle ovulatory disturbances also occur with "eating restraint," a psychological attitude in which women feel they must limit food intake to avoid obesity *(62)*. Women who are classified as highly restrained (based on the Three Factor Eating Questionnaire *[62]*) are very conscious of their food intake, but do not necessarily consume fewer calories than same weight and age-matched controls who are not restrained *(63,64)*. Because maintaining or achieving their desired weight is so important to their emotional well-being, eating carries with it psychological stress for women with eating restraint. Very early, it was shown that women with higher scores on the Eating Restraint Scale of

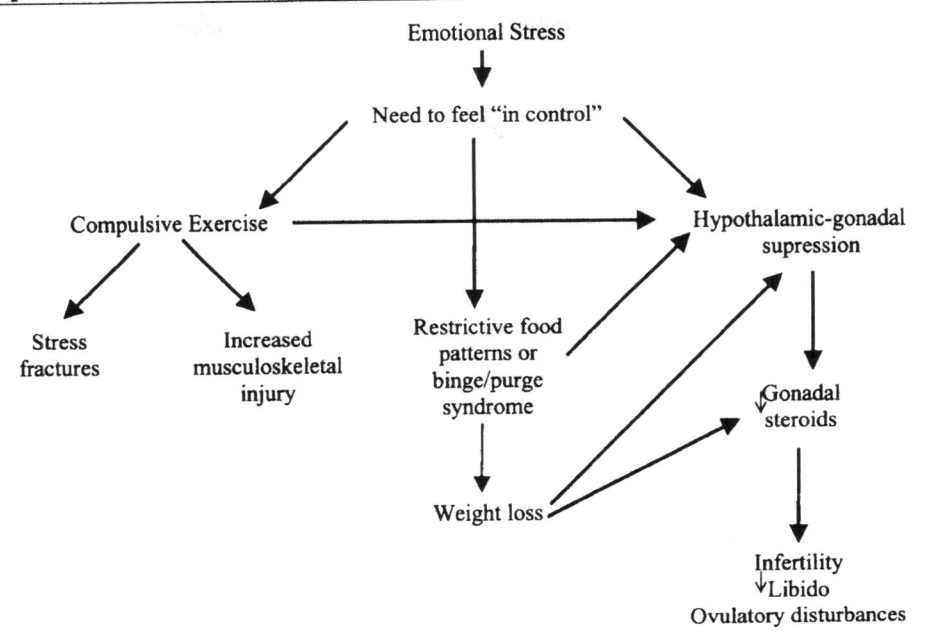

Fig. 3. Interrelationships among multiple factors (stress, compulsive exercise, and restrictive eating) that are causally related to the development of ovulatory disturbances.

the Three Factor Eating Questionnaire were more likely to have short luteal-phase cycles *(65)*. Two recent studies from our laboratory also examined ovulatory function and eating restraint in normal-weight, regularly cycling ovulatory women who varied in their usual activity levels *(66)* and in regularly cycling vegetarian and nonvegetarian women *(67)*. The restraint scale of the Three Factor Eating Questionnaire *(62)* was administered initially, and menstrual cycle characteristics were documented prospectively for at least three *(66)* or six cycles *(67)*, respectively, in each study. In both studies, women in the highest tertile of restraint were significantly more likely than women in the lowest restraint tertile to experience a short luteal phase or anovulatory cycle. These findings could not be attributed to differences in energy intakes, exercise levels, or body mass index (BMI is weight in kg divided by height in m^2) levels. Restrained women did not differ in BMI, weight, energy intake, or activity from the less restrained women in each respective population *(66,67)*. All of the women had consistently normal cycle lengths. Thus, none of these women would have known their cycles were disturbed. They would all have been classified as "eumenorrheic" if ovulation had not been assessed.

It is probable that the effect of eating restraint on ovulatory function is mediated through hypothalamic adaptation pathways. At present, because data examining the potential relationships among cortisol excretion, ovulatory disturbances, and dietary restraint have yet to be published, it is hypothetical that these are hypothalamic adaptive changes. Nonetheless, the evidence that subtle ovulatory disturbances are more common among "highly restrained" eaters, despite similar energy intakes and expenditures, emphasizes that hypothalamic ovulatory disturbances may result from relatively minor psychological as well as physiological stressors.

HYPOTHALAMIC REPRODUCTIVE "MATURATION"

Another variable influencing the ability of the hypothalamic system to respond to stressors is its relative maturity. For example, the majority of menstrual cycles are anovulatory in the first year after menarche *(8)*. However, on average, women do not develop the highest rate of ovulatory cycles (94%) until they are approx 12 yr after menarche *(8)* (or gynecologic age 12). This implies that some are still gynecologically immature. It fits with the adaptation hypothesis that those whose hypothalamic–reproductive axis has not yet become sturdily and regularly ovulatory are more likely than those with mature reproductive patterns to respond to stress with altered reproductive function *(44)*.

One of the first studies documenting the reproductive hormonal characteristics of young athletes showed that both swimmers and controls had short luteal-phase cycles, but in swimmers, the luteal phase was even shorter than in sedentary controls *(68,69)*. Although subject numbers were small, these data confirm the more extensive data of Vollman *(8)* that teenagers are susceptible to subtle disturbances of ovulation. Young runners (gynecologic age < 10 yr, mean chronologic age 20 yr) are also more likely to have disturbed folliculogenesis and decreased estradiol, progesterone, gonadotrophins, and testosterone levels than are gynecologically mature women (gynecologic age > 15 yr, mean chronological age 31 yr) *(70)*. Therefore, data suggest that the combination of more intense training and an immature hypothalamus is potentially additive in suppressing reproduction in young women.

It has already been shown that women of mature gynecologic age who begin exercise or intensify training only experience ovulatory changes. However, evidence suggests, although appropriate experiments to document it conclusively have not been performed, that a woman in her 20s who is only intermittently ovulatory and begins to exercise or intensifies exercise training may well develop cycle as well as ovulatory disturbances. This young woman would likely develop oligomenorrhea or amenorrhea.

Age at menarche has been shown to be influenced by intense exercise training *(71–73)*. Although genetic factors also have a strong influence on menarcheal age *(74,75)*, dancers and gymnasts have delayed menarche compared with their sedentary sisters even though they are genetically very similar. Puberty involves maturation of axillary and pubic hair as well as breast enlargment and maturation. Interestingly, when young athletes are forced (often because of injury) to interupt their gymnastics or dance training, rapid development through one or more Tanner breast stages commonly occurs *(73,76)*.

Women of young gynecologic age have anorexia most frequently. Weight loss and young age may make them more vulnerable to anorexia. In a similar manner they will likely be more prone to exercise effects on ovulatory function, especially if exercise is combined with restricted energy intake or psychological performance pressure from coaches and parents. It is also possible that women experiencing reproductive and ovulatory disturbances in response to stress when younger will be more susceptible to exaggerated stress responses throughout life *(77,78)*.

The pubertal maturation of the breast is primarily dependent on ovarian hormones, with little or no influence of adrenal steroids. By contrast, pubic hair maturation can proceed with the normal adolescent increases in adrenal androgen secretion, without significant increases in ovarian hormones. Discrepancy in the degree of breast maturation compared with pubic hair maturation through the Tanner stages is probably a clue to hypothalamic adaptive changes related to exercise training and/or other stressors. Warren et al. *(73)* reported that pubic hair development occurred at a normal age in young women dancers, yet breast development and age at menarche tended to be delayed. Clinical data from ovarian hormone treatment of male to female transsexuals and observations during a prospective study of puberty suggest that normal breast development to the fully mature Tanner V breast stage will not be reached without adequate exposure to progesterone levels (Prior, unpublished observation).

STRESS INTENSITY

Whether ovulation becomes disturbed partially depends on the intensity of the stress and partly on the rate at which the stress is introduced. For example, all rats responded to "inescapable" shock by suppressed gonadotrophin secretion *(79)*, whereas only some rats are susceptible to the relatively less threatening stress of endurance exercise *(80)*.

Hans Selye coined the term "General Adaptation Syndrome" and published early controlled trials of exercise and energy restriction stress on rats *(1)*. Selye's experiments showed a dramatically different response to gradually increasing exercise compared with rapid imposition of exercise training (or caloric restriction). Animals who started running at 3.5 km/d developed anestrus (the rat equivalent of amenorrhea) with interstitial atrophy, few mature follicles, and increased weight of their adrenal glands. A second group of rats gradually increased exercise intensity to reach 3.5 km/d over 4 wk (Fig. 4). Even though the rats in the second group maintained the same level of exercise intensity as the first group for two of the three months, reproductive function remained normal and ovarian follicle development was appropriate. Similar differences in response were observed in rats treated with rapid "semi-starvation" compared with gradual decreases in caloric intake *(1)*. Selye subsequently showed a similar pattern of reproductive response in rats that were restrained or separated from their cage-mates or siblings. These data suggest that similar mechanisms of hypothalamic adaptation on the reproductive system occur in response to exercise training, weight loss, and psychological stress as well as to illness *(43)*.

In Selye's day, before immunoassays for hormones were available, adrenal gland weights were shown to increase in experimental animals exposed to stressors. Because reproductive disturbances occurred in parallel they were also considered to be "adaptive" and related to a generalized stress response. These observations are consistent with current data showing elevated cortisol levels in women with hypothalamic disturbances of ovulation, oligomenorrhea, and amenorrhea.

The classic animal stress experiments have not been adequately reproduced in humans. However, as will be discussed in more detail below, the data available in humans suggest that a high training intensity and volume can be well tolerated if adequate time for adaptation to that exercise is allowed.

ADAPTATIONS TO EXERCISE TRAINING

Exercise Training Studies in Mature Women

Only a few studies have prospectively documented cycle characteristics with exercise training in mature women. The first prospective documentation, in only one woman, used the elasticity of cervical mucus as a marker of the midcycle estradiol peak to show shortening of the luteal phase associated with an increase in weekly running distance *(2)*. Other early studies showed an increased prevalence of short luteal phase

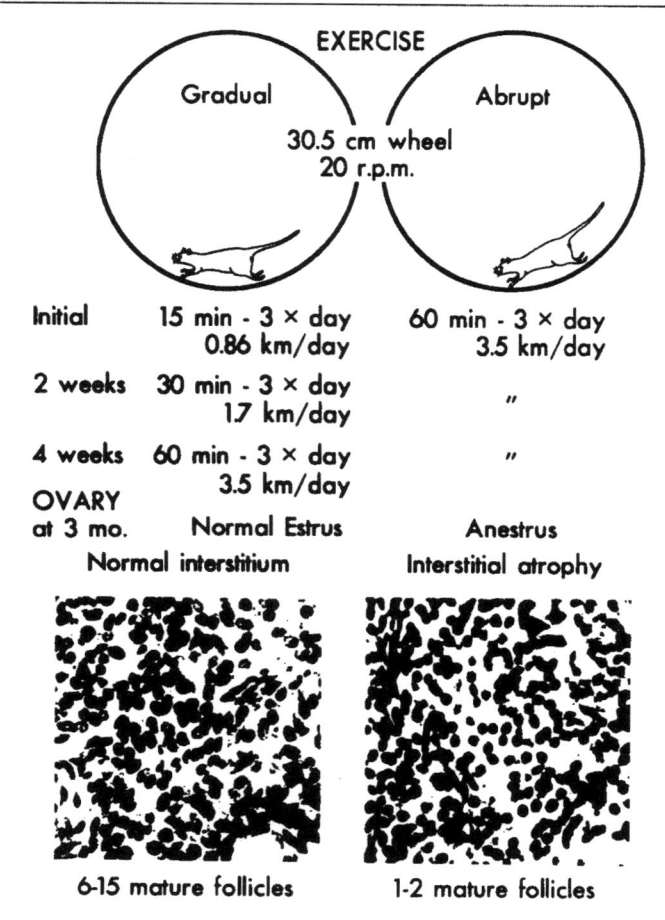

Fig. 4. Illustration of the concept of the "general adaptation syndrome" developed by Hans Selye. Exercise was introduced abruptly or gradually in rats randomized to one or the other group. The photomicrographs show ovulatory adaptation by normal interstitum and follicular development in rats with gradual increase in exercise. Abrupt introduction of exercise led to anestrus (the rat equivalent of amenorrhea), interstitial atrophy, and development of only a few mature follicles. Data redrawn from ref. *1*.

or anovulatory cycles associated with increasing intensity or volume of exercise training *(81,82)*. In a group of 14 gynecologically mature women (gynecologic age > 15 yr, mean chronologic age 35 yr) who had been training for a marathon, only one-third of a total of 48 cycles prior to a marathon (3 cycles/woman) were biphasic (and thus ovulatory) with normal luteal-phase lengths *(82)*. The only difference between nonovulatory and ovulatory cycles appeared to be the length of the usual training run (from approx 2 to 5 miles) *(82)*.

A study of longer duration (14–15 mo) in women not proven to be initially ovulatory showed a decrease in the volume of menstrual blood and lower estradiol levels with marathon training *(83)*. Running activity increased from 24 to 100 km/wk over the study period. Ovulatory characteristics were not examined, however, and the inclusion of participants from 24 to 57 yr *(83)* confounds these outcomes. Nevertheless, in that study and in none of the others to be subsequently described did the women develop amenorrhea, despite rapid increases in running activity/intensity mandated by some protocols.

Three important prospective studies of exercise and reproduction are compared in Table 2. These studies have all sought to establish an influence of exercise training on the reproductive hormonal characteristics of both the follicular and the luteal phases of the cycle and cycle and luteal-phase changes during exercise training: Bullen (26,84), Bonen (3), and Rogol et al. (5). Because of their importance to this discussion, each study is described in detail below.

Bullen and colleagues (26,84) monitored 28 college-aged women residing at a summer camp by measuring hormonal characteristics for two cycles using analysis of daily overnight urines and evening temperatures. These women (whose mean age was 20 yr) were confirmed to be ovulatory prior to entry into the study and were also randomly assigned to either weight-loss or weight-maintenance groups. Running activity increased from 4.5 to 10 miles/d by week 5 of the 8-wk camp. In addition to running 10 miles/d, women also participated in 3 h/d of varied recreational activities. Bullen and colleagues documented that none of the women in the study developed amenorrhea despite their young age and that they were exposed to several stressors, including change of residence, intense and rapidly increasing exercise training, and caloric restriction (in the weight-loss group). Ovulatory disturbances and shortened luteal-phase cycles were common, however, and only 8 of the 28 women ovulated normally in both cycles. The addition of weight loss to the exercise training caused a further significant increase in ovulation disturbances as well as oligomenorrhea in a few women (26,84).

Bonen and colleagues set out to determine whether a dose–response between running mileage/week and reproductive function was operative. In particular, by observing sedentary, mature women who ran at varying exercise loads, they tried to determine whether or not a threshold of exercise intensity was present above which luteal-phase disturbances would begin. Bonen (3) monitored mature women over 2–4 mo who were variously training at <16, 16–32, or 32–48 km/wk. These investigators showed that although there were trends toward shortening of the luteal phase in the first cycle measured after training began, no consistent luteal-phase length changes were documented, nor were there any differences in ovulatory characteristics between women in different intensity groups (3).

As shown in Table 2, the design of the study by Rogol and colleagues (5) was similar to Bonen's, but used VO_2max testing to document the aneorobic threshold as when increased lactate was produced. This assessment was used to increase gradually the exercise intensity to maintain it just below or above the "lactate threshold." This allowed them to document more accurately the exercise load, which was gradually increasing over 1 yr for all participants whose hormone levels were intensively sampled every 4 mo before the next increase in exercise intensity. Rogol et al. (5) also report that neither running intensity nor duration affected ovulatory function in women training for 1 yr at increasing intensities that were maintained either above or below their own adjusted lactate threshold.

Several differences exist between the studies of Bullen and those by Bonen and Rogol, which at least partially explain their discrepant outcomes. The rapid introduction of a high volume of training, and the addition of weight loss (26) in Bullen's protocol provides a greater stress load, and would thus be more likely to lead to ovulatory disturbances than an exercise program alone in older women who remained in their own homes

Table 2
Published Prospective Studies of Exercise Training on Menstrual Cycle and Luteal Length

Author	Bullen et al. (26)	Bonen (3)	Rogol et al. (5)
Total (*n*)	28	57	23
Chronologic age	22 (0.6)	30.0 (1.3)	31.4 (1.3)
Gynecologic age mean (SE)	10 (0.6)	17.1 (1.4)	17.8 (0.9)
Study groups	Exercise + weight maintenance (A) Exercise + weight loss (B) (max of −0.45 kg/wk)	<10 mile/wk for 2 mo (A) <10 mile/wk for 4 mo (B) 10–20 mile/wk for 2 mo (C) 10–20 mile/wk for 4 mo (D) 20–30 mile/wk for 2 mo (E) 20–30 mile/wk for 4 mo (F)	Train at lactate threshold (*n* = 9) Train above lactate threshold (*n* = 8)
Duration of exercise training	2 mo	2–4 mo	1 yr
Exercise schedule	Running 4 mile/d progressing to 10 mile/d by week 5, plus 3.5 h of cycling, tennis, or volleyball	As described above	Start: 6.25 mile/wk Wk 1–20: add 1.25 mile every 2nd wk Wk 20–39: hold at 24 mile/wk Wk 40–end: add 1.25 mile every 2nd wk (max of 40 or 65 mile/wk)
Exercise intensity	70–80% of max aerobic capacity (adjusted each month)	Not reported	6 d/wk ran at lactate threshold 3 d/wk ran at lactate threshold and 3 d/wk ran above lactate threshold
Sampling method	Daily BBT and daily urinary sampling (overnight)	Daily blood samples	Daily blood samples day 9 through end of cycle
Sampling intervals	Continuous	Every second cycle	Every fourth cycle
Luteal length (LL) mean (SE)	Mean LL not available Cycle types during training		Mean LL Control cycle 14.2 (1.5) Run cycle 1 12.6 (1.0) Run cycle 3 14.2 (1.5) (only includes groups B, D, and F) Detrain, cycle 12.1 (1.3) 3 or 5	Mean LL Cycle 1 13.9 (0.6) Cycle 4 13.4 (0.7) Cycle 8 13.8 (0.7) Cycle 12 12.8 (0.7)
		A B	
Study group		25 6	
%Ovulatory		66 63	
%Short Luteal Phase			
%Anovulatory		42 81	
		NA	NA
Additional stressors	Young gynecologic age Weight loss Away from home Intense exercise training		

150

and communities (3,5). In addition, the women in Bullen et al.'s (26) study were significantly younger both in chronological and gynecological age. Another important difference is in design—Bullen and colleagues increased exercise intensity rapidly, whereas the other two studies were more gradual in exercise intensification. Finally, these studies differ in the methods and time-course of monitoring. Bullen and colleagues (26) monitored cycles consecutively and inclusively. In contrast, Bonen (3) and Rogol et al. (5) assessed ovulatory characteristics intermittently every two or every four cycles, respectively. Shortened luteal phase or anovulatory cycles may have been missed because monitoring occurred after one or three cycles of probable adaptation to a new exercise load. Any ovulatory disturbances would have likely occurred in the first cycle following the increase in training volume. By the second or fourth cycle after the increase in intensity/duration of training, adaptation would have occurred, homeostatic balance would be achieved, and normal ovulatory function would have returned.

We, like Bullen et al. (26), have monitored luteal length and ovulation continuously, but over 1 yr in 66 women of varying self-chosen activity levels (4). As described earlier, all women were confirmed to be normally ovulatory on two consecutive cycles prior to study entry. Despite that, over 80% of the women experienced at least one short luteal phase or anovulatory cycle during the year of study. When the average cycle, luteal phase, and two cycles of hormone levels are used as previously reported (4), no differences were found by exercise habit in the number or severity of ovulatory disturbances, or in estradiol and progesterone levels. That was true regardless of whether the women were completing <1 h of aerobic exercise/wk (normally active controls), running more than 1 h/wk, but not training for a specific event (consistent runners), or runners increasing training in preparation for a marathon during the study year (4). The reason for ovulation disturbances that did occur was not initially understood. However, we have subsequently found them to be more prevalent in women scoring high on the Restraint Scale, suggesting they are related to dietary restraint (66,67).

The same study was recently used to compare the characteristics of the premarathon cycle in the marathon-training women with a season-matched cycle in the consistent runners. Exercise training without weight loss can be shown to cause shortening of the luteal phase. The luteal-phase characteristics of the cycle before the marathon were compared in marathon-training women with their own initial and final cycles and the premarathon cycle with a season-matched middle cycle from the consistent runners. Compared to both their own cycles during less-intense training and all of the cycles in the consistent runners, significant shortening of the luteal-phase length before the marathon occurred in the marathon-training women (85).

Hypothalamic adaptation to the runners' baseline exercise probably had occurred before they passed the screening for two consecutive ovulatory cycles and became qualified to enter the study. However, the intensified training before the marathon appears to cause shortening of the luteal phase in the cycle prior to the marathon when their training mileage was the greatest. The detailed dietary, weight, body fat, and hormonal characteristics also monitored before the marathon are being studied for explanations other than exercise training to explain the luteal-phase shortening that was documented. These data all suggest that adaptation to increased exercise, even as intense as training for a marathon, normally occurs with only shortening of the luteal phase in well-nourished, reproductively mature women who have no major emotional distress. In addition, as discussed below, adaptation allows a woman's reproductive system to show a luteal-phase change quite rapidly and then to become normal again.

Observable Changes Prior to Ovulation Disturbances—Molimina

Prior to shortening of the luteal-phase length, which is the first objective change in reproductive function, other observable, but even more subtle changes are commonly reported by mature women who are beginning exercise training. The earliest change with moderate, recreational levels of exercise is a decrease in molimina *(86)*. "Molimina" whose Greek etymology means "to try hard," includes the set of physical and emotional, but not troublesome indicators of the coming menstrual flow. Although the so-called premenstrual syndrome occurs in both ovulatory and nonovulatory cycles, in the truest sense, molimina indicates that ovulation has occurred. Its most accurate differentiating characteristic is the development, during the week before flow, of breast tenderness only on the high sides of the breasts (Prior [1987], unpublished observation). An additional indicator of an ovulatory cycle is the disappearance of elastic cervical mucus after the midcycle estrogen surge. Because progesterone inhibits cervical production of elastic mucus, this time pattern of presence and then disappearance of mucus is also a potential indicator that ovulation has occurred.

However, molimina is often confused with premenstrual syndrome (PMS), which may include only emotional symptoms and is more apt to occur in cycles with high estradiol levels and decreased progesterone productions *(87)*. This early exercise-training-related decrease in molimina could be associated with the minimally decreased follicular-phase estradiol levels that occur early after onset of training *(83)*. Older evidence says that increased emotional sensitivity, fluid symptoms, and appetite in the week before menstruation are all indicative of ovulatory cycles *(88)*.

We asked the question concerning whether exercise would decrease molimina by studying a group of running women who were increasing their exercise training over 6 mo. Exercise training was associated with decreased molimina, especially fluid symptoms and perception of personal stress as well as decreased anxiety despite no change in weight or cycle characteristics *(86)*. Age and weight matched non-exercising women studied in parallel experienced no significant changes in the molimina over the same study period *(86)* (Fig. 5).

Time-Course of Ovulatory Adaptation

With the addition of more strenuous training, endocrine changes progress from decreased molimina to shortened luteal phase. The next and more disturbed cycle is non-ovulatory. This sometimes occurs as training workload increases *(6)*. The sedentary woman whose training and cycle characteristics are shown in Fig. 6 developed severe back pain during the 12th cycle and did not ovulate. It is likely that she developed anovulation because she not only had the stress of the pain to deal with but also what for her was an important worry, that she would be unable to compete in and finish the marathon for which she had trained so hard.

In a woman with well-established normally ovulatory cycles (probably after gynecological age 12), exercise-training adaptive changes do not normally progress to anovulation. However, if an additional stressor is added, such as illness, weight loss, and/or emotional stress (*see* Exercise Training Studies in Mature Women and Reversibility/Adaptation), anovulation may develop. Amenorrhea will usually not develop unless the

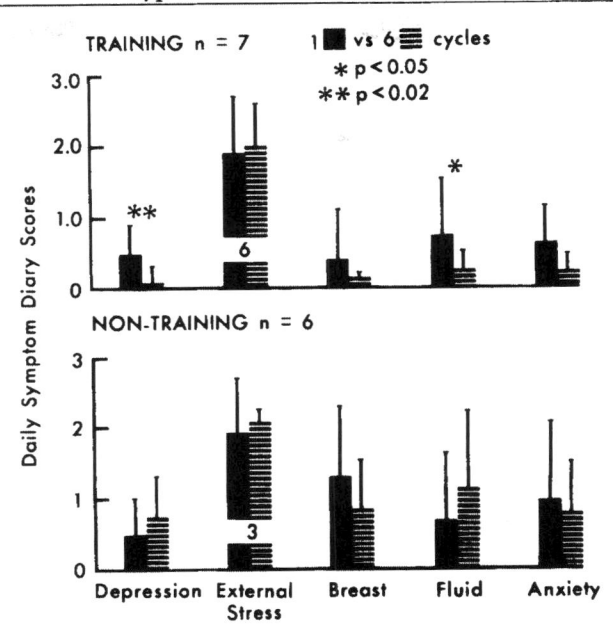

Fig. 5. The progressive changes in moliminal experiences are shown as mean ± SD of daily Menstrual Cycle Diary scores during the 14 d preceding menstrual flow with the first and sixth consecutive menstrual cycle in seven women runners who intensified exercise before a marathon race and in six nontraining women. Nonparametric statistics showed that training women had significantly lower breast symptoms compared with sedentary women during cycle 1 ($p = 0.019$). At cycle 6, the two groups differed in depression ($p = 0.045$), fluid ($p = 0.019$), and breast symptoms ($p = 0.006$). For external stress, the data were available on only six training and three nontraining women. Reprinted with permission from ref. 86.

woman is of young gynecologic age, is not yet sturdily ovulatory, and has stresses in addition to exercise-training, such as eating restraint or psychological stress, energy imbalance, rapid induction of exercise, or rapid weight loss.

Reversibility/Adaptation

A few case studies are useful to illustrate further the progression and reversibility of ovulatory adaptation. Figures 6 and 7 show luteal-phase lengths as documented by semiquantitative BBT *(8)* for 1 yr of consecutive cycles in two mature, normal-weight women. One of these women, as discussed above, was a sedentary woman who trained for and ran a marathon during the year of observation (Fig. 6). The other was a rather lean and compulsive runner who wanted to become pregnant (Fig. 7) *(82)*. The first woman's prospective record indicated alternating cycles showing short luteal-phases (<10 d) and normal luteal-phase lengths with anovulation during the cycle before and of the marathon race. As mentioned above, the pain and worry as well as exercise training likely accounted for anovulatory cycles. A normal luteal-phase length cycle returned when both her emotional stress and her training workload decreased immediately after her successful marathon.

Figure 7 shows prospective documentation of ovulatory characteristics over 1 yr in another woman who was running regularly, but was quite lean and stressed. She showed consistently short luteal-phase cycles early in the year (Fig. 7). In an effort to reverse her

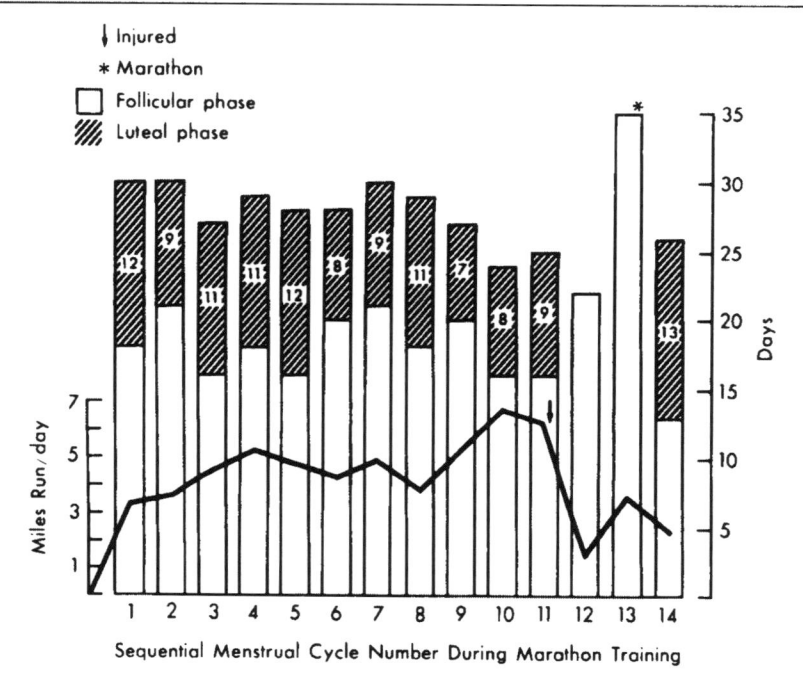

Fig. 6. This bar graph, illustrating cycle lengths as open bars and luteal-phase lengths as crosshatched areas within those bars, shows sequential menstrual cycles during 1 yr of marathon training in a previously sedentary woman. Note the alternating short and normal luteal phases and progression to anovulatory cycles (in cycles #12 and #13) just after the most intense and highest mileage of training just before and in the marathon cycle. When she decreased her training following the marathon, ovulation and her luteal-phase lengths were restored to normal. Reprinted with permission from ref. 82.

secondary infertility, she decreased running for one cycle, but this was emotionally stressful. Inadequate or insufficient luteal-phase characteristics were documented by endometrial biopsy accepted as a cause for her secondary infertility. When she stopped running for approx 6 wk, she became pregnant (before a normal luteal-phase length and appropriate endometrial histology could be documented).

These detailed case histories of two women who monitored their individual exercise and ovulatory characteristics over an extended period of time indicate the rapid hypothalamic adaptation and reversibility of ovulatory disturbances related to exercise training (82). These data have been supported in larger samples of women runners (4,85,89) showing shortened luteal-phase lengths with increased running mileage/intensity and a return to normal luteal length with decreased training volume or at the same exercise load when the stress of the competition is over or adaptation has had time to occur. Animal data also support that endurance exercise training is more likely to influence the first cycle after exercise is initiated rather than later cycles when adaptation has occurred (80). In contrast, perhaps because it is less psychologically stressful, voluntary exercise in rats appears to have no influence on ovulation (90).

Very few data document long-term adaptation to exercise well. As an example, it is useful to observe the second marathon-training year in the woman whose cycles were documented in Fig. 6. The characteristics of the cycle before her second marathon a year after her first are shown in Fig. 8. During the first marathon, she had shown short luteal-

Chapter 8 / Exercise and the Hypothalamus

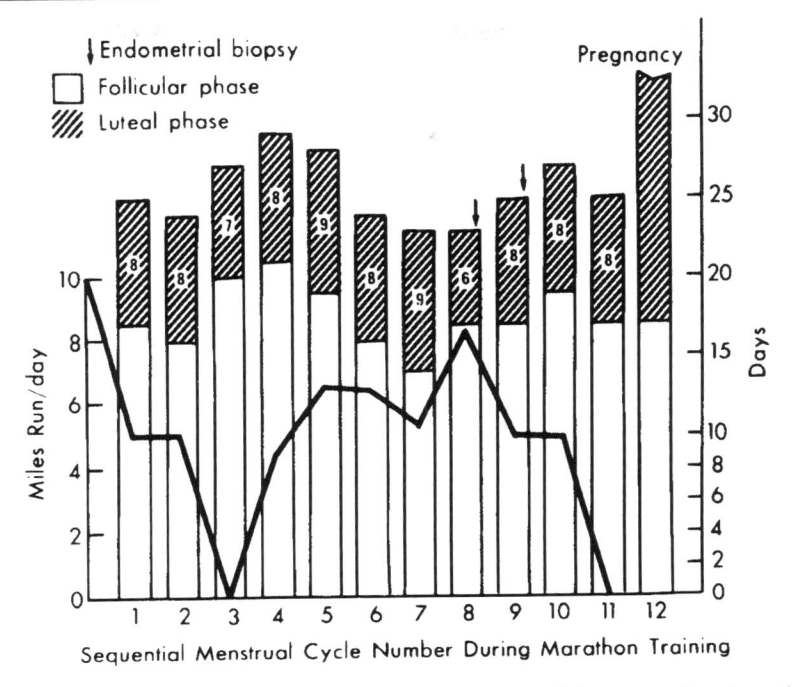

Fig. 7. This bar graph is similar to Fig. 6 and shows the sequential menstrual cycle and ovulatory characteristics in a woman who was training intensely and compulsively. Even with decreased running during the first few cycles, she continued having short luteal-phase cycles. Endometrial biopsies (arrows) were consistent with luteal-phase deficiency. In the middle of cycle 11, she stopped running and became pregnant before a normal luteal phase could be documented. She carried the child to term and delivered a healthy baby. Reprinted with permission from ref. 82.

phase cycles progressing to anovulatory cycles the month prior to (M-1) and of (M) the marathon. In her second marathon, 1 yr later, luteal length remained normal throughout training, even through her training was similar in volume and intensity to her earlier marathon. It appears possible that by the second year she had adapted to the marathon training, which allowed her cycles to maintain normal ovulation. Key in each of these stories is the fact that the woman was basically emotionally healthy and maintained normal body weight without significant weight loss.

In mature women, adaptation to exercise training and reversal to normal commonly occur within one cycle. These adaptive changes of luteal-phase length with increasing exercise training are modeled in Fig. 9. Note that, as in the woman described above who trained for her first marathon, by the end of the year, the model suggests that a level of exercise intensity that had provoked ovulatory disturbances now no longer causes a change from a normal ovulatory cycle.

Bullen's study (26) also demonstrates rapid reversibility when training ceased. Although a few women developed oligomenorrhea as well as disturbances of ovulation, all of the women experiencing ovulatory and cycle disturbances (short luteal phase or anovulatory cycles as well as oligomenorrhea) regained both normal cycle intervals and normal ovulatory function within a few months after the end of the summer training camp (26). Furthermore, it is common for athletic women to become pregnant within months of decreasing their training (and competitive stress), even though they may have

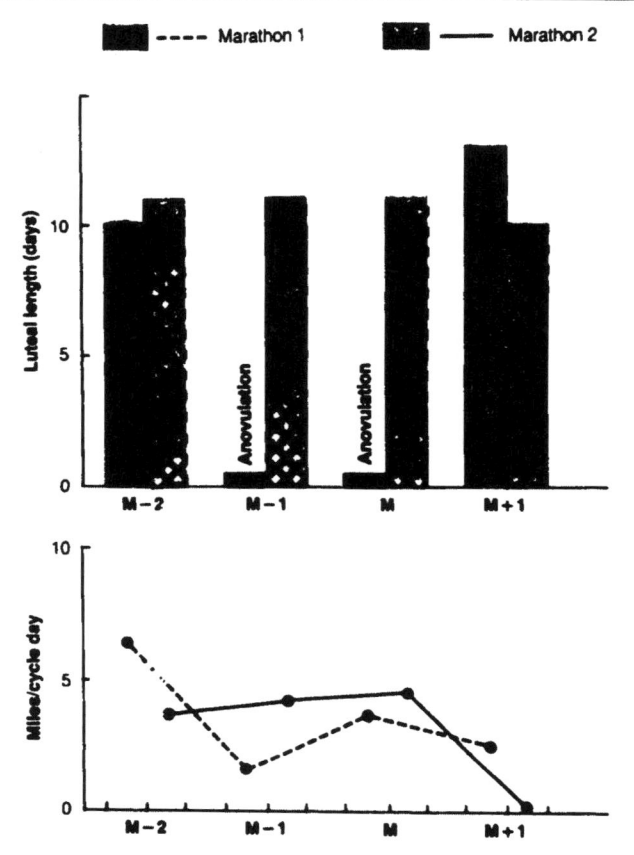

Fig. 8. Luteal-phase lengths during the cycles before and just after a marathon in the first marathon training and race (as shown in Fig. 6) and in a subsequent marathon a year later. During the second marathon, despite similar or increased mileage, there were no luteal-phase disturbances documented. This illustrates reproductive adaptation to the levels of exercise this woman was now performing. Prior et al. Reprinted with permission from *(91a)*.

had several years of anovulatory cycles or amenorrhea *(82,91,92)*. However, in exercising younger women, in whom the hypothalamus has not fully matured, the return to or achievement of normal ovulatory cycles will often take longer.

Although the majority of the data just presented were collected using QBT analyses nearly 15 yr ago, no studies since have closely examined ovulatory characteristics continuously during several months of exercise training. The development of new methods of monitoring ovulation and luteal-phase length (using blood spot progesterone levels *[22]*) should soon allow the nuances of cycle adaptation to be more specifically characterized, and mechanisms and modulating factors more carefully delineated.

CLINICAL APPLICATIONS/TREATMENT

The practical and clinical implications of ovulatory adaptation to exercise training are not the purpose of this chapter. However, it is important that the clinician and coach be alert to document persistent changes in luteal-phase length or any anovulatory cycles. These changes are useful indicators that the exercise training load is excessive for that

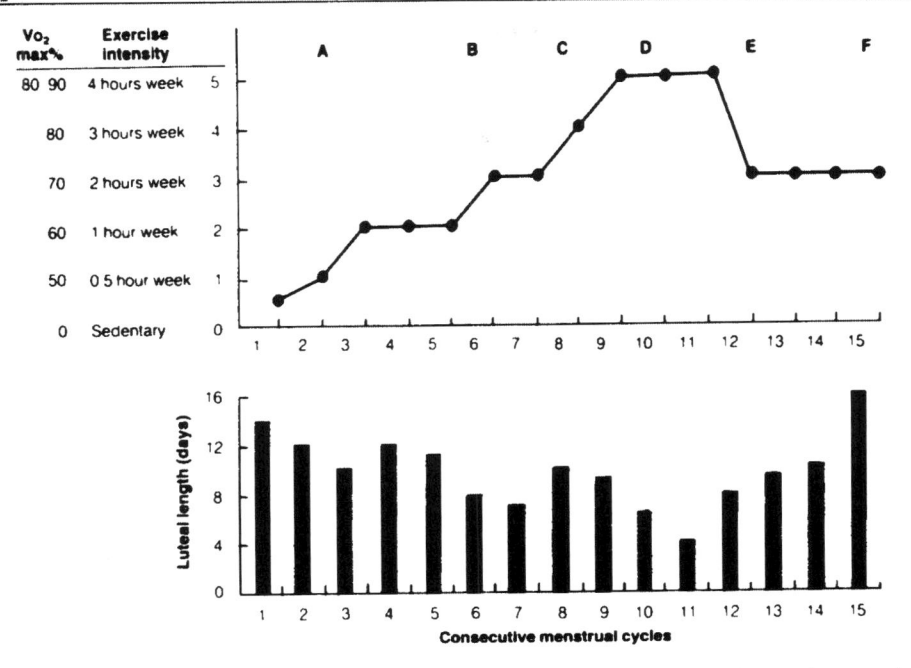

Fig. 9. Theoretical model of the luteal-phase changes that occur over time with increasing exercise in an ovulatory woman who is undergoing exercise training. Note that at the end of the year's sequence of cycles, despite a considerable exercise load, luteal-phase length and ovulation are normal. Prior et al. Reprinted with permission from *(91a)*.

woman's level of hypothalamic reproductive maturation and/or when combined with her other stressors (competitive anxiety, moving, weight loss or eating restraint, or even illness).

If ovulatory disturbances are documented, it is very easy to provide physiological treatment. Persistant ovulatory disturbances should be treated by prescribing either cyclic oral micronized progesterone (300 mg at bedtime) or medroxyprogesterone (10 mg) on d 14–27 of the woman's own cycle *(55,93)*. Although this "treatment" does not directly correct the hypothalamic stressor that led to the disturbances in the first place, feedback to the hypothalamus by progesterone may aid in the maturation process. The most useful function of cyclic progesterone is to provide physiological levels of progesterone, which will cause regular menstrual flow if estradiol levels are normal.

Cyclic medroxyprogesterone, in a randomized, placebo-controlled 1-yr trial, caused a significant 2% increase in spinal bone density in athletic women with abnormal cycles (Fig. 10) *(34)*. In contrast, no prospective controlled study of oral contraceptive use has clearly shown increased bone density, and several large, well-designed studies indicate oral contraceptives may cause skeletal harm *(94)*, especially in young women or primates whose reproductive maturation is incomplete *(95,96)*.

The most important reason for the clinician to know about ovulatory adaptive responses is to teach each woman to observe and understand the menstrual cycle changes she may experience. In this era of "self-help medicine" molimina, quantitative basal temperature recording, and the concepts of adaptation rather than disease are all beneficial to the health-conscious woman.

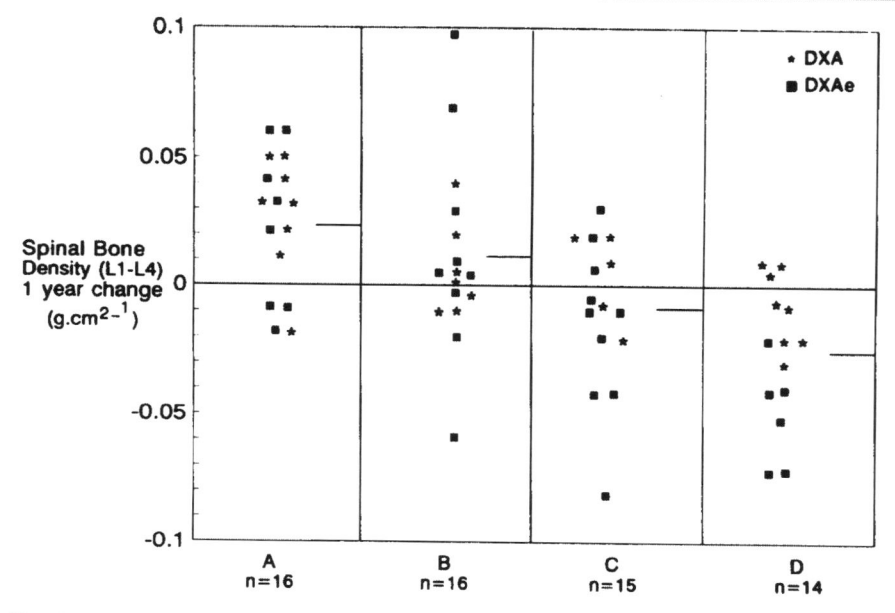

Fig. 10. This data table shows as individual marks the rates of 1-yr spinal bone mineral density change by dual-energy X-ray absorptiometry (DXA) in 61 active women with abnormal menstrual cycles randomized to receive medroxyprogesterone acetate cyclically for 10 d/cycle (MPA) with or without active/calcium therapy or placebo. It shows a significant 2.5% loss of bone in D, the double-placebo group, despite the fact that these women were of normal weight, had good exercise habits, and took an average of 1000 mg/d in their diets. By contrast, women in A who were similar and randomized to receive double-masked therapy with cyclic MPA and an extra 1000 mg of supplemental calcium experienced an average 2% increase in bone density. Reprinted with permission from ref. *34*.

CONCLUSIONS

This chapter has reviewed the subtle adaptation of the reproductive system to increasing exercise training gradually. Evidence suggests that changes in luteal-phase progesterone (and perhaps estradiol) production and duration are the first and the major adaptive response of the hypothalamic–pituitary–ovarian system to increasing exercise intensity. These ovulatory disturbances are commonly perceived by decreases in molimina—this is often seen as both a physical and emotional benefit and will motivate women to continue to exercise. If no additional stressor other than the exercise is present, the luteal-phase changes will reverse to normal in the next cycle, even though the exercise level is maintained.

Although more data are needed, it is likely that these physiological and psychological changes during exercise training are conservative for the individual, are reversible, and cause no long-term harm. However, if luteal-phase defects persist, bone loss occurs *(4)*. In addition, fertility is impaired by luteal-phase defects. Persistence of ovulatory disturbances may be commonly related to the psychological stress of dietary restraint *(66,67)*.

The benefits of exercise for cardiovascular *(97)*, skeletal *(98,99)*, and emotional health *(100)* are well supported, yet the concept persists that exercise causes women major reproductive harm in the form of amenorrhea. In this chapter, we have attempted to erase that perception by viewing the body's responses to exercise training as adaptive. When increasing levels of exercise are introduced gradually, adaptation can occur and the result is a minimal change. Ovulatory disturbances occur normally when initiating a more intense training program or increasing the exercise load, but will reverse rapidly to normal once adaptation has occurred. When taken to an extreme or combined with other psychological or physiological stressors, exercise can, as is always emphasized, become negative. In that circumstance, persistent ovulatory disturbances occur, which depending on the age, nutritional state, and emotional support of the woman, may progress to oligomenorrhea or amenorrhea.

Amenorrhea, although it is uncommonly associated with exercise in mature, ovulatory women, may occur in the face of exercise combined with a negative energy balance or when several stressors coexist, especially in women who have never established regularly ovulatory cycles. Gynecological immaturity is a significant factor in the ability of women to adapt to exercise stress. This implies that caution should be taken in the intensity and rate of exercise training with young athletes.

In summary, although the concept of adaptation to exercise training has been known for 50 years *(1)* and has been applied to women's reproduction for over 16 years *(82)* few well-controlled studies have documented the most subtle evidence of this adaptation: ovulatory disturbances. Much work remains to be done to document the variables that influence the hypothalamic reproductive centers to change their signals and the ovarian as well as adrenal responses to these alterations.

REFERENCES

1. Selye H. The effect of adaptation to various damaging agents on the female sex organs in the rat. Endocrinology 1939;25:615–624.
2. Shangold M, Freeman R, Thysen B, Gatz M. The relationship between long-distance running, plasma progesterone, and luteal phase length. Fertil Steril 1979;32:130–133.
3. Bonen A. Recreational exercise does not impair menstrual cycles: a prospective study. Int J Sports Med. 1992;13:110–120.
4. Prior JC, Vigna YM, Schechter MT, Burgess AE. Spinal bone loss and ovulatory disturbances. N Engl J Med 1990;323:1221–1227.
5. Rogol AD, Weltman A, Weltman JY, Seip RL, Snead DB, Levine S, et al. Durability of the reproductive axis in eumenorrheic women during 1 yr of endurance training. J Appl Physiol 1992;72:1571–1580.
6. Prior JC. Endocrine "conditioning" with endurance training: a preliminary review. Can J Appl Sport Sci 1982;7:149–157.
7. Drinkwater BL, Nilson K, Chesnut CH III, Bremner WJ, Shainholtz S, Southworth MB. Bone mineral content of amenorrheic and eumenorrheic athletes. N Engl J Med 1984;311:277–281.
8. Vollman RF. The menstrual cycle. In: Friedman EA, ed. Major Problems in Obstetrics and Gynecology. W.B. Saunders Company, Toronto, 1977, pp. 11–193.
9. Abraham GE. The normal menstrual cycle. In: Givens JR, ed. Endocrine Causes of Menstrual Disorders. Year Book Medical Publishers, Chicago, 1978, pp. 15–44.
10. Prior JC. Vigna YM, Schulzer M, Hall JE, Bonen A. Determination of luteal phase length by quantitative basal temperature methods: Validation against the midcycle LH peak. Clin Invest Med 1990;13:123–131.
11. Taaffe D, Robinson T, Snow C, Marcus R. High-impact exercise promotes bone gain in well-trained female athletes. J Bone Miner Res 1997;12:255–260.
12. Nielsen HK, Brixen K, Bouillon R, Mosekilde L. Changes in biochemical markers of osteoblastic activity during the menstrual cycle. J Clin Endocrinol Metab 1990;70:1431–1437.
13. Burger HG. Clinical utility of inhibin measurements. J Clin Endocrinol Metab 1993;76:1391–1396.
14. Landgren BH, Unden AL, Diczfalusy E. Hormonal profile of the menstrual cycle in 68 normally menstruating women. Acta Endocrinol 1980;94:89–98.

15. Fraser IS, Baird DT. Endometrial cystic glandular hyperplasia in adolescent girls. J Obstet Gynaecol 1972;79:1009–1013.
16. van Look PF, Lothian H, Hunter WM, Michie EA, Baird DT. Hypothalamic–pituitary–ovarian function in perimenopausal women. Clin Endocrinol. 1977;7:13–31.
17. Cowan LD, Gordis L, Tonascia JA, Jones GS. Breast cancer incidence in women with a history of progesterone deficiency. Am J Epidemiol 1981;114:209–217.
18. Sherman BM, Korenman SG. Hormonal characteristics of the human menstrual cycle throughout reproductive life. J Clin Invest 1974;55:699–706.
19. Sowers MF, Shapiro J, Zhang B. Urinary ovarian and gonadotrophin hormones in premenopausal women with low bone mass. J Bone Miner Res 1995;10(S):M377.
20. Aksel S, Wiebe RH, Tyson JE, Jones GS. Hormonal findings associated with aluteal cycles. Obstet Gynecol 1996;48:598–602.
21. Soules MR, McLachlan RI, Ek M, Dahl KD, Cohen NL, Bremner WJ. Luteal phase deficiency: characterization of reproductive hormones over the menstrual cycle. J Clin Endocrinol Metab 1989;69:804–812.
22. Petsos P, Ratcliffe WA, Anderson DC. Assessment of corpus luteum function by direct radioimmunoassay for progesterone in blood spotted on filter paper. Clin Chem 1985;31:1289–1293.
23. Kassam A, Overstreet JW, Snow-Harter C, De Souza MJ, Gold EB, Lasley BL. Identification of anovulation and transient luteal function using a urinary pregnanediol-3-glucuronide ratio algorithm. Environ Health Perspect 1994;104:408–413.
24. Finn MM, Gosling JP, Tallon DF, Madden AT, Meehan FP, Fottrell PF. Normal salivary progesterone levels throughout the ovarian cycle as determined by a direct enzyme immunoassay. Fertil Steril 1988;50:882–887.
25. Santoro N, Rosenberg J, Adel T, Skurnick JH. Characterization of reproductive hormonal dynamics in the perimenopause. J Clin Endocrinol Metab 1996;81:4,1495–1501.
26. Bullen BA, Skrinar GS, Beitins IZ, VonMering G, Turnbull BA, McArthur JW. Induction of menstrual cycle disorders by strenuous exercise in untrained women. N Engl J Med 1985;312:1349–1353.
27. McNelly M, Soules M. The diagnosis of luteal phase deficiency: a critical review. Fertil Steril 1988;50:1–15.
28. Elking-Hirsch K, Goldziecher JW, Gibbons WE, Besch PK. Evaluation of the ovustick urinary luteinizing hormone kit in normal and stimulated menstrual cycles. Obstet Gynecol 1986;67:450–453.
29. Hinney B, Henze C, Kuhn W, Wuttke W. The corpus luteum insufficiency: a multifactorial disease. J Clin Endocrinol Metab 1996;81:565–570.
30. Prior JC, Vigna YM, Barr SI, Kennedy S, Schulzer M, Li DKB. Ovulatory premenopausal women lose cancellous spinal bone: A five year prospective study. Bone 1996;18:261–267.
31. Hitchcock CL, Bishop C, Prior JC. Modeling ovulation and detecting subclinical ovulatory disturbances. Proceedings from the Society for Menstrual Cycle Research. Chicago, IL, 1997.
32. McCarthy JJ Jr, Rockette HE. A comparison of methods to interpret basal body temperature graph. Fertil Steril 1983;39:640–646.
33. Royston JP, Abrams RM, Higgins MP, Flynn AM. The adjustment of basal body temperature measurements to allow for time of waking. Br J Obstet Gynecol 1980;87:1123–1127.
34. Prior JC, Vigna YM, Barr SI, Rexworthy C, Lentle BC. Cyclic medroxyprogesterone treatment increases bone density: a controlled trial in active women with menstrual cycle disturbances. Am J Med 1994;96:521–530.
35. Prior JC. Physical exercise and the neuroendocrine control of reproduction. Bailleres Clin Endocrinol Metab 1987;1:299–317.
36a. Prior JC. Exercise-associated menstrual disturbances. In: Adashi EY, Rock JA, Rosenwaks Z, eds. Reproductive Endocrinology, Surgery, and Technology. Raven, New York, 1996, pp. 1077–1091.
36b. Prior JC. Hormonal mechanisms of reproductive function and hypothalamic adaptation to endurance training. In: The Menstrual Cycle and Physical Activity. Puhl J, Brown H, eds. Human Kinetics Publishers, Urbana, IL, 1986, pp. 63–75.
37. Petraglia F, Sutton S, Vale W, Plotsky P. Corticotropin-releasing factor decreases plasma luteinizing hormone levels in female rats by inhibiting gonadotrophin-releasing hormone release into hypophysial-portal circulation. Endocrinology 1987;120:1083–1088.

38. Williams CL, Nishihara M, Thalabard JC, Grosser PM, Hotchkiss J, Knobil E. Cortiocotropin-releasing factor and gonadotropin-releasing hormone pulse generator activity in the Rhesus monkey. Neuroendocrinology 1990;52:133–137.
39. Barr SI, Janelle KC, Prior JC. Energy intakes are higher during the luteal phase of ovulatory menstrual cycles. Am J Clin Nutr 1995;61:39–43.
40. Kaplan JR, Adams MR, Clarkson TB, Koritnik DR. Psychological influences on female 'protection' among cynomolgus macaques. Atherosclerosis 1984;53:100–104.
41. Chatterton RT Jr, Kazer RR, Rebar RR. Depletion of luteal phase serum progesterone during constant infusion of cortisol phosphate in the cynomolgus monkey. Fertil Steril 1991;56:547–554.
42. Kowalski W, Chatterton RT, Kazer RR, Wentz AC. The impact of subchronic hypercortisolemia on progesterone metabolism and luteinizing hormone-progesterone axis in the cynomolgus monkey. J Clin Endocrinol Metab 1993;77:1597–1604.
43. Warren MP, Siris ES, Petrovich C. The influence of severe illness on gonadotrophin secretion in the postmenopausal female. J Clin Endocrinol Metab 1977;45:99–104.
44. Nagata I, Koichi K, Katsuyoshi S, Furuya K. Ovulatory disturbances: causative factors among Japanese student nurses in a dormitory. J Adolesc Health 1986;7:1–5.
45. Schweiger V, Laessle R, Schweiger M, Herrmann F, Riedel W, Pirke KM. Caloric intake, stress, and menstrual function in athletes. Fertil Steril 1988;49:447–450.
46. Warren MP. Effects of undernutrition on reproductive function in the human. Endocr Rev 1983;4:363–377.
47. Alvero R, Kimzey L, Sebring N, Reynolds J, Loughran M, Nieman L, et al. Effects of fasting on neuroendocrine function and follicle development in lean women. J Clin Endocrinol Metab 1998;83:76–80.
48. Loucks AB, Verdun M, Heath EM. Low energy availability, not stress of exercise, alters LH pulsatility in exercising women. J Appl Physiol 1998;84:37–46.
49. Barron JL, Noakes TD, Levy W, Smith C, Millar RP. Hypothalamic dysfunction in overtrained athletes. J Clin Endocrinol Metab 1985;60:803–806.
50. Ding JH, Sheckter CB, Drinkwater BL, Soules MR, Bremner WJ. High serum cortisol levels in exercise-associated amenorrhea. Ann Int Med 1988;108:530–534.
51. Berga SL, Daniels TD, Giles DE. Women with functional hypothalamic amenorrhea but not other forms of anovulation display amplified cortisol concentrations. Fertil Steril 1997;67:1024–1030.
52. Loucks AB, Mortola JF, Girton L, Yen SSC. Alterations in the hypothalamic–pituitary–ovarian and hypothalamic–pituitary–adrenal axes in athletic women. J Clin Endocrinol Metab 1989;68:402–411.
53. Cumming DC, Vickovic MM, Wall SR. Defects in pulsatile LH release in normally menstruating runners. J Clin Endocrinol Metab 1985;65:810–812.
54. Constantini NW, Warren MP. Menstrual dysfunction in swimmers: a distinct entity. J Clin Endocrinol Metab 1995;80:2740–2744.
55. Prior JC. Ovulatory disturbances: they do matter. Can J Diagn 1997;February:64–80.
56. Casper RC, Schoeller DA, Kushner R, Hnilicka J, Gold ST. Total daily energy expenditure and activity level in anorexia nervosa. Am J Clin Nutr 1991;53:1143–1150.
57. Graham TE, Viswanathan M, VanDijk P, Bonen A, George JC. Thermal and metabolic responses to cold by men and by eumenorrheic and amenorrheic women. J Appl Physiol 1989;67:282–290.
58. Pertides JS, Meuller GP, Kalogeras KT, Churousos GP, Gold PW, Deuster PA. Exercise-induced activation of the hypothalamic–pituitary–adrenal axis: marked differences in the sensitivity to glucocorticoid suppression. J Clin Endocrinol Metab 1994;79:377–383.
59. Kaye WH, Gwirtsman HE, George DT, Ebert MH, Jimerson DC, Tomai TP, et al. Elevated cerebrospinal fluid levels of immunoreactive corticotropin-releasing hormone in anorexia nervosa: relation to state of nutrition, adrenal function, and intensity of depression. J Clin Endocrinol Metab 1987 64:203–208.
60. Pirke KM, Schwieger V, Strowitzki T, Tuschl RJ, Laessle RG, Broocks A, et al. Dieting causes menstrual irregularities in normal weight women through impairment of luteinizing hormone. Fertil Steril 1989;51:263–268.
61. Suh BY, Liu JH, Berga SL, Quigley ME, Laughlin GA, Yen SS. Hypercortisolism in patinets with functional hypothalamic-amenorrhea. J Clin Endocrinol Metab 1988;66:733–739.
62. Stunkard AJ, Messick S. The Three-Factor Eating Questionnaire to measure dietary restraint, disinhibition and hunger. J Psychosom Res 1985;29:71–83.

63. Laessle RG, Tuschl RJ, Kotthaus BC, Pirke KM. Behavioral and biological correlates of dietary restraint in normal life. Appetite 1989;12:83–94.
64. Tuschl RJ, Platte P, Laessle RG, Stichler W, Pirke KM. Energy expenditure and everyday eating behaviour in healthy young women. Am J Clin Nutr 1990;52:81–86.
65. Schweiger U, Tuschl RJ, Platte P, Broocks A, Laessle RG, Pirke KM. Everyday eating behavior and menstrual function in young women. Fertil Steril 1992;57:771–775.
65a. Prior JC. Reversible reproductive changes with endurance training. In: Endurance in Sport. Shephard RJ, Astrand PO, eds. Blackwell Scientific Publications, Oxford, UK, 1992, pp. 365–373.
66. Barr SI, Prior JC, Vigna YM. Restrained eating and ovulatory disturbances: possible implications for bone health. Am J Clin Nutr 1994;59:92–97.
67. Barr SI, Janelle KC, Prior JC. Vegetarian vs nonvegetarian diets, dietary restraint, and subclinical ovulatory disturbances: prospective 6-mo study. Am J Clin Nutr 1994;60:887–894.
68. Bonen A, Ling WY, MacIntyre KP, Neil R, Mcgrail JC, Belcastro AN. Effects of exercise on the serum concentrations of FSH, LH, progesterone and estradiol. Eur J Appl Physiol 1979;12:15–23.
69. Bonen A, Belcastro AN, Ling WY, Simpson AA. Profile of selected hormones during menstrual cycles of teenage athletes. J Appl Physiol Respir Environ Exerc Physiol 1981;50:545–551.
70. Ronkainen H. Depressed follicle-stimulating hormone, luteinizing hormone, and prolactin responses to the luteinizing hormone-releasing hormone, thyrotropin-releasing hormone, and metoclopramide test in endurance runners in the hard-training season. Fertil Steril 1985;44:755–759.
71. Malina RM, Bouchard C. Growth Maturation and Physical Activity. Human Kinetics Publishers, Champaign, IL, 1991.
72. Rees M. Menarche: when and why. Lancet 1993;342:1375–1376.
73. Warren MP. The effects of exercise on pubertal progression and reproductive function in girls. J Clin Endocrinol Metab 1980;51:1150–1157.
74. Loesch DZ, Huggins R, Rogucka E, Hoang NH, Hopper JL. Genetic correlates of menarcheal age: a multivariate twin study. Ann Hum Biol 1995;22:479–490.
75. Treloar SA, Martin NG. Age at menarche as a fitness trait: non-additive genetic variance detected in a large twin sample. Am J Hum Genet 1990;47:137–148.
76. Frisch RE, Gotz-Welbergen AV, McArthur JW, Albright TE, Witschi J, Bullen BA, et al. Delayed menarche and amenorrhea of college athletes in relation to age of onset of training. JAMA 246, 1981;1559–1563.
77. McEwen BS. Protective and damaging effects of stress mediators. Semin Med Beth Israel Deconess Medical Center 1998;338:171–179.
78. Meaney MJ, Tannenbaum B, Francis D. Early environmental programming; hypothalamic–pituitary–adrenal responses to stress. Semin Neurosci 1994;6:247–259.
79. Rivier C, Rivier J, Vale W. Stress-induced inhibition of reproductive functions: role of endogenous corticotropin-releasing factor. Science 1986;231:607–609.
80. Chatterton RT Jr, Hrycyk L, Hickson RC. Effect of endurance exercise on ovulation in the rat. Med Sci Sports Exerc 1995;27:1509–1515.
81. Bonen A. Alterations in menstrual cycles: effects of exercise. Med Can 1986;41:331–342.
82. Prior JC, Ho-Yeun B, Clement P, Bowie L, Thomas J. Reversible luteal phase changes and infertility associated with marathon training. Lancet 1982;1:269,270.
83. Boyden T, Pamenter R, Stanforth P, Rotkis T, Wilmore J. Sex steroids and endurance running in women. Fertil Steril 1983;39:629–632.
84. Beitins IZ, McArthur JW, Turnbull BA, Skrinar GS, Bullen BA. Exercise induces two types of human luteal dysfunction: confirmation by urinary free progesterone. J Endocrinol Metab 1991; 72:1350–1358.
85. Petit MA, Prior JC, Vigna YM. Neuroendocrine adaptation causes reversible ovulation disturbances with marathon training: prospective controlled study in ovulatory women. ISPNE conference proceedings (abstract), 1998, Trier, Germany.
86. Prior JC, Vigna Y, Sciarretta D, Alojado N, Schulzer M. Conditioning exercise decreases premenstrual symptoms: a prospective, controlled 6-month trial. Fertil Steril 1987;47:402–408.
87. Wang M, Seippel L, Purdy RH, Backstrom T. Relationship between symptom severity and steroid variation in women with premenstrual syndrome: study on serum pregnenolone, pregnenolone sulfate, 5 alpha-pregnane-3,20-dione and 3 alpha-hydroxy-5 alpha-pregnan-20-one. J Clin Endocrinol Metab 1996;81:1076–1082.

88. Magyar DM, Boyers SP, Marshall JR, Abraham GE. Regular menstrual cycles and premenstrual molimina as indicators of ovulation. Obstet Gynecol 1979;53:411–414.
89. Prior JC, Cameron K, Yuen BH, Thomas J. Menstrual cycle changes with marathon training: anovulation and short luteal phase. Can J Appl Sport Sci 1982;7:173–177.
90. Kagabu S, Mamba K, Makita T. No effect of voluntary exercise on ovarian follicle in rats. Exp Anim 1997;46:247–250.
91. Bonen A. Exercise-induced menstrual cycle changes: a functional, temporary adaptation to metabolic stress. Sports Med 1994;17:373–392.
91a. Prior JC, Vigna YM. The short luteal phase: a cycle in transition. Contemporary Ob/Gyn 1985; 25:169–175.
92. Cohen GC, Prior JC, Vigna Y, Pride SM. Intense exercise during the first two trimesters of unapparent pregnancy. Physician Sports Med 1989;17:11–16.
93. Prior JC, Vigna YM, McKay DM. Reproduction for the athletic woman: new understandings of physiology and management. Sports Med 1992;14:190–199.
94. Cooper C, Hannaford P, Croft P, Kay CR. Oral contraceptive pill use and fractures in women: a prospective study. Bone 1993;14:41–45.
95. Polatti F, Perotti F, Filippa N, Gallina D, Nappi RE. Bone mass and long-term monophasic oral contraceptive treatment in young women. Contraception 1995;51:221–224.
96. Register TC, Jayo MJ, Jerome CP. Oral contraceptive treatment inhibits the normal acquisition of bone mineral in skeletally immature young adult female monkeys. Osteoporosis Int 1997;7:348–353.
97. Powell KE, Thompson PD, Caspersen CJ, Kendrick JS. Physical activity and the incidence of coronary heart disease. Ann Rev Public Health 1987;8:253–287.
98. Dalsky GP, Stocke KS, Ehsani AA, Slatopolsky E, Lee WC, Birge S Jr. Weight-bearing exercise training and lumbar bone mineral content in postmenopausal women. Ann Intern Med 1988; 108:824–828.
99. Petit MA, Prior JC, Barr SI. Running and ovulation positively change cancellous bone in premenopausal women. Med Sci Sports Exerc 1999;31:780–787.
100. McCann L, Holmes DS. Influence of aerobic exercise on depression. J Personal Soc Psych 1984;46:1142–1147.

9 Exercise Training in the Normal Female
Effects of Exercise Stress and Energy Availability on Metabolic Hormones and LH Pulsatility

Anne B. Loucks, PhD

CONTENTS

HYPOTHETICAL MECHANISMS OF HYPOTHALAMIC–PITUITARY–GONADAL (HPG) AXIS DISORDERS IN EXERCISING WOMEN
PROSPECTIVE CLINICAL EXPERIMENTS
INTERIM INTERPRETATIONS
ACKNOWLEDGMENTS
REFERENCES

HYPOTHETICAL MECHANISMS OF HYPOTHALAMIC–PITUITARY–GONADAL (HPG) AXIS DISORDERS IN EXERCISING WOMEN

In this field of study, as in others, competing schools of thought have developed to explain the HPG axis disorders observed in exercising women. Of the several early mechanisms proposed, three maintain adherents today in at least a refined version.

Body Composition

In 1974, body composition was offered as an explanation for the amenorrhea observed in anorexia nervosa patients *(1)*. This idea was a refinement of an earlier hypothesis about body weight accounting for the timing of menarche *(2)*. The body composition hypothesis holds that menarche occurs in girls when the amount of energy stored in their bodies as fat rises to a critical 17% of their body weight, and that menstrual function is lost later when their body fat declines to less than a critical 22% of body weight *(1)*.

The body composition hypothesis has been the most widely publicized explanation for menstrual disorders in athletes in the lay community and the most widely embraced by the clinical community, but it is also the least widely accepted within the scientific community. The hypothesis is based entirely on correlations without any supporting experimental evidence *(3)*. Observations of athletes have not consistently verified an association of menstrual status with body composition (e.g., *4*), or have not found the appropriate temporal relationship between changes in body composition and menstrual

From: *Contemporary Endocrinology: Sports Endocrinology*
Edited by: M. P. Warren and N. W. Constantini © Humana Press Inc., Totowa, NJ

function (for reviews, *see* refs. *5–8*). Rather, eumenorrheic and amenorrheic athletes span a common range of body compositions *(9)* leaner than that of eumenorrheic sedentary women. In addition, after the growth and sexual development of prepubertal animals have been blocked by dietary restriction, normal LH pulsatility resumes only a few hours after *ad libitum* feeding is permitted, long before any change in body weight or composition can occur *(10)*.

Despite such criticisms, scientific interest in the body composition hypothesis was renewed with the discovery in 1994 of the adipocyte hormone leptin *(11)*, with the observation of a correlation between leptin levels and body fatness in rodents and humans (e.g., *12*), and with the discovery of leptin receptors on hypothalamic neurons thought to be involved in control of the gonadotropin-releasing hormone (GnRH) pulse generator, which regulates luteinizing hormone (LH) pulsatility *(13)*.

Energy Availability

In 1980, Warren was the first to suggest that menstrual disorders in dancers are disrupted by an "energy drain" *(14)*, but an empirically testable energy-availability hypothesis was first clearly stated in terms of brain energy availability by Winterer et al. in 1984 *(15)*. This hypothesis holds that failure to provide sufficient metabolic fuels to meet the energy requirements of the brain causes an alteration in brain function that disrupts the GnRH pulse generator, although the mechanism of this alteration was unknown.

At the organismal level, the energy availability hypothesis recognizes that mammals partition energy among five major metabolic activities: cellular maintenance, thermoregulation, locomotion, growth, and reproduction *(16)*, and that the expenditure of energy in one function, such as locomotion, makes it unavailable for others, such as reproduction. Considerable observational data from biological field trials support this idea and indicate that the dependence of reproductive function on energy availability operates principally in females (for reviews, *see* refs. *16–19*). Experiments have induced anestrus in Syrian hamsters by food restriction, by the administration of pharmacological blockers of carbohydrate and fat metabolism, by insulin administration (which shunts metabolic fuels into storage), and by cold exposure (which consumes metabolic fuels in thermogenesis) *(16)*. Disruptions of reproductive function were independent of body size and composition. In addition, amenorrhea has been induced in monkeys by training them to run voluntarily for prolonged periods on a motorized treadmill, after which their menstrual cycles were restored by dietary supplementation, without any moderation of their exercise regimen *(20)*.

The energy availability hypothesis is also supported by endocrine observations of athletes. Amenorrheic athletes display low 24 h blood glucose, low 24 h insulin, and high 24 h insulin-like growth factor binding protein-1 (IGFBP-1) *(21)*, loss of the leptin diurnal rhythm *(22)*, and low tri-iodothyronine (T_3) levels in the morning *(23,24)*. All of these abnormalities are signs of energy deficiency. T_3 regulates basal metabolic rate, and low T_3 occurs in numerous conditions, from fasting to cancer, in which dietary energy intake is insufficient to meet metabolic demands. In addition, eumenorrheic and amenorrheic athletes both display low insulin and high IGFBP-1 levels during the feeding phase of the day, as well as low leptin *(22)* and elevated growth hormone levels over 24 h *(21)*. Meanwhile, leptin has been shown to fluctuate in response to fasting, dietary restriction, and overfeeding before any change in adiposity occurs *(25–28)*. Thus, even if leptin does participate in the regulation of the HPG axis, it may communicate information about energy availability rather than energy stores.

Amenorrheic and eumenorrheic athletes report similar stable body weights, despite dietary energy intakes similar to those of sedentary women *(23,29–33)*. That is, they report their dietary energy intakes to be much less than would be expected for an athlete's level of physical activity. This apparent discrepancy between stable body weight and unexpectedly low dietary energy intake is controversial. Since energy intake and expenditure are very difficult to measure accurately, the apparent discrepancy might be an artifact of methodological errors. Some investigators have attributed the apparent discrepancy between energy intake and expenditure in athletic women to underreporting of dietary intake *(34,35)*, for underreporting dietary intake is common in all populations *(36)*. Underreporting does not account for the abnormalities in metabolic substrates and hormones observed in athletes, however. Furthermore, behavior modification and endocrine-mediated alterations of resting metabolic rate operate to stabilize body weight despite dietary energy excess and deficiency *(37)*.

Exercise Stress

The stress hypothesis holds that exercise activates the hypothalamic–pituitary–adrenal axis, which disrupts the GnRH pulse generator by another unknown mechanism. To be meaningfully independent of the energy availability hypothesis, the stress hypothesis must also imply that the adrenal axis is activated by some aspect of exercise other than its energy cost.

Certainly, there are central and peripheral mechanisms by which the adrenal axis can disrupt the ovarian axis *(38)* and prolonged aerobic exercise without glucose supplementation does activate the adrenal axis. Furthermore, Selye *(39)* induced anestrus and ovarian atrophy in rats by abruptly forcing them to run strenuously for prolonged periods. Others, too, have induced anestrus in rats by forced swimming *(40,41)*, by forced running *(42)*, and by requiring animals to run farther and farther for smaller and smaller food rewards *(43,44)*. Elevated cortisol levels observed in such studies were interpreted as signs of stress, and the resulting disruptions of the HPG axis were widely interpreted as evidence that "exercise stress" has a counterregulatory influence on the female reproductive system.

Amenorrheic athletes also display mildly elevated cortisol levels *(21,29,45–47)*, and this observation is the basis for attributing their amenorrhea to stress. Mild hypercortisolism is also associated with amenorrhea in patients with functional hypothalamic amenorrhea *(48)* and anorexia nervosa *(49)*. Nevertheless, it is wise to recognize that cortisol is a glucoregulatory hormone activated by low blood glucose levels.

It is not known whether the adrenal axis mechanisms that disrupt the HPG axis in forced experiments on animals also operate in voluntarily exercising women. Until recently, all animal experiments investigating the influence of the "activity stress paradigm" on reproductive function confounded the stress of exercise with the stress of the method used to force animals to exercise and with energy deficiency. Consequently, to this day, there does not exist any unconfounded experimental evidence that the stress of exercise disrupts the HPG axis. Indeed, glucose supplementation during exercise blunts the usual rise in cortisol in both rats *(50)* and men *(51)*. Thus, the mild hypercortisolism observed in amenorrheic athletes may reflect a chronic energy deficiency rather than exercise stress.

PROSPECTIVE CLINICAL EXPERIMENTS

Experiments Confounding Exercise Stress and Energy Availability

Several investigators have attempted to induce menstrual disorders through chronic exercise training, but most *(52–55)* have applied only a moderate volume of exercise, or the volume of exercise was increased gradually over several months, and diet was uncontrolled or unquantified. In the most recent such study *(55)*, physically trained subjects were selected, and they appear to have been luteally suppressed before the study began *(56,57)*.

Only one experiment has successfully induced menstrual disorders in regularly menstruating women *(58)*. Modeled on Selye's early animal experiments *(39)*, this single successful experiment imposed a high volume of aerobic exercise abruptly, causing a large proportion of menstrual disorders in the first month, and an even larger proportion in the second. Both proportions were greater in a subgroup fed a controlled weight-loss diet than in another subgroup fed for weight maintenance, but even the weight-maintenance subgroup may have been underfed, since behavior modification and endocrine-mediated alterations of resting metabolic rate operate to stabilize body weight despite dietary energy excess and deficiency *(37)*.

Such chronic experiments suffer from practical problems with subject retention and compliance over a period of several months. The outcome variable in such experiments is the menstrual cycle itself, which requires sustained observations over a period of weeks. Short-term experimental protocols have been developed to avoid these difficulties. In these short-term protocols, LH pulsatility is chosen as the outcome variable, because ovarian function is critically dependent on LH pulsatility. Of course, short-term effects on LH pulsatility are not proof of chronic effects on ovarian function, but hypotheses about mechanisms regulating LH pulsatility can be tested in highly controlled short-term experiments, and then chronic effects can be confirmed in prolonged experiments later.

One such short-term experimental protocol found that a combination of increased exercise and dietary restriction disrupts LH pulsatility during the early follicular phase *(59)*. LH pulse frequency during 12 waking hours was lower in four habitually physically active women when their exercise training regimen was increased during a few days of dietary restriction than during dietary supplementation. This experiment did not determine, though, whether LH pulse frequency could be suppressed by exercise without dietary restriction, or whether the stress of exercise had a suppressive effect on LH pulsatility beyond the impact of the energy cost of exercise on energy availability.

Experiments Distinguishing the Independent Effects of Exercise Stress and Energy Availability

For the past several years, we have focused our efforts on experiments that are designed to determine the independent effects of exercise stress and energy availability on the HPG axis *(60–65)*. For these experiments, we defined energy availability operationally as dietary energy intake minus exercise energy expenditure. Conceptually, this corresponds to the amount of dietary energy available for all physiological functions, except exercise. Although not the actual physiological quantity hypothetically affecting the HPG axis at the cellular level, our operational definition in behavioral terms has the advantage of being readily measurable and controllable. We control the dietary energy intake of our subjects by feeding them a commercially available clinical dietary product (Ensure®) of known amount and composition as their only food during the experiments. We also require them to exercise under supervision in our laboratory on a treadmill while we measure and control their energy expenditure until they have expended a predetermined amount of energy. We then defined exercise stress as everything associated with exercise except its energy cost.

Subject selection has been an important factor in our experiments, since we have taken pains to minimize the influence of potentially confounding factors. Healthy, regularly menstruating, habitually sedentary, nonobese, nonsmoking women 18–30 yr of age at least 5 yr past menarche, with no recent history of dieting, weight loss, or aerobic training were recruited. Before being admitted to the study, these volunteers undergo an extensive screening procedure, including written medical, menstrual, dietary, and athletic histories, a physical examination, a 12-lead resting electrocardiogram, a 7-d prospective dietary record, determination of body composition by hydrostatic weighing, and a treadmill test to determine their aerobic capacity. Volunteers were admitted into experiments only if they present no current use of medications including oral contraceptives, no history of heart, liver, or renal disease, diabetes, or menstrual or thyroid disorders. They must also have documented prospective records of menstrual cycles 26–32 d in length for at least the previous 3 mo. They must be 18–30% body fat, with habitual energy intakes between 35 and 55 kcal/kg lean body mass [LBM]/d based on their 7-d diet records, with maximal aerobic capacities <42 mL O_2/kg body wt/min, and they must have been performing <60 min of habitual aerobic activity/wk for the previous 3 mo.

The narrow range of our subjects' menstrual cycle lengths implies that we restrict our subject pool to the central 60% of menstrual cycle lengths in the population, and that from this pool, we choose women whose menstrual cycle lengths are in the least variable 20% of the population *(66)* Thus, if anything, our subjects' reproductive systems are robust against disturbance by commonly occurring environmental and behavioral influences. We can be confident, therefore, that if our treatments disrupt the reproductive systems of these women, they will disrupt the reproductive systems of other women, too. We can also be confident that our subject's metabolism has not been disturbed by any confounding medical conditions or dietary or exercise habits before our treatments are applied.

EXCALIBUR I

Excalibur I *(60)* was designed to investigate whether exercise stress has any suppressive effect on T_3 levels independent of the impact of the energy cost of exercise on energy availability. We were interested in T_3, because it regulates the rate of energy expenditure at rest and because it was known to be suppressed in amenorrheic athletes. We reasoned that if the energy cost of exercise necessitates such major metabolic adjustments as the suppression of reproductive function, then these metabolic adjustments might be reflected in suppressed T_3 levels. At the time, the effect of exercise on T_3 was controversial. In some previous experiments, T_3 levels had risen in exercising subjects, whereas in others it had decreased. We suspected that these conflicts might be owing to a failure to control energy availability.

If the energy availability hypothesis were true and the stress hypothesis were false, then we ought to be able to suppress T_3 levels in habitually sedentary women by requiring them to expend energy in exercise without increasing their energy intake, and we ought also to be able to prevent this suppression by increasing their dietary energy intake in compensation for the exercise energy expenditure. If this effect were there to find, we wanted to make sure we found it. Therefore, we required our subjects to expend a lot of energy. Our experimental design is illustrated in Fig. 1.

We controlled the diet and exercise of six groups of subjects for 4 d in the early follicular phase of the menstrual cycle. On the morning of each treatment day, we drew blood samples that we assayed later for several thyroid hormones.

Two groups of subjects performed no exercise during the treatment period. A second pair of groups performed a large amount of high-intensity exercise (1300 kcal/d at 70% of each individual's aerobic capacity, similar to a half marathon race each day). It took about 3 h for our unconditioned subjects to complete this exercise in 30-min bouts separated by 10-min rest periods. A third pair of groups performed the same amount of exercise at a very low exercise intensity, only 40% of aerobic capacity. It took these women about 5 h each day to complete this exercise treatment.

To one group within each pair of groups, we provided an approximately balanced energy availability of 30 kcal of energy for each kg of their body wt (30 kcal/kg body wt/d, which worked out to about 1750 kcal/d). On the other group, we imposed a low energy availability of only 500 kcal/d (corresponding to about 8 kcal/kg body wt/d). We chose 500 kcal/d, because 600 kcal/d had already been shown to suppress T_3 levels in obese patients *(68)*.

Therefore, one of the groups that expended no energy in exercise consumed 30 kcal/kg body wt/d, whereas the other group consumed only 500 kcal/d. We imposed the same low-energy availability of 500 kcal/d, on one of the groups exercising at high intensity and on one of the groups exercising at low-intensity exercise by feeding them only 500 kcal/d in addition to the 1300 kcal/d that they were expending in exercise. By contrast, we imposed a balanced energy availability of 30 kcal/kg body wt/d on the other exercising groups by feeding them 30 kcal/kg body wt/d in addition to their 1300 kcal/d of exercise energy expenditure.

Thus, we contrasted high and low levels of energy availability (30 vs 8 kcal/kg body wt/d) in women exercising not at all, and in women exercising a great deal both at a low intensity and at a high intensity. We analyzed the resulting T_3 measurements to determine the effect of energy availability by contrasting groups exercising similarly, and we determined the independent effect of exercise stress by contrasting groups exercising differently.

We found that low-energy availability had suppressed T_3 levels by 15%, whereas exercise stress had no effect on T_3 (Fig. 1). T_3 levels were suppressed similarly regardless of whether energy availability was reduced by dietary energy restriction or by exercise energy expenditure. Furthermore, the suppression of T_3 in exercising women was prevented by supplementing their diet in compensation for the energy cost of their exercise. We also found that the suppression of free T_3, T_4, and free T_4 and the elevation of reverse T_3 were all similarly preventable. These findings were consistent with the energy-availability hypothesis and inconsistent with the exercise stress hypothesis.

EXCALIBUR II

Excalibur II *(61)* was designed to reveal whether T_3 levels in exercising women vary in linear proportion to energy availability or are suppressed abruptly at a particular threshold of energy availability. We suspected the existence of a threshold, because most

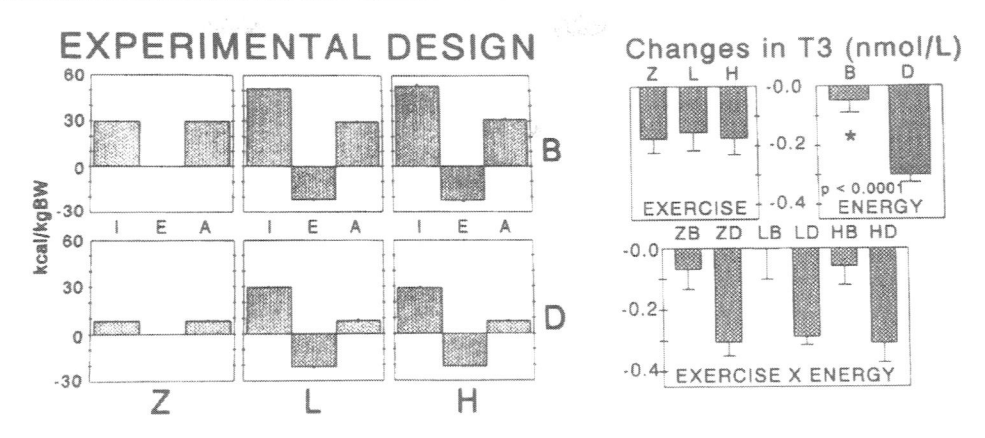

Fig. 1. (Left) Experimental design of Excalibur I. Dietary energy intake (I), energy expenditure during exercise (E), and net energy availability (A) in the 3 × 2 (exercise stress × energy availability) experimental design. Pairs of groups performed zero exercise (Z), 30 kcal/kg of body wt/d (kcal/kg body wt/d) of low-intensity exercise (L), or 30 kcal/kg body wt/d of high-intensity exercise (H). At each exercise treatment level, one group was in approximate energy balance (B), whereas the other was energy-deficient (D). (Where SE bars appear to be missing, the SEs are smaller than a line width.) (Right) Treatment effects on T_3 (nmol/L). Changes (means and internal SE) in response to 4 d of treatments, with achieved significance levels for exercise and energy availability treatments. Z, the two zero-exercise groups; L, the two low-intensity exercise groups; H, the two high-intensity exercise groups; B, the three energy-balanced groups; D, the three energy-deficient groups (67, with permission).

cross-sectional comparisons had been unable to find differences in energy intake or expenditure between eumenorrheic and amenorrheic athletes. We reasoned that such findings would have occurred if the disruption of reproductive function occurred abruptly over a range of energy availability smaller than the habitual ranges of energy intake and expenditure among athletes. If so, then small reductions in energy availability might have little effect on the HPG axis, even though slightly larger reductions might disrupt it. We reasoned further that if the disruption of HPG axis were abrupt, and if the energy availability hypothesis were true, then the suppression of T_3 might also be abrupt. We also knew that the techniques used to measure habitual energy intake and expenditure were not very reliable, but that we could control dietary energy intake and exercise energy expenditure very precisely in the laboratory.

To search for our hypothesized energy availability threshold, we employed a binary search technique. All subjects performed the same high-intensity exercise treatment that we had employed in Excalibur I. This corresponded to an energy expenditure of approx 30 kcal/kg LBM/d. By this time, we had begun normalizing energy by LBM instead of by body weight, since lean tissue is much more metabolically active than adipose tissue. For 4 d in the early follicular phase, we supplemented the diet of a group of subjects in compensation for the energy that they expended in exercise, while not supplementing the dietary energy intake of a second exercising group at all. In this experiment, though, the dietary energy intake of a third group was supplemented by half of the energy expended in exercise, and a decision on which of three supplementations to administer to a fourth group was deferred until the results in the third group were known. If T_3 levels in the third group were suppressed half as much as those in the unsupplemented group,

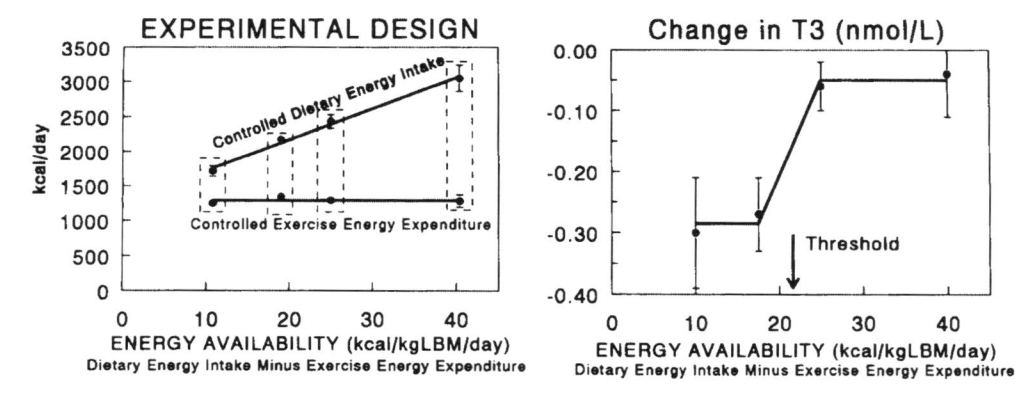

Fig. 2. (Left) Experimental design of Excalibur II. All women performed ~30 kcal/kg LBM/d of supervised aerobic exercise for 4 d, receiving no, one-quarter, one-half, or complete dietary compensation for the energy expended during exercise. **(Right)** Effects of energy availability on T_3. A threshold of energy availability for the maintenance of normal T_3 production was detected between 19 and 25 kcal/kg LBM/d. (*67*, with permission).

then the fourth group would receive the same dietary supplementation as the third group to confirm the implied linearly proportional dependence of T_3 on energy availability. If T_3 levels in the third group were similar to those in the fully supplemented group, then the supplementation of the fourth group would be reduced by half again. If T_3 levels in the third group were similar to those in the unsupplemented group, then the supplementation of the fourth group would be increased by half.

The first group, whose diet was fully supplemented, received a balanced energy availability of 40 kcal/kg LBM/d, but the unsupplemented group received approx 10 kcal/kg LBM/d, and the third group, whose dietary intake was supplemented by only half of their exercise energy expenditure, received 25 kcal/kg LBM/d. The experimental design is illustrated in Fig. 2.

We found that T_3 levels in the third group were not suppressed at all. Therefore, the dietary supplementation of our fourth group was reduced by half so that they received an energy availability of 19 kcal/kg LBM/d. In them, T_3 levels were suppressed as much as they were in the unsupplemented group (Fig. 2). Thus, we found that the suppression of T_3 by low-energy availability occurs abruptly at a threshold of energy availability somewhere between 19 and 25 kcal/kg LBM/d. For our women of average body size and composition, dietary energy intake at that threshold was about 1000 kcal/d.

EXCALIBUR III

In Excalibur III (*62,63*), we moved on to test the exercise stress and energy availability hypotheses as they apply to LH pulsatility. Normal ovarian function depends not on some stable concentration of LH, but rather on the appearance of pulsatile surges of LH concentrations in the blood at regular, approximately hourly, intervals. These pulses correspond to regular secretory bursts of LH from the pituitary gland in response to similar secretory bursts of GnRH from the hypothalamus. The frequency and amplitude of these pulses vary around the menstrual cycle. In sedentary women in the early follicular phase, the pulsatile pattern is characterized as high-frequency and low-amplitude. In regularly menstruating athletes, the pulses are larger in amplitude, and they occur less

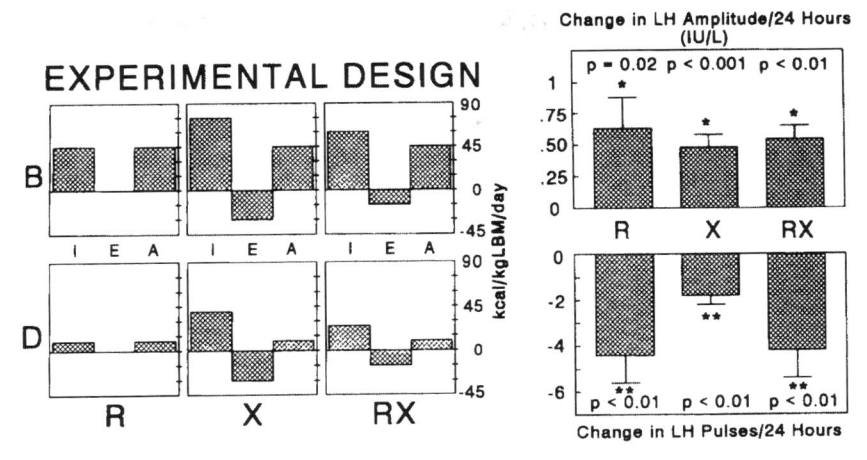

Fig. 3. **(Left)** Experimental design of Excalibur III. Energy availability (A) was defined as dietary energy intake (I) minus exercise energy expenditure (E). Balanced (B = 45 kcal/kg LBM/d) and deficient (D=10 kcal/kg LBM/d) energy availability treatments were administered through extreme dietary energy restriction alone (R), through extreme exercise energy expenditure alone (X: E = 30 kcal/kg LBM/d = 1300 kcal/d at 70% VO_2max), and through the combination (RX) of moderate dietary restriction (I = 25 kcal/kg LBM/d) and moderate exercise energy expenditure (E = 15 kcal/kg LBM/d = 650 kcal/d at 70% VO_2max) for 4 d in the early follicular phase. **(Right)** Effects of low-energy availability on LH pulsatility. Top: Effects on LH pulse amplitude. LH pulse amplitude was increased by all three low-energy availability treatments. Bottom: Effects on LH pulse frequency. LH pulse frequency was reduced by all three treatments (67, with permission).

often, but still at regular intervals. In amenorrheic athletes, LH pulses occur even less often and irregularly *(29)*.

In an experimental design reminiscent of Excalibur I, we investigated whether exercise has any suppressive effect on LH pulsatility beyond the impact of its energy cost on energy availability. The design is illustrated in Fig. 3.

For 4 d in the midfollicular phase of two menstrual cycles, we controlled the energy availability of three groups of women. During one cycle, we administered a balanced energy availability of 45 kcal/kg LBM/d, and during the other cycle, we administered a low-energy availability of 10 kcal/kg LBM/d. One group of subjects performed no exercise during the two treatment periods. A second group performed the same large amount of high-intensity exercise that we had utilized in Excalibur I and II (30 kcal/kg LBM/d). A third group performed half as much exercise (15 kcal/kg LBM/d) and completed their exercise in about 90 min.

We imposed balanced and low energy availabilities on the nonexercising group by feeding them 45 and 10 kcal/kg LBM/day, respectively. We imposed the same balanced and low energy availabilities on the group performing 30 kcal/kg LBM/d of exercise by feeding them 75 and 40 kcal/kg LBM/d, respectively, and we imposed the same energy availabilities on the women exercising 15 kcal/kg LBM/d by feeding them 60 and 25 kcal/kg LBM/d, respectively. Thus, we contrasted energy availability in women exercising not at all, a large amount, and a moderate amount.

At the end of each of these 4-d treatments, we admitted the women to a General Clinical Research Center and drew blood samples from them at 10-min intervals for

24 h. Later, we measured the amount of LH in each sample and used a special statistical computer program to calculate the frequency and amplitude of their LH pulses. We determined the effects of energy availability on these frequencies and amplitudes by contrasting data taken while performing the same exercise at different energy availabilities, and we determined the independent effect of exercise stress by contrasting groups exercising differently at the same energy availabilities.

We found that low-energy availability reduced LH pulse frequency and increased LH pulse amplitude, and that exercise stress had no suppressive effect on LH pulsatility beyond the impact of the energy cost of exercise on energy availability (Fig. 3). LH pulsatility was disrupted regardless of whether energy availability was reduced by extreme energy restriction alone, by extreme exercise energy expenditure alone, or by a combination of moderate dietary energy restriction and moderate exercise energy expenditure. Dietary supplementation prevented the suppression of LH pulsatility by exercise energy expenditure.

Low-energy availability also suppressed plasma glucose, insulin insulin-like growth factor 1 (IGF-1), leptin, and T_3, while raising growth hormone and cortisol levels. All these effects are reminiscent of abnormalities observed in amenorrheic athletes *(21,23,24,29,45–47)*.

Others have shown that short-term fasting also reduces LH pulse frequency in sedentary women during the early follicular phase *(69,70)*. In lean women, ovarian function during the ensuing menstrual cycle is also impaired *(70)*.

EXCALIBUR IV

Excalibur IV *(65)* was designed to reveal whether refeeding reverses the suppression of LH pulsatility in women as quickly as it does in other mammalian species. A single *ad libitum* meal stimulates LH pulses within 2 h in food-restricted female rats *(10,71)* and ewes *(72)*, and in fasted heifers *(73)* and male rhesus monkeys *(74)*. Such observations have been interpreted to imply that the physiological signals produced by a single large meal are sufficient to activate the hypothalamic GnRH neurons that control LH pulsatility *(75)*.

We suspected that the restoration of LH pulsatility by refeeding might be considerably slower in energetically disrupted women than in other mammals, because the human brain requires so much more energy than does the brain of any other mammal. The brain competes against all other tissues of the body for energy, and the adult human brain requires 20% of basal metabolic energy, compared to only 2% for most species and 8% for nonhuman primates *(76)*. Therefore, we suspected that a single meal might not provide enough energy to activate GnRH neurons in energetically disrupted women.

To test this hypothesis stringently, we assayed LH in blood samples drawn from women at 10-min intervals for 48 h during the midfollicular phase, first during 24 h on the 5th d of low energy availability treatments and then during 24 h of aggressive refeeding. A combination of moderate dietary energy restriction (25 kcal/kg LBM/d) and moderate exercise energy expenditure (15 kcal/kg LBM/d) was administered to impose a low-energy availability of 10 kcal/kg LBM/d. The aggressive refeeding regimen was comprised of 15 meals providing 85 kcal/kg LBM/d. Combined with the same exercise treatment, the energy availability during the 24 h of aggressive refeeding was 70 kcal/kg LBM/d.

Compared to measurements of LH pulsatility in 18 other women studied previously in this laboratory under balanced energy availability conditions and at the same phase of the menstrual cycle, low energy availability suppressed LH pulsatility unambiguously in five of the eight subjects treated in this experiment. Their LH pulse frequency was reduced 57% to 8.2 ± 1.5 pulses/24 h, well below the 5th percentile of LH pulse frequencies in energy-balanced women (14.6 pulses/24 h), whereas their LH pulse amplitude was increased 94% to 3.1 ± 0.3 IU/L, well above the 95th percentile of LH pulse amplitudes in energy-balanced women (2.5 IU/L).

Among these women, aggressive refeeding raised LH pulse frequency by only 2.4 ± 1.0 pulses/24 h, still far below the 5th percentile of LH pulse frequency in energy-balanced women. Meanwhile, the unambiguously elevated LH pulse amplitude was completely unaffected (Δ = 0.0 ± 0.4 IU/L) by aggressive refeeding. (Results were similar when all eight subjects were included in the analysis. Aggressive refeeding pushed the group as a whole to, but not past the 5th and 95th percentiles of LH pulse frequency and amplitude, respectively.)

Thus, 24 h of a refeeding protocol much more aggressive than the *ad libitum* refeeding protocols commonly employed in animal experiments had very little restorative effect on LH pulsatility in our energetically suppressed women. This striking difference from other mammalian species may be related to the equally striking difference between the energy requirements of human and other mammalian brains. Investigators should be alert for other differences between humans and other mammals in the dependence of HPG axis function on energy availability.

INTERIM INTERPRETATIONS
Mechanisms

BODY COMPOSITION

We are unaware of any experiments that have determined the independent effect of body composition on the HPG axis. From the experimental data on energy availability, however, it would appear to be more likely that a lean body composition and disruption of the HPG axis are both effects of low-energy availability than that a lean body composition disrupts the HPG axis.

EXERCISE STRESS

Our short-term experiments have demonstrated that exercise stress has no suppressive effect on metabolic hormones and substrates or on LH pulsatility beyond the impact of the energy cost of the exercise on energy availability. This finding appears to contradict the exercise stress hypothesis, although we will not know for sure until we learn the results of more prolonged experiments investigating the independent effects of exercise stress and energy availability on ovarian function. At this time, there are still no experimental data that any stressor has any suppressive effect on the HPG axis beyond the impact of an associated energy cost on energy availability.

ENERGY AVAILABILITY

All the experimental data available at this time suggest that the factor disrupting the HPG axis in physically active women is low energy availability, and that they may be able to prevent or to reverse menstrual disorders by dietary reform without moderating their exercise regimen. This hypothesis will not be confirmed, though, until we have the results of more prolonged experiments investigating the independent effects of exercise stress and energy availability on ovarian function.

CARBOHYDRATE AVAILABILITY

In Excalibur III, the suppression of LH pulse frequency by low-energy availability was actually smaller in exercising women than in nonexercising women with the same low-energy availability (63). This result was unexpected, and it suggests that LH pulsatility might actually depend on a more specific metabolic factor that is easily confused with energy availability, but that is less compromised by exercise energy expenditure than by dietary energy restriction.

Research in other mammals suggests that GnRH neuron activity and LH pulsatility are actually regulated by brain glucose availability (16,19). The adult female human brain oxidizes about 80 g of glucose each day at a continuous rate. This must be provided daily by dietary carbohydrate, because the brain's daily glucose requirement is much greater than can be supplied by liver glycogen (77). Moderate exercise oxidizes as much glucose in an hour.

In the nonexercising women in Excalibur III, low-energy availability owing to dietary energy restriction reduced carbohydrate intake by 77%. This reduction in carbohydrate intake was similar to the 73% increase in carbohydrate oxidation revealed by respiratory gas analysis in the exercising women during the balanced energy availability treatment. By contrast, carbohydrate oxidation increased only 49% in the exercising women under low-energy availability conditions. This alteration in fuel selection conserved almost 70% of the brain's daily glucose requirement. Thus, exercise may compromise brain glucose availability less than dietary energy restriction, and this may account for the smaller disruption of LH pulsatility that we observed in exercising women than in dietarily restricted women.

This speculation is consistent with the 10% lower plasma glucose levels observed in amenorrheic athletes than in regularly menstruating athletes and sedentary women (21). Thus, LH pulsatility may depend on carbohydrate rather than energy availability in women, just as it does in other mammals.

Clinical Implications

Although energy availability appears to be the driving factor in disrupting LH pulsatility, acute refeeding may not restore normal patterns immediately. If athletes are able to prevent or to reverse disruptions of the HPG axis by dietary reform without moderation of their exercise regimen, then the appropriate advice to them is to increase their dietary energy intake, and there is no need to interfere in their endurance, strength, and skill training.

In this regard, it is noteworthy that during our experiments, women reported that they felt hungry during dietary restriction, but not while their energy availability was similarly reduced by exercise energy expenditure. Meanwhile, women whose diets were supplemented in compensation for their exercise energy expenditure reported that they felt overfed and that they had to force themselves to eat when they were not hungry. This observation suggests that appetite may be an inaccurate indicator of energy balance during athletic training, just as thirst is an inadequate indicator of water balance during athletic competition. Athletes may need to eat by discipline rather than appetite during training, just as they drink by discipline rather than thirst during competition.

Other conditions besides exercise have also been thought to disrupt the HPG axis via a stress mechanism, but they, too, impair energy availability. Surgery, burns, and infection, for example, reduce energy availability physiologically. Melancholic depression impairs energy availability psychologically and behaviorally through reduced appetite, decreased emphasis on feeding, and sustained anorexia *(38,78)*. Immobilization stress in animal experiments is accompanied by a 60% suppression of *ad libitum* dietary energy intake *(79)*. Thus, none of these stressors may have any disruptive effect on the HPG axis independent of the impact of their energy cost on energy availability.

Needed Research

More short-term experiments are needed to resolve the ambiguity about whether LH pulsatility depends on energy or glucose availability, to determine whether LH pulsatility, like T_3, is disrupted at a threshold of energy availability, and whether this threshold differs between men and women. Prolonged experiments are needed to confirm that short-term effects on LH pulsatility are predictive of chronic effects on ovarian function. Intervention experiments are needed to confirm that women can prevent or reverse amenorrhea by dietary reform without moderating their exercise regimen. In addition, experiments like ours are needed to test whether other stressors besides exercise have any suppressive effect on LH pulsatility beyond the impact of their energy cost on energy availability.

ACKNOWLEDGMENTS

This research was supported in part by the American Heart Association Ohio Affiliate, NIH Shannon Award 1R55-HD-29547-01, the US Army Medical Research Acquisition Activity (USAMRAA) grant #DAMD 17-95-1-5053, and grant M01-RR-00034 from the General Clinical Research Branch, Division of Research Resources, NIH. The content of the information presented in this chapter does not necessarily reflect the position or the policy of the government, and no official endorsement should be inferred.

REFERENCES

1. Frisch RE, McArthur JW. Menstrual cycles: fatness as a determinant of minimum weight for height necessary for their maintenance or onset. Science 1974;185:949–951.
2. Frisch RE, Revelle R. Height and weight at menarche and a hypothesis of menarche. Arch Dis Child 1971;46:695–701.
3. Schneider JE, Wade GN. Letter to the editor. Am J Physiol 1997;273 (Endocrinol Metab 36):E231,E232.
4. Crist DM, Hill JM. Diet and insulin like growth factor I in relation to body composition in women with exercise-induced hypothalamic amenorrhea. J Am Coll Nutr 1990;9:200–204.
5. Bronson FH, Manning JM. The energetic regulation of ovulation: A realistic role for body fat. Biol Reprod 1991;44:945–950.
6. Loucks AB, Horvath SM. Athletic amenorrhea: a review. Med Sci Sports Exerc 1985;17:56–72.
7. Scott EC, Johnson FE. Critical fat, menarche, and the maintenance of menstrual cycles: a critical review. J Adolesc Health Care 1982;2:249–260.
8. Sinning WE, Little KD. Body composition and menstrual function in athletes. Sports Med 1987;4:34–45.
9. Loucks AB, Horvath SM, Freedson PS. Menstrual status and validation of body fat prediction in athletes. Hum Biol 1984;56:383–392.
10. Bronson FH. Food-restricted, prepubertal, female rats: Rapid recovery of luteinizing hormone pulsing with excess food, and full recovery of pubertal development with gonadotropin-releasing hormone. Endocrinology 1986;118:2483–2487.
11. Zhang Y, Proenca R, Maffei M, Barone M, Leopold L, Friedman JM. Positional cloning of the mouse *obese* gene and its human homologue. Nature 1994;372:425–432.
12. Maffei M, Halaas J, Ravussin E, et al. Leptin levels in human and rodent: measurement of plasma leptin and cb RNA in obese and weight-reduced subjects. Nature Medicine 1995;1:1155–1161.

13. Cheung CC, Clifton DK, Steiner RA. Proopiomelanocortin neurons are direct targets for leptin in the hypothalamus. Endocrinology 1997;138:4489–4492.
14. Warren MP. The effects of exercise on pubertal progression and reproductive function in girls. J Clin Endocrinol Metab 1980;51:1150–1157.
15. Winterer J, Cutler GB Jr, Loriaux DL. Caloric balance, brain to body ratio, and the timing of menarche. Med Hypotheses 1984;15:87–91.
16. Wade GN, Schneider JE. Metabolic fuels and reproduction in female mammals. Neurosci Biobehav Rev 1992;16:235–272.
17. Bronson FH, Heideman PD. Seasonal regulation of reproduction in mammals. In: Knobil E, Neill JD, eds. The Physiology of Reproduction. Raven, New York, NY, 1994, pp. 541–583.
18. Bronson FH, Manning J. Food consumption, prolonged exercise, and LH secretion in the peripubertal female rat. In: Pirke KM, Wuttke W, Schweiger U, eds. The Menstrual Cycle and Its Disorders. Springer-Verlag, Berlin, 1989, pp. 42–49.
19. Wade GN, Schneider JE, Li H-Y. Control of fertility by metabolic cues. Am J Physiol 1996;270 (Endocrinol Metab 33):E1–E19.
20. Cameron JL, Nosbisch C, Helmreich DL, Parfitt DB. Reversal of exercise-induced amenorrhea in female cynomolgus monkeys (Macaca fascicularis) by increasing food intake. Endocrine Society Annual Meeting 1990;285 (Abstract): 1042.
21. Laughlin GA, Yen SSC. Nutritional and endocrine-metabolic aberrations in amenorrheic athletes. J Clin Endocrinol Metab 1996;81:4301–4309.
22. Laughlin GA, Yen SSC. Hypoleptinemia in women athletes: absence of a diurnal rhythm with amenorrhea. J Clin Endocrinol Metab 1997;82:318–321.
23. Myerson M, Gutin B, Warren MP, et al. Resting metabolic rate and energy balance in amenorrheic and eumenorrheic runners. Med Sci Sports Exerc 1991;23:15–22.
24. Loucks AB, Laughlin GA, Mortola JF, Girton L, Nelson JC, Yen SSC. Hypothalamic–pituitary–thyroidal function in eumenorrheic and amenorrheic athletes. J.Clin Endocrinol Metab 1992;75: 514–518.
25. Kolaczynski JW, Considine RV, Ohannesian J, et al. Responses of leptin to short-term fasting and refeeding in humans: a link with ketogenesis but not ketones themselves. Diabetes 1996;45: 1511–1515.
26. Kolaczynski JW, Ohannesian J, Considine RV, Marco C, Caro JF. Response of leptin to short term and prolonged overfeeding in humans. J Clin Endocrinol Metab 1996;81:4162–4165.
27. Weigle DS, Duell PB, Connor WE, Steiner RA, Soules MR, Kuijper JL. Effect of fasting, refeeding, and dietary fat restriction on plasma leptin levels. J Clin Endocrinol Metab 1997;82:561–565.
28. Jenkins AB, Markovic TP, Fleury A, Campbell LV. Carbohydrate intake and short-term regulation of leptin in humans. Diabetologia 1997;40:348–351.
29. Loucks AB, Mortola JF, Girton L, Yen SSC. Alterations in the hypothalamic-pituitary-ovarian and hypothalamic–pituitary–adrenal axes in athletic women. J Clin Endocrinol Metab 1989;68:402–411.
30. Drinkwater BL, Nilson K, Chesnut CH III, Bremner WJ, Shainholtz S, Southworth MB. Bone mineral content of amenorrheic and eumenorrheic athletes. N Engl J Med 1984;311:277–281.
31. Kaiserauer S, Snyder AC, Sleeper M, Zierath J. Nutritional, physiological, and menstrual status of distance runners. Med Sci Sports Exerc 1989;21:120–125.
32. Marcus R, Cann C, Madvig P, et al. Menstrual function and bone mass in elite women distance runners. Endocrine and metabolic features. Ann Intern Med 1985;102:158–163.
33. Nelson ME, Fisher EC, Catsos PD, Meredith CN, Turksoy RN, Evans WJ. Diet and bone status in amenorrheic runners. Am J Clin Nutr 1986;43:910–916.
34. Edwards JE, Lindeman AK, Mikesky AE, Stager JM. Energy balance in highly trained female endurance runners. Med Sci Sports Exerc 1993;25:1398–1404.
35. Wilmore JH, Wambsgans KC, Brenner M, et al. Is there energy conservation in amenorrheic compared with eumenorrheic distance runners? J Appl Physiol 1992;72:15–22.
36. Mertz W, Tsui JC, Judd JT, et al. What are people really eating? The relation between energy intake derived from estimated diet records and intake determined to maintain body weight. Am J Clin Nutr 1991;54:291–295.
37. Leibel RL, Rosenbaum M, Hirsch J. Changes in energy expenditure resulting from altered body weight. N Engl J Med 1995;332:621–628.
38. Rivier C, Rivest S. Effect of stress on the activity of the hypothalamic-pituitary-gonadal axis: peripheral and central mechanisms. Biol Reprod 1991;45:523–532.

39. Selye H. The effect of adaptation to various damaging agents on the female sex organs in the rat. Endocrinology 1939;25:615–624.
40. Asahina K, Kitahara F, Yamanaka M, Akiba T. Influences of excessive exercise on the structure and function of rat organs. Jpn J Physiol 1959;9:322–326.
41. Axelson JF. Forced swimming alters vaginal estrous cycles, body composition, and steroid levels without disrupting lordosis behavior or fertility in rats. Physiol Behav 1987;41:471–479.
42. Chatterton RT Jr, Hartman AL, Lynn DE, Hickson RC. Exercise-induced ovarian dysfunction in the rat. Proc Soc Exp Biol Med 1990;193:220–224.
43. Manning JM, Bronson FH. Effects of prolonged exercise on puberty and luteinizing hormone secretion in female rats. Am J Physiol 257 (Regul Integrative Comp Physiol 1989;26):R1359–R1364.
44. Manning JM, Bronson FH. Suppression of puberty in rats by exercise: effects on hormone levels and reversal with GnRH infusion. Am J Physiol 260 (Regul Integrative Comp Physiol 1991;29):R717–R723.
45. De Souza MJ, Maguire MS, Maresh CM, Kraemer WJ, Rubin KR, Loucks AB. Adrenal activation and the prolactin response to exercise in eumenorrheic and amenorrheic runners. J Appl Physiol 1991;70:2378–2387.
46. De Souza MJ, Luciano AA, Arce JC, Demers LM, Loucks AB. Clinical tests explain blunted cortisol responsiveness but not mild hypercortisolism in amenorrheic runners. J Appl Physiol 1994;76:1302–1309.
47. Ding J-H, Scheckter CB, Drinkwater BL, Soules MR, Bremner WJ. High serum cortisol levels in exercise-associated amenorrhea. Ann Intern Med 1988;108:530–534.
48. Suh BY, Liu JH, Berga SL, Quigley ME, Laughlin GA, Yen SSC. Hypercortisolism in patients with functional hypothalamic-amenorrhea. J Clin Endocrinol Metab 1988;66:733–739.
49. Gold PW, Gwirtsman H, Avgerinos PC, et al. Abnormal hypothalamic-pituitary-adrenal function in anorexia nervosa: pathophysiologic mechanisms in underweight and weight-corrected patients. N Engl J Med 1986;314:1335–1342.
50. Slentz CA, Davis JM, Settles DL, Pate RR, Settles SJ. Glucose feedings and exercise in rats: glycogenous, hormone responses, and performance. J Appl Physiol 1990;69:989–994.
51. Tabata I, Ogita F, Miyachi M, Shibayama H. Effect of low blood glucose on plasma CRF, ACTH, and cortisol during prolonged physical exercise. J Appl Physiol 1991;71:1807–1812.
52. Bonen A. Recreational exercise does not impair menstrual cycles: A prospective study. Int J Sports Med 1992;13:110–120.
53. Boyden TW, Pamenter RW, Stanforth P, Rotkis T, Wilmore JH. Sex steroids and endurance running in women. Fertil Steril 1983;39:629–632.
54. Bullen BA, Skrinar GS, Beitins IZ, et al. Endurance training effects on plasma hormonal responsiveness and sex hormone excretion. J Appl Physiol 1984;56:1453–1463.
55. Rogol AD, Weltman A, Weltman JY, et al. Durability of the reproductive axis in eumenorrheic women during 1 year of endurance training. J Appl Physiol 1992;72:1571–1580.
56. Loucks AB, Cameron JL, De Souza MJ. Subject assignment may have biased experimental results. J Appl Physiol 1993;74:2045,2046.
57. Rogol AD, Evans WS, Weltman JY, Veldhuis JD, Weltman AL. Reply to "Subject assignment may have biased experimental results." J Appl Physiol 1993;74:2046–2047.
58. Bullen BA, Skrinar GS, Beitins IZ, von Mering G, Turnbull BA, McArthur JW. Induction of menstrual disorders by strenuous exercise in untrained women. N Engl J Med 1985;312:1349–1353.
59. Williams NI, Young JC, McArthur JW, Bullen B, Skrinar GS, Turnbull B. Strenuous exercise with caloric restriction: effect on luteinizing hormone secretion. Med Sci Sports Exerc 1995;27:1390–1398.
60. Loucks AB, Callister R. Induction and prevention of low-T3 syndrome in exercising women. Am J Physiol 264 (Regul Integrative Comp Physiol 1993;33):R924–R930.
61. Loucks AB, Heath EM. Induction of low-T_3 syndrome in exercising women occurs at a threshold of energy availability. Am J Physiol 266 (Regul Integrative Comp Physiol 1994;35):R817–R823.
62. Loucks AB, Heath EM. Dietary restriction reduces luteinizing hormone pulse frequency during waking hours and increases luteinizing hormone pulse amplitude during sleep in young menstruating women. J Clin Endocrinol Metab 1994;78:910–915.
63. Loucks AB, Verdun M, Heath EM. Low energy availability, not stress of exercise, alters LH pulsatility in exercising women. J Appl Physiol 1998;84:37–46.
64. Loucks AB, Brown R, King K, Thuma JR, Verdun M. A combined regimen of moderate dietary restriction and exercise training alters luteinizing hormone pulsatility in regularly menstruating young women. Endocrine Society Annual Meeting 1995, p. 558, Abstract #P3-360.

65. Loucks AB, Verdun M. Slow restoration of LH pulsatility by refeeding in energetically disrupted women. Am J Physiol (Regulatory, Integrative Comp Physiol) 1998;44:R1218–R1226.
66. Treloar AE, Boynton RE, Behn BG, Brown BW. Variation of the human menstrual cycle through reproductive life. Int J Fertil 1967;12:77–126.
67. Loucks AB. The reproductive system. In: Bar-Or O, Lamb DR, Clarkson PM, eds. Perspectives in Exercise Science and Sports Medicine, vol. 9, Exercise and the Female—A Life Span Approach. Cooper Publishing, Carmel, IN, 1996, pp. 42–71.
68. O'Brian JT, Bybee DE, Burman KD, Osburne RC, Ksiazek MR, Wartofsky L, et al. Thyroid hormone homeostasis in states of relative caloric depression. Metabolism 1980;29:721–727.
69. Olson BR, Cartledge T, Sebring N, Defensor R, Nieman L. Short-term fasting affects luteinizing hormone secretory dynamics but no reproductive function in normal-weight sedentary women. J Clin Endocrinol Metab 1995;80:1187–1193.
70. Alvero R, Kimzey L, Sebring N, et al. Effects of fasting on neuroendocrine function and follicle development in lean women. J Clin Endocrinol Metab 1998;83:76–80.
71. Bronson FH, Heideman PD. Short-term hormonal responses to food intake in peripubertal female rats. Am J Physiol 1990;259 (Regul Integrative Comp Physiol 28):R25–R31.
72. Foster DL, Ebling FJ, Micka AF, et al. Metabolic interfaces between growth and reproduction. I. Nutritional modulation of gonadotropin, prolactin, and growth hormone secretion in the growth-limited female lamb. Endocrinology 1989;125:342–350.
73. McCann JP, Hansel W. Relationships between insulin and glucose metabolism and pituitary-ovarian functions in fasted heifers. Biol Reprod 1986;34:630–641.
74. Parfitt DB, Church KR, Cameron JL. Restoration of pulsatile luteinizing hormone secretion after fasting in rhesus monkeys (*Macaca mulatta*): Dependence on size of the refeed meal. Endocrinology 1991;129:749–756.
75. Schreihofer DA, Renda F, Cameron JL. Feeding-induced stimulation of luteinizing hormone secretion in male Rhesus monkeys is not dependent on a rise in glucose concentration. Endocrinology 1996;137:3770–3776.
76. Grande F. Energy expenditure of organs and tissues. In: Kinney JM, ed. Assessment of Energy Metabolism in Health and Disease. Ross Laboratories, Columbus, OH, 1980, pp. 88–92.
77. Bursztein S, Elwyn DH, Askanazi J, Kinney JM, ed. Energy Metabolism, Indirect Calorimetry, and Nutrition. Williams & Wilkins, Baltimore, MD, 1989, p. 146.
78. Chrousos GP, Gold PW. The concepts of stress and stress system disorders. Overview of physical and behavioral homeostatsis. JAMA 1992;267:1244–1252.
79. Shibasaki T, Yamauchi N, Kato Y, et al. Involvement of corticotropin-releasing factor in restraint stress-induced anorexia and reversion of the anorexia by somatostatin in the rat. Life Sci 1988;43:1103–1110.

10 Adrenergic Regulation of Energy Metabolism

Michael Kjær, MD, PhD and Kai Lange, MD

CONTENTS

INTRODUCTION
ADRENERGIC RESPONSES TO ACUTE EXERCISE
MOTOR CONTROL AND REFLEX INFLUENCE ON ADRENERGIC RESPONSE
ADRENERGIC ACTIVITY AFTER PHYSICAL TRAINING
HEPATO-SPLANCHNIC GLUCOSE PRODUCTION AND ADRENERGIC ACTIVITY
ADRENERGIC EFFECT ON SKELETAL MUSCLE CARBOHYDRATE METABOLISM
SYMPATHOADRENERGIC ACTIVITY AND FAT METABOLISM
SUMMARY
REFERENCES

INTRODUCTION

During exercise, energy turnover increases and adrenergic mechanisms play an important role in this regulation. In addition, increased adrenergic activity during exercise also results in an increased heart rate and in an enhanced force of myocardial contraction as well as in vasoconstriction in the splancnic circulation, in the kidneys, and in noncontracting muscles. These circulatory changes favors a redistribution of blood flow to exercising muscle as well as an increased cardiac output (1). Furthermore, the adrenergic activity stimulates sweat glands and thereby influences thermoregulation, and it causes an increased contractility of skeletal muscle as well as influences exercise-induced suppression of components of the human immune system. In the present chapter, it is demonstrated how adrenergic activity can influence substrate mobilization and utilization both directly and indirectly via secretion of hormones.

ADRENERGIC RESPONSES TO ACUTE EXERCISE

Adrenergic activity can be assessed both by direct measurements of electrical activity in superficial sympathetic nerves and by measurement of circulating norepinephrine and epinephrine in the blood. The direct recording of sympathetic activity can be performed to resting muscle only, but during exercise of, e.g., the arms, sympathetic activity to the resting leg muscle has been shown to increase with progressively increasing intensity of arm exercise *(2)*. In addition to these measurements, a correlation has been found between sympathetic nerve activity and plasma levels of norepinephrine *(3)*. Although a correlation between circulating norepinephrine and direct recordings of sympathetic nerve activity from the peroneal nerve has been demonstrated during exercise, the increase in sympathetic outflow to the various regions of the body differs somewhat during exercise. During exercise, using methods to measure norepinephrine spillover, it has been demonstrated that the increase in sympathetic activity during exercise is dominated by an increased sympathetic activity directed toward active muscle. During two-legged exercise, approx 50% of all circulating norepinephrine is released from sympathetic nerve endings in active muscle. Furthermore, when arm exercise is added to leg exercise, the norepinehrine spillover from active leg muscle also increases despite unchanged work output and unchanged blood flow to the leg muscles *(4)*.

In addition to norepinephrine released from sympathetic nerve endings, epinephrine is released from the adrenal medulla in response to sympathetic neural activity during exercise. The circulating epinephrine is responsible for the major adrenergic effect on energy metabolism during exercise compared with norepinephrine. In the present chapter, the adrenergic effect on carbohydrate and fat metabolism will be discussed, but epinephrine *per se* has been shown also to increase protein metabolism in isolated electrically stimulated rat muscle *(5)*.

The levels of circulating free norepinephrine and epinephrine increase with exercise intensity expressed by the percentage of maximal individual performance ($\%VO_2$max). This holds true both during prolonged exercise as well as in response to short-term intermittent exercise and to intense weight training. The increase in plasma norepinephrine and epinephrine occurs rapidly in arterial blood, and it has been calculated that the half-life of epinephrine is around 2–3 min during exercise. Circulating levels of catecholamines can only be considered as overall markers of symphatoadrenergic activity and are influenced not only by secretion, but also by clearance of the hormone. Whereas clearance of norepinephrine is difficult to determine on a whole-body level owing to the fact that it is extracted at two levels in series, namely both the lung and the systemic organs *(6)*, the turnover of epinephrine can be studied in humans, using a radiolabeled tracer. It has been shown that whole-body clearance of epinephrine increases by 15% at low exercise intensities and decreases around 20% below basal levels after more intense exercise *(7)*. However, since the increase in plasma epinephrine seen during dynamic exercise in humans is 5- to 10-fold, these changes are caused by increases in secretion from the adrenal medulla rather than by changes in clearance. Among the major contributors to epinephrine clearance are the hepatosplancnic area and the kidneys.

MOTOR CONTROL AND REFLEX INFLUENCE ON ADRENERGIC RESPONSE

In experiments using partial neuromuscular blockade to weaken the muscle force and thereby increase the motor center activity needed to produce a certain force output, it was found that exercise-induced increases in levels of circulating catecholamines were augmented compared to control experiments with saline infusion (8). These findings are supported by experiments in paralyzed cats where direct stimulation of the subthalamic locomotor areas in the brain resulted in adrenergic hormonal responses similar to the ones seen during voluntary exercise (9). Together, these experiments support the view that motor center activity can directly stimulate sympathoadrenergic activity during exercise directly and independently of feedback from contracting muscle. That central factors linked to exercise intensity are not sufficient to elicit a maximal adrenergic response can be demonstrated in different ways. When exercising a small muscle group (e.g., one knee extensor) even at maximal intensity, only a small catecholamine response can be observed (4). Furthermore, when maximal work output was reduced by more than 60% with a neuromuscular blockade (tubocurarine), despite subjects working at the highest possible effort, adrenergic responses were far from maximal (10). In addition to central factors, peripheral neural feedback can be demonstrated using lumbar epidural anesthesia in doses sufficiently high to block impulses in thin afferent nerves, but preserving motor nerves and the ability to perform exercise to the highest possible degree. During static exercise, but not during dynamic exercise, catecholamine responses were inhibited when afferent responses were absent (11,12). Interestingly, both ACTH and β-endorphin responses during submaximal exercise were abolished during epidural anesthesia (11,13). In support of a role of afferent nerves in adrenergic responses, plasma catecholamines increased in response to direct stimulation of these nerve fibers in cats (14). An alternative model to study feedback mechanisms during exercise is to use patients with metabolic deficiencies. Both in myophosphorylase (McArdles disease) and phosphofructokinase deficiency and in mitochondrial myopathy, an excessive neuroendocrine response and exaggerated mobilization of extramuscular substrate (glucose and free fatty acid [FFA]) was found, most likely a coupling toward the oxidative demands of the muscle cell rather than to the oxidative capacity of the working muscle (15–17).

ADRENERGIC ACTIVITY AFTER PHYSICAL TRAINING

Vigorous endurance training will reduce the catecholamine response to a given absolute workload (18), whereas neither sympathetic nerve activity nor norepinephrine levels at maximal workloads differ between individuals with different training status (19). This supports the view that physical training does not alter the capacity of the sympathetic nervous system, but that responses to submaximal exercise are linked closely to the relative rather than to the absolute workload (20). Surprisingly, however, it has in a 24-h study been found that highly trained individuals had a higher catecholamine release over the day compared with sedentary individuals (21). Epinephrine response in trained individuals vs sedentary has been shown to be enlarged when stimulated by a variety of stimuli, such as hypoglycemia, caffeine, glucagon, hypoxia, and hypercapnia (20,22–25). This indicates that the capacity to secrete epinephrine from the adrenal medulla improves with training. In rats who underwent 10 wk of intense swim training, the adrenal medullary volume and the adrenal content of epinephrine were larger in trained rats compared with controls who were either weight matched, sham-trained, or cold-stressed (26). Although these findings indicate that the improved secretion capacity of epinephrine is a result of training, this will most likely require several years of training. In well-trained athletes who underwent hypoglycemia before and 4–5 wk after an injury that resulted in inactivity, epinephrine responses did not change with this short-lasting alteration in activity level *(27)*. However, still it is interesting that endocrine glands apparently are able to adapt to physical training and alter their secretion capacity, similar to other tissues like muscle and heart.

HEPATO-SPLANCHNIC GLUCOSE PRODUCTION AND ADRENERGIC ACTIVITY

During intense exercise the rise in hepatic glucose production was parallel with a rise in plasma catecholamine levels *(28–30)*. In addition, in models where electrically induced cycling was used in spinal cord-injured individuals with impaired sympathoadrenergic activity, hepatic glucose production was abolished *(31)*.

In swimming rats, the removal of the adrenal medulla reduced the hepatic glycogenolysis *(32)*, as well as the exercise-induced increase in hepatic glucose production in running rats *(33)*. However, most studies have been unable to demonstrate any effect of epinephrine on liver glycogen breakdown during exercise *(34–37)*. In running dogs, evidence has been provided that epinephrine may play a minor role in liver glucose output late during exercise *(38)* probably owing to an increased gluconeogenic precursor level. Furthermore, adrenalectomized individuals maintain a normal rise in hepatic glucose production during exercise *(39)*, and only when epinephrine is infused in these patients, hepatic glucose production was augmented during the early stages of exercise (unpublished observation).

Direct stimulation of liver nerves caused an increase in hepatic glycogenolysis, and the hypothesis has been put forward that liver nerves are important for the exercise-induced rise in liver glucose output. In contrast to this, surgical or chemical denervation of the liver in various species did not reduce the exercise-induced increment in hepatic glucose production *(32,33,40,41)*, which indicates that sympathetic liver nerves are not essential during exercise. In humans, the role of liver nerves and epinephrine has been studied with application of local anesthesia around the sympathetic celiac ganglion innervating liver, pancreas, and adrenal medulla *(42)*. Pancreatic hormones were standardized by infusion of somatostatin, glucagon, and insulin. During blockade, the exercise induced epinephrine response was inhibited by up to 90%, and presumably liver nerves were also blocked, but this did not diminish the glucose production response to exercise. This indicates that sympathoadrenergic activity is not responsible for an exercise-induced rise in splanchnic glucose output. In further support of this hypothesis, the exercise induced increase in liver glucose production was identical in liver-transplanted patients compared to healthy control subjects as well as in kidney-transplanted patients who received a similar hormonal and immunosuppressive drug treatment as liver-transplanted patients *(43)*. Liver-transplanted patients were investigated approx 8 mo after surgery, and no sign of reinnervation occurred in any of the patients as judged by the content of norepinephrine in liver biopsies *(44)*. Finally, in recent experiments in exercising dogs who underwent a selective blockade of hepatic α- and β-receptors, it was demonstrated that circulating norepinephrine and epinephrine do not participate in the stimulation of glucose production during intense exercise *(45,46)*. Taken together, sympathetic liver nerves or circulating norepinephrine play no role in glucose mobilization from the liver during exercise, and circulating epinephrine only plays a minor role during intense exercise and late during prolonged exercise.

ADRENERGIC EFFECT ON SKELETAL MUSCLE CARBOHYDRATE METABOLISM

Muscle contractions *per se* increase glucose uptake, and humoral factors can modify this *(47)*. Insulin and contractions have a synergistic effect on glucose uptake with contractions *(48)*, whereas epinephrine has been demonstrated to decrease glucose clearance in running dogs *(49)*. In addition to this, femoral arterial infusion of epinephrine into an exercising leg in humans caused a reduction in the normal exercise-induced glucose uptake *(50)*. More recently, it has been shown that in adrenalectomized individuals performing leg cycling for 45 min at 50% VO_2max followed by 15 min at 85% VO_2max, the rise in glucose uptake during exercise was reduced when epinephrine was infused to substitute plasma epinephrine levels normally observed during exercise (unpublished observation). The mechanism behind this is at present unknown, but could be related to an enhanced glycogenolysis, increased intramuscular glucose concentration, or altered uptake of FFA, all changes that can influence glucose uptake.

It has been shown that adrenergic activity can enhance the glycogen breakdown in muscle during contraction both in exercising animals *(51)* and in humans *(50,52)*. However, those studies often used supraphysiological doses of epinephrine, and later studies in humans using lower doses have only been able to demonstrate a higher activation of phosphorylase, but could not demonstrate any marked increase in glycogen breakdown *(53)*. Noradrenergic activity probably does not play any role in muscle glycogenolysis, since unilateral hindlimb sympathectomy did not diminish glycogen breakdown in swimming rats *(54)*.

SYMPATHOADRENERGIC ACTIVITY AND FAT METABOLISM

Lipolysis in fat tissue is enhanced by β-adrenergic activity, and catecholamine responsiveness of β-adrenergic receptors in adipose tissue is increased after acute exercise *(55)*. By the use of microdialysis of subcutaneous abdominal tissue, it was demonstrated that nonselective β-adrenoceptor blockade inhibited the exercise-induced increase in dialysate levels of glycerol *(56)*. Although this indicates a role for adrenergic activity in fat metabolism during exercise, the relative role between sympathetic nerve activity and circulating norepinephrine/epinephrine is currently not known. Intravenous infusion of epinephrine in resting humans caused an increase in lipolytic activity as determined by microdialysis of subcutaneous adipose tissue, an effect that was desensitized by repeated epinephrine infusions *(57)*. The direct role of sympathetic nerve activity on adipose tissue has recently been adressed using microdialysis, and it was found that during hand-grip exercise, the increase in umbilical glycerol release was attenuated in spinal cord-injured individuals with impaired sympathetic nerve activity when compared with healthy control individuals *(58)*. It should be noted that this very moderate type of stress was not able to document any increase in lipolysis in the clavicular region. Furthermore, in a recent study, glycerol output in subcutaneous abdominal adipose tissue was found to be lower during prolonged arm-cranking in spinal cord-injured individuals compared with controls performing a similar relative workload (unpublished observation). Taken together, indices are provided that sympathetic nerves to adipose tissue stimulate lipolysis directly during exercise. If regional differences (visceral vs subcutaneous fat) exist in responsiveness of the adipose tissue toward increased sympathetic activity, this could play an important role in the treatment of adipositas.

Not only adipose tissue, but also intramuscular fat can be stimulated by catecholamines, and both lipoprotein lipase (LPL) and hormon-sensitive lipase (HSL) play important roles in this regulation (59). HSL might be under control by both contractions and epinephrine, and it has recently been shown that activation of HSL and glycogen phosphorylase occurs in parallel in adrenalectomized individuals who receive infusion with epinephrine during exercise (unpublished observation). This could indicate that mobilization of intramuscular triglycerid and glycogen occurs simultaneously stimulated by adrenergic activity, and that choice of substrate for energy production takes place at another level.

SUMMARY

Physical exercise causes an increase in adrenergic activity that can be determined both by changes in plasma catecholamines and in intraneural sympathetic activity. Release of norepinephrine from contracting muscles and release of epinephrine from the adrenal medulla are major contributors to high levels of plasma catecholamines. Both feed-forward stimulation from motor centers in the brain and afferent impulses from working muscles stimulate sympathoadrenergic activity, and a coupling to oxidative demands of the working muscle is likely. Long-term physical training increases the size and secretory capacity of the adrenal medulla, which may improve exercise capacity. Sympathoadrenergic activity only plays a minor role in regulation of hepatic glucose release, but via depressing insulin secretion and influencing target tissue adrenergic activity improves glycogen and fatty acid mobilization.

REFERENCES

1. Rowell LR. Human Circulation Regulation During Physical Stress. Oxford University Press, New York, 1986.
2. Victor R, Seals DR, Mark AL. Differential control of heart rate and sympathetic nerve activity during dynamic exercise: insigth from direct intraneural recordings in humans. J Clin Invest 1987; 79:508–516.
3. Searls DR, Victor RG, Mark AL. Plasma norepinephrine and muscle sympathetic discharge during rhythmic exercise in humans. J Appl Physiol 1988;65:940–944.
4. Savard G, Richter EA, Strange S, Kiens B, Christensen NJ, Saltin B. Norepinephrine spillover from skeletal muscle during exercise in humans: role of muscle mass. Am J Physiol 1989;257: H1812–H1818.
5. Nie ZT, Lisjo S, Åstrand PO, Henriksson J. In-vitro stmulation of the rat epitrochlearis muscle II. Effects of catecholamines and nutrients on protein degradation and amino acid metabolism. Acta Physiol Scand 1989;135:523–529.
6. Esler M, Jennings G, Korner P, Blomberry P, Sacharias N, Leonard P. Measurement of total and organ-specific norepinephrine kinetics in humans. Am J Physiol 1984;247:E21–E28.
7. Kjær M, Christensen NJ, Sonne B, Richter EA, Galbo H. Effect of exercise on epinephrine turnover in trained and untrained male subjects. J Appl Physiol 1985;59:1061–1067.
8. Kjær M, Secher NH, Bach FW, Galbo H. Role of motor center activity for hormonal changes and substrate mobilization in exercising man. Am J Physiol 1987;253:R687–R695.
9. Vissing J, Iwamoto GA, Rybicki KJ, Galbo H, Mitchell JH. Mobilization of glucoregulatory hormones and glucose by hypothalamic locomotor centers. Am J Physiol 1989;257:E722–E728.
10. Galbo H, Kjær M, Secher NH. Cardiovascular, ventilatory and catecholamine responses to maximal dynamic exercise in partially curarized man. J Physiol 1987;389:557–568.
11. Kjær M, Secher NH, Bach FW, Sheikh S, Galbo H. Hormonal and metabolic responses to exercise in humans: effect of sensory nervous blockade. Am J Physiol 1989;257:E95–E101.

12. Kjær M, Secher NH, Bach FW, Galbo H, Reeves DR, Mitchell JH. Hormonal, metabolic and cardiovascular responses to static exercise in man: influence of epidural anesthesia. Am J Physiol 1991;261:214–220.
13. Klokker M, Kjær M, Secher NH, Hanel B, Worm L, Kappel M, et al. Natural killer cell response to exercise in humans: effect of hypoxia and epidural anesthesia. J Appl Physiol 1995;78:709–716.
14. Vissing J, Iwamoto GA, Fuchs IE, Galbo H, Mitchell JH. Reflex control of gluregulatory exercise responses by group III and IV muscle afferents. Am J Physiol 1994;266:R824–R830.
15. Vissing J, Lewis SF, Galbo H, Haller RG. Effect of deficient muscular glycogenolysis on extramuscular fuel production in exercise. J Appl Physiol 1992;72:1773–1779.
16. Vissing J, Galbo H, Haller R. Paradoxically enhanced glucose production during exercise in humans with blocked glycolysis due to muscle phosphofructokinase deficiency. Neurology 1996;47:766–771.
17. Vissing J, Galbo H, Haller RG. Exercise fuel mobilization in mitochondrial myopathy: a metabolic dilemma. Ann Neurol 1996;40:655–662.
18. Winder WW, Hagberg JM, Hickson RC, Ehsani AA, McLane JA. Time course of sympathoadrenergic adaptation to endurance exercise training in man. J Appl Physiol 1978;45:370-374.
19. Svedenhag J. The sympathoadrenal system in physical conditioning. Acta Physiol Scand 1985;125, suppl. 543:1–74.
20. Kjær M, Bangsbo J, Lortie G, Galbo H. Hormonal response to exercise in man: influence of hypoxia and physical training. Am J Physiol 1988;254:R197–R203.
21. Dela F, Mikines KJ, Linstow M, Galbo H. Heart rate and plasma catecholamines during 24 hour everyday life in trained and untrained men. J Appl Physiol 1992;73:2389–2395.
22. Kjær M, Mikines KJ, Christensen NJ, Tronier B, Vinten J, Sonne B, et al. Glucose turnover and hormonal changes during insulin-induced hypoglycemia in trained humans. J Appl Physiol 1984;57:21–27.
23. Kjær M, Farrel PA, Christensen NJ, Galbo H. Increased epinephrine response and inaccurate glucoregulation in exercising athletes. J Appl Physiol 1986;61:1693–1700.
24. Kjær M, Galbo H. The effect of physical training on the capacity to secrete epinephrine. J Appl Physiol 1988;64:11–16.
25. LeBlanc J, Jobin M, Cote J, Samson P, Labri A. Enhanced metabolic response to caffeine in exercise-trained human subjects. J Appl Physiol 1985;59:832–837.
26. Stallknecht B, Kjær M, Ploug T, Maroun L, Ohkuwa T, Vinten J, et al. Diminished epinephrine response to hypoglycemia despite enlarged adrenal medulla in trained rats. Am J Physiol 1990;259:R998–R1003.
27. Kjær M, Mikines KJ, Linstow M, Nicolaisen T, Galbo H. Effect of 5 weeks detraining on epinephrine response to insulin induced hypoglycemia in athletes. J Appl Physiol 1992;72:1201–1205.
28. Kjær M, Kiens B, Hargreaves M, Richter EA. Influence of active muscle mass on glucose homeostasis during exercise in humans. J Appl Physiol 1991;71:552–557.
29. Marliss EB, Simantirakis E, Miles PDG, Purnon C, Gougeon R, Field CJ, et al. Gluregulatory and hormonal responses to repeated bouts of intense exercise in normal male subjects. J Appl Physiol 1991;71:924–933.
30. Sigal R, Fisher SF, Halter JB, Vranic M, Marliss EB. The roles of catecholamines in gluregulation in intense exercise as defined by the islet cell clamp technique. Diabetes 1996;45:148–156.
31. Kjær M, Pollack SF, Mohr T, Weiss H, Gleim GW, Bach FW, et al. Regulation of glucose turnover and hormonal responses during exercise: electrical induced cycling in tetraplegic humans. Am J Physiol 1996;271:R191–R199.
32. Richter EA, Galbo H, Holst JJ, Sonne B. Significance of glucagon for insulin secretion and hepatic glycogenolysis during exercise in rats. Horm Metab Res 1981;13:323–326.
33. Sonne B, Mikines KJ, Richter EA, Christensen NJ, Galbo H. Role of liver nerves and adrenal medulla in glucose turnover of running rats. J Appl Physiol 1985;59:1640–1646.
34. Arnall DA, Marker JC, Conlee RK, Winder WW. Effect of infusing epinephrine on liver and muscle glycogenolysis during exercise in rats. Am J Physiol 1986;250:E641–E649.
35. Carlson KI, Marker JC, Arnall DA, Terry ML, Yang HT, Lindsay LG, et al. Epinephrine is unessential for stimulation of liver glycogenolysis during exercise. J Appl Physiol 1985;58:544–548.
36. Marker JC, Arnall DA, Conlee RK, Winder WW. Effect of adrenodemedullation on metabolic responses to high intensity exercise. Am J Physiol 1986;251:R552–R559.

37. Winder WW, Arogyasami J, Yang HT, Thompson KG, Nelson A, Kelly KP, et al. Effects of glucose infusion in exercising rats. J Appl Physiol 1988;64:2300–2305.
38. Moates JM, Lacy DB, Goldstein RE, Cherrington AD, Wasserman DH. The metabolic role of the exercise induced increment in epinephrine in the dog. Am J Physiol 1988;255:E428–E436.
39. Hoelzer DR, Dalsky GP, Schwartz NS, Clutter WE, Shah SD, Holloszy JO, et al. Epinephrine is not critical to prevention of hypoglycemia during exercise in humans. Am J Physiol 1986;251: E104–E110.
40. Wasserman DH, Williams PE, Lacy DB, Bracy D, Cherrington AD. Hepatic nerves are not essential to the increase in hepatic glucose production during muscular work. Am J Physiol 1990;259: E195–E203.
41. Wasserman DH, Cherrington AD. Regulation of extramuscular fuel sources during exercise. In: Rowell LB, Shepherd JT, eds. Handbook of Physiology. Bermedica Production, Columbia, MD, 1996, pp. 1036–1074.
42. Kjær M, Engfred K, Fernandes A, Secher NH, Galbo H. Regulation of hepatic glucose production during exercise in man: role of sympathoadrenergic activity. Am J Physiol 1993;265:E275–E283.
43. Kjær M, Keiding S, Engfred K, Rasmussen K, Sonne B, Kirkegård P, et al. Glucose homeostasis during exercise in humans with a liver or kidney transplant. Am J Physiol 1995;268:E636–E644.
44. Kjær M, Jurlander J, Keiding S, Galbo H, Kirkegaard P, Hage E. No reinnervation of hepatic sympathetic nerves after liver transplantation in human subjects. J Hepatol 1994;20:97–100.
45. Coker RH, Krishna MG, Brooks Lacy D, Allen EJ, Wasserman DH. Sympathetic drive to liver and nonhepatic splanchnic tissue during heavy exercise. J Appl Physiol 1997;82:1244–1249.
46. Coker RH, Krishna MG, Brooks Lacy D, Bracy DP, Wasserman DH. Role of hepatic alpha- and beta-adrenergic receptor stimulation on hepatic glucose production during heavy exercise. Am J Physiol 1997;273:E831–E838.
47. Richter EA. Glucose utilization. In: Rowell LB, Shepherd JT, eds. Handbook of Physiology 1997, Bermedica Production, Columbia, MD, 1996, pp. 912–951.
48. Ploug T, Galbo H, Richter EA. Increased muscle glucose uptake during contractions: no need for insulin. Am J Physiol 1984;247:E726–E731.
49. Issekutz B. Effect of epinephrine on carbohydrate metabolism in exercising dogs. Metabolism 1985;34:457–464.
50. Jansson E, Hjemdahl P, Kaijser L. Epinephrine-induced changes in muscle carbohydrate metabolism during exercise in male subjects. J Appl Physiol 1986;60:1466–1470.
51. Richter EA, Ruderman NB, Gavras H, Belur ER, Galbo H. Muscle glycogenolysis during exercise: dual control by epinephrine and contractions. Am J Physiol 1982;242:E25–E32.
52. Spriet LL, Ren JM, Hultman E. Epinephrine infusion enhances glycogenolysis during prolonged electrical stimulation. J Appl Physiol 1988;64:1439–1444
53. Chesley A, Hultman E, Spriet LL. Effects of epinephrine infusion on muscle glycogenolysis during intense aerobic exercise. Am J Physiol 1995;268:E127–E134.
54. Richter EA, Galbo H, Christensen NJ. Control of exercise induced muscular glycogenolysis by adrenal medullary hormones in rats. J Appl Physiol 1981;50:21–26.
55. Wahrenberg H, Engfeldt P, Bolinder J, Arner P. Acute adaptation in adrenergic control of lipolysis during physical exercise in humans. Am J Physiol 1987;253:E383–E390.
56. Arner P, Kriegholm E, Engfeldt P, Bolinder J. Adrenergic regulation of lipolysis in situ at rest and during exercise. J Clin Invest 1990;85:893–898.
57. Stallknecht B, Bülow J, Frandsen E, Galbo H. Desensitization of human adipose tissue to adrenaline stimulation studied by microdialysis. J Physiol 1997;500:271–282.
58. Karlsson AK, Elam M, Friberg P, Biering-Sørensen F, Sullivan L, Lönnroth P. Regulation of lipolysis by the sympathetic nervous system: a microdialysis study in normal and spinal cord injured subjects. Metabolism 1997;46:388–394.
59. Oscai LB, Essig DA, Palmer WK. Lipase regulation of muscle triglyceride hydrolysis. J Appl Physiol 1990;69:1571–1577.

11 Energy Balance and Weight Control (Male and Female)
Endocrine Considerations

*Gilbert W. Gleim, PhD, FACSM, FACN
and Beth W. Glace, MS*

Contents

INTRODUCTION
THE THYROID HORMONES
WEIGHT REGULATION IN PREPUBESCENT AND PUBESCENT GIRLS
ENDOCRINE CONSIDERATIONS AND SEX HORMONES IN MEN
GROWTH HORMONE (GH)
THE EFFECT OF CHANGES IN ENERGY BALANCE
    AND EXERCISE ON ENDOCRINE FUNCTION
ENDOCRINE CONSIDERATIONS AND ENERGY BALANCE
    IN POSTMENOPAUSAL WOMEN
LEPTIN
REFERENCES

INTRODUCTION

Evolution in all species is dependent to a large degree on metabolic efficiency. If energy intake does not at least equal energy utilization, growth and reproduction are not possible. Because *Homo sapiens* have been subjected to these same forces for millions of years, availability of energy will profoundly influence behavior and activity. Environmental and supply factors today make energy surplus a real possibility for most humans. Indeed, unless dietary habits are controlled and physical activity is a steady component of daily life, an energy surfeit is likely. It is estimated that one-third of all Americans are 20% over ideal body weight. This stress is not without effects on multiple hormonal systems in the body. There are situations where energy expenditure exceeds supply, and adjustments to this stress can result in extreme changes in hormone activity and metabolic rate. Alternatively, extreme changes in hormone activity and metabolic rate can cause energy expenditure to exceed supply. Some of these changes are significant threats

From: *Contemporary Endocrinology: Sports Endocrinology*
Edited by: M. P. Warren and N. W. Constantini © Humana Press Inc., Totowa, NJ

to normal health and may impact well-being for long periods following the caloric challenge. This chapter attempts to make sense of the current literature addressing the interaction of energy balance and various hormone systems in the body.

THE THYROID HORMONES

Thyroid hormone function represents a complex physiological system that is sensitive to overfeeding, underfeeding, carbohydrate ingestion, hormone metabolism, and plasma protein binding. The manifestation of changes in thyroid hormone function may follow several weeks of dietary changes, but may not be apparent from alterations in short-term dietary modification. Study of thyroid hormone function in humans subjected to dietary challenges has thus been difficult.

The major thyroid hormones triiodothyronine (T_3) and thyroxine (T_4) are formed from iodinated thyroglobulin in the thyroid gland. Their release from the gland is regulated by the anterior pituitary hormone, thyroid-stimulating hormone (TSH), whose release in turn is regulated by the hypothalamic hormone, thyrotropin-releasing hormone. The effect of an abrupt increase in T_4 in humans is an increase in basal metabolic rate, but the maximal effect is not evident until a week and half after administration. Thyroxine has a negative feedback on the secretion of TSH. Secretion of T_4 from the thyroid gland is much greater than secretion of T_3, although peripheral conversion of T_4 to T_3 is profound. Although T_3 is more potent in its effect on metabolism than T_4, it persists in the blood for a shorter period of time. Peripheral metabolism of T_4 is adjusted to energy intake and energy consumption, and conversion is altered only when there is an imbalance in energy *(1)*.

Resting metabolic rate (RMR) changes with changes in energy balance, but these changes do not always parallel changes in thyroid hormone status. In periods of high-energy intake and high-energy expenditure that are balanced, there may be no change in thyroid hormones.

What must also be considered in the overall equation of metabolic rate is alterations in sympathetic nervous system activity. Increases in energy expenditure that lead to a caloric deficit are not associated with changes in norepinephrine levels, but will result in decreases in thyroid hormone levels. If challenges are not too great, RMR may remain the same. Alternatively, a decrease in energy expenditure with a concomitant decrease in caloric intake is associated with decreased norepinephrine levels and a decrease in RMR with no change in thyroid hormone levels *(2)*. Only an increase in energy intake with increases in energy expenditure promotes an increase in RMR.

Another important player in the balance of thyroid hormone is the amount of carbohydrate in the diet. Decreased carbohydrate intake in the diet results in decreases in circulating T_3 levels, and if carbohydrate levels are supplemented sufficiently during overall caloric restriction, T_3 levels can be maintained *(3)*. Such changes in circulating levels of T_3 are related to both the peripheral conversion of T_3 to rT_3 *(4)* and to changes in the levels of thyroid binding proteins *(5)*. Nevertheless, in a study of obese women, a low-calorie diet supplemented with higher carbohydrate content resulted in less of a fall in T_3, but similar declines in RMR *(6)*.

Exercise has been associated with acute increases in TSH levels that are intensity-dependent *(7)*, but these increases did not result in any acute changes in T_3 or T_4. The apparent increase in hypothalamo–pituitary activity (illustrated by TSH levels) that occurs is likely to be related to increased sympathetic activity, which is profoundly intensity-dependent. With respect to exercise, it is therefore important to distinguish between short-term releasing hormone activity and the long-term effects on thyroid hormone levels and RMR.

WEIGHT REGULATION IN PREPUBESCENT AND PUBESCENT GIRLS

Modifications in energy metabolism and endocrine homeostasis in girls are of much concern to the practitioner. The reproductive system in this population is extremely sensitive to changes in caloric intake, and physical and emotional stress. Adolescent girls are particularly vulnerable to perturbed eating patterns; anorexia nervosa is observed most often in girls between the ages of 12 and 20 yr (8).

The first indication of endocrine disturbances in adolescent girls is altered pubertal progression (9). Genetic and environmental factors contribute to the onset of pubertal development. Ballet dancers have often served as models when studying endocrine function as it relates to energy balance, since they typically begin dancing at a young age and continue training throughout adolescence. Additionally, dancers often voluntarily limit food intake, with caloric intakes <1000 calories daily (10).

Young dancers exhibit delayed skeletal growth, accentuated long bone growth, and depressed weight for height, perhaps owing to suppression of gonadotropin-releasing hormone pulsation, which in turn suppresses leutinizing hormone (LH) (11). Although age at pubarche may be normal in dancers, Tanner scores for breast development indicate a marked delay in thelarche, which then progresses rapidly during periods of relative inactivity, such as during vacations.

Mean menarcheal age has increased during the last century (12,13), probably as a result of decreased activity and improved nutrition. Although menarche is typically related to the mother's age of menarche, leanness (14) and years of training (15) delay the onset of menses, overriding the genetic determinants. Girls with early menarche are likely to be fatter than those with late menarche (16,17), and dietary fat intake has been positively associated with early menarche (18). Leptin, an appetite-regulating hormone, is associated with both an increased body fatness and a decline in the age at menarche (19), underscoring the relationship between body fat and reproductive ability.

Onset of menses occurs at a later age in girls who participate in sports (18). Each year of athletic training prior to menarche delays onset of menstruation by approx 5 mo (19). Although some have suggested an absolute threshold for body fat and cyclicity, it appears that there is significant individual variation and that other factors, such as chronic exercise and changes in regional fat storage sites, affect menstrual regulation (20).

Secondary amenorrhea is common in girls with restricted food intake (11,21) and is marked by a return to a premenarcheal endocrine pattern, with suppressed LH and low T_4 levels (11,22). It has been postulated that these mechanisms represent a form of energy conservation (23) and may serve to decrease the likelihood of an unsustainable pregnancy. Inadequate energy intake relative to expenditure may stimulate the hypothalamic–pituitary–adrenal axis and reduce the activity of the hypothalamic–pituitary–ovarian axis (24). Collectively, the data indicate that the physical stress of training and the caloric drain it imposes strongly influence sexual maturation and cyclicity, and these effects are similar to those seen in nutritional deprivation (25).

```
        ┌─────────────────────┐
        │     Leaness         │
        │  Physical Activity  │
        │  Caloric Restriction│
        └─────────────────────┘
                   │
                   ▼
```

Altered Pubertal Progression
  Normal Pubarche
  Delayed Thelarche
  Delayed Menarche
  Secondary Amenorrhea
         ▼
Low Estrogen Exposure
         ▼
Poor Bone Mineralization
         ▼
Increased Risk Of
  Stress Fractures
  Injury
  Osteoporosis

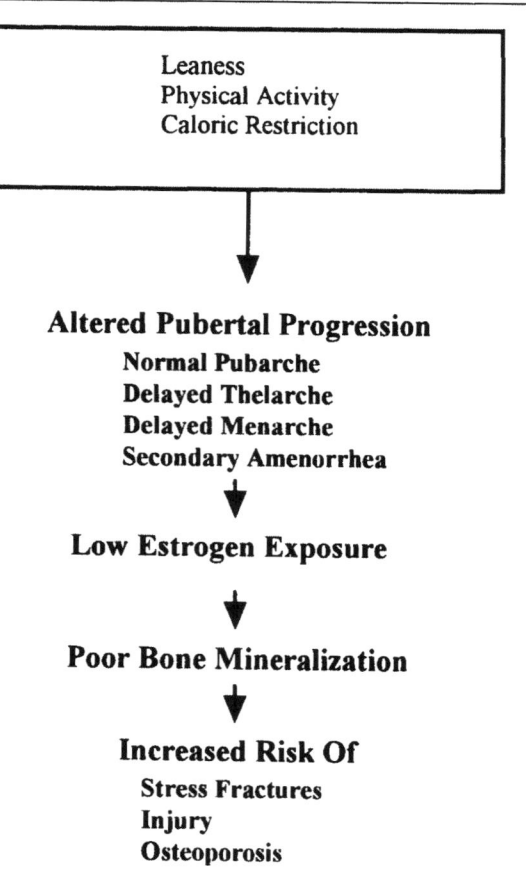

Fig. 1. Energy balance affects pubertal progression and bone mineralization.

The repercussion of delayed menarche may be insufficient accrual of bone during the second decade of life. Estradiol levels correlate with bone density of the spine and wrist *(26)*. Hypercortisolism, often observed in similar clinical scenarios, such as anorexia nervosa, may contribute to the poor bone mineralization observed in girls with delayed menarche or with secondary amenorrhea. The glucocorticoids promote osteoporosis via altered vitamin D metabolism and calcium absorption and decreased collagen synthesis *(27)*.

Approximately 50% of skeletal mass is accrued during adolescence *(28)*, and hypoestrogenism at this critical period of development may lead to premenopausal osteopenia *(29)* and to an increased risk of stress fractures and injury *(26)*, and may increase the risk of osteoporosis later in life. Long-term estrogen deficiency during adolescence results in impaired bone mineral density as determined by absorptiometry methods *(30)*. If left untreated, bone mineral density remains stable or declines during the teen years in hypoestrogenic girls, indicating a relative loss of density (Fig. 1).

ENDOCRINE CONSIDERATIONS AND SEX HORMONES IN MEN

The normal gonadal hormone axis in males is demonstrated in Fig. 2. The Leydig and Seroli cells, which are responsible for viable spermatogenesis, are under the regulation

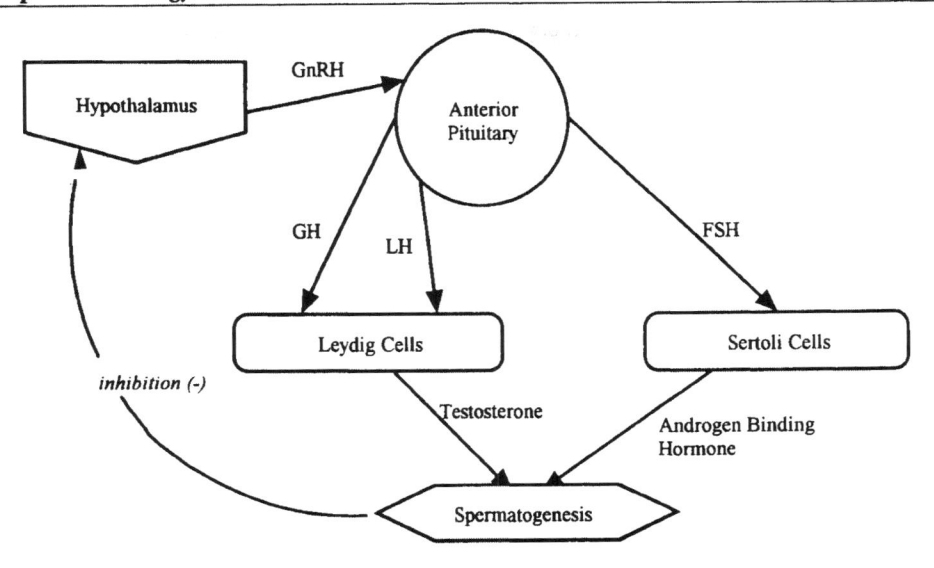

Fig. 2. HPG axis in men.

of follicle-stimulating hormone (FSH), LH, and growth hormone (GH). Regulation of these hormones is by the releasing factors of the hypothalamus. Testosterone, made by the Leydig cells, has a negative feedback on gonadal-releasing hormone from the hypothalamus.

Malnutrition has a profound effect on the pituitary–gonadal axis in men. The pituitary LH response may be normal or absent, and LH elevations are related to Leydig cell insufficiency, with low serum testosterone levels. FSH elevations are thought to be owing to Leydig cell dysfunction as well *(31)*. Levels do seem to be regulated to some extent by body weight and obesity, which were positively correlated to plasma testosterone and FSH in male twins. Fat intake was also associated with testosterone levels *(32)*. Six weeks of a lacto-ovo vegetarian diet were observed to cause minor decreases in testosterone levels without changes in endurance performance in endurance athletes *(33)*. An apparently independent effect of aging on Leydig cell function and number can also result in diminished levels of testosterone, resulting in loss of bone mass *(34)*. Short-term food restriction (1000 kcal/d deficit) accompanied by intense physical training resulting in a weight loss of 12% over 8 wk decreased serum testosterone and LH levels, but increased sex hormone binding globulin. Following 5 wk of refeeding and recovery, normal levels of all hormones were re-established *(35)*. Taken together, these findings indicate that male gonadal function is certainly not inert to metabolic challenges, although it would appear that the system is well designed to recover function and the metabolic challenges must be severe in order to have a significant impact.

Although alterations in the male gonadal hormone axis have been observed with chronic and acute exercise, long-term dysfunction resulting from exercise training has rarely if ever been documented. The authors are unaware of any reports of male infertility from exercise training which does not employ exogenous hormone supplementation. Statistically significant changes may be observed, but these do not appear to have important biological significance.

Ultramarathoning and exercise of over 3 h of duration have been shown to decrease serum testosterone levels, whereas shorter-term exercise is usually associated with increased levels of testosterone *(36)*, an effect that is apparently independent of hemoconcentration and a result of gonadotropin stimulation *(37)*.

An endurance training program of 40 wk in previously untrained men enhanced testicular hormone response to exercise and was without effect on resting levels *(38)*. Nevertheless, chronically trained marathoners had a deficiency in the release of hypothalamic gonadotropin-releasing hormone, thought to be induced by daily elevations of gonadal steroids from bouts of daily exercise *(39)*. A higher basal FSH concentration has been observed in trained vs untrained subjects, which was suggested as "compensated hypogonadism," even though serum testosterone levels were normal on a control day *(40)*. Weight lifting is associated with increases in testosterone levels, and fat intake was positively associated with testosterone levels as well *(41)*. Finally, in a comparison of cyclists, marathoners, and controls, it was observed that cyclists had decreased sperm motility during the competitive season, but this normalized during the off season and was found to be similar between marathoners and controls. Changes in the cyclists were thought to be owing to the physical factors of the bicycle seat and not to any changes caused by metabolic stress *(42)*.

In conclusion, male reproductive hormone function is relatively resistant to metabolic perturbations of even chronic, severe exercise, but not those of chronic alterations nutrition. Malnutrition will eventually decrease male hormone function, and fat intake appears to be related to testosterone levels.

GROWTH HORMONE (GH)

GH is a protein hormone secreted by the anterior pituitary gland. Its release is stimulated by the hypothalamic-releasing factor (GH-releasing hormone, GHRH) and inhibited by somatostatin, also a product of the hypothalamus and pancreas. The net effect of GH is to increase protein synthesis, but it does so by stimulating the production of somatomedins made by the liver and possibly kidney and muscle. GH promotes the development of bones and cartilage during youth, and increases protein synthesis and mobilization of fatty acids while inhibiting glucose utilization by promoting glycogen deposition in adulthood. Without the presence of insulin, GH's action are severely curtailed because of insulin's role in promoting amino transport into cells. Alternatively, excessive levels of GH may cause such an elevation of blood glucose that a pituitary diabetes results, requiring enormous production of insulin by the liver to maintain blood glucose within normal ranges.

Release of GH is pulsatile, and this complicates its accurate measurement. Twenty-four-hour measurements are the most accurate way to measure GH secretion. The most potent stimulus for GH stimulation is chronic protein malnutrition, and these elevations respond briskly to protein refeeding. Healthy men consuming a diet supplying 75% of daily energy requirements for 6 d experienced no changes in GH levels with diets that were high in fat or carbohydrate, even though the high-fat diet spared more nitrogen *(43)*. Alternatively, a 96-h fast increased GH levels in normal men, but not obese men *(44)*, indicating that sufficient caloric restriction may be a potent enough stimulus for increased GH secretion. This is confirmed by observations that spontaneous release of GH is reduced in obese and short-term fasted obese subjects *(45)*.

Energy Intake During Menstrual Cycle

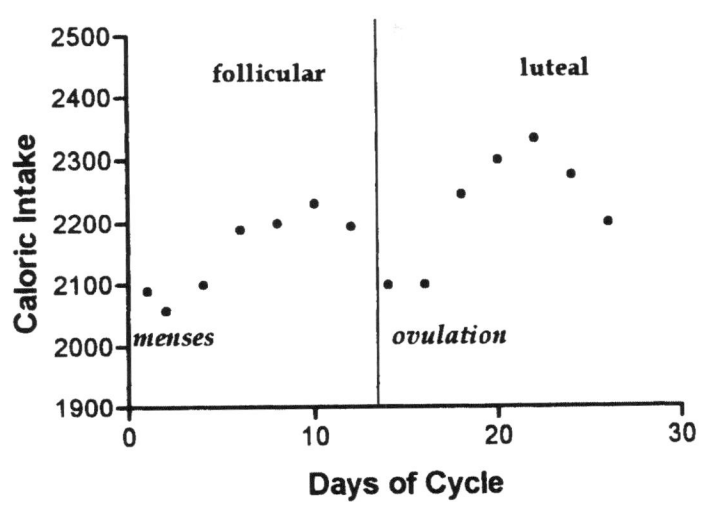

Fig. 3. HPG axis in women. Negative energy balance may reduce GnRh pulse generation, which in turn reduces frequency of LH surges and suppresses follicular and luteal development.

Exercise is a stimulus for GH release and is related to some degree to intensity, with less fit individuals having a greater response than fit individuals *(46)*. Obese subjects have a reduced GH response to exercise as well as dietary restriction.

Protein and amino acid administration (oral or iv) of >250 mg/kg is associated with increased GH release *(47,48)*. However, it is unlikely that in normal exercising individuals, chronic high protein intake will result in increased levels of GH. A more likely cause for any increased body mass from such diets is the increase in total calories afforded by high protein supplements.

Premenopausal Women

The menstrual cycle can be considered biphasic. The follicular phase follows the onset of menstruation, and is characterized by increasing levels of estrogen secreted by a maturing follicle, which in turn increase FSH and LH. After ovulation, the follicle releases large amounts of estrogen and progesterone and the corpus luteum rapidly degenerates. Estrogen and progesterone levels fall during the luteal phase, stimulating the onset of menstrual flow once again *(49)*.

ENDOCRINE EFFECTS ON ENERGY BALANCE

Food intake is affected by menstrual cycle phase. Caloric intake rises during the midluteal and midfollicular phases *(50)*, with the greatest intakes during the luteal phase. Intake is lowest at the onset of menses and immediately postovulation (Fig. 3). Neither menstrual symptoms nor illnesses explain the observed variations in intake. Estrogen transiently acts as an appetite suppressant: caloric intake is lowest when estrogen levels are rising *(51,52)*. Progesterone has been suggested to act as an estrogen antagonist, indirectly stimulating appetite. Other hormones known to affect body weight and composition via increased food intake are prolactin and GH. Prolactin increases fat compartments, whereas GH increases lean body weight *(53)*.

Patterns of food intake also change over the menstrual cycle. Women experiencing premenstrual syndrome tend to increase both total calories and the carbohydrate content of their diets in the late luteal phase. Carbohydrate-rich meals may decrease the dysphoria commonly seen in women suffering from premenstrual syndrome (PMS), presumably owing to a serotonin-mediated effect *(54)*. Pharmacologically-enhanced serotonin release in women with PMS results in decreased food and carbohydrate intake and normalizes mood *(55)*, suggesting that the increased food intake seen in the luteal phase may be part of a regulatory mechanism that serves to alleviate mood disturbances.

Energy expenditure in women is subject to endocrine regulation. Lasting changes in spontaneous exercise after hormonal manipulation are seen in rodents, and the altered exercise patterns are apparent even when weight has stabilized *(56)*. Basal metabolic rate varies significantly over the menstrual cycle, reaching a low approx 5 d prior to ovulation and peaking approx 1 wk prior to menstruation *(57)*.

THE EFFECT OF CHANGES IN ENERGY BALANCE AND EXERCISE ON ENDOCRINE FUNCTION

A number of risk factors have been identified as predisposing women to the development of menstrual irregularities. Animal studies suggest that females may more closely regulate food intake and body weight than males. Female rats markedly increase food intake in response to a calorically dilute diet; males show less precision in long-term weight control when faced with regulatory challenges. The differences between genders in eating and body weight regulation appear to be owing to estrogen *(58)*.

Effect of Changes in Energy Expenditure

Rigorous exercise training, if engaged in abruptly, often results in endocrine dysfunction in previously normal women. Untrained women who begin strenuous exercise programs may experience suppression of the LH surge and ovulation *(59)*. Athletic amenorrhea is characterized by reduced frequency of pituitary LH surges secondary to insufficient GNRH pulse generation in the hypothalamus, with complete absence of follicular and luteal development *(60)*. Athletic amenorrhea may be seen as one indication of overtraining syndrome *(23)*. More gradual introduction of training regimens appears less likely to result in reproductive alterations in previously normal menstruating women *(61,62)*. See Fig. 4.

Luteal function may be suppressed in trained eumenorrheic women. Follicular phase is frequently lengthened, and luteal phase shortened, in exercising women *(24,63)*. These changes are marked by reduced progesterone. Laughlin and Yen demonstrated that LH pulse frequency was most affected in amenorrheic athletes compared to eumenorrheic athletes and was negatively correlated to cortisol and insulin levels, suggesting that the GNRH/LH pulse generator activity reduction may in part result from the central inhibiting effects of corticotropin-releasing factor *(64)*.

Effects of "Energy Drain"

Menstrual dysfunction may result from chronic "energy drain." Hunter-gatherers display lower ovarian function and conception rates during yearly cycles of food scarcity

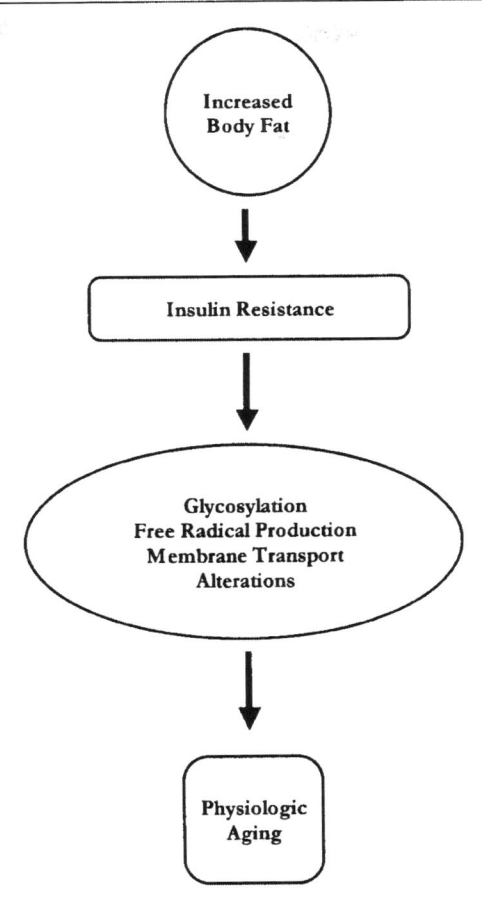

Fig. 4. Proposed relationship between obesity and aging. Adapted from ref. 92, with permission.

(65). Limiting food intake in sedentary women can induce amenorrhea *(66)* and alter LH pulse frequency *(67)*. It has also been noted that weight loss results in an increased formation of 2-methoxy estrone, a biologically inactive catechol *(68)*, which may bind to estrogen receptors and exert an antiestrogenic effect.

It appears that the effect of energy restriction or energy expenditure on menstrual function is relative to the woman's initial endocrine status. Anovulatory women and those with luteal phase insufficiency *(69)* are more likely to cease to menstruate if energy balance is altered. Although low body weight in conditions, such as anorexia nervosa, or in healthy subjects *(70)* may result in loss of menstruation, there does not appear to be an absolute threshold for body fat for normal ovarian function. Body fat of amenorrheic women is often similar to that of eumenorrheic women *(64)*, and it has been suggested that each woman has a genetically determined set point for body fatness *(71)*. This concept was supported by a case report by Duek et al., which utilized nutritional intervention and a slight reduction in exercise training in the treatment of an amenorrheic collegiate runner. The runner's body mass index was similar to that of her eumenorrheic counterparts, but her body fat was lower. During the 15-wk intervention, her daily caloric intake was increased, and her daily caloric expenditure decreased slightly. Serum cortisol decreased and LH pulsatility normalized as body fatness increased from 8 to 14% via a 2-kg increase in body weight. After 3 mo at the higher body weight, the athlete spontaneously resumed menses while continuing to compete at a national level *(72)*.

Effect of Diet Composition

The evidence suggests that diet composition as well as total calories may affect endocrine function in premenopausal women. High-fat diets are associated with increased estrogen levels in serum and urine *(73)*. Decreased dietary fat has been shown to lower serum estrone sulfate *(74)* and plasma estradiol *(75)*. Low-fat diets are often also high-fiber diets, and it may be the dietary fiber that affects estrogen metabolism, via alterations in intestinal metabolism and reabsorption *(76)*. Protein restriction has also often been noted in amenorrheic athletes *(64,77,78)*.

Effect of Weight Loss in Obese Women

Obesity is associated with menstrual irregularity and can lessen fertility *(79)*, perhaps owing to hyperinsulinemia *(80)*. Weight loss in a group of obese women with menstrual dysfunction resulted in an improvement in ovulation rate in 80% of the women, and approx 30% conceived. These changes occurred concomitantly with a reduction in plasma insulin and cortisol. Women with android-type obesity are more likely to develop menstrual irregularity than those with gynoid-type obesity *(81)*. Weight loss may be an effective and inexpensive treatment option in these obese infertile women.

ENDOCRINE CONSIDERATIONS AND ENERGY BALANCE IN POSTMENOPAUSAL WOMEN

Body weight and composition are altered during the postmenopausal period. Body weight and body mass index increase during the perimenopausal period and remain significantly higher after menopause. These changes have not been explained by alterations in dietary intake or energy expenditure *(82)*. The distribution of body fat is changed at menopause. The proportion of fat over the gynoid area decreases, whereas android fat distribution increases *(83)*. Android fat distribution is associated with hyperinsulinemia and hypersensitivity of the hypothalamic–pituitary–adrenal axis *(84)*. Women with visceral fat accumulation exhibit elevated cortisol and androgens, and depressed GH. The combined effect of elevated cortisol and insulin, and depressed estrogen and GH is that of fat accretion *(85)*.

Although hormone-replacement therapies may moderate bone mineral losses *(86)*, they do not lessen the amount of weight gained during menopause. These hormones may alter the typical pattern of postmenopausal adipose by attenuating the accumulation of lipid in central fat depots, however *(87)*. Hormone replacement therapy was found to attenuate the gain of fat in the abdominal region following an exercise program in older women *(88)*. Progesterone stimulates lipoprotein lipase activity or fat storage in the femoral regions, whereas estradiol enhances lipolysis *(89)*. Provision of these hormones to postmenopausal women then alters the pattern of weight gain.

Low-Calorie Diets and Aging

Body fat increases with age. The gain in fat content approximates 12 kg between the age of 25 and 55 yr in sedentary men *(90)*. Muscle mass may actually decrease during

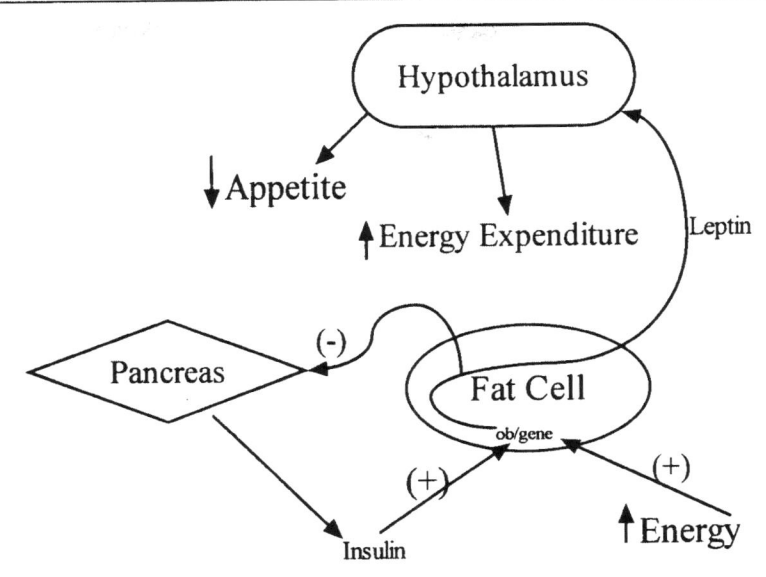

Fig. 5. Theoretical effects of leptin on hypothalmic regulation of body weight. Increased levels of leptin result in appetite suppression and increased energy expenditure.

this period, thus lowering basal energy requirements *(91)*. The incidence of many diseases that plague modern acculturated countries appears to be related in part to diet *(92)*. Disorders, such as diabetes and hypertension, are affected by body fatness. Although Western cultures typically see increased body fatness with age, more primitives societies do not *(93)*. These societies also have a reduced incidence of diabetes and hypertension. It has been suggested that many of the disorders associated with aging are related to insulin resistance *(94)*, and insulin resistance is often accentuated by obesity *(91)*.

Caloric restriction has been shown to lengthen life-span in animal models. Food-restricted rodents exhibit improved immune function, glucose tolerance, and cardiovascular health as compared to *ad libitum*-fed animals *(95)*. Enhanced longevity appears to be owing to lower fasting glucose and insulin levels *(96)*. Decreased insulin requirements may in turn decrease glycosylation *(97)*, free radical formation *(98)*, renal sodium retention *(99)*, and membrane transport alterations *(100)*, all of which contribute to the aging process. Studies in humans are limited, since it is difficult to manipulate experimentally human food intake over a lifetime. One such study was conducted in Biosphere 2, a closed environmental space. Persons sealed in Biosphere 2 ate a reduced-calorie, nutrient-rich diet for 2 yr. Significant weight loss was observed, with concomitant decreases in insulin, glucose, glycosylated hemoglobin, and blood cholesterol, changes known to decrease risk of the chronic diseases of adulthood *(101)*. These results indicate that aging processes may be retarded in food-limited humans via alterations in glucocorticoid physiology. *See* Fig. 5.

LEPTIN

The plasma protein leptin is the product of the *obese* gene *(ob)*, and defects in this gene in mice have been associated with obesity *(102)*. Furthermore, in obese mice that were homozygous for the *ob* gene defect *(ob/ob)*, the injection of the *ob* gene product profoundly reduced food intake and increased energy expenditure. Since that time, a number of studies have examined the role of leptin in human obesity and energy expenditure.

Expression of the (*ob*) gene on adipose tissue of humans is evident in humans, and the gene is overexpressed in the adipose tissue of obese humans *(103)*. The magnitude of this increase was 79% by comparison to nonobese subjects and 75% higher in female obese than male obese subjects. Consistent with this observation is the fact that leptin levels are elevated in obese subjects compared to nonobese subjects and also higher in women than in men *(104–107)* even when corrected for fat mass.

Theoretically, increasing leptin levels have an effect on the hypothalamus, so that appetite is suppressed and energy expenditure is increased (Fig. 5). Weight loss in obese subjects is associated with decreases in leptin levels, but baseline levels of leptin and changes in leptin levels are not predictive of success or maintenance of weight loss *(108)*. Obesity is associated with hyperinsulinemia and increased leptin levels, and insulin may regulate leptin release by fat cells, whereas leptin diminishes insulin secretion by pancreatic β-cells *(109)*. The counterregulatory nature of this relationship makes teleologic sense, but does not gain sufficient support from the published literature to warrant its acceptance. One possibility is that obese individuals have a reduced transport of leptin into the cerebrospinal fluid (CSF), and this may impede its hypothalamic effects *(110)*.

Cross-sectional studies of pre- and postmenopausal women have demonstrated that leptin levels corrected for fat mass decline after menopause. This fact, along with the decreased leptin levels in men, suggests that androgens may have a suppressive effect on leptin levels *(105)*.

Exercise training has a suppressive effect on leptin levels *(111,112)*. By partial correlation analysis, it can be shown that the changes in leptin levels are independent of the changes in weight and insulin that occur with exercise training, but these factors are clear covariates of leptin changes *(111)*. It has further been demonstrated that exercise training has greater suppressive effects on leptin levels in women than men *(112)*. It is not difficult to reconcile these changes in leptin as being consistent with energy deficits, which are likely to occur from exercise training. In an energy-challenged individual, the beneficial adaptation would be to increase appetite and decrease energy expenditure, opposite to those of a normal system responding to increased leptin levels from overfeeding.

REFERENCES

1. Danforth ES, Burger AG. The impact of nutrition on thryroid hormone physiology and action. Ann Rev Nutr 1989;9:201–227.
2. Woo R, O'Connell M, Horton E, Danforth ES. Changes in resting metabolism with increased intake and exercise. Clin Res 1985;33:712.
3. Serog P, Apfelbaum M, Autissier N, Baigts F, Brigant L, Kortza A. Effects of slimming and composition of diets on VO$_2$ and thyroid hromones in healthy subjects. Am J Clin Nutr 1982;35:24–35.
4. Pasquali R, Parenti M, Mattioli L, Capelli M, Cavazzini G, Sorrenti G, et al. Effect of dietary carbohydrates during hypocaloric treatment of obesity on peripheral thyroid hormone metabolism. J Endocrinol Invest 1982;5:47–52.
5. Welle S, O'Connell M, Danforth ES, Cambell R. Increased free triiodothyronine and thyroid hormone binding protein concentrations during carbohydrate overfeeding. J Clin Endocrinol 1984;33:837–839.
6. Mathieson RA. Walberg JL, Gwazdauskas FC, Hinkle DE, Gregg JM. The effect of varying carbohydrate content of a very-low-caloric diet on resting metabolic rate and thyroid hormones. Metabolism 1986;35:394–398.
7. Galbo H, Hummer L, Petersen IB, Christensen NJ, Bie N. Thyroid and testicular hormone responses to graded and prolonged exercise in man. Eur J Appl Physiol 1977;36:101–107.

8. Katz JL. Anorexia Nervosa. In: Brodoff BN, Bleicher SJ, eds. Diabetes Mellitus and Obesity. William and Wilkins, Baltimore, MD, 1982, pp. 310–321.
9. Frisch RE, Gotz-Welbergen AV, McArthur JW, Albright T, Witschi J, Bullen B, et al. Delayed menarche and amenorrhea of college athletes in relation to age at onset of training. JAMA 1981;246(14):1559–1563.
10. Benson J, Gillien DM, Bourdet K, Loosli AR. Inadequate nutrition and chronic caloric restriction. Phys Sports Med 1985;13(10):79–90.
11. Warren MP. The effects of exercise on pubertal progression and reproductive function in girls. J Clin Endocrinol Metab 1980;51(5):1150–1157.
12. Singh L, Thapar M. Age at menarche among the Bhotias of Mana Valley. Anthropol Anz 1983; 41(4):259–262.
13. Wyshak G. Secular changes in age at menarche in a sample of US women. Ann Hum Biol 1983;10(1):75–77.
14. Warren MP, Brooks-Gunn J. Delayed menarche in athletes: the role of low energy intake and eating disorders and their relation to bone density. In: Laron Z, Rogol A, eds. Hormones and Sport. Raven, New York, 1989.
15. Nelson ME. Diet and bone status in amenorrheic runners. Am J Clin Nutr 1986;43:910.
16. Stark O, Peckam CS, Moynihan C. Weight and age at menarche. Arch Dis Child 1989;64(3):383–387.
17. Linholm C, Hagenffeldt K, Hagman J. A nutrition study in elite juvenile gymnasts. Acta Paediatr 1995;84(3):273–277.
18. Merzenich H, Boeing J, Wahrendorf J. Dietary fat and sports activity as determinants for age at menarche. Am J Epidemiol 1993;138(4):217–224.
19. Matkovik V, Ilich JZ, Skugor M, Badenhop NE, Goel P, Clairmont A, et al. Leptin is inversely related to age at menarche in human females. J Clin Endocrinol Metab 1997;82(10):3239–3245.
20. Snow RC, Barbieri RL, Frisch RE. Estrogen 2-hydroxylase oxidation and menstrual function among elite oarswomen. J Clin Endocrinol Metab 1989;69(2):369–376.
21. Vigersky RA, Anderson AE, Thompson RH, Loriaux DL. Hypothalamic dysfucntion in secondary amenorrhea associated with simple weight loss. N Engl J Med 1977;297:1141–1145.
22. Warren MP, Vande Wiele RL. Clinical and metabolic features of anorexia nervosa. Am J Obstet Gynecol 1973;117:435–449.
23. Dueck CA, Manore MM, Matt KS. Role of Energy Balance in Athletic Menstrual Dysfunction. Int J Sports Nutr 1996;6:24–40.
24. Loucks AB, Mortola JF, Girton L, Yen SSC. Alterations in the hypothalamic–pituitary–ovarian and the hypothalamic–pituitary–adrenal axis in athletic women. J Clin Endocrinol Metab 1989;68: 402–411.
25. Kulin HE, Bwibo N, Mutie D, Santner SJ. The effect of chronic childhood malnutrition on pubertal growth and development. Am J Clin Nutr 1982;36(3):527–536.
26. Warren MP, Brooks-Gunn J, Fox RP, Lancelot C, Newman D, Hamilton WG. Lack of bone accretion and amenorrhea: evidence for a relative osteopenia in weight-bearing bones. J Clin Endocrinol Metab 1991;72:847–853.
27. Warren MP, Shane E, Lee MJ, Lindsay R, Dempster DW, Warren LF, et al. Femoral head collapse associated with anorexia nervosa in a 20 year old ballet dancer. Clin Orthop Rel Res 1990;251:171–176.
28. Glastre C, Braillon P, David L, Meunier PJ, Delmar PD. Measurement of bone mineral content of the lumber spine by dual energy x-ray absorptiometry in normal children: correlations with growth parameters. J Clin Endocrin Metab 1990;70(8):1330–1333.
29. Lloyd T, Buchanan JR, Bitzer S, Waldman CJ, Myers C, Ford BG. Interrelationships of diet, athletic activity, menstrual status and bone density in collegiate women. Am J Clin Nutr 1987;46:681–684.
30. Emans SJ, Grace E, Hoffer FA, Gundberg C, Ravnikar V, Woods ER. Estrogen deficiency in adolescents and young adults: impact on bone mineral content and effects of estrogen replacement therapy. Obstet Gynecol 1990;76:585–592.
31. Smith SR, Chhetri MK, Johanson J, Radfar N, Migeon CJ. The pituitary-gonadal axis in men with protein-calorie malnutrion. J Clin Endocrinol Metab 1975;41:60–69.
32. Bishop DT, Meikle AW, Slattery ML, Stringham JD, Ford MH, West DW. The effect of nutritional factors on sex hormone levels in male twins. Genet Epidemiol 1988;5:43–59.
33. Raben A, Kiens B, Richter EA, Rasmussen IB, Svenstrup B, Micic S, et al. Serum sex hormones and endurance performance after a lacto-ovo vegetarian and mixed diet. Med Sci Sports Exerc 1992;24:1290–1297.

34. Seeman E. Osteoporosis in men: epidemiology, pathophysiology and treatment possibilities. Am J Med 1993;95(suppl 5A):22s–28s.
35. Nindl BC, Friedl KE, Frykman PN, Marchitelli LJ, Shippee RL, Patton JF. Physical performance and metabolic recovery among lean, healthy men following a prolonged energy deficit. Int J Sports Med 1997;18:317–324.
36. Guglielmini C. Paolini AR, Conconi F. Variations of serum testerone concentrations after physical exercises of different duration. Int J Sports Med 1984;5:246–249.
37. Cumming DC, Brunsting LA III, Strich G, Ries AL, Rebar RW. Reproductive hormone increases in response to acute exercise in men. Med Sci Sports Exerc 1986;4:369–373.
38. Fellman N, Coudert J, Jarrige J-F, Bedu M, Denis C, Boucher D, et al. Effects of endurance training on the androgenic response to exercise in man. Int J Sports Med 1985;6:215–219.
39. MacConnie SE, Barkan A, Lampman RM, Schork MA, Beitins IZ. Decreased hypothalamic gonadotropin-releasing hormone secretion in male marathon runners. N Engl J Med 1986;315:411–417.
40. Vasankari TJ, Kujala UM, Heinonen OJ, Huhtaniemi IT. Effects of endurance training on hormonal responses to prolonged physical exercise in males. Acta Endocrinol 1993;129:109–113.
41. Volek JS, Kraemer WJ, Bush JA, Incledon T, Boetes M. Testosterone and cortisol in relationship to dietary nutrients and resistance exercise. J Appl Physiol 1997;82:49–54.
42. Lucia A, Chicharro JL, Perez M, Serratosa L, Bandres F, Legido JC. Reproductive function in male endurance athletes: sperm analysis and hormonal profile. J Appl Physiol 1996;81:2627–2636.
43. McCarger LJ, Clandinin MT, Belcastro AN, Walker K. Dietary carbohydrate-to-fat ratio: influence on whole-body nitrogen retention, substrate utilization, and hormone response in healthy male subjects. Am J Clin Nutr 1989;49:1169–1178.
44. Riedel M, Hoeft B, Blum WF, von zur Muhlen A, Brabant G. Pulsatile growth hormone secretion in normal-weight and obese men: differential metabolic regulation during energy restriction. Metabolism 1995;44:605–610.
45. Rasmussen MH, Juul A, Kjems LL, Skakkebaek NE, Hilsted J. Lack of stimulation of 24-hour growth hormone release by hypocaloric diet in obesity. J Clin Endocrinol Metab 1995;80:796–801.
46. Galbo H. Hormonal and Metabolic Adaptation to Exercise. George Thieme Verlag, New York, NY, 1983, pp. 40–45.
47. Besset A, Bonardet A, Rondouin G, Descomps B, Passouant P. Increase in sleep related GH and Prl: secretion after chronic arginine aspartate administration in man. Acta Endocrinol 1989;99:18–23.
48. Buckler JM. The relationship between changes in plasma growth hormone levels and body temperature occurring with exercise in man. Biomedicine 1973;19:193–197.
49. Barr SI. Women, nutrition and exercise: A review of athletes' intakes and a discussion of energy balance in active women, Prog Food Nutr Sci 1987;11:307–361.
50. Lissner L, Stevens J, Levitsky D, Rasmussen KM, Strupp BJ. Variations in energy intake during the menstrual cycle: implications for food-intake research. Am J Clin Nutr 1988;48:956–962.
51. Dalvit SP. The effect of the menstrual cycle on patterns of food intake. Am J Clin Nutr 1981;34:1811–1815.
52. Lyons PM, Truswell AS, Mira M, Vizzard J, Abraham SF. Reduction of food intake in the ovulatory phase of the menstrual cycle. Am J Clin Nutr 1989;49:1164–1168.
53. Byatt JC, Staten NR, Salsgiver WJ, Kostelc JG, Collier RJ. Stimulation of food intake and weight gain in mature female rats by bovine prolactin and bovine growth hormone. Am J Physiol 1993;264(6):E986–992.
54. Wurtman JJ. Depression and weight gain: the serotonin connection. J Affect Disord 1993;29:183–192.
55. Brzezinski A, Wurtman J, Wurtman R, Gleason R, Greenfield J, Nader T. D-Fenfluramine suppresses the increased calorie and carbohydrate intakes and improves the mood of women with premenstrual depression. Obstet Gynecol 1990;76:298–301.
56. Mook DG, Kenney NJ, Roberts S, Nussbaum AI, Rudier WI III. Ovarian-adrenal interactions in regulation of body weight by female rats. J Comp Physiol Psychol 1972;81:198–211.
57. Solomon SJ, Kurzer MS, Calloway DH. Menstrual cycle and basal metabolic rate in women. Am J Clin Nutr 1982;36:611–616.
58. Nance DM, Gorski RA. Sex hormone dependent alterations in responsiveness to caloric dilution. Physiol Behav 1977;19(5):679–683.
59. Bullen BA, Skrinar GS, Beitins IZ, Von Mering G, Turnbull BA, McArthur JW. Induction of menstrual disorders by strenuous exercise in untrained women. N Engl J Med 1985;312:1349–1353.

60. Loucks AB. Effects of exercise training on the menstrual cycle: existence and mechanisms. Med Sci Sports Exerc 1990;22(3):275–280.
61. Bullen BA, Skrinar GS, Beitins IZ, Carr DB, Reppert SM, Dotson CO, et al. Endurance training effects on plasma hormonal responsiveness and sex hormone excretion. J Appl Physiol: Respir Environ Exerc Physiol 1984;56:1453–1463.
62. Rogol AD, Weltman A, Weltman JY, Seip RL, Snead DB, Levine S, et al. Durability of the reproductive axis in eumenorrheic women during 1 yr of endurance training. J Appl Physiol 1992;72(4):1571–1580.
63. Bonen A, Belcastro AN, Ling WY, Simpson AA. Profiles of selected hormones during menstrual cycles of teenage athletes. J Appl Physiol: Respir Environ Exerc Physiol 1981;50(3):545–551.
64. Laughlin GA, Yen, SSC. Nutritional and endocrine-metabolic aberrations in amenorrheic athletes. J Clin Endocrinol Metab 1996;81:4301–4309.
65. Kurzer MS, Calloway DH. Effects of energy deprivation on sex hormone patterns in healthy menstruating women. Am J Physiol 1986;251:e483–488.
66. Loucks AB, Heath EM, Law T Sr, Verdun M, Watts JR. Dietary restriction reduces luetinizing hormone (LH) pulse frequency during waking hours and increases LH pulse amplitude during sleep in young menstruating women. J Clin Endocrinol Metab 1994;78:910–915.
67. Fishman J, Boyer RM, Hellman L. Influence of body weight on estradiol metabolism in young women. J Clin Endocrinol Metab 1975;41:989–991.
68. Van Der Walt L, Wilmsen EN, Jenkins T. Unusual Sex Hormone Patterns among desert-dwelling hunter-gatherers. J Clin Endocrinol Metabol 1978;46:658–663.
69. Pirke KM, Schweiger U, Brooks A, Tuschl RJ, Laessle RG. Luteinizing hormone and follicle stimulating hormone secretion patterns in female athletes with and without menstrual disturbances. Clin Endocrinol (Oxford) 1990;33(3):345–353.
70. Fichter MM, Pirke K-M, Holsboer F. Weight loss causes neuroendocrine disturbances: experimental study in healthy starving subjects. Psych Res 1986;17:61–72.
71. Carlberg KA, Buckman MT, Peake GT, Riedesel ML. Body composition of oligo/amenorrheic athletes. Med Sci Sports Exerc 1983;15(3):215–217.
72. Duek CA, Matt KS, Manore MM, Skinner JA. Treatment of athletic amenorrhea with a diet and training intervention program. Int J Sports Nutr 1996;6:24–40.
73. Longcope C, Gorbach S, Goldin B, Woods M, Dwyer J, Morrill A, et al. The effect of a low fat diet on estrogen metabolism. J Clin Endocrinol Metab 1987;64(6):1246–1250.
74. Woods MN, Gorbach SL, Longcope C, Goldin BR, Dwyer JT, Morrill-LaBrode A. Low-fat, high-fiber diet and serum estrone sulfate in premenopausal women. Am J Clin Nutr 1989;49(6):1179–1183.
75. Goldin BR, Adlercreutz H, Gorbach SL, Woods MN, Dwyer JT, Conlon T, et al. The relationship between estrogen levels and diets of Caucasian American and Oriental immigrant women. Am J Clin Nutr 1986;44(6):945–953.
76. Aldercreutz H, Fotsis T, Bannwart C, Hamalainen E, Bloigu S, Ollus A. Urinary estrogen profile determination in young Finnish vegetarian and omnivorous women. J Steroid Biochem 1984;24(1):289–296.
77. Brooks SM, Sanborn CF, Albrecht BH, Wagner WW. Diet in athletic amenorrhea. Lancet 1984;March 10:559,560.
78. Slavin J, Lutter J, Cushman S. Amenorrhea in vegetarian athletes. Lancet 1984;June 30:1474,1475.
79. Clark AM, Ledger W, Galletly C, Tomlinson L, Blaney F, Wang X, et al. Weight loss results in significant improvement in pregnancy and ovulation rates in annovulatory obese women. Hum Reprod 1995;10(10):2705–2712.
80. Hollmann M, Runnenbaum B, Gerhard I. Effects of weight loss on the hormonal profile in obese, infertile women. Hum Reprod 1996;11(9):1884–1981.
81. Hollmann M, Runnebaum B, Gerhard I. Impact of waist-hip-ratio and body-mass-index on hormonal and metabolic parameters in young, obese women. Int J Obes Relat Metab Disord 1997;21(6):476–483.
82. Pasquali R, Casimirri F, Labate AM, Tortelli O, Pascal G, Anconetani B, et al. Body weight, fat distribution and the menopausal status in women. Int J Obes Relat Metab Disord 1994;18(9):614–621.
83. Ley CJ, Lees B, Stevenson JC. Sex- and menopause-associated changes in body-fat distribution. Am J Clin Nutr 1992;55:950–954.
84. Bjorntorp P. Neuroendocrine abnormalities in human obesity. Metab 1995;44(S2):38–41.
85. Bjorntorp P. The regulation of adipose tissue distribution in humans. Int J Obes Relat Metab Disord 1996;20(4):291–302.

86. Grady D, Rubin SM, Pettiti BD, Fox CS, Black D, Ettinger B, et al. Hormone replacement therapy to prevent disease and prolong life in postmenopausal women. Ann Intern Med 1992;117:1016–1037.
87. Reubinoff BE, Wurtman J, Rojansky N, Adler D, Stein P, Schenker JG, et al. Effects of hormone replacement therapy on weight, body composition, fat distribution, and food intake in early postmenopausal women: a prospective study. Fertil Steril 1995;64(5):963–968.
88. Kohrt MW, Ehsani AA, Birge SJ. HRT preserves increases in bone mineral density and reductions in body fat after a supervised exercise program. J Appl Physiol 1998;84(5):1506–1512.
89. Rebuffe-Scrive M. Steroid hormones and distribution of adipose tissue. Acta Med Scand Suppl 1988;723:143–146.
90. Stamford BA. Exercise and the elderly. In: Holloszy J, ed. Exercise and Sport Science Reviews. Williams & Wilkins, Philadelphia, PA, 1988, pp. 341–379.
91. Evans WJ, Cyr-Campbell D. Nutrition, exercise, and healthy aging. J Am Diet Assoc 1997;97(6): 632–638.
92. Pruess HG. Effects of glucose/insulin perturbations on aging and chronic disorders of aging: the evidence. J Am Coll Nutr 1997;16(5):397–403.
93. Tuomilehto J, Zimmet P, Taylor R, Bennett P, Kanakaanpaa J, Wolf E. A cross-sectional ecological analysis of blood pressure and its determinants in eleven Pacific populations. J Am Coll Nutr 1989;8(2):151–165.
94. Masoro EJ, McCarter RJM, Katz MS, McMahon CA. Dietary restriction alters characteristics of glucose fuel use. J Gerontol 1992;47:B202–208.
95. Masoro EJ. Assessment of nutritional components in prolongation of life and health by diet. Proc Soc Exp Biol Med 1990;193:31–34.
96. Masoro EJ. Antiaging action of caloric restriction: endocrine and metabolic aspects. Obes Res 1995;3(s2):241s–247s
97. Cerami A, Vlassare H, Brownlee M. Glucose and aging. Sci Am 1987;256:90–96.
98. Gallaher DD, Csallany AS, Shoeman DW, Olson JM. Diabetes increases excretion of urinary malonaldehyde conjugates in rats. Lipids 1993;28:663–666.
99. DeFronzo RA, Ferinimmi E. Insulin resistance: a multifaceted sydrome reponsible for NIDDM, obesity, hypertension, dyslipidemia and athersclerotic cardiovascular disease. Diabetes Care 1991;14:173–194.
100. Flack JM, Showers JR. Epidemiologic and clinical aspects of insulin resistance and hyperinsulinemia. Am J Med 1991;s1a:11s–21s.
101. Walford RL, Weber L, Panov S. Caloric restriction and aging as viewed from Biosphere 2. Receptor 1995;5(1):29–33.
102. Hallaas J, Gajiwala KS, Maffei M, Cohen SL, Chait BT, Rabinowitz D, et al. Weight-reducing effects of the plasma protein encoded by the obese gene. Science 1995;269:543–546.
103. Lonnqvist F, Arner P, Nordfors L, Schalling M. Overexpression of he obese (ob) gene in adipose tissue of human obese subjects. Nature Med 1995;9:950–953.
104. Havel PJ, Kasim-Karakas S, Mueller W, Johnson PR, Gingrich RL, Stern JS. Relationship of plasma leptin to plasma insulin and adiposity in normal weight and overweight women: effects of dietary fat content and sustained weight loss. J Clin Endocrinol Metab 1996;81:4406–4413.
105. Rosenbaum M, Nocolson M, Hirsch J, Heymsfield SB, Gallagher D, Chu F, Leibel RL. Effcts of gender, body composition, and menopause on plasma concentrations of leptin J Clin Endocrinol Metab 1996;81:3424–3427.
106. Bennett FI, McFarlane-Anderson N, Wilks R, Luke A, Cooper RS, Forrester TE. Leptin concentration in women is influenced by regional distribution of adipose tissue. Am J Clin Nutr 1997;66: 1340–1344.
107. Kennedy A, Gettys TW, Watson P, Wallace P, Ganaway E, Pan Q, et al. The metabolic significance of leptin in humans: gender-based differences in relationship to adiposity, insulin sensitivity, and energy expenditure. J Clin Endocrinol Metab 1997;82:1293–1300.
108. Wing RR, Sinha MK, Considine RV, Lang W, Caro JF. Relationship between weight loss maintenance and changes in serum leptin levels. Horm Metab Res 1997;28:698–703.
109. Ramesar X, Rafecas I, Fernandez-Lopez JA, Alemany M. Is leptin an insulin counter-regulatory hormone? FEBS Lett 1997;402:9–11.

110. Caro JF, Kolaczynski JW, Nyce MR, Ohannesian JP, Opentanova I, Goldman WH, et al. Decreased cerebrospinal-fluid/serum leptin ration in obesity: a possible mechanism for leptin resistance. Lancet 1996;348:159–161.
111. Pasman WJ, Westerterp-Plantenga MS, Saris WHM. The effect of exercise training on leptin levels in obese males. Am J Physiol 1998;274:E280–E286.
112. Hickey MS, Houmard JA, Considine RV, Tyndall GL, Midgette JB, Gavigan KE, et al. Gender-dependent effects of exercise training on serum leptin levels in humans. Am J Physiol 1997;272: E562–E566.

12 Hormonal Regulation of Fluid Homeostasis During and Following Exercise

Charles E. Wade, PhD

CONTENTS
    INTRODUCTION
    MODULATING FACTORS
    HORMONE RESPONSES
    FLUID AND ELECTROLYTE REGULATION
    SUMMARY
    REFERENCES

INTRODUCTION

The focus of this chapter will be the role of the endocrine system in the maintenance of fluid and electrolyte homeostasis during and following exercise. The approach will be to describe hormone responses to exercise, define the routes by which fluids and electrolytes are lost and replaced during and following exercise, and identify the roles of various hormones in these processes. A number of previous reviews address these issues (1–10). In the present chapter, these reviews will be used to build a foundation. The chapter's primary emphasis will be on new findings and their impact on our understanding of the function of the endocrine system in fluid and electrolyte homeostasis during and following exercise.

MODULATING FACTORS

In the maintenance of fluid and electrolyte balance, the hormones of interest are vasopressin, natriuretic peptides, the renin–angiotensin–aldosterone (RAA) axis, and catecholamines. Each of these hormonal systems is modified in response to exercise. During exercise, the circulating concentrations of these hormones may be the product of metabolism, changes in secretion, and volume of distribution. The discussion here will focus on the product of these factors in circulating concentrations.

From: *Contemporary Endocrinology: Sports Endocrinology*
Edited by: M. P. Warren and N. W. Constantini © Humana Press Inc., Totowa, NJ

Exercise is a broad term covering a wide range of physical activities. For this reason, the specific type and duration of exercise will often be mentioned in the presentation. Of primary importance is an understanding of the definitions of workload in assessing the response of hormones. Absolute workload is the level of work being performed, such as running on a treadmill at a set speed at a given inclination. For individuals at this absolute workload, the resulting level of oxygen consumption would be highly variable, with the variability a function of the relative fitness of each person. Thus, in order to compare exercise among individuals, relative workloads are employed. That is, workload is expressed as a percentage of the maximum absolute workload, the maximum oxygen consumption, or the maximum heart rate of the individual subject. Use of the percentage of maximal workload allows comparison among subjects. This is especially true for evaluating the response of hormones to exercise *(2,11)*.

Exercise Workload

The responses to exercise of the hormone systems to be discussed are closely coupled to the amount of relative work performed. There are three basic response patterns of hormones to acute exercise. The first is a linear response to relative workload. This is seen in the response of atrial natriuretic peptide (ANP) to progressive increases in workload (Fig. 1). With an increase in the level of exercise, there is a proportional increase in the circulating concentration of this hormone. The second pattern is a log-rhythmic/exponential increase in the level of hormones in response to exercise. This is seen in the RAA system where, with increasing workloads, concentrations increase at a progressively faster rate (Fig. 1). Finally, the third pattern is a threshold response. Beyond a set level of exercise, there is a linear increase in concentration. This is seen for vasopressin (AVP) (Fig. 1). The threshold response is often associated with the onset of anaerobic metabolism, at about 70% of maximum workload, and is thus termed the anaerobic threshold *(12)*. These three patterns are typical of the hormonal responses to exercise when these responses are evaluated as a function of relative workload *(11–13)*.

Exercise Duration

The duration of exercise may greatly influence the magnitude of hormonal responses to exercise *(4)*. Exercise duration may have a greater influence on the levels of hormones attained than the intensity of exercise. For example, the levels of aldosterone after acute maximal exercise increases by two to three times resting levels, whereas after 2 h of submaximal exercise, the values are increased by over three times basal levels with the increase persisting for over 24 h *(14–16)*. Further, hormone concentrations may vary in a bimodal manner over exercise of an extended duration. From the initiation of a marathon run, ANP concentrations were increased sixfold during the first 10 km of the race, but at the end, levels were only elevated twofold (Fig. 2) *(17)*. The duration of the exercise thus is a major consideration in the modulation of endocrine responses *(18)*.

Training

Training may also impact endocrine responses to exercise. For most hormones, the response to an absolute workload is attenuated following training. Further, for a number of hormones the response to the same relative workload is attenuated or potentiated with training. This does not appear to be the case for those hormones modulating fluid and electrolyte homeostasis during exercise *(11)*. Plasma catecholamine concentrations are

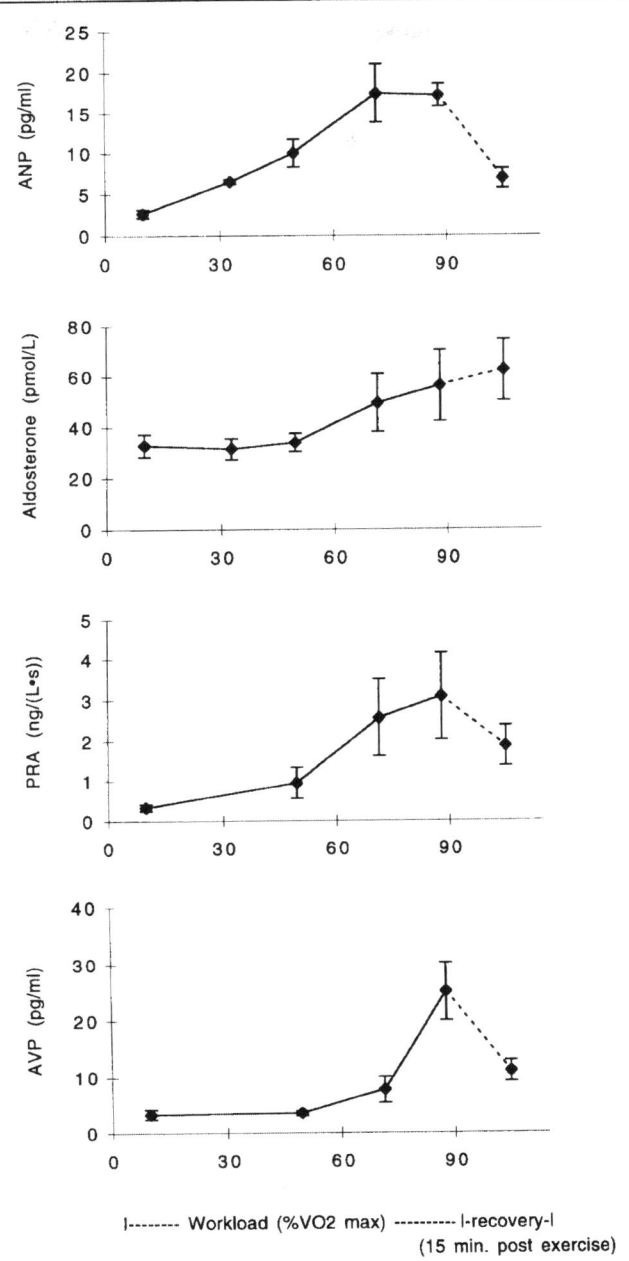

Fig. 1. Plasma concentrations of atrial natriuretic peptide (ANP), aldosterone, renin activity (PRA), and vasopressin (AVP) in response to increasing workloads (0, 33, 49, 71, and 88% of maximum oxygen uptake) on bicycle ergometer in five male subjects. The dashed line represents the change over 15 min of recovery (redrawn from Tanaka et al., ref. 46).

not altered at the same relative workload of 70% of maximum following training (19,20). Training does not affect the response of vasopressin, renin activity, or aldosterone to the same relative workload (21–24). Thus, in consideration of the response of those hor-

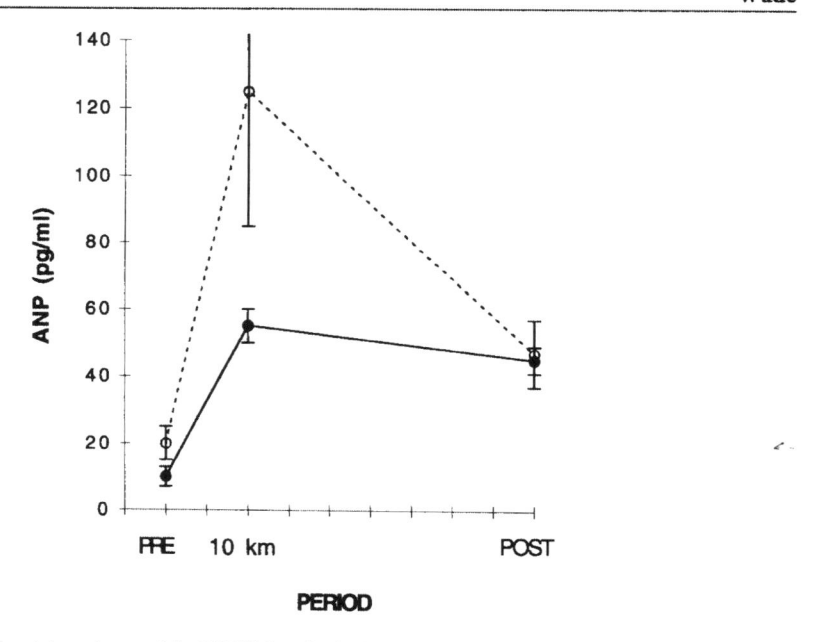

Fig. 2. Plasma atrial natriuretic peptide (ANP) levels during a marathon race. Samples were obtained prior to the start of the race, at 10 km, and at the end. The subjects were young (24–34 yr of age; solid line) and middle-aged (41–55 yr of age; dashed line) individuals who had undergone regular exercise training for the event (redrawn from Freund et al., ref. *17*).

mones important in the regulation of fluid and electolyte status, the training level does not appear to be as important a factor as the relative intensity and duration of exercise.

Other Modulating Factors

A number of other factors can influence the response of hormones to exercise. These include the mode of exercise and the body position in which exercise is performed *(9,25)*, environmental factors *(26,27)*, age (Fig. 2) and gender of the subjects *(17,26,28–30)*, and a variety of medical/physical conditions *(26,31–33)*. In addition, reported differences in hormonal concentrations in response to exercise can also, in part, be explained by the differing methods of hormone determination used.

HORMONE RESPONSES

After consideration of the factors mentioned above in modulating the response of the endocrine system to exercise, response among individuals is relatively consistent for those hormones important in the regulation of fluid and electrolyte homeostasis *(6,11,13)*.

Catecholamines

The catecholamines of interest are norepinephrine and epinephrine *(20,34)*. These hormones are closely coupled regarding their actions and are often referred to as the sympathoadrenal system. Norepinephrine is predominately released from the sympathetic nervous system, whereas epinephrine is derived from the adrenal medulla. In response to exercise, there is a progressive increase in norepinephrine from a resting level of 1.2–3.0 nmol/L to levels as high as 12.0 nmol/L at maximal exercise *(1,18,34)*.

Chapter 12 / Hormonal Regulation of Fluid Homeostasis

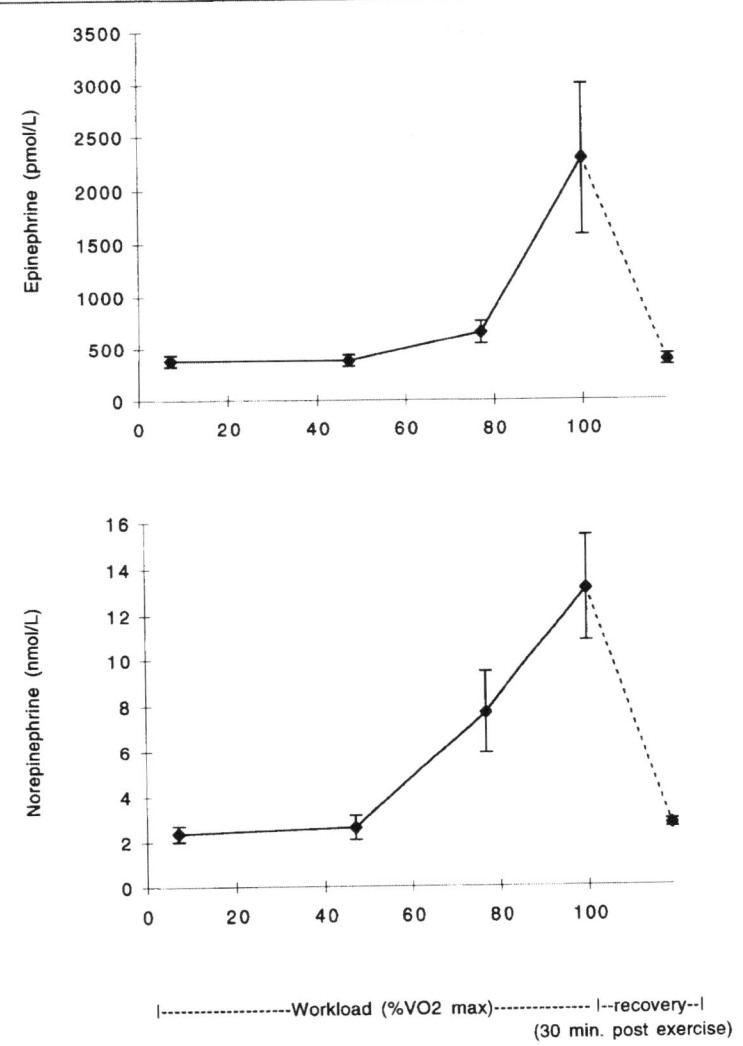

Fig. 3. Plasma concentrations of epinephrine and norepinephrine during progressive increases in workload during treadmill running and through 30 min of recovery (redrawn from Galbo et al., ref. *18*).

Resting concentrations of epinephrine are 380–655 pmol/L. With maximal exercise, epinephrine concentrations can attain levels up to 3300 pmol/L. For both of these hormones, there is a progressive elevation in concentration as workload is increased (Fig. 3). Following exercise, these increases are not sustained, and resting concentrations are achieved within 30 min after exercise.

Catecholamines are rapid responders to exercise. Acute, short-duration maximal exercise can elicit a significant increase in norepinephrine and epinephrine levels *(11)*. This rapid onset suggests that the levels are primarily regulated via neural release mediated by activation of the sympathetic nervous system. The exact tissue type from which the increase in circulating norepinephrine is derived is not clear. Although spillover from active muscle during exercise appears to be the primary contributor, the kidneys are possibly another source *(10,34,35)*. In addition, alteration in the ratio of norepinephrine to epinephrine, favoring a greater proportional increase in the release of epinephrine from the adrenal medulla during exercise, suggests possible hypothalamic mediation in the response to exercise.

Vasopressin

Vasopressin is produced in the hypothalimus and stored in the posterior pituitary *(36)*. Vasopressin is also referred to as antidiuretic hormone (ADH). Resting levels of vasopressin are 1–4 pg/mL. Following maximal exercise, concentrations range from 4 to 24 pg/mL *(6,37,38)*. During submaximal exercise, an increase in vasopressin is not observed until a workload above 70% is attained (Fig. 1). At low workloads (25% of maximum), a decrease may occur *(13)*. The increase in vasopressin may persist for over 60 min following maximal exercise *(37)*.

The stimulus for the increase in vasopressin during exercise could be the increase in plasma osmolality and reduction in blood volume *(37,38)*. Recent work by Montain et al. *(39)* assessed the regulation of vasopressin during exercise. Subjects performed 20 min of exercise up to 65% of maximum on a treadmill following various levels of dehydration: 0, 3, and 5% of body weight. At rest, the concentration of vasopressin increased in a graded manner with hypohydration. The response of vasopressin to exercise was independent of hydration status, since the increase was proportional to the change in plasma osmolality. Therefore, during exercise, the increase in plasma osmolality appears to be the primary mediator of the increase in vasopressin independent of the status of blood volume. The independence of the increase in osmolality and reduction in blood volume during exercise in the regulation of vasopressin is similar to that observed during dehydration alone *(40)*.

Natriuretic Peptides

A number of peptides have been shown to elicit a natriuretic effect *(41–44)*. These include ANP, brain natriuretic peptide (BNP), and urodilatin. All of these hormones have been suggested to be altered by exercise.

ATRIAL NATRIURETIC PEPTIDE (ANP)

ANP has been shown to be increased with exercise *(45)*. ANP increases with exercise from a resting level of 10–40 to 100 pg/mL following acute maximal exercise *(13,45,46)*. Of note is the transitory response of this hormone to exercise of extended duration (Fig. 2) *(45,47,48)*. Although initial concentrations are increased in a progressive manner dependent on the level of the workload, values return to resting levels over time. When ANP levels are increased with acute exercise, basal levels are attained within 1 h of completion of exercise *(46)*.

The transient nature of the ANP response during exercise appears to be coupled with alterations in cardiovascular function *(45,48)*. ANP release is stimulated by an increase in atrial pressure, which occurs at the onset of exercise *(49)*. However, as exercise progresses, atrial pressure decreases owing to the redistribution of blood flow (cardiovascular drift) to meet demands to compensate for the increase in body temperature *(50)*. Kaka et al. *(51)* recently reported an increase in ANP in subjects completing a 20-km run within 3 h. Over the course of exercise, there was no change in ANP from resting levels of 6 pmol/L. However, if the subjects ingested water over the course of the

Chapter 12 / Hormonal Regulation of Fluid Homeostasis

exercise, there was a 3.4-fold increase in ANP levels. The increase in ANP concentration with water intake would support the hypothesis that the reduction in the course of extended exercise was altered by hydration status and subsequent redistribution of blood flow *(52)*. The ANP response to volume changes during exercise appears to be mediated by physical effects on the heart rather than by neural inputs. In patients who had cardiac transplants, the increase in ANP during exercise on a cycle ergometer for 45 min was accentuated compared to the ANP increase in control subjects *(53)*. Resting ANP levels in patients with heart transplants were higher, 105 pg/mL, compared to control subjects, 31 pg/mL. In response to exercise, ANP levels increased to about 200 pg/mL in patients with transplants, a 90% increase. In controls, a 22% increase was noted. These findings suggest that in normal subjects with innervated hearts, there may be an inhibition of ANP release at rest and in response to exercise. Supporting this hypothesis [*see* Brain Natriuretic Peptide (BNP)], Tanka et al. *(54)* found the response of ANP to exercise to be potentiated in the presence of β-blockade in patients with hypertension.

Sodium intake may affect the ANP response to exercise *(55,56)*. In normal subjects on a low-sodium diet (40 mmol/d), performance of graded exercise on a bicycle ergometer at a maximum of 150 W resulted in an increase in ANP from 42 to 59 pg/mL. When the subjects were on a high-sodium diet (300 mmol/d), concentrations increased from 72 to 119 pg/mL with the same exercise. The increase in ANP concentrations with exercise appears to be potentiated by a chronic high-sodium intake.

BRAIN NATRIURETIC PEPTIDE (BNP)

BNP, which is markedly different in sequence from ANP, was originally identified in the porcine brain from which it attained its name *(42)*. Higher concentrations were subsequently identified in the hearts of both pigs and humans *(42,57)*. Thus, BNP and ANP are colocated in the heart and appear to have similar actions—natriuretic and hypotensive activities—when infused in rats *(42)*. Wambach and Koch *(56)* found BNP levels to be unchanged from resting levels of 28 pg/mL with graded exercise on a bicycle ergometer to 150 W in subjects when they were on a low-sodium diet. While the subjects were on a high-sodium diet, exercise resulted in an increase from 32 to 45 pg/mL. Hydration status may also modulate the BNP response to exercise. Kata et al. *(51)* found no difference in BNP levels following a 20-km run if the subjects were not allowed access to water. However, if water was provided during the run, BNP levels increased from a resting level of 5 to 20 pg/mL following exercise. Values remained elevated through 15 min of recovery, but were not different from basal levels after 60 min. Tanka et al. *(58)* reported that BNP was not altered from resting levels of 1.5 pg/mL with graded exercise on a bicycle ergometer by healthy subjects. Of note was that in hypertensive subjects, BNP concentrations were elevated at rest compared to controls and increased from resting levels of 4.8–9 pg/mL with the same level of exercise. In both populations, ANP levels were increased with exercise. Basal BNP levels were reached within 20 min following exercise. Similar findings were noted by Nishikimi et al. *(33)* in normal and hypertensive subjects performing exercise on a bicycle ergomenter in a supine position at up to 80 W. BNP levels were increased in the hypertensive subjects at rest, 14 pg/mL, compared to normal subjects, 6 pg/mL. With exercise, no change was noted in normal subjects, but in hypertensive subjects, BNP increased to 19 pg/mL. Both groups had significant increases in ANP concentration. In all subjects, resting levels for BNP and ANP were attained within 10 min following exercise. In hypertensive subjects, the increase in BNP with exercise was correlated with the initial basal level. The authors suggest that the regulation of ANP and BNP in response to exercise occurs by different mechanisms, and that the stimulation of BNP may depend on the underlying pathophysiology of hypertension *(33)*. This conclusion is supported by further work of Tanka et al. *(54)*, who studied the BNP and ANP response to exercise in hypertensive subjects with and without β-adenoreceptor blockade (bisoprolol 5 mg/d). At rest, there was no difference in ANP or BNP levels between treatments. With bicycle ergometer exercise up to 75 W, both ANP and BNP were increased. There was no difference in the BNP response with or without blockade. The ANP response was accentuated with β-blockade resulting in a fourfold greater response. Thus, the β-adrenergic system appears to attenuate the release of ANP in response to exercise, but does not modulate the response of BNP. Therefore, the regulation of BNP in response to exercise in hypertensive subjects is, in part, modulated by factors other than those affecting ANP.

URODILATIN

Urodilatin, a renal peptide, has recently been suggested to play a role in the regulation of sodium balance via a natriuretic action *(43)*. In subjects with mildly impaired left ventricular function, exercise on a bicycle ergometer at 50 W did not alter the rate of urinary urodilatin excretion though ANP was elevated by 130%. Kentsch et al. *(59)* also found no change in urodilatin excretion following exercise in patients with mildly impaired left ventricular function. The absence of change of urodilatin excretion suggests that urodilatin is probably not contributing to the regulation of sodium balance during exercise.

ADRENOMEDULLIN

Adrenomedullin has been reported to have significant natriuretic and diuretic effects when administered to dogs *(44,60)*. In humans, adrenomedullin plasma concentrations are increased in diseases associated with an increase in blood volume *(32,61)*. Further, in these conditions, the adrenomedullin levels are correlated with ANP and BNP concentrations as well as with the extent of the illness. In normotensive subjects, adrenomedullin levels were found not to change with exercise at 80 W on a supine bicycle ergometer *(33)*. In subjects with hypertension, although basal levels were increased compared to normal subjects, there still was no significant response to exercise.

RAA System

The RAA system is closely coupled and often appears to respond as a unit to exercise. Renin is released from the juxtaglomerular apparatus of the kidneys and converts angiotensinogen to angiotensin I *(62)*. In the lungs, angiotensin I (A-I) is transformed by angiotensin-converting enzyme (ACE), producing angiotensin II (A-II). A-II stimulates the release of aldosterone from the adrenal gland. This cascade is activated during exercise and plays a major role in the maintenance of fluid and electrolyte homeostasis.

Plasma renin activity (PRA) at rest ranges from 0.15 to 0.55 ng AI/(L · s). Values of 1.11–1.67 ng AI/(L · s) are reported following maximal exercise *(2,6,12,34,46)*. The increase in PRA is noted at submaximal workloads >60–70% of maximum *(12)*. The duration of the exercise may also be a factor. With the increase in PRA during exercise, there is a correlated increase in A-II *(34)*. At rest, the levels of A-II are 15–25 ng/L.

Concentrations of 130–160 ng/L are attained with maximal exercise. With exercise, there is an increase in the circulating concentrations of aldosterone, which may, in part, be mediated by the increase in A-II. Aldosterone concentrations are increased from resting concentrations of 80–830 to 250–3330 pmol/L following maximal exercise *(6,14,46)*. Elevated levels of aldosterone may persist for days after the end of exercise depending on water and sodium intake *(15,16,63)*.

The primary activator of the RAA system during exercise is the sympathetic nervous system. Stimulation of the release of renin is modulated by changes in renal sympathetic nerve activity resulting in an increase in local norepinephrine *(34)*. This is supported by pharmacological blockade of the β-receptors attenuating the response of the renin-angiotensin system to exercise *(64–66)*. During exercise, the increase in renin activity is correlated with the increase in norepinephrine concentration in the renal vein *(34)*. Further, the renin response may be modulated by negative feedback owing to elevated levels of A-II or vasopressin *(62,67)*.

The increase in aldosterone with exercise is assumed to be mediated by the increase in A-II in response to activation of the renin-angiotensin system *(6,7,67)*. However, inhibition of ACE does not attenuate the increase in aldosterone with maximal exercise in healthy subjects *(14)*. Other factors may influence the response of aldosterone to exercise, such as sodium intake, potassium balance, and levels of adrenocorticotropic hormone (ACTH) *(68)*. Of note are recent studies regarding the effect of reductions in blood volume on the response of aldosterone to exercise. Zappe et al. *(69)* reduced blood volume by administration of a diuretic, which reduced plasma volume, but did not alter plasma osmolality. Resting levels of aldosterone were increased from 720 to 2770 pmol/L with the reduction in plasma volume. In response to exercise on a cycle ergometer at 60% for 60 min, aldosterone levels increased to 1470 pmol/L in the euhydrated state and to 4740 pmol/L with a reduced plasma volume of 12%. Thus, with exercise in the presence of a reduction in blood volume, there was a potentiation of the response of aldosterone to exercise. In another study, Montain et al. *(39)* reduced volume by dehydration, thus raising plasma osmolality and sodium levels. Resting aldosterone levels were increased by dehydration from about 890 to 1890 pmol/L in the presence of a 5% reduction in blood volume (assumed to represent a 9% decrease in plasma volume). With 50 min of treadmill exercise at 65% of maximum, aldosterone levels were increased to 1390 pmol/L euhydrated and to 2440 pmol/L after dehydration. Thus, in the presence of volume reduction and increases in plasma sodium and osmolality, the response to exercise is not potentiated. Further, plasma aldosterone concentrations are increased long after the end of exercise *(15,16)*. The increase in aldosterone at this time may be associated with reductions in plasma osmolality and sodium concentrations owing to ingestion of water to replace total body water (TBW) losses *(15,16,63)* (Fig. 4). Therefore, the interaction of a number of regulating factors, not just the renin-angiotensin system, appears to be mediating the response of aldosterone.

FLUID AND ELECTROLYTE REGULATION

A number of systems act in concert to regulate fluid and electrolyte homeostasis during and following exercise. This is a classic case of balance between the mechanisms of loss and the mechanisms of conservation and replacement.

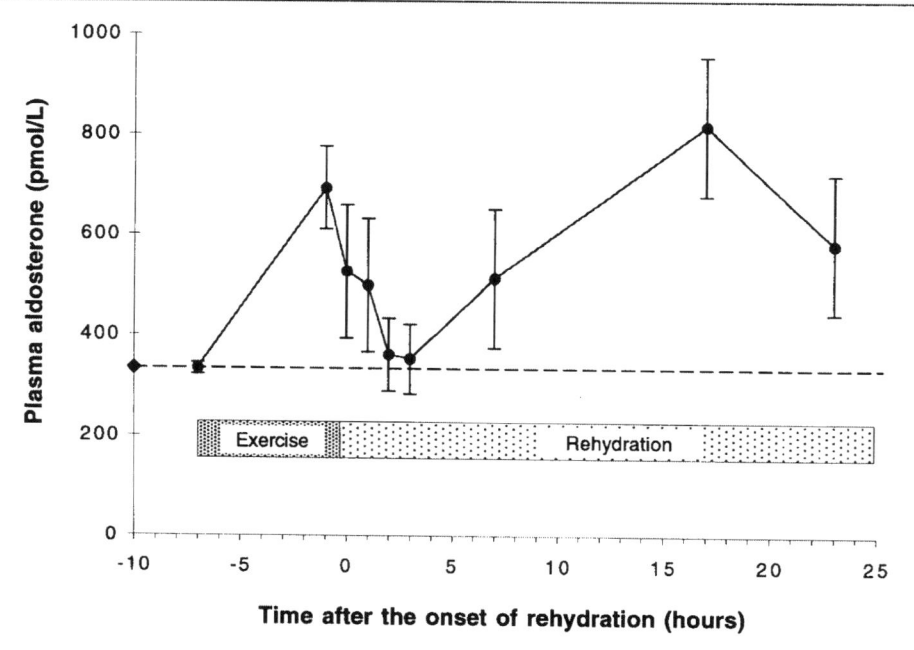

Fig. 4. Response of plasma aldosterone to submaximal exercise for 6 h in the heat and over the subsequent 23 h with rehydration (redrawn from Takamata et al., ref. *16*).

Total Body Water

Over the course of exercise, there is a reduction in TBW that is tolerated until the completion of exercise *(26)*. The decrease in TBW during exercise is equivalent to weight loss and, during long-duration exercise, may attain levels >5% of body weight *(70,71)*. This represents a fluid loss in a human weighing 70 kg on the order of 3000 to 4000 mL or about 7% of TBW. A reduction in TBW by as little as 2% of body weight may lead to a significant detriment in exercise performance *(27,72)*. Even with free access to water in the course of exercise at a moderate level (70% of maximum), the rate of fluid loss is about 1000 mL/h. This loss in the presence of water available for ingestion is referred to as a "voluntary dehydration" *(73,74)*. The level of voluntary dehydration represents about 20–30% of the fluid loss, since supplemental intake in the course of exercise replaces about 70–80%. Thus, a level of dehydration is tolerated during the conduct of exercise, but fluid losses are usually replaced over the following 24 h *(6,15,16,63)*. Recently, the degree of weight loss, and thus the reduction in TBW, during competitive running has tended to be reduced owing to increased emphasis on adequate hydration to attenuate thermal complications.

Although TBW is decreased during exercise, this loss does not appear to be equally distributed among the fluid compartments of the body. Over the course of exercise, there is a redistribution of fluids, resulting in a reduction in plasma volume *(75–77)*. The decrease in plasma volume during maximal exercise is on the order of 8–12%. This equates to a reduction in blood volume of 5–7%. This blood volume reduction is accompanied by a redistribution of blood flow, which is highly dependent on blood volume status and may impact work performance *(50)*. The decrease in blood volume is compensated for by an increase in cardiac output and redistribution of blood flow to meet the metabolic requirements and thermal loads of various tissues *(50,78,79)*. This redistribution of blood flow is owing to alterations of local vascular resistance, in part mediated by hormones, such as catecholamines, A-II, and vasopressin *(67,80–82)*.

Sweat Loss

The primary loss of fluids occurs owing to sweating necessitated to handle the increased thermal load incurred during exercise *(83)*. The level of sweat loss in individuals is highly variable, and is influenced by level of training and prior adaptation or acclimation to a hot environment *(83–85)*. The rate of fluid loss owing to sweating may be as high as 1500 mL/h *(71,73,74)*. The rate of sweating may be hormonally mediated specifically by vasopressin *(86,87)*. An increase in circulating vasopressin is postulated to modulate the rate and composition of sweat during exercise, since injection of vasopressin in the area of the sweat glands results in such changes *(86)*. However, during exercise, the rate of sweating and subsequent changes in plasma osmolality and blood volume—the primary mediators of vasopressin—are closely coupled *(38,41,78,79)*. This makes the role of vasopressin in the regulation of sweat production difficult to delineate. Further, sweat rate has been reported to be unchanged or reduced with β-blockade, providing no definitive answer regarding the role of sympathoadrenal hormones *(88,89)*.

Accompanying the loss of fluid in sweat is the loss of electrolytes *(83–85,90,91)*. The concentration of electrolytes in sweat may vary greatly: sodium 20–135 mmol/L, potassium 3–35 mmol/L, and chloride 10–100 mmol/L *(83,90,91)*. At these concentrations, the loss of electrolytes in sweat is significant. For example, although the overall concentration of sodium in sweat is lower than the levels observed in plasma at a sweat rate of 1500 mL/h with the sodium concentration being 60 mmol/L, the rate of loss would be 90 mmoL/h or 3% of total body sodium. There is variability regarding the rate of sodium loss in sweat as a result of the degree of training of the subjects, level of heat acclimation, and duration of exercise since the composition of sweat has been shown to be decreased by exercise training and repeated exposure to heat *(76,84,85)*. This alteration in the composition of sweat has been postulated to be in part mediated by aldosterone *(85,92)*.

Fluid and Electrolyte Intake

Ingestion is the primary mechanism for replacing fluids and electrolytes lost during exercise *(74,93,94)*. During performance of long-duration exercise with free access to fluids, approx 80% of the loss of total body water is replaced by intake *(71,93)*. The extent to which loss is replaced is, in part, dependent on the composition of the fluid ingested *(93,94)*. In humans, the replacement of electrolytes does not appear to be subjectively sensed, but is the result of the normal intake of food. However, recent work by Takamata et al. *(16)* suggests that salt appetite may be increased 6–23 h after exercise. This increase in salt appetite is associated with a reduction in plasma osmolality and sodium concentration owing to fluid replacement with water. Thus, the replacement of electrolyte loss may be coupled with hunger and an increase in salt appetite, but this has not been fully evaluated in relation to the consequences of exercise.

The loss of fluids is replaced by the subsequent ingestion of liquids, which is modulated by thirst *(95–97)*. Following exercise, there is an increase in thirst: the subjective sensation to seek and drink fluids. The resulting increase in fluid intake, stimulated by thirst, may persist for hours after exercise *(16)*. Although the loss in TBW is not immediately replaced, the TBW reduction is usually replenished within 24 h *(15,16,63)*. Thirst is regulated by a variety of factors, such as an increase in plasma osmolality (hypertonicity) and a reduction in blood volume *(95)*. With sustained exercise, there is an increase in plasma osmolality and reduction in blood volume *(6,7,77)*. There is, however, a conflict that may, in part, explain the voluntary dehydration observed during exercise *(73,74)*. In the course of exercise, if water is ingested, blood volume is maintained. However, water is hypotonic and could lead to a reduction in plasma osmolality, thus attenuating thirst. This hypothesis is supported by the work of Nose et al. *(98,99)*, who found that replacement of the volume of fluid lost as sweat with water led to a decrease in plasma osmolality and sodium concentration associated with a subsequent reduction in the urge to drink and an increase in urine output. Takamata et al. *(16)* found thirst to be attenuated immediately after exercise when fluid was provided, yet increased again 15 h later though plasma osmolality was reduced. This period was associated with an increase in aldosterone and presumably A-II. Hormones, such as A-II, have also been shown to stimulate thirst directly *(97,100)*. Intracerebroventricular injection of BNP into conscious rats suppresses thirst, and ANP administered by the same route attenuates the thirst response evoked by A-II *(101–104)*. Thus, during and following exercise, there are circumstances associated with changes in blood volume and plasma osmolality that alter hormone levels, potentiate thirst, and lead to rectification of the loss in fluids.

The ingestion of fluids during exercise has been advocated to improve performance *(27,72)*. As noted earlier, a moderate level of dehydration will be tolerated without an adverse effect on performance. However, at some level of reduction in TBW, performance will be compromised. Some studies have suggested that replacement of fluid losses by drinking will not influence performance *(93,105)*. To assess the effects of fluid intake on performance, Robinson and colleagues *(105)* had subjects perform 1 h of cycling with and without fluid intake. Sweat rate was similar under both conditions, though with access to fluid, body weight loss was reduced by 60%. Further, plasma osmolality and sodium concentration were greater in the absence of water intake, but did not result in differences in plasma concentrations of vasopressin or A-II. Others have shown hypohydration to impair performance at even low levels of hypohydration *(27,72,93,106)*. Further, rehydration blunts ANP, PRA, and vasopressin responses to exercise, making the roles of these hormones difficult to assess *(52,107)*. These reductions in hormone levels, probably owing to a maintenance of vascular volume, may, in part, be the result of the act of drinking stimulating an oral-pharyngeal reflex that suppresses circulating concentrations of vasopressin and renin activity independent of changes in plasma osmolality or blood volume *(108,109)*. However, it appears from the majority of the data that the maintenance of adequate hydration status during extended periods of exercise facilitates performance and attenuates the increase in hormone levels and the necessity of fluid conservation *(27,93)*.

Renal Function

Renal function is altered by exercise *(6,37,110–113)*. Although changes in renal function play a negligible role in fluid and electrolyte homeostasis during exercise, after exercise, these changes are important. Renal function is the major mechanism by which electrolytes are conserved following exercise. Changes in renal function are regulated by a number of hormones altered by exercise *(6,8,10)*. A basic understanding of the function of the kidneys in fluid and electrolyte homeostasis is necessary to appreciate the role of the endocrine system.

RENAL BLOOD FLOW (RBF)

The kidneys may be thought of as performing based on what is delivered to them. At rest, about 20% of the cardiac output flows to the kidneys. Therefore, RBF is on the order of 1000 mL/min. During exercise, RBF is reduced *(50,114)*. The degree of reduction appears to be related to the intensity and duration of the exercise *(8,10,34)*. During light to moderate exercise (<50% of maximum), there is minimal change in RBF. At higher work intensities, the extent of the reduction of RBF is proportional to the intensity of the workload. With maximal exercise, the magnitude of the reduction ranges from 40 to 60%. Suzuki et al. *(115)* found RBF to be reduced by 53% in subjects following maximal exhaustive exercise on a bicycle ergometer. The decrease in RBF persisted during recovery, being reduced by 21% of resting values 60 min after exercise. Since arterial perfusion pressure is maintained during exercise and recovery, the decrease in RBF is owing to an increase in renal vascular resistance, specifically vasoconstriction of the afferent arterioles of the glomeruli presumably mediated by sympathetic nerve inputs and circulating norepinephrine *(10,34,115–117)*. Therefore, during exercise, the reduction in RBF results in a decrease in the volume of fluid, and thus the quantity of electrolytes that is presented to be handled by the kidneys and subsequently excreted.

GLOMERULAR FILTRATION RATE (GFR)

Glomerular filtrate, the fluid that is filtered across the glomerulus, is plasma devoid of those constituents that have a molecular weight greater than approx 50,000. The composition of this ultrafiltrate, in terms of electrolytes, can be assumed to be equal to that of plasma. Changes in GFR occurring with exercise are also related to the intensity and duration of the workload. Poortmans and coworkers *(118)* recently evaluated the change in GFR during the performance of acute exercise. Subjects performed at a maximal speed over distances ranging from 100 to 3000 m. During the shorter runs, 800 m and less, GFR was not altered. At the longer distances, a reduction was noted with a 40% decline during the 3000-m run. The change in GFR was from a resting level of about 158 to 118 mL/min at the end of exercise. Thus, although all efforts were at maximal, the decrease in GFR appeared to be dependent on the duration of the exercise. In general, at exercise levels of <50% of maximal, a reduction in GFR is not reported even with prolonged exercise *(10)*. However, with greater exercise workloads, there is a reduction in GFR, which may result in decreases to levels 50–70% of resting values, which may persist after completion of exercise.

The decrease in GFR during maximal exercise is often less pronounced than the decrease observed for RBF. This difference leads to an increase in the filtration fraction (FF) during exercise. The FF is the percentage of renal plasma flow (RPF) that becomes glomerular filtrate. The increase in FF during maximal exercise is on the order of 15–20%. With exercise at moderate to high workloads, there is an increase in the filtration fraction in spite of a decrease in RPF. The decrease in RPF is proportional to the reduction in RBF. For example, in subjects performing moderate exercise on a bicycle ergometer, RPF was decreased by 17%, but GFR was reduced by 7% with a resulting increase in FF of 14% *(119)*. Thus, there is an increase in the glomerular hydrostatic pressure owing to selective vasoconstriction of the efferent arterioles mediated by the levels of A-II *(10)*. There may also be increased permeability of the glomerular membrane, allowing more protein across with accompanying fluid, though the resulting effect on the GFR should be minimal *(112,113)*. Therefore, although a greater proportion of the RPF is filtered during exercise, there is a net reduction in RPF owing to the decrease in RBF.

URINE FLOW RATE

The product of the changes in renal hemodynamics during exercise is a reduction in the quantity of fluid delivered to the kidney and a subsequent decrease in fluid loss via urine. During light exercise, there is no change or a possible increase in urine flow rate *(13,111)*. In response to moderate to heavy exercise, urine flow rate may be reduced by 20–60% from normal levels in a euhydrate subject of 0.8–1.5 mL/min. Thus, during exercise, renal production of urine is decreased, resulting in the conservation of water. During exercise, the 60% decrease in urine loss accounts for a conservation of water on the order of <60 mL/h. However, in light of the magnitude of the losses of water incurred during exercise (1000–1500 mL/h), the contribution of renal conservation would appear to be of limited benefit during exercise, but may be a factor during recovery *(6,8,10)*.

The primary endocrine factor modulating the excretion of urine is the reduction in GFR during exercise mediated by norepinephrine via increased sympathetic nerve activity *(34,50,117)*. This reduced fluid delivery results in a reduction in urine excretion. However, these changes are acute and often rectified within 30 min of completion of exercise when there is still a reduced urine flow *(110)*.

Logic would suggest a role for vasopressin during exercise in the conservation of water *(36–38)*. However, there is an increase in the excretion of free water during exercise possibly owing to changes in the concentration gradient across the kidney resulting from redistribution of renal blood flow or inhibition of the actions of vasopressin possibly by prostaglandins *(8,10,37)*. An exact mechanism for this observation has yet to be identified. Following exercise, though vasopressin levels are lower than during exercise, these values are often still elevated, possibly mediating the retention of water by the kidneys seen after exercise *(15,16)*.

EXCRETION OF ELECTROLYTES

At a resting GFR of 150 mL/min, a volume equivalent to total body water would be filtered in 5–6 h. Since the initial filtrate has concentrations of electrolytes similar to plasma, if electrolytes are not handled efficiently by the kidney, there could be significant electrolyte losses. Though 0.8–1.5 mL/min of urine is produced, the concentration of key electrolytes is small in that there is a net reabsorption of over 90% of the filtered load. This reabsorption is in part hormonally mediated and is increased during and following exercise *(6,110)*. Although the total amount of electrolytes delivered to the kidney is reduced during exercise owing to a decrease in GFR, there is an increase in the reabsorption of electrolytes, compensating for losses in sweat *(15,16,112)*. This increase in reabsorption is, in part, mediated by aldosterone *(15,16)*. Following heavy daily exercise, there is a persistent elevation in plasma levels of aldosterone, which inversely correlates with the excretion of sodium *(15)*. Thus, over the period of recovery from exercise, reabsorption of sodium is increased possibly via the actions of aldosterone *(15,16,62,120)*.

SUMMARY

With the onset of exercise, there are increases in a number of hormones—specifically catecholamines, natriuretic peptides, vasopressin, and the RAA axis—which are involved in the regulation of fluid and electrolyte homeostasis. The actions of these hormone during exercise are not clear. However, following exercise, these hormones play a role in the correction of the fluid and electrolyte losses incurred during exercise by stimulating fluid intake and reducing renal excretions. The action of the hormones on fluid and electrolyte homeostasis may persist for hours after completion of exercise.

REFERENCES

1. Galbo H. Hormonal and Metabolic Adaptation to Exercise. Thieme-Stratton, New York, NY, 1983.
2. Viru A. Hormones in Muscular Activity. CRC, Boca Raton, FL, 1985.
3. Francesconi RP. Endocrinological responses to exercise in stressful environments. In: Pandolf KB, ed. Exercise and Sports Science Reviews. Macmillian, New York, NY, 1988, pp. 255–284.
4. Sutton, JR, Farrett P. Endocrine responses to prolonged exercise. In: Lamb DR, Murray R, eds. Perspectives in Exercise Science and Sports Medicine, vol. 1, Prolonged Exercise. Benchmark, Carmel, IN, 1988, pp. 153–212.
5. Terblanche SE. Recent advances in hormonal response to exercise. Comp Biochem Physiol 1989;93B:727–739.
6. Wade CE, Freund BJ, Claybaugh JR. Fluid and electrolyte homeostasis during and following exercise: Hormonal and non-hormonal factors. In: Claybaugh JR, Wade CE, eds. Hormonal Regulation of Fluids and Electrolytes: Environmental Effects. Plenum, New York, 1989, pp. 1–44.
7. Wade CE, Freund BJ. Hormonal control of blood volume during and following exercise. In: Lamb DR, Gisolfi CV, eds. Perspectives in Exercise Science and Sports Medicine, vol. 3, Fluid Homeostasis During Exercise. Benchmark, Carmel, IN, 1990, pp. 207–241.
8. Zambraski EJ. Renal regulation of fluid homeostasis during exercise. In: Gisolfi CV, Lamb DR, eds. Perspectives in Exercise Science and Sports Medicine, vol. 3, Fluid Homeostasis During Exercise. Benchmark, Carmel, IN, 1990, pp. 247–276.
9. Wade CE. Hormonal control of body fluid volume. In: Buskirk ER, Puhl SM, eds. Body Fluid Balance: Exercise and Sport. CRC, Boca Raton, FL, 1996, pp. 53–73.
10. Zambraski EJ. The kidney and body fluid balance during exercise. In: Buskirk ER, Puhl SM, eds. Body Fluid Balance: Exercise and Sport. CRC, Boca Raton, FL, 1996, pp. 75–95.
11. Viru A. Plasma hormones and physical exercise: A review. Int J Sports Med 1992;13:201–209.
12. Gleim GW, Zabetakis PM, DePasquale EE, Michelis MF, Nicholas JA. Plasma osmolality, volume, and renin activity at the "anaerobic threshold." J Appl Physiol 1984;56:57–63.
13. Freund BJ, Shizuru EM, Hashiro GM, Claybaugh JR. Hormonal, electrolyte, and renal responses to exercise are intensity dependent. J Appl Physiol 1991;70:900–906.
14. Wade CE, Ramee SR, Hunt MM, White CJ. Hormonal and renal responses to converting enzyme inhibition during maximal exercise. J Appl Physiol 1987;63:1796–1800.
15. Wade CE, Hill LC, Hunt MM, Dressendorfer RH. Plasma aldosterone and renal function in runners during a 20-day road race. Eur J Appl Physiol 1985;54:456–460.
16. Takamata A, Mack GW, Gillen CM, Nadel ER. Sodium appetite, thirst, and body fluid regulation in humans during rehydration without sodium replacement. Am J Physiol 1994;266:R1493–R1503.
17. Freund BJ, Claybaugh JR, Hashiro GM, Buono M, Chrisney S. Exaggerated ANF response to exercise in middle-aged vs. young runners. J Appl Physiol 1990;69:1607–1614.
18. Galbo H, Holst JJ, Christensen NJ. Glucagon and plasma catecholamine responses to graded and prolonged exercise in man. J Appl Physiol 1975;38:70–75.
19. Kjaer M, Secher NH, Galbo H. Physical stress and catecholamine release. Baillieres Clin Endocrinol Metabl 1987;1:279–298.
20. Svedenhag J. The sympatho-adrenal system in physical conditioning. Acta Physiol Scand Suppl 1985;125:3–73.

21. Melin B, Eclache JB, Geelen G, Annat G, Allevard AM, Jarsallion E, Zebid A, et al. Plasma AVP, neurophysin, renin activity and aldosterone during submaximal exercise performed until exhaustion in trained and untrained men. Eur J Appl Physiol 1980;44:141–151.
22. Geysant A, Geelen G, Denis C, Allevard AM, Vincent M, Jarsallion E, et al. Plasma vasopressin, renin activity and aldosterone: effect of exercise and training. Eur J Appl Physiol 1981;46:557–568.
23. Greenleaf JE, Sciaraffa D, Shvartz E, Keil LC, Brock PJ. Exercise training hypotension: implications for plasma volume, renin, and vasopressin. J Appl Physiol 1981;51:298–305.
24. Freund BJ, Claybaugh JR, Dice MS, Hashiro GM. Hormonal and vascular fluid responses to maximal exercise in trained and untrained males. J Appl Physiol 1987;63:669–675.
25. Wolf JP, Nguyen NU, Dumoulin G, Berthelay S. Plasma renin and aldosterone changes during twenty minutes' moderate exercise. Eur J Appl Physiol 1986;54:602–607.
26. Buskirk ER, Puhl SM, eds. Body Fluid Balance: Exercise and Sport. CRC, Boca Raton, FL, 1996.
27. Sawaka MN, Montain SJ, Latzka WA. Body fluid balance during exercise-heat exposure. In: Buskirk ER, Puhl SM, eds. Body Fluid Balance: Exercise and Sport. CRC, Boca Raton, FL, 1996, pp. 139–157.
28. De Souza MJ, Maresh CM, Maguire MS, Kraemer WJ, Flora-Ginter G, Goetz KL. Menstrual and plasma vasopressin, renin activity, and aldosterone exercise responses. J Appl Physiol 1989;67: 736–743.
29. Fortney SM. Hormonal control of fluid balance in women during exercise. In: Buskirk ER, Puhl SM, eds. Body Fluid Balance: Exercise and Sport. CRC, Boca Raton, FL, 1996, pp. 231–258.
30. Stachenfeld NS, Gleim GW, Zabetakis PM, Nicholas JA. Fluid balance and renal response following dehydrating exercise in well-trained men and women. Eur J Appl Physiol 1996;72:468–477.
31. Schneider SH, Vitug A, Ananthakrishnan R, Khachadurian AK. Impaired adrenergic response to prolonged exercise in type I diabetes. Metabolism 1991;40:1219–1225.
32. Nishikimi T, Saito Y, Kitamura K, Ishimitsu T, Eto T, Kangawa K, et al. Increased plasma levels of adrenomedullin in patients with heart failure. J Am Coll Cardiol 1995;26:1424–1431.
33. Nishikimi T, Morimoto A, Ishikawa K, Saito Y, Kangawa K, Matsuo H, et al. Different secretion patterns of adrenomedullin, brain natriuretic peptide during exercise in hypertensive and normotensive subjects. Clin Exp Hyperten 1997;19:503–518.
34. Tidgren B, Hjemdahl P, Theodorsson E, Nussberger J. Renal neurohormonal and vascular responses to dynamic exercise in humans. J Appl Physiol 1991;70:2279–2286.
35. Peronnet F, Beliveau L, Boudreau G, Trudeau F, Brisson G, Nadeau R. Regional catecholamine removal and release at rest and exercise in dogs. Am J Physiol 1988;254:R663–R672.
36. Weitzman R, Kleeman CR. Water metabolism and neurohypophyseal hormones. In: Maxwell MH, Kleeman CR, eds. Clinical Disorders of Fluid and Electrolyte Metabolism. McGraw-Hill, New York, 1980, pp. 531–645.
37. Wade CE, Claybaugh J. Plasma renin activity, vasopressin concentration, and urinary excretory responses to exercise in men. J Appl Physiol 1980;49:930–936.
38. Wade CE. Response, regulation, and actions of vasopressin during exercise: A review. Med Sci Sports Exerc 1984;16:506–511.
39. Montain SJ, Laird JE, Latzka WA, Sawka MN. Aldosterone and vasopressin responses in the heat: hydration level and exercise intensity effects. Med Sci Sports Exerc 1997;29:661–668.
40. Wade CE, Keil LC, Ramsay DJ. Role of volume and osmolality in the control of plasma vasopressin in dehydrated dogs. Neuroendocrinology 1983;37:349–353.
41. Weidmann P, Hasler L, Gnadinger MP, Lang RE, Uehlinger DE, Shaw S, et al. Blood levels and renal effects of atrial natriuretic peptide in normal man. J Clin Invest 1986;77:734–742.
42. Sudoh T, Kangawa K, Minamino N, Matsuo H. A new natriuretic peptide in porcine brain. Nature 1988;332:78–81.
43. Gerzer R, Drummer C. Is the renal natriuretic peptide urodilatin involved in the regulation of natriuresis? J Cardiovasc Pharmacol 1993;22 (Suppl 2):S86,S87.
44. Ebara T, Miura K, Okumura M, Matsuura T, Kim S, Yukimura T, et al. Effect of adrenomedullin on renal hemodynamics and function in dogs. Eur J Pharmacol 1994;263:69–73.
45. Freund BJ, Wade CE, Claybaugh JR. Effects of exercise on atrial natriuretic factor: Implications to fluid homeostasis. Sports Med 1988;6:364–376.
46. Tanaka G, Shindo M, Gutkowska J, Kinoshita A, Urata H, Ikeda M, et al. Effect of acute exercise on plasma immunoreactive-atrial natriuretic factor. Life Sci 1986;39:1685–1693.

47. Pastene J, Germain M, Allevard AM, Gharib C, Lacour J-R. Water balance during and after a marathon running. Eur J Appl Physiol 1996;73:49–55.
48. Nose H, Takamata A, Mack GW, Kawabata T, Oda Y, Hashimoto S, et al. Right atrial pressure and ANP release during prolonged exercise in a hot environment. J Appl Physiol 1994;76:1882–1887.
49. Kanstrup IL, Marving J, Gadsbøll N, Lønborg-Jensen H, Høilund-Carlsen PF. Left ventricle haemodynamics and vasoactive hormones during graded supine exercise in healthy male subjects. Eur J Appl Physiol 1995;72:86–94.
50. Rowell LB. Human cardiovascular adjustments to exercise and thermal stress. Physiol Rev 1974;54:75–159.
51. Kaka S, Mudambo MT, Coutie W, Rennie MJ. Plasma arginine vasopressin, atrial natriuretic peptide and brain natriuretic peptide responses to long-term field training in the heat: effects of fluid ingestion and acclimatization. Eur J Appl Physiol 1997;75:219–225.
52. Freund BJ, Claybaugh JR, Hashiro GM, Dice MS. Hormonal and renal responses to water drinking in moderately trained and untrained humans. Am J Physiol 1988;254:R417–R423.
53. Saini J, Geny B, Brandenberger G, Mettauer B, Wittersheim G, Lampert E, et al. Training effects on the hydromineral endocrine responses of cardiac transplant patients. Eur J Physiol 1995;70:226–233.
54. Tanka M, Ishizaka Y, Ishiyama Y, Kato J, Kida O, Kitamura K, et al. Chronic effect of β-adrenoceptor blockade on plasma levels of brain natriuretic peptide during exercise in essential hypertension. Hypertens Res 1996;19:239–245.
55. Cuneo RC, Espiner EA, Nicholls MG, Yandle TG, Joyce SL, Gilchrist NL. Renal, hemodynamic, and hormonal responses to atrial natriuretic peptide infusions in normal man, and effect of sodium intake. J Clin Endocrinol 1986;63:946–953.
56. Wambach G, Koch J. BNP plasma levels during acute volume expansion and chronic loading in normal men. Clin Exper Hypertens 1995;17:619–629.
57. Sudoh T, Minamino N, Kangawa K, Matsuo H. Brain natriuretic peptide-32: N-terminal six amino acid extented form of brain natriuretic peptide identified in porcine brain. Biochem Biophys Res Commun 1988;155:726–732.
58. Tanka M, Ishizaka Y, Ishiyama Y, Kato J, Kida O, Kitamura K, et al. Exercise-induced secretion of brain natriuretic peptide in essential hypertension and normal subjects. Hypertens Res 1995;18:159–166.
59. Kentsch M, Otter W, Drummer C, Peinke V, Theisen K, Müller-Esch et al. The dihydropyridine calcium channel blocker BAY t 7207 attenuates the exercise induced increase in plasma ANF and cyclic GMP in patients with mildly impaired left ventricular function. Eur J Clin Pharmacol 1995;49:177–182.
60. Jougasaki M, Wei C, Aarhus LL, Heublein DM, Sandberg SM, Burett JC. Renal localization and actions of adrenomedullin: a natriuretic factor. Am J Physiol 1995;268:F657–F663.
61. Ishimitsu T, Nishikimi T, Saito Y, Kitamura K, Eto T, Kangawa K, et al. Plasma levels of adrenomedullin, a hypotensive peptide, in patients with hypertension and renal failure. J Clin Invest 1994;94:2158–2161.
62. Reid IA, Ganong WF. Control of aldosterone secretion. In: Genest J, Koiw E, Kuchel O, eds. Hypertension: Pathophysiology and Treatment. McGraw-Hill, New York, 1977, pp. 265–292.
63. Wade CE, Dressendorfer RH, O'Brien JC, Claybaugh JR. Renal function, aldosterone, and vasopressin excretion following repeated long distance running. J Appl Physiol 1981;50:709–712.
64. Zambraski EJ, Tucker MS, Lakas CS, Grassl SM, Scanes CG. Mechanisms of renin release in exercising dog. Am J Physiol 1984;246:E71–E76.
65. Hespel P, Lijnen P, Vanhees L, Fagard R, Amery A. Beta-adrenoceptors and the regulation of blood pressure and plasma renin during exercise. J Appl Physiol 1986;60:108–113.
66. Bouissou P, Richalet J-P, Galen FX, Lartigue M, Larmignat P, Devaux F, et al. Effect of β-adrenoceptor blockage on renin-aldosterone and a-ANF during exercise at altitude. J Appl Physiol 1989;67:141–146.
67. Fagard R, Lijnen P, Amery A. Effects of angiotensin II on arterial pressure, renin and aldosterone during exercise. Eur J Appl Physiol 1985;54:254–261.
68. Morris DJ. The metabolism and mechanism of action of aldosterone. Endocr Rev 1981;2:234–247.
69. Zappe DH, Helyar RG, Green HJ. The interaction between short-term exercise training and diuretic-induced hypovolemic stimulus. Eur J Physiol 1996;72:335–340.

70. Pugh LGCE, Corbett JL, Johnson RH. Rectal temperature, weight loss and sweat rates in marathon running. J Appl Physiol 1967;23:347–352.
71. Rogers G, Goodman C, Rosen C. Water budget during ultra-endurance exercise. Med Sci Sports Exerc 1997;29:1477–1481.
72. Swaka MN, Franceconi RP, Young AJ. Influence of hydration level and body fluids on exercise performance in the heat. J Am Med Assoc 1988;252:1165–1169.
73. Greenleaf JE, Sargent F. II. Voluntary dehydration in man. J Appl Physiol 1965;20:719–724.
74. Greenleaf JE. The consequences of exercise on thirst and fluid intake. In: Ramsay DJ, Booth DA, eds. Thirst. Springer-Verlag, London, 1991, pp. 412–421.
75. Convertino VA, Keil LC, Bernauer EM. Plasma volume, osmolality, vasopressin, and renin activity during graded exercise in man. J Appl Physiol 1981;50:123–128.
76. Convertino VA, Keil LC, Greenleaf JE. Plasma volume, renin and vasopressin responses to graded exercise after training. J Appl Physiol 1983;54:508–514.
77. Harrison MH. Effects of thermal stress and exercise on blood volume in humans. Physiol Rev 1985;65:149–201.
78. Fortney SM, Wenger CB, Bove JR, Nadel ER. Effect of blood volume on sweating rate and body fluids in exercising humans. J Appl Physiol 1981;51:1594–1600.
79. Fortney SM, Wenger CB, Bove JR, Nadel ER. Effect of hyperosmolality on control of blood flow and sweating. J Appl Physiol 1984;57:1688–1695.
80. Mitchell JH. Neural control of the circulation during exercise. Med Sci Sports Exer 1990;22:141–154.
81. Stebbins CL. Reflex cardiovascular response to exercise is modulated by circulating vasopressin. Am J Physiol 1992;263:R1104–R1109.
82. Stebbins CL, Symons JD. Vasopressin contributes to the cardiovascular response to dynamic exercise. *Am. J. Physiol.* 1993;264:H1701–H1707.
83. Sato K. The physiology, phamacology and biochemistry of the eccrine sweat gland. Rev Physiol Biochem Pharm 1977;79:51–131.
84. Daly C, Dill DB. Salt economy in humid heat. Am J Physiol 1937;118:285–289.
85. Kirby CR, Convertino VA. Plasma aldosterone and sweat sodium concentrations after exercise and heat acclimation. J Appl Physiol 1986;61:967–970.
86. Fasciolo JC, Totel GL, Johnson RE. Antiduretic hormone and human eccrine sweating. J Appl Physiol 1969;27:303–307.
87. Gibiniski K, Kozbowski S, Chwalbinksa-Moneta J, Giec L, Zmudzinski J, Markiewicz A. ADH and thermal sweating. Eur J Appl Physiol 1979;42:1–13.
88. Allen JA, Jenkinson DJ, Roddie IC. The effect of beta-adrenoceptor blockade on human sweating. Br J Pharmacol 1972;47:487–497.
89. Mack GW, Shannon LM, Nadel ER. Influence of beta-adrenergic blockage on the control of sweating in humans. J Appl Physiol 1986;61:1701–1705.
90. Robinson RJ, Robinson AH. Chemical composition of sweat. J Appl Physiol 1954;205:79–89.
91. Verde T, Shephard J, Corey P, Moore R. Sweat composition in exercise and in heat. J Appl Physiol 1982;53:1540–1545.
92. Collins KJ. Action of exogenous aldosterone on the secretion and compostion of drug-induced sweat. Clin Sci 1969;30:207–313.
93. Coyle EF, Hamilton M. Fluid replacement during exercise; effects on physiological homeostasis and performance. In: Lamb DR, Gisolfi CV, eds. Perspectives in Exercise Science and Sports Medicine, vol. 3, Fluid Homeostasis During Exercise. Benchmark, Carmel, IN, 1990, pp. 281–303.
94. Nadel ER, Mack GW, Nose H. Influence of fluid replacement beverages on body fluid homeostasis during exercise and recovery. In: Lamb DR, Gisolfi CV, eds. Perspectives in Exercise Science and Sports Medicine, vol. 3, Fluid Homeostasis During Exercise. Benchmark, Carmel, IN, 1990, pp. 181–206.
95. Rolls BJ, Rolls ET. Thirst—Problems in the Behaviorial Sciences, Gray J, ed., Cambridge University Press, Cambridge, 1982.
96. Stricker EM, Verbalis JG. Hormones and behavior: The biology of thirst and sodium appetite. Am Scientist 1988;76:261–267.
97. Szczepanska-Sadowska E. Hormonal inputs to thirst. In: Ramsay DJ, Booth DA, eds. Thirst. Springer-Verlag, London, 1991, pp. 110–130.

98. Nose H, Mack GW, Shi V, Nadel ER. Role of osmolality and plasma volume during rehydration in humans. J Appl Physiol 1988;65:325–331.
99. Nose H, Mack GW, Shi X, Nadel ER. Involvement of sodium retention hormones during rehydration in humans. J Appl Physiol 1988;65:332–336.
100. Fitzsimons JT, Simons BJ. The effect on drinking in the rat of intravenous angiotensin, given alone or in combination with other stimuli of thirst. J Physiol London 1969;203:45–57.
101. Masotto C, Negro-Vilar A. Inhibition of spontaneous or angiotensin II-stimulated water intake by atrial natriuretic factor. Brain Res Bull 1985;15:523–536.
102. Yamada T, Nakao K, Morii N, Itoh H, Shiono S, Sakamoto M, et al. Central effect of atrial natriuretic polypeptide on angiotensin II-stimulated vasopressin secretion in conscious rats. Eur J Pharmacol 1986;125:453–456.
103. Itoh H, Nakao K, Katsuura G, Morii N, Shino S, Yamada T, et al. Atrial natriuretic polypeptides: structure-activity relationship in the centralaction—a comparison of their antidipsogenic actions. Neurosci Lett 1987;74:102–106.
104. Itoh H, Nakao K, Yamada T, Shirakami G, Kangawa K, Minamino N, et al. Antidipsogenic action of a novel peptide, brain natriuretic peptides in rats. Eur J Pharmacol 1989;150:193–196.
105. Robinson TA, Hawley JA, Palmer GS, Wilson GR, Gray DA, Noakes TD, et al. Water ingestion does not improve 1-h cycling performance in moderate ambient temperatures. Eur J Appl Physiol 1995;71:153–160.
106. Walsh RM, Noakes TD, Hawley JA, Dennis SC. Impaired exercise performance time at low levels of dehydration. Int J Sports Med 1992;15:392–398.
107. Follenius M, Candas V, Bothorel B, Brandenberger G. Effect of rehydration on atrial natriuretic peptide release during exercise in the heat. J Appl Physiol 1989;66:2516–2521.
108. Thrasher TN, Nistal-Herrera JF, Keil LC, Ramsay DJ. Satiety and inhibition of vasopressin secretion after drinking in dehydrated dogs. Am J Physiol 1981;240:E394–E401.
109. Geelen G, Keil LC, Kravik SE, Wade CE, Thrasher TN, Barnes PR, et al. Inhibition of plasma vasopressin after drinking in dehydrated humans. J Appl Physiol 1984;247:R968–R971.
110. Castenfors J. Renal function during exercise. Acta Physiol Scand Suppl 1967;70:1–44.
111. Kachadorian WA, Johnson RE. Renal responses to various rates of exercise. J Appl Physiol 1970;28:748–752.
112. Poortmans JR. Exercise and renal function. Sports Med 1984;1:125–153.
113. Poortmans JR, Vanderstraeten J. Kidney function during exercise in healthy and diseased humans. Sports Med 1994;18:419–437.
114. McAllister RM. Adaptation in control of blood flow with training: splanchic and renal blood flows. Med Sci Sports Exerc 1997;30:375–381.
115. Suzuki M, Sudoh M, Matsubara S, Kawakami K, Shiota M, Ikawa S. Changes in renal blood flow measured by radionuclide angiography following exhausting exercise in humans. Eur J Appl Physiol 1996;74:1–7.
116. Baer PG, McGiff JC. Hormonal systems and renal hemodynamics. Annu Rev Physiol 1980;42:589–601.
117. Johnson MD, Barger AC. Circulating catecholamines in control of renal electrolyte and water excretion. Am J Physiol 1981;240:F192–F199.
118. Poortmans JR, Mathieu N, De Plaen P. Influence of running different distances on renal glomerular and tubular impairment in humans. Eur J Appl Physiol 1996;72:522–527.
119. Svarstad E, Iversen BM, Ofstad J. Extended measurement of glomerular filtration rate and effective renal plasma flow in ambulatory patients. Scand J Urol Nephrol 1995;29:375–382.
120. Costill DL, Branam G, Fink W, Nelson R. Exercise induced sodium conservation: Changes in plasma renin and aldosterone. Med Sci Sports 1976;8:209–213.

13 Diabetes and Exercise

*Stephen H. Schneider, MD
and Pushpinder S. Guleria, MD*

CONTENTS

    INTRODUCTION
    EFFECTS OF EXERCISE ON GLYCEMIC CONTROL
    MECHANISM BY WHICH EXERCISE AFFECTS GLYCEMIC CONTROL
    EXERCISE IN NORMAL INDIVIDUALS
    EXERCISE AND TYPE 1 DIABETES
    EXERCISE AND CARDIOVASCULAR DISEASE
    EXERCISE AND HYPERTENSION
    EXERCISE AND DYSLIPIDEMIA
    EXERCISE AND OBESITY
    ROLE OF EXERCISE IN PREVENTION OF TYPE 2 DM
    TYPE OF EXERCISE
    INTENSITY AND DURATION OF EXERCISE NECESSARY
        FOR IMPROVED INSULIN SENSITIVITY
    RISKS OF EXERCISE IN PATIENTS WITH DIABETES
    SUMMARY
    REFERENCES

INTRODUCTION

Ancient Indian physicians first noted the association of diabetes and a sedentary lifestyle, and physicians of the 18th, 19th, and early 20th centuries have recognized the therapeutic usefulness of exercise in the treatment of this disease (1–3). In many quarters, the role of exercise in the treatment of diabetes was so widely accepted that when insulin became available, exercise, along with insulin and diet, was considered one of the three cardinal elements in its management. Because insulin resistance in skeletal muscle (4) characterizes Type 2 diabetes mellitus (DM), there has been considerable interest in the possibility that physical training, by enhancing insulin sensitivity, might improve a key underlying defect of Type 2 DM. Also, evidence that the risk of myocardial infarction is reduced in trained individuals may be of particular importance to diabetic patients. Finally, there is now strong evidence that regular physical exercise protects against the development of Type 2 DM in high-risk populations *(5–7)*. These considerations have led to an increased interest in the effects of exercise and how it can best be used for patients with the metabolic abnormalities of diabetes.

EFFECTS OF EXERCISE ON GLYCEMIC CONTROL

The effects of exercise on carbohydrate metabolism are complex and involve type, intensity, and duration of exercise, changes in body composition, alterations in other behaviors, such as food intake, degree of insulin deficiency, and a complex time-course of the glucose–insulin response. In the study by Schneider et al. *(8)*, an important observation was that glucose tolerance was improved at 12, but not at 72 h after a single moderate exercise bout, unrelated to any effects of the trained state *per se*. The findings of improved levels of HbA1C during exercise training, but unchanged glucose tolerance assessed more than 3 d after the last exercise bout confirm the importance of the subacute effects of exercise in improved glucose control *(9)*. Since then, a number of investigators have shown prolonged effects of a single exercise bout on subsequent glucose disposal *(10–16)*. Burstein et al. *(17)* showed that even after physical training of >6 mo, improved insulin sensitivity reverts to baseline within days after the last exercise bout. These observations suggest that many of the effects of regular exercise are owing to the cumulative effects of individual exercise bouts and are independent of the "trained state" or changes in body composition. Quantitatively similar conclusions in healthy subjects suggest that this phenomenon is universal *(17,18)*. Regular exercise at least every other day will result in lower average blood glucose and glycohemoglobin concentrations with unchanged or decreased levels of plasma insulin. A number of controlled studies have now demonstrated long-term beneficial effects on the metabolic abnormalities of Type 2 diabetes by regular physical activity *(14)*. It is likely that in addition to the effects mentioned above, long-term exercise programs that lead to important changes in body composition are likely to result in additional and more long-lasting improvements in carbohydrate metabolism.

MECHANISM BY WHICH EXERCISE AFFECTS GLYCEMIC CONTROL

The mechanism of increased glucose uptake during and after exercise is not well understood. An increase in blood flow to the muscle during activity may account for much of the acute increase in glucose uptake, but the effects of exercise persist long after the increase in blood flow has returned to normal. Since glucose transport is the major rate-limiting step in glucose utilization, regulation of this system must play an important role in exercise *(19)*. Recently, several studies have demonstrated that exercise can increase the number of insulin receptors *(20)* and the number and intrinsic activity of glucose transporter proteins present in plasma membrane of skeletal muscle *(21–24)*.

It is now widely accepted that obesity and Type 2 DM are associated with insulin resistance. Although in nondiabetic individuals exercise has little effect on glucose tolerance, Bjorntorp et al. *(25)* demonstrated that insulin levels decrease after exercise, but glucose levels remain unchanged, suggesting improved insulin sensitivity. Saltin et al. *(26)* randomized 100 men with "chemical" diabetes into dietary advice alone or diet and 60 min of physical training. Both groups demonstrated similar improvements in oral glucose tolerance, but only the diet plus exercise groups had decreased insulin levels. In more recent studies, Milkins et al. *(27)* have shown that a single bout of exercise increases the sensitivity and responsiveness of insulin-stimulated glucose uptake in untrained persons. In addition, physically trained subjects have increased insulin action when studied 15 h after their last training session compared with untrained subjects. Even when studied 5 d after their last training session, insulin responsiveness remains increased compared with untrained subjects, suggesting that there is a long-term adaptive increase in whole-body response to insulin with training. Several other studies later showed increased insulin sensitivity and responsiveness in physically trained patients (28–32).

When studied by the hyperinsulinemic-euglycemic clamp technique, both normal persons and patients with Type 2 DM show a 30–35% increase in insulin-stimulated glucose disposal after physical training. This increase of insulin sensitivity is mainly owing to increased uptake in skeletal muscle, because no changes were observed in hepatic glucose output. In a study by Bogardus et al. (32) comparing the effect of a very low-caloric diet with the same diet plus a physical training program in noninsulin-dependent diabetes mellitus (NIDDM), the physically trained group had a significant increase in insulin-stimulated glucose disposal rates. The group treated by diet alone had no change after 3 mo of treatment. The increase in insulin-stimulated glucose disposal in the group treated by diet and physical training was entirely owing to an increase in nonoxidative glucose disposal, presumably reflecting increased glycogen synthesis.

The increase in insulin sensitivity and responsiveness associated with physical activity is rapidly lost when exercise is discontinued. Burstein et al. (17) found that much of the effect is lost within 60 h, and others have found that the effect is no longer present after 5–7 d of inactivity.

EXERCISE IN NORMAL INDIVIDUALS

In normal individuals, exercise rarely results in major alterations in blood glucose levels despite the large increase in glucose utilization by skeletal muscle. In the postprandial state, hepatic glucose output is matched closely to peripheral glucose utilization to maintain euglycemia during exercise. A complex hierarchy of hormonal responses regulates the maintenance of plasma glucose during exercise. With the onset of activity, activation of the α-adrenergic system results in inhibition of insulin release from the pancreas. This results in an increased rate of lipolysis in the periphery as well as a stimulation of hepatic glucose output. As glucose levels begin to fall, glucagon levels rise, further stimulating hepatic glucose output. Finally, as plasma glucose drops toward hypoglycemic levels, epinephrine is released, further stimulating hepatic glucose production and enhancing lipolysis in the periphery. The resultant increased availability of free fatty acids for muscle metabolism helps to restrain the rate of glucose utilization. Studies have shown that when one of these mechanisms fail, the others can largely compensate. Thus, multiple defects are necessary for hypoglycemia to develop, except under the most extreme conditions.

EXERCISE AND TYPE 1 DIABETES

The beneficial effect of exercise in Type 1 diabetes is less clear. Although long-term studies are few, it appears that physical training is not consistently associated with improved glucose control. On the other hand, a study of 10 patients over an 8-mo period by Peterson et al. (33) suggests that it is possible to obtain a sustained decrease in HbA1C with exercise in selected patients. Schneider et al. (34) noted a mild initial improvement in glucose control in 25 Type 1 patients trained for more than 3 mo that was lost by the third month of observation, despite continued adherence to the exercise regimen. It is likely that the relatively high incidence of hypoglycemia related to exercise in Type 1 diabetes results in increased carbohydrate intake and decreased insulin dosage and that this largely compensates for the effect of exercise on enhancing glucose disposal.

The relatively high incidence of exercise-related hypoglycemia in Type 1 diabetes is related to a number of factors *(35)*. In individuals taking insulin subcutaneously, the normal suppression of insulin secretion during exercise does not occur, resulting in a relative hyperinsulinemia. In addition, exercise can accelerate the absorption of insulin injected over the exercising muscle. This effect is important only for the short-acting insulins when exercise occurs within 1–2 h after injection. For patients with Type 1 diabetes, a blunted glucagon response to hypoglycemia is common after more than 5 yr of the disease. Finally, patients with long-standing diabetes can develop a blunted epinephrine response to exercise, which may be exacerbated in patients who have been in very tight glucose control. The retained glucagon and epinephrine response in Type 2 diabetes explains the lower incidence of exercise-related hypoglycemia in this group, even when they are insulin-treated. The ability to secrete glucagon in Type 2 compared to Type 1 patients probably also accounts for the increased risk for hypoglycemia in the latter, especially in the presence of nonselective β-blockers. Nevertheless, exercise-related hypoglycemia certainly occurs in patients with Type 2 diabetes treated with insulin or oral agents. Avoiding exercise-related hypoglycemia is often difficult and is one of the major reasons for the disappointing results of exercise as a means of improving glucose control in Type 1 diabetes. Short-acting insulin should be injected away from areas in which underlying muscle will be used in the next 1–2 h (i.e., avoiding the thigh if bicycling). Insulin dose can be reduced in anticipation of planned exercise, but this needs to be worked out on a highly individualized basis. In general, reductions of 30–50% in the appropriate insulin dose can be anticipated with more than 30 min of moderate activity. The use of the newer very short-acting insulins may be particularly useful by avoiding excessive insulin levels during periods of increased activity between meals. More commonly, hypoglycemia is avoided by consuming snacks of rapidly absorbable carbohydrate. Fifteen to 30 g taken during every 30 min of exercise are generally adequate to prevent hypoglycemia. In addition to the acute episodes of hypoglycemia during exercise many patients will experience delayed episodes of hypoglycemia occurring from 6–10 h after a brisk exercise bout. Such episodes can be severe and may occur in the early morning hours following the evening exercise. Such events may be related to an increased concentration of glucose transporters. Postmeal snacks of slowly absorbed carbohydrates and protein at bedtime may be helpful in preventing these episodes.

In addition to hypoglycemia, some patients with Type 1 diabetes will experience episodes of postexercise "paradoxical" hyperglycemia. This occurs in two situations. Individuals who exercise at near-maximal exertion often experience a transient rise in plasma glucose levels. This results from the rapid release of glucose from the liver secondary to glycogenolysis with a minimal increase in peripheral glucose utilization. Treatment of this self-limited hyperglycemia with insulin should be avoided. A more difficult problem is the increase of plasma glucose and occasionally ketones during brisk exercise in patients with severe insulin deficiency. Under these circumstances, hepatic production of glucose and ketones is disproportionate to the increase in peripheral utilization. Such situations are often identified by a fasting plasma glucose >300 mg/dL. Postprandial glucose levels cannot be used as a marker of insulin deficiency. Many of these patients will be mildly dehydrated as well. Such patients should be adequately insulinized prior to participating in an exercise activity.

EXERCISE AND CARDIOVASCULAR DISEASE

A large number of retrospective studies have confirmed that physical activity is associated with a lower incidence of coronary artery disease in different populations *(36–39)*. However, such studies are subject to many confounding factors, such as diet, genetic constitution, and level of stress. Ideally, the effects of exercise on cardiovascular risk should be examined by randomizing sedentary individuals into exercise and control groups and following them longitudinally. Studies of this type in healthy or diabetic individuals are scarce. A recent meta-analysis of 27 studies of habitual physical activity supports a beneficial effect in the primary prevention of coronary artery disease *(40)*. In many, but not all, protection from coronary artery disease was independent of traditional risk factors, such as smoking, hypercholesterolemia, and hypertension.

Blair et al. *(41)* classified subjects not by habitual activity, but by a direct measure of physical fitness on a treadmill test. They found that there is a graded association between physical fitness and mortality owing to cardiovascular disease for both men and women even after adjustment for other risk factors. Kohn et al. *(42)* in their study of 8715 men with impaired glucose tolerance and mild Type 2 diabetes also found that those who were physically fit had a lower age-adjusted mortality rate particularly for cardiovascular disease. However, fitness is a complex measure that involves a strong genetic component and thus may diverge from measures of physical activity. In addition, almost all of the survey tools used to estimate activity have been developed for and validated in nondiabetic populations, and few data are available specifically on patients with diabetes.

In addition to beneficial effects of exercise in primary prevention of coronary artery disease, studies of cardiac rehabilitation programs tend to confirm a beneficial effect of physical activity following a myocardial infarction. Three meta-analyses suggested up to a 25% reduction in mortality over a 1- to 3-yr period *(43–45)*, largely owing to a decrease in the risk for sudden death.

EXERCISE AND HYPERTENSION

Essential hypertension is commonly associated with Type 2 DM. In long-term exercise programs in the general population, physical training is associated with a modest (5–10 mmHg) decrease in systolic and diastolic blood pressures *(46)*. In the study by Schneider et al. *(34)*, a modest but significant decrease in systolic blood pressure of 5 mm was noted in a group with Type 2 diabetes. Improvements are most likely to be noted in insulin-resistant hyperinsulinemic patients *(47,48)*. Both resting pressure and the blood pressure response to exercise at a constant absolute workload are reduced in trained subjects. It is likely that the blood pressure responses to stress and integrated blood pressure levels across the day are improved to a greater degree than resting levels, but this has not been demonstrated for diabetics.

EXERCISE AND DYSLIPIDEMIA

The lipid abnormalities commonly associated with diabetes include elevated levels of triglyceride-rich lipoproteins and in Type 2 (but not Type 1) diabetes, decreased levels of high-density lipoprotein (HDL) cholesterol. The most consistent effect of regular exercise is a decrease in plasma triglyceride levels, which often fall by up to 30%. Changes in low-density lipoprotein (LDL) cholesterol have not been consistently demonstrated, but exercise does appear to diminish the concentration of a small, dense subclass of LDL that may be more strongly associated with atherosclerotic cardiovascular disease *(49)*. Effects are greatest in more insulin-resistant hypertriglyceridemic patients.

Some of the effects of exercise on triglyceride levels are transient and mirror effects of carbohydrate metabolism. Improved triglyceride clearance correlated with an acute increase in lipoprotein lipase activity in some studies. Triglyceride levels measured within 12 h of the last bout of exercise were found to be decreased by ~25%, but triglyceride concentrations returned to baseline after 72 h in the study by Schneider et al. *(34)*. Triglyceride lowering was also observed in the 6-yr Malmo Study *(7)*. Most studies have failed to demonstrate significant increases in HDL cholesterol, even when triglycerides are decreased. The major exception is the 1-yr study of Vanninen et al. *(50)* in which HDL cholesterol levels rose and stayed higher for the entire year of study. In nondiabetic populations, increased HDL cholesterol is found only with intense exercise performed over a prolonged period of time. The poor exercise capacity of many patients with Type 2 diabetes and the resulting modest levels of physical activity achieved may explain, in part, the apparent lack of an effect. No effect of exercise on lipoprotein (a) concentrations has been demonstrated.

EXERCISE AND OBESITY

Exercise can be an effective adjunct to diet in achieving weight loss. Wing *(51)* has shown that a combination of diet and exercise improves weight loss in persons with Type 2 DM and allows for greater reduction in the dose of hypoglycemic medications. Exercise may also offset the effect of caloric restriction on energy expenditure. Exercise has consistently been one of the strongest predictors of maintenance of weight loss *(52)*. When weight reduction is a major goal, exercise for 5–6 d/wk is probably necessary. The goal is to burn 250–300 cal/exercise session, but this may be difficult to achieve in many patients with Type 2 diabetes because of their poor levels of fitness. Rhythmic aerobic exercises are recommended for weight loss. On the other hand, a number of studies have shown that lean body mass is a major predictor of basal metabolic rate. It has been proposed, but not yet proven, that resistance training could have an important place in weight maintenance by increasing lean body mass independent of a change in body mass index (BMI).

Exercise alone is not an effective weight loss tool. A compensatory increase in appetite and a subsequent decrease in spontaneous activity often balance the increased caloric expenditure. Nevertheless, the beneficial effects of exercise in a weight-reducing regimen are often underestimated. Increased lean body mass often obscures the effective loss of body fat. In addition, there are studies that suggest a disproportionate loss of intra-abdominal fat when exercise is part of a weight reduction program. Finally, exercise improves many of the cardiovascular risk factors associated with obesity through an effect independent of body composition.

ROLE OF EXERCISE IN PREVENTION OF TYPE 2 DM

Although obesity is generally regarded as the major risk factor for development of Type 2 diabetes, decreased physical activity independent of obesity has also been identified as an important predictor of the disease. Taylor (53) found that in Melanesian and Indian men in the Fiji Islands, the occurrence of Type 2 DM was twice as high in sedentary as in physically active men, an effect that could not be ascribed to differences in body weight (54).

Insulin resistance, visceral adiposity, and hyperinsulinemia all play a key role in the development of Type 2 DM. Regular exercise by its beneficial effects on these parameters could help reduce the risk of Type 2 diabetes in this unusually sedentary population (55). In addition to a sedentary lifestyle, it is possible that there is an abnormality in many Type 2 patients, which results in a decreased aerobic exercise capacity. Most studies have shown VO_2max of 15–20% less than control groups with a similar lifestyle. Interestingly, decreased exercise capacity of a similar degree has been demonstrated in high-risk individuals prior to the development of overt diabetes. Also, patients with diabetes may have a higher percentage of fast-twitch to slow-twitch fibers and a reduced capillary and mitochondrial density compared to controls. Thus, a reduced aerobic exercise capacity may be an early defect in individuals destined to develop Type 2 diabetes, which may contribute to a limited lifestyle. In contrast, in Type 1 diabetes, no decrease in maximal oxygen uptake can be demonstrated. Exercise capacity is only decreased in these patients when insulin deficiency results in significant glycogen depletion.

Several studies have shown that exercise, by reversing insulin resistance, might delay the progression to overt Type 2 diabetes (56). Helmrich et al. (5), in a study of University of Pennsylvania alumni, reported that 500 cal of additional leisure-time activity were associated with a 6% decrease in the age-adjusted risk for developing Type 2 diabetes during the subsequent 15 yr. This study was limited to men, but the results were confirmed in a study by Manson et al. (6) of 87, 253 female nurses followed for 8 yr. Subjects who engaged in vigorous physical activity (enough to work up a sweat) at least once a week had a significantly lower risk of developing Type 2 DM than those who exercised less often and less vigorously.

In another prospective study of 21, 271 US male physicians followed up for up to 5 yr who exercised vigorously at least once a week, a similar effect was demonstrated (57). In this study, however, a significant effect of frequency of exercise was also found. As in Nurses' study (6), correlation for other known risk factors for Type 2 DM did not affect the conclusion that regular, vigorous exercise at least once a week has an independent protective effect against development of Type 2 DM.

Kawate et al. (58) compared Japanese living in Hiroshima with those who had migrated to Hawaii. Despite a similar genetic background, the prevalence of diabetes was nearly double in the Japanese living in Hawaii than in those living in Hiroshima. This was correlated with a decreased frequency of physical activity in the Japanese Hawaiians. Increased physical activity, independent of other risk factors, such as obesity, hypertension, and a family history of Type 2 DM, has a protective effect (57,59).

Most recently, two large prospective studies confirm a protective effect of exercise. In the Da Quing study in China, a program of modest physical activity reduced the incidence of diabetes over a 6-yr period by almost 50% in a large group of high-risk patients (60). Eriksson and Lindgarde (7) studied the effect of home exercise in people with impaired glucose tolerance and noted that over a 5-yr period, 10.6% of exercising persons developed diabetes compared with 28.6% in sedentary control group. These studies strongly support the notion that persons at a high risk for development of Type 2 DM should maintain a high level of physical activity.

TYPE OF EXERCISE

The American Diabetes Association (ADA) clinical practice recommendations for exercise provide a good starting point for developing a personalized exercise program *(61)*. To perform activity adequate to enhance insulin sensitivity, exercises using large muscle groups that can be maintained for prolonged periods and that are aerobic in nature are preferred. Typical examples include walking, jogging, swimming, cycling, crosscountry skiing, rowing, dancing, skating, stair climbing, and various endurance game activities. For a given level of energy expenditure, the health-related benefits appear to be independent of the mode of aerobic activity.

A number of small studies have shown that resistance exercise improves glucose tolerance and insulin sensitivity in the absence of changes in VO_2max *(62–64)*. The magnitude of effect is similar to that seen in programs using aerobic exercise and does not depend on a reduction of fat mass *(63)*. Fluckey et al. *(65)* studied the effect of a single high-volume resistance session on 17 subjects, 7 with Type 2 diabetes. Resistance exercise resulted in unchanged glucose tolerance in the face of a decrease in plasma insulin levels. Durak et al. *(66)* have studied the effects of 10 wk of resistance training three times a week on eight men with Type 1 diabetes. They found a decrease in HbA1C from 6.9 to 5.8% associated with a fall in self-monitored glucose levels and plasma triglycerides in the absence of changes in VO_2max. Improvements in hypertension and lipid levels have been demonstrated as well.

INTENSITY AND DURATION OF EXERCISE NECESSARY FOR IMPROVED INSULIN SENSITIVITY

The intensity and duration of exercise necessary to improve insulin sensitivity are not entirely clear. Virtually all of the larger studies on the effects of training on glucose disposal have used intensities of 50% or more of VO_2max, and prospective studies of lower-intensity exercise over longer periods are lacking.

Studies by King et al. *(67)* have raised the possibility that programs using relatively modest levels of physical activity may result in improvements in healthy subjects similar to those of more intense regimens. It should be noted, however, that the "modest" intensity groups exercised at ~50% VO_2max, which is within the current guidelines.

Older studies suggest that a level of activity approaching 50% VO_2max for 20–30 min may be required to improve subsequent intravenous glucose tolerance *(68)*. This is consistent with observations suggesting that some glycogen depletion is necessary to trigger a subsequent enhancement of glucose disposal, although the mechanism by which this signal is transduced remains unknown.

Of equal importance to exercise intensity and duration is the issue of exercise frequency. Many of the metabolic benefits of exercise are related to the summed effects of individual exercise bouts. This suggests that regular exercise on at least an every other day schedule is necessary for sustained improvements in carbohydrate metabolism.

RISKS OF EXERCISE IN PATIENTS WITH DIABETES

Although there are some potential risks for a patient with diabetes entering an exercise program, in general it is possible to devise a safe and effective exercise regimen for most patients. Before starting an exercise program, all patients with Type 2 DM should have a complete history and physical examination, with particular attention to identifying any long-term complications of diabetes that may affect exercise safety or tolerance (69). The most feared risk of exercise is that of sudden death. Fortunately, this is an extremely rare event. An exercise stress test is recommended for all patients >35 yr of age who intend to start a program of moderate or vigorous exercise. This test will help identify previously undiagnosed ischemic heart disease and abnormal blood pressure response to exercise. A dilated fundoscopic examination to identify proliferative retinopathy, a neurologic examination to determine sensory and autonomic neuropathy, and urine testing for microalbuminuria should also be performed.

Musculo-skeletal injuries are quite common during exercise, especially at higher exercise intensities. Beginning the exercise session with a warmup of low-intensity aerobic exercise and stretching for 5–10 min can reduce such injuries. Musculo-skeletal injuries are more common in patients with sensory neuropathy.

Patients with microvascular disease may also be at increased risk. Although retinal hemorrhage is rare in the presence of background retinopathy, it may occur when proliferative disease is present. Shear forces from rapid head movements, direct trauma to the eye, and activities that involve valsalva-type maneuvers often precede such events. Monitored exercise at an intensity that keeps the systolic pressure <200 mmHg is rarely associated with retinal hemorrhage, so that a safe level of activity can be identified for most patients. Similarly, up to a third of patients will develop postexercise proteinuria, which may persist for up to 24 h. It remains unclear whether this response, which is proportional to the increment in systolic blood pressure, predicts the development of subsequent nephropathy. Long-term studies have not identified exercise as a risk factor for the development of diabetic renal disease.

For patients treated with insulin or oral hypoglycemic agents, exercise may cause hypoglycemia during exercise or in the postexercise period unless precautions are taken. These include more frequent blood glucose monitoring, use of carbohydrate snack before, during, and after exercise, and avoiding exercise at time of peak insulin action.

SUMMARY

Regular exercise has become an integral part of the prescription for Type 2 diabetic patients, since it improves insulin sensitivity and results in lower average blood glucose concentrations. Physical training results in an increase in insulin-stimulated glucose disposal and improved glucose control in Type 2 diabetes. However, the increase in insulin sensitivity is rapidly lost if exercise is not performed on a regular basis. Exercise may also be most effective way to delay or prevent the development of Type 2 diabetes. This may be partly owing to the high incidence of exercise-related hypoglycemia in insulin-dependent diabetics. Fitness is associated with a lower incidence of coronary artery disease in diabetic patients. Although exercise has a modest beneficial effect on hypertension and dyslipidemia, protection from coronary artery disease is greater than can be explained by improvement in these factors alone. Exercise, however, is not without risks for patients with diabetes. Patients need to be instructed regarding adjustment in their dietary intake and antidiabetic therapy prior to start of an exercise regimen. Also, before an exercise program is started, a detailed history and physical examination should be carried out to determine the presence and extent of chronic complications of diabetes, especially proliferative retinopathy and sensory neuropathy. An exercise stress may be indicated in selected patients to rule out significant coronary artery disease.

REFERENCES

1. Rollo J. (1798) Cases of Diabetes Mellitus: with the Results of the Trials of Certain Acids and Other Substances in the Cure of the Lues Venerea, 2nd ed. Dilly, London, 1798.
2. Allen FM, Stillan E, Fitz R. Total dietary regulation in the treatment of diabetes. In: Exercise. Monograph. Rockefeller Institute, New York;11:1919, chapter 5.
3. Lawrence RH. The effects of exercise on insulin action in diabetes. Br Med J 1926;1:648.
4. DeFronzo RA. Lilly lecture 1987. The triumvirate: B-cell, muscle, liver—a collusion responsible for NIDDM. Diabetes 1988;37:667.
5. Helmrich SP, Ragland DR, Leang RW, Paffenbarger RS. Physical activity and reduced occurrence of noninsulin dependent diabetes mellitus. N Engl J Med 1991;325:147–152.
6. Manson JE, Rimm EB, Stanofer MJ, Colditz GA, Willet WC, Krolewski AS, et al. Physical activity and the incidence of non-insulin dependent diabetes mellitus in women. Lancet 1991;338:774–778.
7. Eriksson KF, Lindgarde F. Prevention of type II (noninsulin dependent) diabetes mellitus by diet and physical exercise: the six year Malmo feasibility study. Diabetologia 1991;34:891–898.
8. Schneider SH, Amorosa LF, Khachadurian AK, Ruderman NB. Studies on the mechanism of improved glucose control during exercise in type 2 (non-insulin dependent) diabetes. Diabetologist 1984;26:355–360.
9. Ruderman NE, Ganda OP, Johansen K. The effect of physical training on glucose tolerance and plasma lipids in maturity onset diabetes. Diabetes 1979;28:89–91.
10. Bjorntorp P, de Jonge K, Sjostrom L, Sullivan L. The effect of physical training on insulin production in obesity. Metabolism 1970;19:631.
11. Israel RG, Davidson PC, Albrink MJ, Krall JM. Exercise effects on fitness, lipids, glucose tolerance and insulin levels in young adults. Arch Phys Med Rehab 1981;62:336–341.
12. Fahlen M, Stenberg J, Bjorntorp P. Insulin secretion in obesity after exercise. Diabetologia 1971;8: 141–144.
13. Bjorntorp P. Effect of exercise and physical training on carbohydrate and lipid metabolism in man. Adv Cardiol 1976;18:158–166.
14. Schneider, SH. Long-term exercise programs. In: The Health Professional's Guide to Diabetes and Exercise. Ruderman N, and Devlin JT, eds. American Diabetes Association, Alexandria VA, 1995, pp. 123–132.
15. Devlin JT, Hirshman M, Horton ED, Horton ES. Enhanced peripheral and splanchnic insulin sensitivity in NIDDM men after a single bout of exercise. Diabetes 1987;36:434–439.
16. Rogers MA, Yamamoto C, King DS, Hagberg JM, Ehasani AA, Holloszy JO. Improvement in glucose tolerance after 1 week of exercise in patients with mild NIDDM. Diabetes Care 1988;11:613–618.
17. Burstein R, Polychronakos C, Toews CJ, MacDougall JD, Guyda HJ, Posner BI. Acute reversal of enhanced insulin action in trained athletes. Diabetes 1985;34:750–760.
18. Heath GW, Gavin JR, Hinderliter JM, Hagberg JM, Bloomfield SA, Holloszy JO. Effects of exercise and lack of exercise on glucose tolerance and insulin sensitivity. J Appl Physiol 1983;55:512–517.
19. Goodyear LJ, Smith RJ. Exercise and diabetes. In: Joslin's Diabetes, 13th ed. Kahn CR, Weir GC, eds. Lea and Febiger, Boston, 1994, pp. 451–459.
20. Dohm GL, Sinha MK, Caro JF. Insulin receptor binding and protein kinase activity in muscles of trained rats. Am J Physiol 1987;252:E170–E175.
21. Douen AG, Ramlal T, Klip A, et al. Exercise induced increase in glucose transporters in plasma membranes of rat skeletal muscle. Endocrinology 1989;124:449–454.
22. King PA, Hirshman MF, Horton ED, Horton ES. (1989) Glucose transport in skeletal muscle membrane vesicles from control and exercised rats. Am J Physiol 1989;257:C1128–C1134.

23. Klip A, Marette A, Dimitrakoudis P, Ramlal T, Giacda A, Shi ZQ, Vranic M. Effect of diabetes on glucoregulation. Diabetes Care 1992;15. (Suppl. 4):1742–1766.
24. Rodnick Ki, Holloszy JO, Mondon CE, James DE. Effects of exercise training on insulin-regulatable glucose transporter protein levels in rat skeletal muscle. Diabetes 1990;39:1425–1429.
25. Bjorntorp P, DeJounge K, Sjostrom L, Sullivan L. Physical training in human obesity. II. Effects of plasma insulin in glucose intolerant subjects without marked hyperinsulinemia. Scand J Clin Invest 1973;32:41–45.
26. Saltin B, Lindgarde F, Houston M, Horlin R, Nygaard E, Gad P. Physical training and glucose tolerance in middle-aged men with chemical diabetes. Diabetes 1978;28:30–32.
27. Milkins KJ, Sonne B, Tronier B, Galbo H. Effects of acute exercise and detraining on insulin action in trained men. J Appl Physiol 1989;66:704.
28. DeFronzo RA, Ferrannini E, Koivisto V. New concepts in the pathogenesis and treatment of non-insulin dependent diabetes mellitus. Am J Med 1983;74:52.
29. Sato Y, Iguchi A, Sakamoto N. Biochemical determination of training effects using insulin clamp technique. Horm Metab Res. 1984;16:483.
30. Yki-Jarvinen H, Kovisto VA. Effects of body composition on insulin sensitivity. Diabetes 1983;32:965.
31. Rosenthal M, Haskell WL, Solomon R, et al. Demonstration of a relationship between level of physical training and insulin stimulated glucose utilization in normal humans. Diabetes 1983;32:408.
32. Bogardus C, Ravussin E, Robbins DC, et al. Effects of physical training and diet therapy on carbohydrate metabolism in patients with glucose intolerance and non-insulin dependent diabetes mellitus. Diabetes 1984;33:311.
33. Peterson CM, Jones RL, Dupuis A, et al. Feasibility of improved blood glucose control in patients with insulin dependent diabetes mellitus. Diabetes Care 1979;2:329–335
34. Schneider SH, Khachadurian AK, Amorosa LF, Clemow L, Ruderman NB. Ten-year experience with an exercise-based outpatient life-style modification program in the treatment of diabetes mellitus. Diabetes Care 1992;15:1800–1810.
35. Wasserman DH, Zinman B. Fuel homeostasis. In: The Health Professional's Guide to Diabetes and Exercise. Ruderman N, Devlin JT, eds. American Diabetes Association, Alexandria, VA, 1995, pp. 29–47.
36. Kahn HA. The relationship of reported coronary heart disease mortality to physical activity of work. Am J Public Health 1963;53:1058–1067.
37. Taylor HL, Klepetar E, Keyes A, Parlin W, Blackburn H, Puchner T. Death rates among physically active and sedentary employees of the railroad industry. Am J Public Health 1962;52:1697–1707.
38. Brunner D, Manelis G, Modan M, Levin S. Physical activity at work and the incidence of myocardial infarction, angina pectoris, and death due to ischemic heart disease: an epidemiologic study in Israeli collective settlements (Kubbutzim). J Chronic Dis. 1974;27:217–233.
39. Frank CW, Weinblatt E, Shapiro S, Savier RV. Physical inactivity as a lethal factor in myocardial infarction among men. Circulation 1966;34:1022–1032.
40. Berlin JA, Colditz GA. A meta analysis of physical activity in the prevention of coronary heart disease. Am J Epidemiol 1990;132:612–628.
41. Blair SN, Kohl HW, Paffenbarger RS, Clark DG, Cooper KH, Gibbons LW. Physical fitness and all cause mortality: a prospective study of healthy men and women. J Am Med Assoc 1989;262:2395–2401.
42. Kohn HW, Gordon NF, Villegas JA, Blair SN. Cardiorespiratory fitness, glycemic status, and mortality risk in men. Diabetes Care 1992;15:184–192.
43. May GS, Eberlein KA, Furberg CD, Passarnani ER, DeMets DL. Secondary prevention after myocardial infarction: a review of long-term trials. Prog Cardiovasc Dis. 1982;24:331–362.
44. O'Connor GT, Buring JE, Yusaf S, Guldhaber SZ, Olmstead EM, Barger RS, et al. (1989) An overview of randomized trials of rehabilitation with exercise after myocardial infarction. Circulation 1989;80:234–244.
45. Oldridge NB, Guyait GH, Fischer ME, Rimm AA. Cardiac rehabilitation with exercise after myocardial infarction. JAMA 1988;260:945–950.
46. Tipton CM. Exercise training and hypertension: an update. In: Exercise and Sport Sciences Reviews vol. 19. Holloszy, John O., ed. Williams & Wilkins, 1991, Philadelphia, PA, pp. 462,463.
47. Krotkiewski M, Mandrousask K, Sjostrom L, SuDivan L, Wetterquist H, Bjorntor P. Effects of long term physical training on body fat, metabolism and BP in obesity. Metabolism 197;28:650–658.

48. Rocchini AP, Katch V, Schork A, Kelch RP. Insulin and blood pressure during weight loss in obese adolescents. Hypertension 1987;10:267–273.
49. Houmard JA, Bruno NJ, Bruner RK, McCammon MR, Israel RG, Barakal HA. Effects of exercise training on chemical composition of plasma LDL. Atheroscler Thromb 1994;14:325–330.
50. Vanninen E, Uusitupa M, Siitonen O, Laitinen J, Lansimies E. Habitual physical activity, aerobic capacity and metabolic control in patients with newly diagnosed type II diabetes mellitus: effect of a one year diet and exercise intervention. Diabetologia 1991;35:340–346.
51. Wing RR. Behaviour change, weight loss, and physiological improvements in type II diabetic patients. J Consult Clin Psychol 1985;53:111–122.
52. Wing RR. Behavioral Strategies for weight reduction in obese type II diabetic patients. Diabetes Care 1989;12:139–144.
53. Taylor R. Physical activity and prevalence of diabetes in Melanesian and Indian men in Fiji. Diabetologia 1984;27:578–582.
54. Franz MJ. Exercise and diabetes. In: Components of Diabetes Care/The Therapeutic Regimen. Haire-Joshu D, ed. Mosby Year Book, St. Louis: pp. 80–118.
55. Dowse GK, Zimmet PZ, Gareeboo H, et al. Abdominal obesity and physical activity are risk factors for NIDDM and impaired glucose tolerance in Indian, Creole, and Chinese Mauricians. Diabetes Care 1991;14:271.
56. Kriska AM, Blair SN, Pereira MA. The potential role of physical activity in the prevention of non-insulin dependent diabetes mellitus: The epidemiological evidence. Exerc Sports Sci Rev 1991;22:121.
57. Manson JE, Nathan DM, Krolewski AS, Stampfer MJ, Willett WC, Hennekens CH. A prospective study of exercise and incidence of diabetes among U.S. male physicians. JAMA 1992;268:63–67.
58. Kawate R, Yamakido M, Nishimoto Y, et al. Diabetes mellitus and its vascular complications in Japanese migrants on the island of Hawaii. Diabetes Care 1979;2:161.
59. Frisch RE, Wyshak G, Albright TE, et al. Lower prevalence of diabetes in female former college athletes compared with non-athletes. Diabetes 1986;35:1101.
60. Pan X, Li G, Hu YH, et al. Effects of diet and exercise in preventing NIDDM in people with impaired glucose tolerance. The Da Qing IGT and Diabetes Study. Diabetes Care 1997;20:537–544
61. American Diabetes Association Clinical Practice Recommendations 1999;22(Suppl. 1):s49–s53.
62. Szczypaczewska M, Nazar K, Kaciwba-Uscilko H. Glucose tolerance and insulin response to glucose load in body builders. Int J Sports Med 1989;10:34–37.
63. Miller WJ, Sherman WM, Ivy JL. Effect of strength training on glucose tolerance and after glucose insulin response. Med Sci Sports Exerc 1984;16:539–543.
64. Smutok MA, Reece C, Goldberg AP, Kokkinos PF, Dawson P, Shulman R, et al. (1989) Strength training improves glucose tolerance similar to jogging in middle-aged men (Letter). Med Sci Sports. Exerc 1989;21 (Suppl. 2):S33.
65. Fluckey JD, Hickey MS, Brambrink JK, Hart KK, Alexander K, Craig BW. Effect of resistance exercise on glucose tolerance in normal and glucose intolerant subjects. J Appl Physiol 1994;77:1087–1092.
66. Durak EP, Jovanovic-Peterson L, Peterson CM. Randomized crossover study of effect of resistance training on glycemic control, muscular strength and cholesterol in type I diabetic men. Diabetes Care 1990;13:1039–1043.
67. King AC, Haskell WL, Taylor CB, Kraemer HC, DeBusk RF. Home-based exercise training in healthy older men and women. JAMA 1991;266:1535–1542.
68. Maehlum S, Pruett EDR. Muscular exercise and metabolism in male juvenile diabetics. Scand J Clin Lab Invest 1973;32:149–153.
69. Horton ES. Exercise in patients with non-insulin-dependent diabetes mellitus. In: Diabetes Mellitus. LeRoith D, Taylor SI, Olefsky JM, eds. Lippincott-Raven Publishers, Philadelphia, 1996, pp. 638–643.

14 Hormonal Regulations of the Effects of Exercise on Bone

Positive and Negative Effects

Philip D. Chilibeck, PhD

CONTENTS

INTRODUCTION
NEGATIVE EFFECTS OF EXERCISE ON HORMONAL REGULATION OF BONE
POSITIVE EFFECTS OF EXERCISE ON HORMONAL REGULATION OF BONE
DIRECTIONS FOR FUTURE RESEARCH
SUMMARY
REFERENCES

INTRODUCTION

Exercise is generally thought to have a positive effect on bone; numerous studies indicate that bone mass is increased with training. Increasing physical activity levels throughout the life-span has been recommended for preventing the development of osteoporosis [1]. It has become evident, however, that too much exercise in combination with deficient energy intake may be detrimental to bone in some individuals. This may be owing to hormonal changes that occur when the body attempts to conserve energy or when an individual is under excess stress.

The Negative Effects of Exercise on Hormonal Regulation of Bone section of this chapter covers the negative effects of high levels of exercise on hormones that regulate bone metabolism. In females, adequate estrogen levels are necessary for maintenance of skeletal integrity. The secretion of estrogen is reduced with extremes of exercise training. A number of studies indicate that this may be prevented if dietary intake is sufficient to compensate for energy expenditure. Testosterone may be similarly affected in males, again with detrimental effects on the skeleton. Extreme exercise training may also have effects on the calciotropic hormones, but results of studies are mixed, with some indicating negative effects and some indicating positive effects on bone.

The Positive Effects of Exercise on Hormonal Regulation of Bone section of this chapter covers the positive effects that exercise may have on the hormones that affect

From: *Contemporary Endocrinology: Sports Endocrinology*
Edited by: M. P. Warren and N. W. Constantini © Humana Press Inc., Totowa, NJ

bone mass. Exercise and estrogen may have synergistic effects on bone (i.e., their combined influences may be greater than the addition of their influences alone). Exercise may also stimulate the release of anabolic hormones (testosterone, growth hormone, insulin-like growth factor), and these may have positive effects on bone. Finally, exercise may have a positive effect on the calciotropic hormones to increase calcium balance and prevent bone resorption.

NEGATIVE EFFECTS OF EXERCISE ON HORMONAL REGULATION OF BONE

Negative Effects of Exercise on Reproductive Hormone Status

ESTROGEN AND PROGESTERONE

Adequate estrogen and progesterone production is necessary for maintenance of bone mineral status in women. Estrogen has several effects that lead to positive influences on bone: It increases the efficiency of intestinal absorption of calcium *(2)*, and it affects bone-resorbing and bone-forming cells (osteoclasts and osteoblasts) to suppress bone turnover *(3)*. The effects of progesterone on bone are not as well understood, but it may increase bone formation by influencing osteoblastic activity, or it may play a role in the coupling of bone resorption with formation *(4)*. Although exercise is generally thought to be of benefit to bone, excessive exercise may have negative effects on reproductive hormone status in some females.

Athletic Amenorrhea. Intense training in some female athletes may lead to development of amenorrhea with decreases in progesterone and estrogen production, and a corresponding decrease in bone mineral content *(5)*. Athletic amenorrhea is most common in sports that require lower body mass or activities that involve subjective judgment, including long-distance running *(5)*, gymnastics *(6)*, rowing *(7)*, figure skating *(8)*, and ballet *(9)*. For some of these athletes, local positive effects of weight-bearing exercise or muscle pull on bone may override the negative effect of decreased estrogen and progesterone. Amenorrheic or oligomenorrheic gymnasts have elevated bone mass at most sites compared to amenorrheic runners and eumenorrheic controls *(6,10)*, and amenorrheic rowers have higher lumbar spine bone mass compared to amenorrheic runners and dancers *(7)*. Amenorrheic dancers may *(11)* or may not *(9)* have an elevated bone mass at weight-bearing sites. Amenorrheic dancers have an increase in stress fractures *(12)*, implying that weight-bearing exercise may not have a protective effect. Most studies of amenorrheic runners indicate a decrease in bone density, even at weight-bearing sites *(13)*, and this is associated with an increased rate of stress fracture *(14,15)*.

Etiology of Athletic Amenorrhea. The development of amenorrhea with exercise training has been attributed to many factors, but the leading candidates are: 1) a decreased energy availability owing to greater energy expenditure of exercise than dietary energy intake, or 2) abnormal levels of stress hormones (i.e., cortisol) owing to chronic stress of exercise. Both factors may negatively effect gonadotropin-releasing hormone pulse generation at the hypothalamus, which in turn results in decreased release of follicle-stimulating and leutenizing hormone from the anterior pituitary. The evidence for both hypotheses has recently been outlined by Loucks et al. *(16)* (Figs. 1 and 2). The "low energy availability" hypothesis is supported by findings that amenorrheic and eumenorrheic athletes in general have lower dietary energy intakes than expected for their activity levels *(17,18)* and that amenorrheic athletes have endocrine

Chapter 14 / Effects of Exercise on Bone

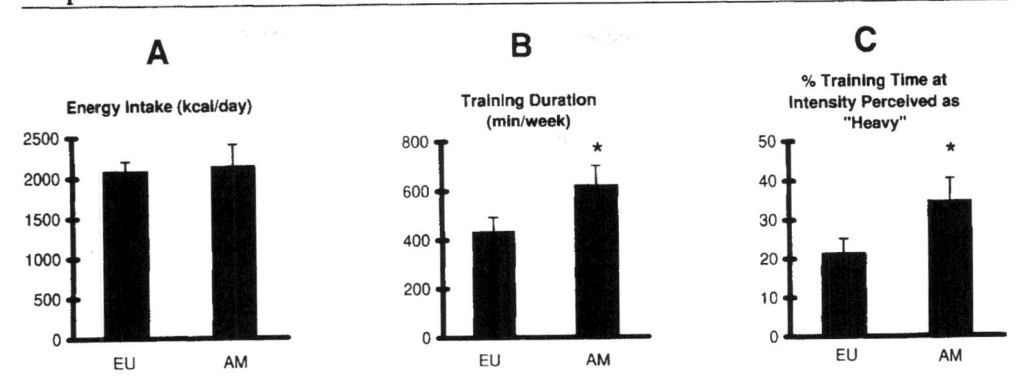

Fig. 1. EU = eumenorrheic athletes; AM = amenorrheic athletes. This is one form of experimental evidence for the "low energy availability" hypothesis proposed by Loucks et al. *(16)* in the development of amenorrhea with exercise training. For an equivalent level of energy intake, amenorrheic athletes were found to have a greater training volume and intensity when compared to eumenorrheic athletes (data taken from ref. *17*). This implies that amenorrheic athletes have a lower energy availability (where energy availability = energy intake – energy expenditure). *Amenorrheic means are significantly different from eumenorrheic means ($p < 0.05$).

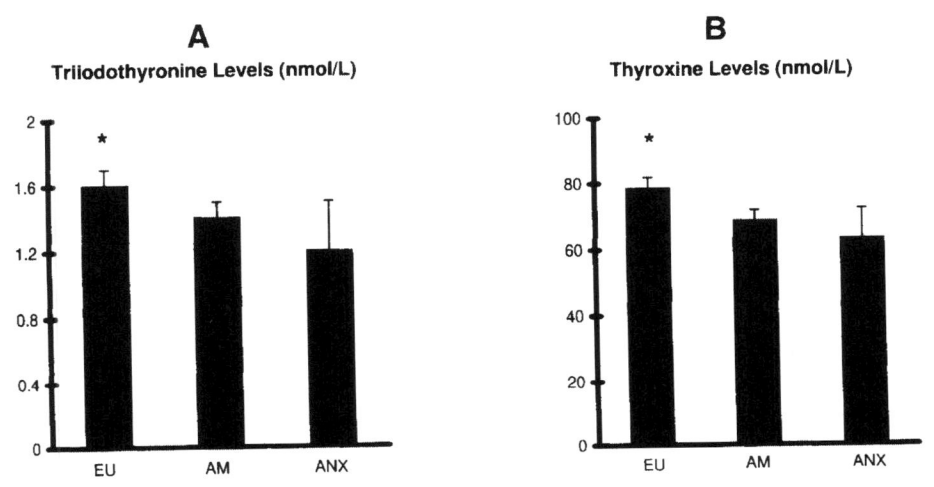

Fig. 2. EU = eumenorrheic athletes; AM = amenorrheic athletes; ANX = anorexics. This is a second form of experimental evidence for the "low energy availability" hypothesis proposed by Loucks et al. *(16)* in the development of amenorrhea with training. Amenorrheic athletes have endocrine profiles (altered thyroid status) similar to a group of subjects (anorexics) characterized by chronic energy deficiencies (data taken from refs. *17* and *20*). *Eumenorrheic means are significantly different from amenorrheic and anorexic means ($p < 0.05$).

profiles (i.e., altered thyroid status *[17,19]*) similar to groups characterized by chronic energy deficiencies *(20)*. The "stress hormone" hypothesis is supported by findings that amenorrheic athletes have alterations in the hypothalamic–pituitary–adrenal axis *(21,22)* and that alterations in either corticotropin-releasing hormone or cortisol levels in animals negatively affect gonadotropin secretion *(23,24)*. In support of the "low energy availability" hypothesis, it has recently been demonstrated that short-term induction of menstrual cycle changes with exercise can be prevented by adequate dietary compensation *(16)*. It is therefore suggested that athletes may be able to reverse menstrual disorders by increasing their dietary energy intake, without decreasing their exercise levels *(16)*.

Treatment and Reversal of Athletic Amenorrhea. Amenorrheic athletes have been able to reverse menstrual disorders and increase bone mass successfully by reducing training volume and increasing consumption of calcium *(25,26)* or by taking hormone-replacement therapy *(27)*. With resumption of menses in these athletes, bone mineral density increased by an average of 6–14% over 15.5–30 mo at the lumbar spine *(25–28)* and 4% over 24–30 mo for the femoral neck *(27)*. The frequency of stress fractures in one report was also reduced following reversal of menstrual disorders *(26)*. The greatest increase in bone mineral density was in those athletes that gained weight *(25,26,28)*, implying that they had achieved a more positive energy balance. Despite these increases, however, bone density still remained below control levels in many of the formerly amenorrheic athletes *(25,28)*. Recently, a follow-up of 8 yr duration determined that despite return of normal menses or use of oral contraceptives, the bone mass of former oligomenorrheic or amenorrheic athletes remained below normal *(29)*. This suggests that early treatment and reversal of menstrual disorders may be necessary to prevent an irreversible bone loss *(29)*.

Testosterone

Just as excessive exercise may affect reproductive hormone status in females, excessive exercise may negatively affect testosterone levels in males *(30,31)*. Adequate testosterone levels in males may be necessary for intestinal calcium absorption *(32)*, and for stimulation of osteoblasts and bone formation *(33)*.

Similar to the etiology for disruption of the hypothamic–pituitary–gonadal axis in females, disruption in this axis with excessive exercise in males may be owing to decreased energy availability *(31)* or production of stress hormones *(34,35)*. When caloric balance is shifted to allow for increased body weight, testosterone levels are returned to normal *(31)*.

In contrast to studies of females, with males there is less evidence for a link between reductions of reproductive hormones and a corresponding reduction in bone mass. Testosterone levels are altered with excessive training in a number of studies *(30,31)*, and excessive training is associated with reduced bone mass in others *(36,37)*; however, in studies in which bone mass was reduced, testosterone levels were found to be normal *(36,37)*. We are aware of only one case study where excessive training was associated with hypogonadism, decreased bone mass, and skeletal fragility in a single male subject *(38)*. Treatment of this subject with clomiphene citrate (an analog of the nonsteroid estrogen, chlororrianisene) simulated gonadotropin secretion, and testosterone levels returned to normal *(38)*. Further research is needed to determine if other male athletes with low testosterone levels may be at a risk of losing bone mass and developing skeletal fracture.

Negative Effect of Exercise on Calciotropic Hormones

The calciotropic hormones (parathyroid hormone, calcitonin, and to an extent, 1,25-dihydroxyvitamin D_3 [vitamin D]) are involved in the maintenance of optimal blood calcium levels, which is vital for the regulation of neuromuscular excitability. Low blood calcium levels stimulate the secretion of parathyroid hormone from the parathyroid gland. Parathyroid hormone stimulates osteoblasts to release a factor that stimulates osteoclastic bone resorption, causing movement of calcium from bone to blood *(39)*. Calcitonin, a much less powerful hormone, has an opposing effect. Calcitonin is released from cells of the thyroid gland (which are distinct from the cells that release thyroxine and triiodothyronine) in response to high blood calcium levels and inhibits the release of calcium from bone. The major hormone-like action of vitamin D is a stimulation of active intestinal calcium absorption. Excessive exercise may alter the regulation of the calciotropic hormones, with a negative effect on bone mineral homeostasis. The effects of excessive exercise on parathyroid hormone, calcitonin, and vitamin D metabolism are covered in the following sections.

NEGATIVE EFFECTS OF EXERCISE ON PARATHYROID HORMONE

The response of parathyroid hormone to acute exercise bouts is quite variable with studies reporting an increase in release *(40)*, a decrease in release *(41)*, and no change *(42)*. Although parathyroid hormone increases bone resorption *(39)*, in some cases, it may paradoxally have an anabolic effect on bone *(43)*. Whether parathyroid hormone has catabolic or anabolic effects may depend on the amount released and whether its release is continuous or intermittent. Continuous release of parathyroid hormone induces bone loss, whereas intermittent administration may increase bone mass through stimulation of osteoblasts *(44)*. The responses of bone to changes in parathyroid hormone levels with exercise training have therefore been inconsistent, with some studies demonstrating positive effects on bone and some demonstrating negative effects. The studies demonstrating negative effects are discussed below, with studies demonstrating positive effects discussed in the Parathyroid Hormone section.

Chronic high-intensity exercise training may cause an increase in the continuous release of parathyroid hormone *(40)*, and this may negatively affect bone mass in individuals who overexercise. The continuous release may be related to alterations in catecholamine levels with chronic exercise training. Catecholamines stimulate parathyroid hormone release in animal experiments *(45)*, and release of parathyroid hormone correlates with the intensity *(46)* or volume *(40)* of exercise. Assuming that catecholamine release is greater with higher exercise intensities and volumes, this could be a mechanism by which parathyroid hormone is continuously released with repeated exercise bouts. Two longitudinal exercise training studies have found reductions in bone mineral density and elevations in bone turnover associated with elevations in basal parathyroid hormone levels *(47,48)*. Training in both studies could be described as moderate in intensity and is the type of training usually associated with increases in bone mass. Indeed, one of the studies found a decrease in parathyroid hormone with further training and an increase in bone mass *(48)*. As bone turns over in a cycle of resorption and formation, initial measurements may have occurred during the bone resorption phase of the cycle. The influence of elevated basal parathyroid hormone levels on bone mass as a result of training is still unclear, since elevated parathyroid hormone levels with training have also been associated with increases in bone mass *(49)*. More work is needed in this area to clarify these relationships.

Aside from changes in basal parathyroid hormone levels, excessive training may also alter the set point for which parathyroid hormone is released in response to changes in blood calcium levels. Grimston et al. *(42)* assessed the changes in parathyroid hormone release in response to exercise or exercise combined with calcium ingestion in groups of female runners with normal and low bone mineral density. The osteopenic group had an elevated parathyroid hormone release compared to the group with normal bone mineral density, implying that the set point for parathyroid hormone release was altered in the osteopenic group. There was also a negative correlation between parathyroid hormone release and bone mineral density in this group. It is suggested that low estrogen levels that may have been present in some female runners may amplify the effect of parathyroid hormone on bone turnover, as it does in postmenopausal women *(50)*. More study is needed on the effects of excessive training and the relationship between altered estrogen levels and the set point of parathyroid hormone release.

NEGATIVE EFFECTS OF EXERCISE ON CALCITONIN AND VITAMIN D

A limited number of studies have shown that excessive endurance training in female athletes may result in alterations in calcitonin release and vitamin D levels. Grimston et al. *(42)* demonstrated that female runners characterized by low bone mass had decreased calcitonin release in response to elevated blood calcium levels following exercise, which differed from subjects with normal bone mass, who had increased calcitonin release. This may prevent the beneficial effect of calcitonin on preventing bone resorption in the subset of runners with low bone mass.

Vitamin D levels were found to be lower in runners with low bone mass in one study comparing amenorrheic athletes to eumenorrheic athletes and controls *(14)*, although levels were still within a normal range. It is not clear whether this lowered vitamin D level would significantly alter intestinal calcium absorption and contribute to the lower bone mass of amenorrheic athletes.

POSITIVE EFFECTS OF EXERCISE ON HORMONAL REGULATION OF BONE

Interactions Between Exercise and Estrogen for Increasing Bone Mass

Exercise and estrogen replacement have been shown to be successful therapies for increasing bone mass in postmenopausal women. Recently, it has been shown that when the two are combined, their effects on some bone sites may be synergistic (i.e., greater than the addition of each therapy alone). This implies that exercise may augment the effects of estrogen or vice versa. In postmenopausal women, exercise and estrogen replacement therapy have an additive *(51)* or synergistic *(52)* effect on bone mass of the spine and a synergistic effect on whole-body bone mass *(51,52)*. Animal studies have demonstrated either additive *(53)* or synergistic *(54)* effects with the two therapies. The exact mechanism by which exercise and estrogen synergistically increase bone mass is unknown.

Effects of Exercise on Anabolic Hormones

A number of anabolic hormones have been shown to increase following acute exercise sessions, and basal levels may be elevated in response chronic training. These anabolic hormones include testosterone and growth hormone. Insulin-like growth factor 1 (IGF-1), or somatomedin may also be considered an anabolic hormone that increases with exercise; however, its synthesis in the liver or other sites, including bone, may be mediated by growth hormone *(55)*. Each of these anabolic hormones have been shown to stimulate bone growth or formation by proliferation or activation of osteoblasts

Table 1
Effects of Anabolic Hormones on Bone and the Influence of Exercise[a]

Hormone	Effect of hormone on bone	Effect of exercise on hormone level
Estrogen	⇑ Ca^{2+} absorption *(2)*; ⇓ bone turnover *(3)*	Extreme training with low energy intake: ⇓ release *(5–9, 11–14, 17–19)*
Progesterone	⇑ bone formation *(4)*; couples formation to resorption *(4)*	Same as above
Testosterone	⇑ Ca^{2+} absorption *(32)*; ⇑ bone formation *(33)*	Extreme training: ⇓ release *(30,31)* Acute exercise ⇑ Release *(58, 61, 63)* Chronic exercise ⇑ Release *(63, 70)* or ⇔ *(76)*
Growth hormone	⇑ Bone formation *(56)*; ⇑ production of active form of vitamin D *(84)*	Acute exercise ⇑ Release *(60, 62, 65, 66)* Chronic exercise: ⇔ *(76)*
IGF-1	⇑ Bone formation *(57, 78)*	Acute exercise ⇑ Release *(60, 62, 65, 66)* Chronic exercise ⇑ Release *(67, 69)* or ⇔ *(76, 77)*

[a]References to individual points are shown in parentheses. Abbreviations: ⇑ = increase; ⇓ = decrease; ⇔ = no change; IGF-1 = insulin-like growth factor.

(33,56,57). This section will review the effects of acute and chronic exercise on release of anabolic hormones and the resultant effect on bone mineral.

ACUTE EFFECTS OF EXERCISE ON ANABOLIC HORMONES AND BONE METABOLISM

Single exercise sessions may result in increases in blood levels of anabolic hormones in both men and women (Table 1). In men, a single bout of weight-lifting exercise has been shown to result in increases in testosterone *(58)*, growth hormone *(58,59)*, and IGF-1 *(60)* levels. A single bout of cycle ergometer exercise similarly results in elevations of testosterone *(61)*, growth hormone, and IGF-1 *(62)*. The response occurs in young and old men, but seems to be attenuated with aging *(59)*. Increased testosterone levels have been attributed to hemoconcentration *(58)*, increased testicular production *(61)*, and reductions in clearance rates from hepatic and adipose tissue *(60)*. Increased production of IGF-1 has not always followed the same pattern as growth hormone changes *(60,62)*; therefore, their release may be independent. Similar responses to acute exercise occur in women. In response to a single bout of weight-lifting, increases have been noted in blood testosterone *(63)*, growth hormone *(64)*, and IGF-1 *(65)* levels. Increases in testosterone levels in females have been attributed to production by the adrenal cortex *(63)*.

A single study has related the increases in anabolic hormones with acute exercise to changes in markers of bone turnover *(66)*. In a group of men and women, arterial and venous blood was sampled during and following repeated one-leg, knee-extension exercise. Exercise resulted in an increase in arterial serum concentrations of growth hormone, and there was an exercise-induced uptake of growth hormone over the thigh and a release of IGF-1. Levels of biomarkers for bone formation and resorption were increased during exercise. This release of anabolic hormones and increase of bone turnover may result in increased bone synthesis with training, but firm conclusions can only be drawn from longitudinal study of these responses.

EFFECTS OF EXERCISE TRAINING ON ANABOLIC HORMONES AND BONE MASS

Cross-sectional studies suggest that the higher bone mass of some chronically trained athletic groups may be related to higher basal levels of anabolic hormones. Young strength-trained women were shown to have higher bone mass and higher levels of IGF-1 concentrations than aerobically trained women and sedentary controls (67). Among aerobically trained females, testosterone levels were found to be a significant determinant of bone density, independent of estrogen levels (68). Finally, endurance-trained postmenopausal women were found to have higher bone mineral density adjusted for body weight, along with higher IGF-1 levels and a trend toward higher growth hormone levels than sedentary controls (69). Although cross-sectional and correlative studies cannot imply cause and effect relationships, results suggest that various forms of training may lead to enhancement of basal anabolic hormone levels and stimulation of bone formation.

Longitudinal studies have demonstrated that basal levels of testosterone are elevated in males following 2 yr of training (70). Luteinizing and follicle-stimulating hormones were also elevated, suggesting that training may have influences at the pituitary or hypothalamic levels, which led to the increase in testosterone levels (70). Baseline testosterone levels were also found to be higher following 2 mo of resistance training in females when compared to nonexercised controls (63). It was suggested that increased testosterone levels may have been owing to either gonadal or adrenal responses (63).

Various longitudinal training studies geared toward increasing bone mass have been designed with protocols based on those found to increase anabolic hormone levels optimally during acute exercise sessions. Studies of acute exercise sessions have shown that the anabolic hormone response is greater during resistance training sessions that involve the greatest total work (i.e., a greater training volume) in both male (65,71) and female (65) subjects. Based on this finding, one longitudinal study compared the effects of two training routines in young females: one where all exercises were combined on one training day, and another where exercises were split between successive training days (72). The authors hypothesized that the routine with all exercises combined on one day would produce a greater training effect, since the total work performed was greater within single exercise sessions. This routine produced a greater increase in legs' lean mass (72), but changes in bone mineral mass with both routines were not significant, most likely owing to the relatively short (20-wk) training duration (73).

When total work output during acute weight-lifting sessions is held constant, the anabolic response is greater with sessions that employ higher loads and a lower frequency (repetitions) of movement than sessions that employ lower loads and a higher frequency of movements (74). Specifically, sessions that involved exercises consisting of seven repeated lifts of heavy loads produced greater increases in growth hormone release than sessions that involved an equivalent amount of work, but 21 repeated lifts of loads that were one-third as heavy (74). A recent longitudinal 12-mo training study compared the effects of training on bone using almost identical training protocols (exercises involving 8 lifts of heavy loads vs exercises involving 20 lifts of lighter loads) (75).

The high-load, low-movement frequency training was found to result in significant increases in bone mass, but the low-load, high-movement frequency training had no effect on bone mass *(75)*. Thus, it has been shown that training using protocols known to enhance anabolic hormone secretion optimally result in enhancement of bone mineral synthesis.

One drawback to the abovementioned longitudinal studies is that changes in bone mass and changes in basal levels of anabolic hormones were not measured in combination. Studies in humans combining both measurements have demonstrated that beneficial effects of training on bone mass can be realized without changes in anabolic hormones. Sixteen weeks of resistance training of elderly men produced significant increases in femoral neck bone mineral density without changes in levels of testosterone, growth hormone, and IGF-1 *(76)*. Likewise, 27 wk of gymnastics training of young women produced significant increases in lumbar spine bone mineral density without a change in serum IGF-1 levels *(77)*. One elaborate study of rats was more successful, demonstrating a beneficial effect of training on anabolic hormone level and bone *(78)*. Following 9 wk of treadmill running, exercised female rats had higher levels of serum IGF-1, bone-specific IGF-1, and long-bone formation rate compared to nonexercised controls. IGF-1 concentrations in both long-bone and vertebral extracts were highly correlated with their respective bone formation rates as measured by histomorphology. This indicates that IGF-1, locally produced in stressed bone, may be a mediator between increased mechanical strain and the signal for increased bone formation *(78)*.

Positive Effects of Exercise on Calciotrophic Hormones

PARATHYROID HORMONE

Parathyroid hormone stimulates bone resorption to maintain homeostasis when blood calcium levels are low *(39)*. With chronic exercise training, parathyroid hormone levels may be lowered. This has been associated with higher bone mineral values: Cross-sectionally, male and female endurance-trained athletes have been found to have lower serum parathyroid hormone levels associated with higher bone mineral density when compared to inactive controls *(69,79)*. Rats endurance-trained by treadmill exercise also have lower parathyroid hormone levels and higher bone mass compared to untrained rats *(80)*. The mechanism for the lowering of parathyroid hormone levels with training is not known.

In contrast to the above studies, an increase in basal levels of parathyroid hormone has been found following a resistance training program that increased bone mineral density in postmenopausal women *(49)*. As mentioned in The Negative Effects of Exercise on Parathyroid Hormone section, parathyroid hormone may have anabolic effects on bone through stimulation of osteoblasts, if released in an intermittent fashion *(44)*. Further research is needed to determine the exact direction of changes in basal parathyroid hormone levels in response to different training protocols and whether these changes can be considered beneficial or detrimental to bone.

CALCITONIN AND VITAMIN D

Few studies have looked at the effects of exercise on calcitonin levels. One study showed that calcitonin levels increased in response to exercise *(41)*; this may prevent bone resorption. However, chronic exercise training does not appear to alter serum calcitonin levels *(69)*.

Exercise training may have beneficial effects on vitamin D levels, resulting in increased intestinal calcium absorption and increased bone mass (Table 2). Cross-sectional studies indicate that vitamin D levels may be elevated in endurance-trained *(69)* and resistance-trained *(81)* individuals. This is associated with a higher bone mass in these individuals compared to inactive controls *(69,82)*. Rats trained by treadmill exercise have an increase in vitamin D levels, increased calcium balance, increased intestinal calcium absorption efficiency, and increased bone mass compared to untrained rats *(80,83)*. Increases in growth hormone release with exercise training *(69)* may simulate the production of the active form of vitamin D *(84)*.

DIRECTIONS FOR FUTURE RESEARCH

Extremes of exercise training produce negative effects on bone owing to decreases in estrogen (in females) or testosterone (in males) production. Short-term studies have shown that alterations in hormonal release can be prevented if adequate dietary energy intake is maintain during periods of heavy exercise *(16)*. Longer-term studies need to be performed to determine whether increasing energy availability can prevent reductions in reproductive hormones that may occur with participation in large amounts of exercise.

Another area open for research is assessment of precise treatments that may reverse athletic amenorrhea. Cross-sectional studies on small numbers of subjects have indicated that reduction in training volume and weight gain may reverse amenorrhea *(25,26)*, but larger-scale studies would be beneficial. Although hormone replacement therapy has been shown to increase bone mass in amenorrheic athletes *(27)*, the effects of treatment with low-dose oral contraceptives have not been tested, although it has been recommended *(85)*.

There is an abundance of studies that have compared the effects of different exercise regimes on anabolic hormones during acute exercise sessions; however, few investigators have compared the effects of different training regimes on long-term changes in bone mass within the same study *(75)*. Research is needed to develop exercise prescriptions for optimal enhancement of long-term hormone profiles that result in bone formation.

SUMMARY

Extremes of exercise training may negatively affect hormonal profiles that influence bone mass. Dietary energy compensation for energy expended during exercise has been shown to prevent changes in reproductive hormone profiles in the short term. Longer-term studies are needed to assess whether increased dietary intake can prevent the occurrence of amenorrhea without a decrease in training volumes.

When hormone replacement therapy is administered to postmenopausal women and combined with exercise training, estrogen and exercise may act synergistically to increase bone mass at some skeletal sites. At other sites, the effects of estrogen and exercise are additive.

The effects of exercise on the calciotropic hormones are mixed. Parathyroid hormone may be increased or decreased with exercise training. Parathyroid hormone stimulates bone resorption, but intermittent release may stimulate bone formation. Tightly controlled animal experiments demonstrate a decrease in parathyroid hormone and an increase in vitamin D with training, resulting in positive calcium balance and increased bone mass.

Table 2
Effects of Calciotropic Hormones on Bone and the Influence of Exercise[a]

Hormone	Effect of hormone on bone	Effect of exercise on hormone level
PTH	⇑ Bone resorption when continuously released *(39)*; ⇑ Bone formation when intermittently released *(44)*	Acute exercise: ⇑ *(40)*, ⇓ *(41)*, ⇔ *(42)* Chronic exercise ⇔ *(47–49)* or ⇓ *(48, 69, 79, 80)*
Calcitonin	⇓ Bone resorption	Extreme training: ⇓ *(42)* Acute exercise: ⇑ *(41)* Chronic exercise: ⇔ *(69)*
Vitamin D	⇑ Ca^{2+} absorption	Extreme training: ⇓ *(14)* Chronic exercise ⇑ *(69, 80, 81, 83)*

[a]References to individual points are shown in parentheses. Abbreviations: PTH = parathyroid hormone; ⇑ = increase; ⇓ = decrease; ⇔ = no change;

Resistance training involving high volumes of work within single sessions and heavy loads may optimally stimulate release of anabolic hormones (testosterone, growth hormone, and IGF), but the long-term effects of changes in hormone profiles and their effects on bone have not been studied in detail.

REFERENCES

1. Blimkie CJR, Chilibeck PD, Davison KS. Bone mineralization patterns: reproductive endocrine, calcium and physical activity influences during the lifespan. In: Bar-Or O, Lamb D, Clarkson P, eds. Perspectives in Exercise Science and Sports Medicine: Exercise and the Female—A Life Span Approach, vol. 9. Cooper Publishing Group, Carmel, NJ, 1996; pp. 73–145.
2. Heaney RP, Recher RR, Stegman MR, Moy AJ. Calcium absorption in women: relationship to calcium intake, estrogen status and age. J Bone Miner Res 1989;4:469–475.
3. Yeh JK, Liu CC, Aloia JF. Additive effect of treadmill exercise and 17 beta-estradiol replacement on prevention of tibial bone loss in adult oveariectomized rat. J Bone Miner Res 1993;8:677–683.
4. Prior JC. Progesterone as a bone-trophic hormone. Endocr Rev 1990;11:386–398.
5. Drinkwater BL, Nilson K, Chesnut CH, Bremner WJ, Shainholtz S, Southworth MB. Bone mineral content of amenorrheic and eumenorrheic athletes. N Engl J Med 1984;311:277–281.
6. Robinson TL, Snow-Harter C, Taaffe CR, Gillis D, Shaw J, Marcus R. Gymnasts exhibit higher bone mass than runners despite similar prevalence of amenorrhea and oligomenorrhea. J Bone Miner Res 1995;10:26–35.
7. Wolman RL, Clark P, McNally E, Harries M, Reeve J. Menstrual state and exercise as determinants of spinal trabecular bone density in female athletes. BMJ 1990;301:516–518.
8. Slemenda C, Johnston CC. High impact activities in young women: site-specific bone mass effects among female figure skaters. Bone Miner 1993;20:125–132.
9. Warren MP, Brooks-Gunn J, Fox RP, Lancelot C, Newman D, Hamilton WG. Lack of bone accretion and amenorrhea: evidence for a relative osteopenia in weight-bearing bones. J Clin Endocrinol Metab 1991;72:847–853.
10. Fehling PC, Alekel L, Clasey J, Rector A, Stillman RJ. A comparison of bone mineral densities among female athletes in impact loading and active loading sports. Bone 1995;17:205–210.
11. Young N, Formica C, Szmukler G, and Seeman E. Bone density at weight-bearing and nonweight-bearing sites in ballet dancers: the effects of exercise, hypogonadism, and body weight. J Clin Endocrinol Metab 1994;78:449–454.
12. Warren MP, Brooks-Gunn J, Hamilton LH, Warren LF, Hamilton WG. Scoliosis and fractures in young ballet dancers. Relation to delayed menarche and secondary amenorrhea. N Engl J Med 1986;314:1348–1353.

13. Rencken ML, Chesnut CH, Drinkwater BL. Bone density at multiple skeletal sites in amenorrheic athletes. JAMA 1996;276:238–240.
14. Marcus R, Cann C, Madvig P, Minkoff J, Goddard M, Bayer M, et al. Menstrual function and bone mass in elite women distance runners. Ann Intern Med 1985;102:158–163.
15. Myburgh KH, Hutchins J, Fataar AB, Hough SF, Noakes TD. Low bone density is an etiologic factor for stress fractures in athletes. Ann Intern Med 1990;113:754–759.
16. Loucks AB, Verdun M, Heath EM. Low energy availability, not stress of exercise, alters LH pulsatility in exercising women. J Appl Physiol 1998;84:37–46.
17. Harber VJ, Petersen SR, Chilibeck PD. Thyroid hormone concentrations and muscle metabolism in amenorrheic and eumenorrheic athletes. Can J Appl Physiol 1998;23:293–306.
18. Wilmore JH, Wambscans KC, Brenner M, Broeder CE, Paijmans I, Volpe JA, et al. Is there energy conservation in amenorrheic compared with eumenorrheic distance runners? J Appl Physiol 1992;72:15–22.
19. Loucks AB, Laughlin GA, Mortola JF, Girton L, Nelson JC, Yen SSC. Hypothalamic–pituitary–thyroidal function in eumenorrheic and amenorrheic athletes. J Clin Endocrinol Metab 1992;75:514–518.
20. Harber VJ, Petersen SR, Chilibeck PD. Thyroid hormone concentrations and skeletal muscle metabolism during exercise in anorexic females. Can J Physiol Pharmacol. 1997;75:1197–1202.
21. Ding J, Sheckter CB, Drinkwater BL, Soules M, Bremner WJ. High serum cortisol levels in exercise-associated amenorrhea. Ann Intern Med 1988;108:530–534.
22. Loucks AB, Mortola JF, Girton L, Yen SSC. Alterations in the hypothalamic–pituitary–ovarian and the hypothalamic–pituitary–adrenal axes in athletic women. J Clin Endocrinol Metab 1989; 68:402–411.
23. Mann DR, Jackson GG, Blank MS. Influence of adrenocoritcotropin and adrenalectomy on gonadotropin secretion in immature rats. Neuroendocrinology 1982;34:20–26.
24. Olster DH, Ferin M. Corticotropin-releasing hormone inhibits gonadotropin secretion in the ovariectomized rhesus monkey. J Clin Endocrinol Metab 1987;65:262–267.
25. Drinkwater BL, Nilson K, Ott S, Chesnut CH. Bone mineral density after resumption of menses in amenorrheic athletes. J.A.M.A 1986;256:380–382.
26. Linberg JS, Powell RR, Hunt MM, Ducey DE, Wade CE. Increased vertebral bone mineral in response to reduced exercise in amenorrheic runners. West J Med 1987;146:39–42.
27. Cumming DC. Exercise-associated amenorrhea, low bone density, and estrogen replacement therapy. Arch Intern Med 1996; 56:2193–2195.
28. Jonnavithula S, Warren MP, Fox RP, Lazaro MI. Bone density is compromised in amenorrheic women despite return of menses: a 2-year study. Obstet Gynecol 1993;81: 669–674.
29. Keen AD, Drinkwater BL. Irreversible bone loss in former amenorrheic athletes. Osteoporois Int 1993;7:311–315.
30. Wheeler GD, Wall SR, Belcastro AN, Cumming DC. Reduced serum testosterone and prolactin levels in male distance runners. JAMA 1984;252:514–516.
31. Strauss RH, Lanese RR, Malarkey WB. Weight loss in amateur wrestlers and its effect on serum testosterone levels. J.A.M.A 1985;254:3337,3338.
32. Hope WG, Ibarra MJ, Thomas ML. Testosterone alters duodenal calcium transport and longitudinal bone growth rate in parallel in the male rat. Proc Soc Exp Biol Med 1992;200:536–541.
33. Kasperk CH, Wergedal JE, Farley JR, Linkhart TA, Turner RT, Baylink DJ. Androgens directly stimulate proliferation of bone cells in vitro. Endocrinology 1989;124:1576–1578.
34. Cumming DC, Quigley ME, Yen SS. Acute suppression of circulating testosterone levels by cortisol in men. J Clin Endocrinol Metab 1983;57:671–673.
35. Gambacciani M, Yen SS, Rasmussen DD. GnRH release from the mediobasal hyothalamus: in vitro inhibition by corticotropin-releasing factor. Neuroendocrinology 1986;43:533–536.
36. Hetland ML, Haarbo J, Christinsen C. Low bone mass and high bone turnover in male long distance runners. J Clin Endocrinol Metab 1993;77:770–775.
37. MacDougall JD, Webber CE, Martin J, Ormerod S, Chesley A, Younglai EV, et al. Relationship among running mileage, bone density, and serum testosterone in male runners. J Appl Physiol 1992;73:1165–1170.
38. Burge MR, Lanzi RA, Skarda ST, Eaton RP. Idiopathic hypogonadotropic hypogonadism in a male runner is reversed by clomiphene citrate. Fertil Steril 1997;67:783–785.
39. McSheehy PM, Chambers TJ. Osteoblast-like cells in the presence of parathyroid hormone release soluble factor that stimulates osteoblastic bone resorption. Endocrinology 1986;119:1654–1659.

40. Ljunghall S, Joborn H, Roxin LE, Skarfors WT, Wide LE, Lithell HO. Increase in serum parathyroid hormone levels after prolonged physical exercise. Med Sci Sports Exerc 1988;20:122–125.
41. Aloia JF, Rasulo P, Deftos LJ, Vaswani A, Yeh JK. Exercise-induced hypercalcemia and the calciotropic hormones. J Lab Clin Med 1985;106:229–232.
42. Grimston SK, Tanguay KE, Gundberg CM, Hanley DA. The calciotropic hormone response to changes in serum calcium during exercise in female long distance runners. J Clin Endocrinol Metab 1993;76:867–872.
43. Hodsman AB, Fraher LJ, Ostbye T, Adachi JD, Steer BM. An evaluation of several biochemical markers for bone formation and resorption in a protocol utilizing cyclical parathyroid hormone and calcitonin therapy for osteoporosis. J Clin Invest 1993;91:1138–1148.
44. Dempster DW, Cosman F, Parisien M, Shen B, Lindsay R. Anabolic actions of parathyroid hormone on bone. Endocr Rev 1993;14:690–709.
45. Brown EM, Hurwitz S, Aurbach GD. Beta adrenergic stimulation of cyclic AMP content and parathyroid hormone release from isolated bovine parathyroid cells. Endocrinology 1977;100:1609–1702.
46. Salvesen H, Johansson AG, Foxdal P, Wide L, Piehl-Aulin K, Ljunghall S. Intact serum parathyroid hormone levels increase during running exercise in well-trained men. Calcif Tissue Int 1994;54:256–261.
47. Rockwell JC, Sorensen AM, Baker S, Leahey D, Stock JL, Michaels J, et al. Weight training decreases vertebral bone density in premenopausal women: a prospective study. J Clin Endocrinol Metab 1990;71:988–993.
48. Bloomfield SA, Mysiw WJ, Jackson RD. Bone mass and endocrine adaptations to training in spinal cord injured individuals. Bone 1996;19:61–68.
49. Nelson ME, Fiaterone MA, Morganti CM, Trice I, Greenberg RA, Evans WJ. Effects of high-intensity strength training on multiple risk factors for osteoporotic fractures. JAMA 1994;272:1909–1914.
50. Boucher A, D'Amour P, Hamel L, Fugere P, Gascon-Barre M, Lepage R, et al. Estrogen replacement decreases the set point of parathyroid hormone stimulation by calcium in normal postmenopausal women. J Clin Endocrinol Metab 1989;68:831–836.
51. Kohrt WM, Snead DB, Slatopolsky E, Birge J. Additive effects of weight-bearing exercise and estrogen on bone mineral density in older women. J Bone Miner Res 1995;10:1303–1311.
52. Notelovitz M, Martin D, Tesar R, Khan FY, Probart C, Fields C, et al. Estrogen therapy and variable-resistance weight training increase bone mineral in surgically menopausal women. J Bone Miner Res 1991;6:583–589.
53. Yeh JK, Liu CC, Aloia J. Additive effect of treadmill exercise and 17-estradiol replacement on prevention of tibial bone loss in adult ovariectomized rat. J Bone Miner Res 1993;8:677–683.
54. Cheng MZ, Zaman G, Rawlinson SCF, Suswillo RFL, Lanyon LE. Mechanical loading and sex hormone interactions in organ cultures of rat ulna. J Bone Miner Res 1996;11:502–511.
55. Mathews LS, Norstedt G, Palmiter RD. Regulation of insulin-like growth factor 1 gene expression by growth hormone. Proc Natl Acad Sci USA 1986;83:9343–9347.
56. Kassem M, Blum W, Risteli J, Mosekilde L, Eriksen EF. Growth hormone stimulates proliferation and differentiation of normal human osteoblast-like cells in vitro. Calcif Tissue Int 1993;52:222–226.
57. Schmid C, Guler HP, Rowe D, Froesch ER. Insulin-like growth factor I regulates type 1 procollagen messenger ribonucleic acid steady state levels in bone of rats. Endocrinology 1989;125:1575–1580.
58. Kraemer RR, Kilgore JL, Kraemer GR, Castracane VD. Growth hormone, IGF-1 and testosterone responses to resistive exercise. Med Sci Sports Exerc 1992;24:1346–1352.
59. Craig BW, Brown R, Everhart J. Effects of progressive resistance training on growth hormone and testosterone levels in young and elderly subjects. Mech Age Dev 1989;49:159–169.
60. Kraemer WJ, Marchitelli L, Gordon SE, Harman E, Dziados JE, Mello R, et al. Hormonal and growth factor responses to heavy resistance exercise protocols. J Appl Physiol 1990;69:1442–1450.
61. Cumming DC, Brunsting LA, Strich G, Ries AL, Rebar RW. Reproductive hormone increases in response to acute exercise in men. Med Sci Sports Exerc 1986;18:369–373.
62. Cappon J, Brasel JA, Mohan S, Cooper DM. Effect of brief exercise on circulating insulin-like growth factor 1. J Appl Physiol 1994;76:2490–2496.
63. Cumming DC, Wall SR, Galbraith MA, Belcastro AN. Reproductive hormone responses to resistance exercise. Med Sci Sports Exerc 1987;19:234–238.
64. Kraemer RR, Heleniak RJ, Tryniecki JL, Kraemer GR, Okazaki NJ, Castracane VD. Follicular and luteal phase hormonal responses to low-volume resistive exercise. Med Sci Sports Exerc 1995;27:809–817.

65. Kraemer WJ, Gordon SE, Fleck SJ, Marchitelli LJ, Mello R, Dziados JE, et al. Endogenous anabolic hormonal and growth factor responses to heavy resistance exercise in males and females. Int J Sports Med 1991;12:228–235.
66. Brahm H, Pielhl-Aulin K, Saltin B, Ljunghall S. Net fluxes over working thigh of hormones, growth factors and biomarkers of bone metabolism during short lasting dynamic exercise. Calcif Tissue Int 1997;60:175–180.
67. Davee AM, Rosen CJ, Adler RA. Exercise patterns and trabecular bone density in college women. J Bone Miner Res 1990;5:245–250.
68. Buchanan JR, Myers C, Lloyd T, Leuenberger P, Demers LM. Determinants of peak trabecular bone density in women: the role of androgens, estrogen, and exercise. J Bone Miner Res 1988;3:673–680.
69. Nelson ME, Meredith CN, Dawson-Hughes B, Evans WJ. Hormone and bone mineral status in endurance-trained and sedentary postmenopausal women. J Clin Endocrinol Metab 1988;66:927–933.
70. Hakkinen K, Pakarinen A, Alen M, Kauhanen H, Komi PV. Neuromuscular and hormonal adaptations in athletes to strength training in two years. J Appl Physiol 1988;65:2406–2412.
71. Gotshalk LA, Loebel CC, Nindl BD, Putukian M, Sebastianelli WJ, Newton RU, et al. Hormonal responses of multiset versus single-set heavy-resistance exercise protocols. Can J Appl Physiol 1997;22:244–255.
72. Calder AW, Chilibeck PD, Webber CE, Sale DG. Comparison of whole and split weight training routines in young women. Can J Appl Physiol 1994;19:185–199.
73. Chilibeck PD, Calder A, Sale DG, Webber CE. Twenty weeks of weight training increases lean tissue mass but not bone mineral mass or density in healthy, active young women. Can J Physiol Pharmacol 1996;74:1180–1185.
74. Vanhelder WP, Radomeski MW, Goode RC. Growth hormone responses during intermittent weight lifting exercise in men. Eur J App. Physiol 1984;53:31–34.
75. Kerr D, Morton A, Dick I, Prince R. Exercise effects on bone mass in postmenopausal women are site-specific and load-dependent. J Bone Miner Res 1996;11:218–225.
76. Ryan AS, Treuth MS, Rubin MA, Miller JP, Nicklas BJ, Landis DM, et al. Effects of strength training on bone mineral density: hormonal and bone turnover relationships. J Appl Physiol 1994;77:1678–1684.
77. Nichols DL, Sanborn CF, Bonnick SL, Ben-Ezra V, Gench B, DiMarco NM. The effects of gymnastics training on bone mineral density. Med Sci Sports Exerc 1994;26:1220–1225.
78. Yeh JK, Aloia JF, Chen M, Ling N, Koo H-C, Millard WJ. Effect of growth hormone administration and treadmill exercise on serum and skeletal IGF-1 in rats. Am J Physiol 1994;266:E129–E135.
79. Brahm H, Strom H, Piehl-Aulin K, Mallmin H. Ljunghall S. Bone metabolism in endurance trained athletes: a comparison to population-based controls based on DXA, SXA, quantitative ultrasound, and biochemical markers. Calcif Tissue Int 1997;61:448–454.
80. Yeh JK, Aloia, JF. Effect of physical activity on calciotropic hormones and calcium balance in rats. Am J Physiol 1990;258:E263–E268.
81. Bell NH, Godsen RN, Henry DP, Shary J, Epstein S. The effects of muscle-building exercise on vitamin D and mineral metabolism. J Bone Miner Res 1988;3:369–373.
82. Colletti LA, Edwards J, Gordon L, Shary J, Bell NH. The effects of muscle-building exercise on bone mineral density of the radius, spine, and hip in young men. Calcif Tissue Int 1989;45:12–14.
83. Yeh JK, Aloia JF, Yasumura S. Effect of physical activity on calcium and phosphorus metabolism in the rat. Am J Physiol 1989;256:E1–E6.
84. Spanos D, Barett D, MacIntyre I, Pike JW, Safilian EF, Houssler MR. Effect of growth hormone on vitamin D metabolism. Nature 1978;273:246–247.
85. Shangold M, Rebar RW, Colston A, Schiff I. Evaluation and management of menstrual dysfunction in athletes. JAMA 1990;263:1665–1669.

15 The Role of Exercise in the Attainment of Peak Bone Mass and Bone Strength

Shona L. Bass and Kathryn H. Myburgh, PhD

CONTENTS

INTRODUCTION
EXERCISE AND BONE MASS IN ADULT PREMENOPAUSAL WOMEN
THE OSTEOTROPHIC EFFECT OF EXERCISE DURING GROWTH
CONCLUSION
REFERENCES

INTRODUCTION

Peak bone mass is the maximal lifetime amount of bone tissue accrued in individual bones and the whole skeleton. Recent research has shown that peak bone mass may be a more important determinant of low bone density and risk of fracture in old age than age-related bone loss [1]. Therefore, maximizing the attainment of peak bone mass is now considered to be an important component of osteoporosis prevention strategies. There is a large variation in the normal range for peak bone mass that is influenced by both genetic and environmental factors. Exercise may be the most important modifiable environmental factor that can increase peak bone mass. The osteotrophic effect of exercise has been shown to depend on the time in life exposure occurs and the type of loading. Exercise may not always be beneficial however, since athletic primary and secondary amenorrhea may lead to either a failure to gain bone or bone loss.

The majority of studies that have investigated the effect of exercise on the skeleton have used bone density as the outcome measure. Changes in bone geometric structure and internal architecture, however, may significantly affect bone strength with or without significant changes in bone density. Very little is known about the surface-specific and geometric-specific effects of physical loading on the skeleton during growth and adulthood. The chapter will review how exercise may influence the attainment of peak bone mass and bone strength at different ages. It begins with a brief discussion of the measuring techniques and nomenclature commonly used in the field.

Measuring Techniques and Nomenclature

Osteoporotic fractures are a measurable event. In contrast, bone strength and the risk of fracture are not easily determined *(1)*. Bone strength is influenced by the quality of the bone. There are many factors that contribute to bone quality, and these include bone geometry, trabecular architecture, accumulation of microfractures, bone density, the accumulation of cement lines, cortical porosity, and microheterogeneity of mineralization *(2)*. Of these characteristics, bone density is the most easily measured using noninvasive procedures and is strongly correlated with bone strength and fracture risk *(3)*. Bone density can account for up to 80% of the variance in the in vitro ultimate compressive strength or ultimate stress of bone *(4)*. Therefore, bone density is used as a surrogate measure of the breaking strength of bone, and to assess bone fragility, efficacy of a treatment, fracture risk, and the rate of bone gain and loss *(1)*.

There are various techniques available to determine the amount of mineral in the skeleton. Skeletal weight and the chemical composition of bones were measures commonly used before the introduction of techniques, such as dual-energy X-ray absorptiometry (DXA) and quantitative computed tomography (QCT). DXA and QCT estimate the mineral content of the skeleton, which can be expressed as either a mass or a density. Bone mass is the amount of mineral in grams (g) unadjusted for size. Areal bone density is the bone mass divided by the projected area of the region (grams per square centimeter, g/cm^2). Although areal bone density only adjusts for the width and length of a bone (not depth), it is the unit most commonly reported in the literature. Volumetric bone density is the bone mass divided by the volume of the region (gram per cubic centimeter, g/cm^3). DXA provides a measure of bone mass and areal density. Approximations of volumetric bone density can be obtained by using equations that estimate the volume of the vertebra and femoral neck *(5)*. This estimate is termed bone mineral apparent density (BMAD). QCT measures bone mass and volumetric bone density of a cross-sectional slice of bone rather than the whole bone, such as with DXA. QCT can also differentiate between trabecular and cortical bone.

The term "density" without a clarifying prefix can be misleading, because it does not distinguish between areal or volumetric bone density. This lack of clarity can often lead to misinterpretation of data, because it tends to dismiss the limitations and assumptions associated with each measure. Adding to this confusion is the assumption that volumetric bone density provides a measure of "true density." The true density of a tissue is the mass of a substance per unit length, area, or volume of its own bulk *(6)*. In bone tissue, this is the density of bone excluding marrow space, and Haversian and medullary cavities. Areal and volumetric bone density, as measured by either DXA or QCT, include the marrow spaces in trabecular bone and the medullary cavity in cortical bone. They are therefore not measures of true density, but rather of "apparent density" because the tissue that is measured is not all bone *(6)*.

Also misleading is the notion that bone density increases with age and size. This misunderstanding originates from the use of areal bone density measures (g/cm^2) that do not correct for bone depth. Therefore, areal bone density measures will be higher in a larger compared to a smaller bone of the same true density. This is because the areal measure (cm^2) does not account for changes that occur to volume (cm^3). It has been demonstrated that true bone density does not increase with age or size, that is, the chemical composition of the skeleton remains constant during growth and adulthood *(7–12)*. Trotter and Hixon reported that the percentage ash weight of the total skeleton increased with age during the fetal period, after which there was no further trend *(12)*. This implies that the mineral composition of bone is constant from early childhood to old age. It has also been shown that volumetric bone density is constant with age and size. Dunnill et al. showed that vertebral size increased from birth to young adulthood, but the density of the vertebra was constant, because there was a proportional increase in bone size and bone mass *(9)*. This constancy in volumetric bone density has been confirmed by Kroger et al. *(10)* for the femoral neck, by Schonau et al. *(11)* for the distal radius, and by Lu et al. *(7)* for the mid-femoral shaft.

The distinction between the measures of bone mass and areal and volumetric bone density is important in the comparison of individuals with different stature or bone size. This is particularly pertinent in the comparisons of males to females, individuals from different racial origins, and children in different stages of growth and maturation. Further, it is important to acknowledge that an increase or decrease in areal or volumetric bone density is not a change in the chemical composition of bone, but rather a change in total bone length, bone size, cortical thickness, and/or the biomechanical organization of the trabecular structure *(6,11)*.

Bone Modeling and Remodeling

The skeleton is an active organ that undergoes change throughout life through the processes of modeling and remodeling. Bone modeling refers to the sculpturing of bone (size, shape, and spatial location) through the synthesis of new bone on some surfaces and resorption of bone at other surfaces in response to extraneous factors, such as mechanical strains. Modeling involves the addition of bone, without prior resorption, and therefore, it does not depend on any biological coupling between osteoclasts and osteoblasts *(13)*. It can affect cortical (periosteal and endocortical) and trabecular surfaces; it can increase, but not decrease the periosteal perimeter, cortical thickness, and cortical bone mass; it can only thicken, but not reduce trabeculae. The majority of bone modeling occurs during the growing years, and limited modeling can occur following skeletal maturation *(14)*.

Bone remodeling replaces fatigue-damaged bone (or "turns bone over") in a biologically coupled activation–resorption–formation sequence requiring the coordination of different bone cells in a specific sequence (basic multicellular unit). Remodeling acts throughout life on periosteal, Haversian, endocortical, and trabecular surfaces. Except on the periosteal surface, remodeling does not usually make more bone than is resorbed—bone is either removed or is conserved *(15)*.

At the periosteal surface, remodeling affects bone geometry and has been shown to influence bone strength and the ability to withstand fractures in vitro *(16)*. During aging, bone mass is accrued slowly on the periosteal surface and resorbed on the endocortical surface. In females, this process is not concomitant, that is, less bone mass is accrued on the periosteal surface compared to that being resorbed on the endocortical surface *(17,18)*. This results in a slightly larger bone (cross-sectional diameter) with a relatively thinner cortex. This redistribution of bone can preserve the bone's moment of inertia and resistance to bending under torsional loads. Early studies used cadaver specimens for these investigations, but more recently, the cross-sectional geometry of the forearm was measured in vivo with computed tomography (CT) *(19)*. These results showed that despite the 20–30% lower radial and ulnar bone mass in older women, ulnar width, total bone area, and moment of inertia were greater in older women. Therefore, bone strength is a complex interaction among bone mass, size, shape, and structural organization. All of these are influenced by age, hormonal milieu, and mechanical loading.

When Is Peak Bone Mass Achieved?

Total body calcium increases from 25 g at birth to reach peak bone mass of about 1300 g in adulthood *(12,20,21)*. The changes in calcium content during growth are large and occur quickly, whereas the changes in adulthood are small and occur slowly (Fig. 1). Peak bone mass is the term used to describe the maximal lifetime amount of bone tissue accrued in individual bones and the whole skeleton. It is the consequence of the net accrual of bone mass during childhood and adolescence, and the balance between accrual and resorption in the adult premenopausal period *(22)*. Approximately 80–85% of peak bone mass has been accrued by the time menarche has occurred. About half of this is achieved during prepubertal growth (~10–12 yr), and the other half is achieved very rapidly in the 2–4 yr of pubertal growth *(23–25)*. Bone mass accrual continues slowly after puberty and contributes a further 15–20% to the peak bone mass. Although it is well accepted that bone mass continues to be accrued after linear growth has ceased (at about 16 yr in females), there is still debate about when peak bone mass is achieved. There have been reports that peak bone mass may be achieved from as early as 17–18 yr to as late as 35 yr *(26–33)*.

Evidence that bone mass was still being accrued after the cessation of linear growth was reported by Trotter and Hixon *(12)*. They also reported that the maximal skeletal weight occurred at about 20 yr of age, after which there was a rapid decline *(12)*. In contrast, Teegarden et al. showed that there was still a 4% increase in total bone mass after the early 20s *(30)*. The results from other cross-sectional studies also suggest that peak bone mass is achieved in the third decade *(32,33)*.

These conflicting results about when peak bone mass is achieved may be because the results of one site are not representative of the entire skeleton or different sites within the skeleton. Theintz et al. showed no increase in bone density at the femoral neck or the lumbar spine after 17–19 yr of age *(29)*. Matkovic et al. also reported that the majority of peak bone mass had been achieved by late adolescence or young adulthood, except at the distal forearm, which occurred at 22 yr *(31)*. In contrast Mazess and Barden reported that peak bone mass may be achieved later in adulthood. They reported small differences in bone density between women aged 20–24 and women aged 30–34: lumbar spine was 3% higher in the older cohort, but no differences were noted in the femur *(32)*. These data are similar to that reported by Rodin et al. *(33)*. Although these data indicate that different sites within the skeleton acquire peak bone mass at different ages, there is still considerable debate regarding when peak bone mass is achieved at a particular skeletal site. This may be in part because the results of cross-sectional studies can be influenced by differences that may exist between the cohorts *(34)*.

The results of prospective studies support the notion that peak bone mass may be achieved later rather than earlier in adulthood. Parsons et al. followed subjects aged 18–21 yr for 1 yr *(35)*, and Bennell et al. also studied subjects aged 17–26 yr for 1 yr *(36)*. Both studies showed approx 2.2% increases in total body bone mass in the female subjects. In a longer study, 156 women were followed for up to 5 yr, and peak bone mass

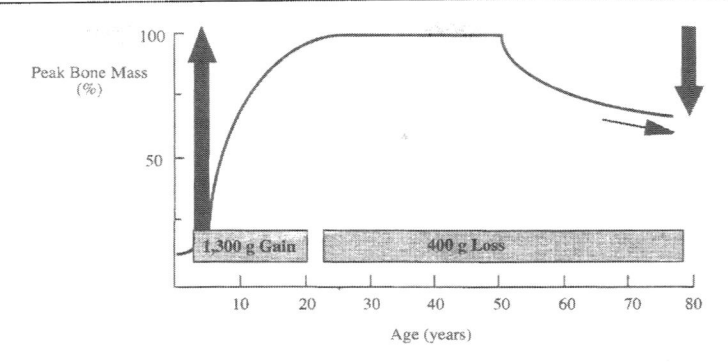

Fig. 1. The 1300 g of calcium that is accrued during growth is approximately three times the age-related loss (~400 g) and is several times more rapid (adapted from ref. *44*).

was reported to be achieved between 28 and 30 yr of age *(34)*. Although the change in bone density was determined over approx 3-1/2 yr, the results were extrapolated and expressed as a rate of change per decade: therefore, the estimated increases of 4.8% at the forearm, 5.9% at the lumbar spine, and 12.5% for total body bone mass in the third decade may be overestimated.

There is also debate about how long peak bone mass is maintained before bone loss begins. Bone loss may occur from the femoral neck and spine shortly after peak bone density has been achieved. Matkovic et al. reported that the bone density of the proximal femur was about 15% lower in older premenopausal women compared to younger premenopausal women *(31)*. This decline appeared to occur shortly after peak bone density had been achieved, since maximal values were found in 17-yr-old females. However, Bonjour et al. reported that at the spine adolescents (aged 14–19 yr; $n = 24$) had 10% higher trabecular bone density than young adults (25 to 35 yr; $n = 24$) *(26)*.

Not all studies report a statistically significant decline in bone density with age during the premenopausal period *(34,37,38)*. The maintenance of bone mass in the lumbar spine and femoral neck has been reported in longitudinal studies in the fourth decade *(32,37)*. The inconsistency reported in the literature might be a reflection of cross-sectional and short-term prospective studies predicting long-term changes in bone mass. Individual variation within the cohorts may also explain these conflicting results. This individual variation in the rate of change and direction of change in bone mass was highlighted by Mazess and Barden *(32)*, who reported that there was no detectable relationship between age and bone mass in a large group of subjects aged 20–39 yr. However, 63 subjects decreased spine bone density by more than 2%, whereas 100 subjects showed change of <2% in either the positive or negative direction and a further 68 subjects gained more than 2% *(32)*.

In summary, there is consensus that the majority of bone mass is accrued during the pre- and peri-pubertal years and that bone mass continues to be accrued at a slower rate in the postpubertal years. There is still no consensus about when peak bone mass is achieved and how long it is maintained. There is consensus, however, that the skeleton should not be considered as a single functioning entity. Rather, the timing of the attainment of peak bone mass and bone loss are site-specific phenomena, which also vary between individuals. This heterogeneity between individuals is likely to be the result of the interaction between genetic and environmental determinants influencing the attainment of peak bone mass.

The Genetic Determinants of Peak Bone Mass

There is a wide normal range in peak bone density. The variance in peak lumbar spine bone density is ± 20% of the mean *(1)*. Twin and family studies have shown that 60–90% of the variation in bone density between individuals is genetically determined *(39–41)*. In large family studies that included investigation of both genetic and environmental influences, there was a greater influence of shared genetics than shared environment *(42,43)*. It has also been found that the genetic effect may be greater at the lumbar spine (up to 90%) than the femoral neck (up to 70%) *(44)*.

A finding that is clinically important is that premenopausal women with a maternal family history of osteoporosis have low bone density *(45)* and perimenopausal women with a family history of hip fracture also have low bone density *(46)*. This familial association may also be site-specific; for instance, daughters of mothers with hip fractures had low bone density at the hip, whereas daughters of mothers with spine fractures had low bone density at the spine *(44,47)*. These results support the notion that low peak bone density may be a more important contributor to the low bone density reported in patients with fracture than age-related bone loss *(1)*. It is often accepted that similarities between mothers and daughters are through common genes, but within families, environmental factors, such as nutrition and habitual exercise, may also be very similar and, if not accounted, for may lead to an overestimate of the genetic effect on bone density. Twin studies account in part for a common environment. A higher correlation reported between monozygotic twins than dizygotic twins for spine bone density supports the finding of a strong genetic effect on bone density *(48,49)*.

The genes that are responsible for regulating bone density have not been identified *(50)*. It has been suggested that there are likely to be multiple genes with small effects rather than a few genes with large effects *(51)*, and that those influencing peak bone mass may be independent of those influencing the rate of postmenopausal bone loss *(52)*. Most of the studies attempting to identify genes related to osteoporosis have taken the approach of assessing candidate genes that are likely to be associated with bone, rather than searching the entire genome for alleles that are shared by affected persons *(53)*. Relatively early studies indicated that allelic variation in the vitamin D receptor gene (VDR) may account for a proportion of the genetic variance *(54)*, but these findings have not been consistently reproduced *(55–58)*. A recent study of 143 members of 7 families who had a high proportion of osteopoenic family members suggests that a single gene may be regulating bone mass and that it is not the VDR gene *(59)*. Several genes that may regulate bone density, either independently or in combination, are the estrogen receptor, calcitonin, transforming growth factor β, interleukin-6, $β_3$-adrenergic receptor, and collagen type I (COLIA1 and COLIA2) *(50,53)*.

Although a large proportion of the variance in bone density may be genetically determined, environmental factors also account for a clinically important proportion of the variance *(60)*. These influences may not be independent, since it has been suggested that there is a common genetic control of both muscle mass and bone mass that may also be influenced by exercise *(61)*. This interaction of genetic and environmental determinants of bone density has recently been reviewed *(61,62)*.

EXERCISE AND BONE MASS IN ADULT PREMENOPAUSAL WOMEN

The Osteotrophic Effect of Exercise in Adult Premenopausal Women

The above discussion highlights the large variance in bone density between individuals and the fact that a large proportion of this variance is genetically determined. Therefore, the effect of exercise on bone mass in young adult women may be less important than previously thought. This issue can be investigated by comparing the bone density of subjects with differing levels of habitual physical activity. Early studies supported the role of exercise in the improvement of bone mass. For instance, there were large bilateral differences between the dominant and nondominant arms in tennis players *(63–65)*. The reported bilateral differences in competitive club players were between 8 and 13%, and even larger differences were reported in the professional players. These data seemed to imply that the effects of regular exercise on bone density could be considerable. However, cross-sectional data of mature athletes do not give an indication of whether the adaptation occurred in childhood or adulthood. Therefore, to investigate the effects of exercise on adult bone mass, a longitudinal approach is required.

The effect of aerobic exercise on bone density in the adult has been extensively reviewed, and the following consensus has been reached: early cross-sectional studies were confounded by sampling bias and led to the belief that exercise in the adult could lead to large increases in bone density (up to 20%). In contrast, intervention studies tended to show mixed results ranging from small increases (2–3%) to no change or even bone loss *(66–68)*.

The osteotrophic effect of weight training has also been extensively investigated. The rationale for weight training having a greater osteotrophic effect than a jogging or walking program was that weight training places a greater load on the skeleton. There have been inconsistent results from weight training studies ranging from 4 to 24 mo *(69–73)*. Some of these studies reported small, but statistically significant changes of 1–2%; others showed no change in bone mass or bone loss (Fig. 2). Snow-Harter et al. conducted an 8-mo intervention trial on a group of 31 healthy premenopausal women (mean age 20 yr) who were randomly assigned to either a control group or progressive training in either jogging or weight training *(73)*. There were small, but statistically significant increases in lumbar spine bone density in the runners and weight trainers compared to the controls who did not change (1.3 ± 1.6% and 1.2 ± 1.8% mean ± SD for runners and weight trainers, respectively, relative to their own baseline, compared with a statistically insignificant decline of –0.8% in controls). No significant changes were reported in any group for the femoral neck. Friedlander et al. *(69)* reported that the change in lumbar spine bone density after 2 yr of aerobics and weight training in adult women (aged 28 yr) was similar to that found by Snow-Harter et al. *(73)* after 8 mo (1.3%), indicating the possibility of a plateau in the adaptation to exercise. The femoral neck increased by 0.5 ± 0.5% with weight training in this study, and this was significantly different from a group of women who only did stretching exercises and who lost 1.9 ± 1.0% ($p < 0.05$). Less encouraging results have been reported in slightly older premenopausal women in response to weight training. Gleeson et al. reported that women aged 30–40 yr gained only 0.8% lumbar spine bone density (not significant) after 12 mo of weight training *(70)*. Similar results were reported by Lohman et al. after 18 mo of weight training *(71)*. In some cases, weight training was associated with bone loss: Rockwell et al. reported a

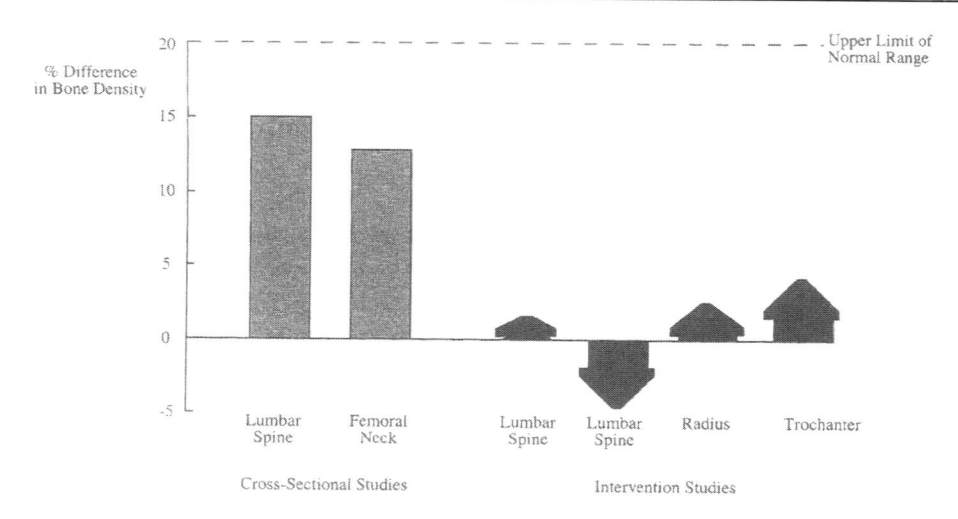

Fig. 2. The results of cross-sectional studies show that adult athletes participating in high-impact sports have high lumbar spine and femoral neck bone density compared with healthy nonactive controls. In contrast, intervention studies in adults show that high-impact exercise results in very small gains, or even losses, in bone density. This suggests that selection bias, lifetime sports participation, or a combination of both may have influenced the results of cross-sectional studies. Data presented is a representation of the results of several studies *(72–74,78,79)*.

4% loss in lumbar spine bone density and no gain in femoral neck bone mass over 1 yr of training *(72)*.

The osteotrophic effect on the skeleton of high- and low-impact loading has also been investigated. Kerr et al. randomized 56 subjects to a high- or low-impact exercise group *(74)*. Only one side of the body was loaded, so each individual acted as her own control. The low-impact, high-repetition group completed 3 × 20 repetitions and the high-impact, low-repetition group completed 3 × 8 repetitions. Both groups exercised 3x/wk for 12 mo. Increases were found in the high-impact, low-repetition group at the trochanter (1.7 ± 4.1 vs –0.1 ± 2.1% exercise and control respectively, $p < 0.05$), Wards triangle (2.3 ± 4.0 vs 0.8 ± 5.2%, $p < 0.05$), and ultradistal radial site (2.4 ± 4.3% vs –1.4 ± 2.3%, $p < 0.01$). There was no increase at the femoral neck or other radial sites. There were no changes at any site (relative to baseline) in the low-impact, high-repetition group except at the midradius (0.1 ± 1.4 vs –1.0 ± 2.3%, exercise and controls respectively, $p < 0.01$).

Bassey and Ramsdale also reported similar results in their high-impact exercise intervention study *(75)*. Premenopausal women were randomized into high-impact or low-impact exercise classes for 6 mo. The high-impact group did intermittent brief bouts of high-impact exercise (jumping and skipping) that accounted for 5–10% of their exercise class. In addition, this group jumped (double footed) on average 33 times/d; this was equivalent to the ground force of twice the body weight. The control group participated in low-impact aerobics and completed approx 20 wall pushes at home. The high-impact group showed an increase at only one site (3.4% at the trochanter, $p < 0.01$), whereas the control showed no change at any site. There was a trend for change at the femoral neck between the test and control groups ($p < 0.06$), but there was no change at the spine, Wards triangle, or the radius. In both groups, leg extensor power, coordination, and balance increased significantly (~10–15%). Of particular interest was that at the end of the test period, the control group crossed over to the high-impact exercise regimen. After a further 6 mo, they had increased their bone mass at the trochanter by a similar amount compared with the initial exercise group (4%).

Sports where impact loading is high may also lead to increased bone density *(76,77)*. Higher bone density has been reported in athletes who play volleyball and basketball *(78)*, and in college gymnasts *(79,80)*. Volleyball and basketball players had 11 and 7% higher lumbar spine bone density than nonathletes, whereas calcaneal density was 21 and 29% higher, respectively. College gymnasts had lumbar spine bone density 8% higher and femoral neck bone density 15% higher than sedentary controls. These results suggest that high-impact loading can lead to greater increases in bone density during adulthood than any other form of exercise. Although this may be the case, it should be remembered that first the results could be affected by selection bias, and second, it cannot be determined from these studies what proportion of these benefits was gained from exercise during childhood and adolescence, and what proportion was gained from exercise in adulthood.

In summary, the participation of premenopausal women in exercise regimes, such as aerobic training, weight training, or high-impact exercise, is likely to lead to small increases in bone density (up to 3%). The greatest osteotrophic response appeared to be associated with the high-impact exercise regimens. Not all studies, however, resulted in increased bone density. In some instances, there was no detectable osteotrophic effect, and at times there was bone loss. Standard deviations two to five times greater than the mean indicate that there is also considerable variation in the individual response within each cohort. This suggests that within a group, some individuals may have a greater osteotrophic response from the same loading regime than others, and this should be investigated in future studies.

The clinical relevance of exercise in the prevention of osteoporosis lies in the reduction of fracture risk late in life. It is generally accepted that a 10% increase in bone density is associated with halving the risk of femoral neck fracture *(81,82)*. Moderate exercise of any type in adulthood is unlikely to result in large increases in bone mass, and limited evidence suggests that the benefits are not maintained once the exercise program has stopped *(68,83)*. The role of exercise during adulthood in the prevention of osteoporosis should not, however, be dismissed. A long-term commitment to an active lifestyle, including exercise that places a mechanical load on the skeleton, through the pre-, peri-, and postmenopausal years may help reduce fracture risk by reducing bone loss and indirectly by reducing the risk of falling by improving muscular strength, coordination, and balance.

The Effect of Menstrual Irregularity on Bone Density

Hypogonadism is an important "risk factor" for osteoporosis. The rapid loss of bone mass following menopause illustrates that normal levels of circulating estrogen play an important role in maintenance of adult bone density. Indeed, low estrogen status at any age will result in rapid bone loss, as has been reported in patients with early oophorectomy *(84)* or anorexia-induced amenorrhea *(85–87)*. Athletic amenorrhea was considered to be less overtly pathological because of the reversibility of this condition. However, research in the mid-1980s and subsequent research confirmed the long-term risk of osteopoenia associated with athletic amenorrhea *(88–94)*.

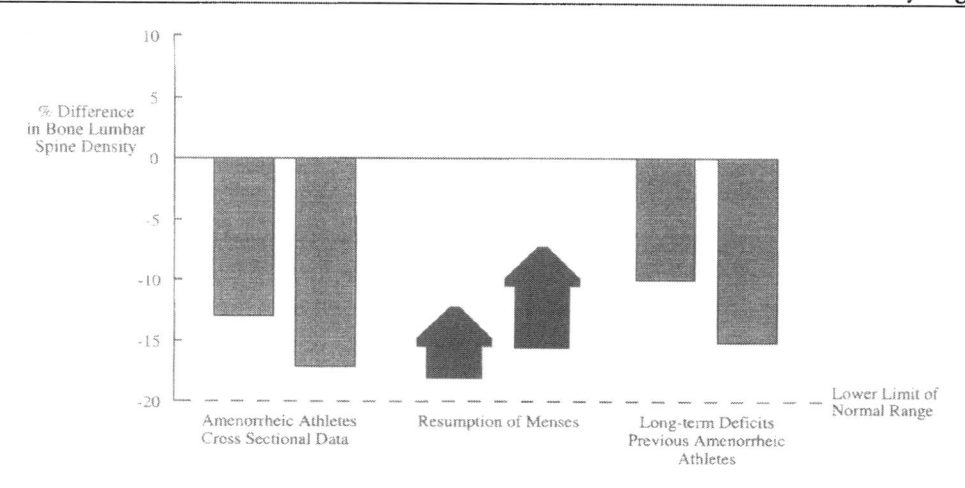

Fig. 3. Relative to eumenorrheic athletic controls, current amenorrheic athletes have very low lumbar spine bone density. This low bone density is the result of the hypoestrogenic state associated with amenorrhea. The gains in lumbar spine bone density immediately following resumption of menses are significant. However, long-term studies show that despite the resumption of menses, for up to 10 yr the remaining deficits are still substantial (a partial influence of genetic predisposition to low bone density in these athletes should not be excluded). Data presented is a representation of the results of several studies *(37,89,91,96,113,122)*.

The reduced bone density reported in athletes with amenorrheic could be caused by either a failure to gain bone mass, bone loss, or a combination of both. Insufficient gain in bone mass may occur in athletes with primary amenorrhea, whereas bone loss occurs in athletes with secondary amenorrhea. The decrements in bone density are seen relative to both sedentary peers and eumenorrheic athletic controls *(95–98)*. The skeletal site most affected by menstrual dysfunction is the lumbar spine, a site containing a large proportion of trabecular bone *(90,91,99–101)*. The deficit in bone density relative to eumenorrheic athletes has been reported to be as high as 20% (Fig. 3) *(91)*. Up to 4% of trabecular bone can be lost in the first year of secondary amenorrhea, and bone loss has been reported to continue for at least 2 yr *(102)*. The mechanism for bone loss is thought to be owing to increased bone resorption in response to the decrease in circulating estrogen associated with amenorrhea.

It has been reported that oligomenorrhea is also associated with low bone density *(94,103,104)*, despite no episodes of amenorrhea *(94)*. There appears to be a relationship between bone density and the severity of current and previous menstrual history expressed either by category *(105)*, the estimated number of cycles per year since menses *(106)*, or the number of cycles per year since age 13 yr *(94)*. This is also likely to be a result of lower circulating estrogen, even though levels may not be as low as in postmenopausal or frankly amenorrheic women. It has also been suggested that more subtle hormonal disturbances may affect bone mass, even when menses is regular. It has been reported that women with more than one short luteal phase per year or anovulatory cycles may lose bone mass owing to decreased progesterone secretion *(107,108)*. Despite these results, the role of progesterone in the maintenance of bone density remains controversial. There are reports that progesterone does not influence bone loss, and others suggest that the contribution of a concurrent decrease in estrogen cannot been excluded as the cause of bone loss *(109,110)*. De Souza et al. followed exercising women for 3 mo and reported that luteal-phase insufficiency was associated with decreased progesterone, but not decreased bone density, whereas reduced estrogen production in the follicular phase, despite regular menses, was associated with lower bone density *(110)*.

Athletes who participate in sports requiring leanness have a higher incidence of menstrual irregularities *(111)*, as do athletes who began to train strenuously before menarche *(112)*, who had a delayed age of menarche *(95,98)*, and who have the most intense training regimens *(113)*. Other risk factors include vegetarianism, increased stress, and a history of menstrual irregularity prior to beginning exercise training *(114)*. The effect of these risk factors on menstrual irregularity seems to be cumulative, since athletes with three or more risk factors have the highest incidence of menstrual irregularity *(113)*.

Although osteoporotic fractures are a distant event that may occur in old age, the immediate negative effect for athletes is a higher incidence of stress fractures. Low bone density has been associated with an increased risk of stress and nontraumatic fractures in athletes *(115–118)*. The results of a cross-sectional study has shown that athletes with stress fractures had lower bone density than athletes who have never had a bone injury *(116)*. Bennell et al. conducted a 12-mo prospective study of 46 female track and field athletes, 10 of whom sustained a stress fracture during the study period *(119)*. The female stress fracture group had lower total body bone mass and lumbar spine and foot bone density. In a subgroup of athletes who had tibial stress fracture, the tibia–fibula bone density on the injured side was on average 8.1% lower than the nonfracture group ($p < 0.01$). Of interest was that although the stress fracture group had lower bone density than the nonfracture group, their lower limb bone density was still higher than age-matched controls.

Can Exercise Offset Bone Loss Associated with Menstrual Dysfunction?

Numerous studies have shown that amenorrheic athletes have lower bone density at the spine, a predominantly trabecular site, and either high or normal bone density at the weight-bearing sites. A popular explanation for this trend is that exercise may offset the negative effects of amenorrhea at the weight-bearing sites. This may not be the case, however, because first, trabecular sites are more at risk of early bone loss (because of the large surface area), and cortical sites, later bone loss. Second, the bone density of the weight-bearing sites is likely to be higher than the nonweight-bearing sites (because of previous loading) before exposure to estrogen deficiency occurred.

In support of this notion, Pearce et al. reported lower bone density at the weight bearing sites in ballet dancers with longer time periods of oligomenorrhea *(120)*. In this cross-sectional study, bone density was correlated negatively with the duration of menstrual irregularity at the weight-bearing and nonweight-bearing sites. The dancers were divided into those with menstrual irregularity <40 mo (<40) and those with menstrual irregularity >40 mo (>40). The bone density of dancers <40 was higher than controls at the weight-bearing sites, and normal at the nonweight-bearing sites. In contrast, the bone density of the dancers >40 was normal at the weight-bearing sites and low at the nonweight-bearing sites. Therefore, the data suggest that the bone density at the nonweight-bearing sites was normal and became lower, whereas the bone density at the weight-bearing sites started high and became normal as the duration of hypogonadism increased.

It has also been suggested that more high-impact exercise may offer protection from menstrual irregularity at the weight-bearing sites. In a group of figure skaters with a substantial history of menstrual irregularity, bone density was only enhanced in the lower limbs, and not in the lumbar spine *(121)*, but Robinson et al. reported that gymnasts had higher bone density at all sites compared with runners who had a similar incidence of menstrual dysfunction (20 and 23% higher at the lumbar spine and femoral neck in the gymnasts compared to runners respectively) *(79)*. It is possible, however, that the gymnasts' higher bone density was not owing to a protective effect of exercise during the time period of menstrual irregularity, but rather may have been the result of exercise loading prior to the exposure of estrogen deficiency. Only longitudinal studies can clarify these issues.

The Effect of Menses Resumption on Bone Density in Previously Amenorrheic Athletes

Bone loss occurs with the hypoestrogenic state of athletic amenorrhea, but is bone gained when menses returns? Gains in lumbar spine bone density (6–7%/yr) have been shown in the year or two immediately following resumption of menses in previously amenorrheic athletes (Fig. 3) *(89,90)*. These gains, however, did not appear to be sufficient to eliminate or ameliorate the original deficits in bone density compared with eumenorrheic athletes. Others reported that the bone density of amenorrheic runners whose menses returned after lifestyle changes increased by about 6% in the first year and 3% in the second year, with no further increase in the third year. The bone density of these athletes was still below the controls at the end of 3 yr *(102)*. A more long-term study investigated changes in bone density over a period of between 3 and 5 yr in subjects with a prior history of menstrual irregularity who had been menstruating regularly for 11.7 ± 7.9 yr at follow-up *(37)*. Subjects were between 29 and 46 yr of age and, therefore, somewhat older than those in the previous studies. Despite these longer periods of time following resumption of menses, lumbar spine bone density did not appear to be fully restored. There was still a 14% deficit in lumbar spine bone density of the runners with prior oligo/amenorrhea relative to their sedentary controls. Keen and Drinkwater have also reported that despite 6–10 yr of either normal menses and/or use of oral contraceptives, former oligo/amenorrheic athletes (38 ± 1.6 yr of age) continued to have low bone density at the lumbar spine (–15%) compared to athletic controls who had always menstruated *(122)*. These data suggest that there is irreversible bone loss in athletes with former menstrual irregularity (Fig. 3). It should be kept in mind, however, that this notion relies on the assumption that the amenorrheic athletes had "normal" bone density before menstrual irregularity occurred. A cohort design is required to address this question accurately, where normally menstruating athletes become amenorrheic and then regain menses. This study is unlikely to be conducted, since it has been recommended that treatment of amenorrhea must be initiated early, perhaps within the first 2 yr, to prevent or reverse the associated bone loss *(88)*.

One possible treatment for athletic amenorrhea is hormone replacement therapy in the form of oral contraceptives. The effectiveness of hormonal therapies in the treatment of athletic amenorrhea is unknown. To date, there have been only one retrospective clinical study and one randomized clinical trial investigating the effect of estrogen replacement therapy and oral contraceptive use on bone density in young women with hypothalamic amenorrhea. Cummings et al. reported that estrogen replacement therapy for 24–30 mo increased vertebral and femoral neck bone density by 8 ± 1.2 and 4.1 ± 0.3%, respectively, in 8 amenorrheic runners *(123)*. In contrast, five amenorrheic runners who did not agree to take estrogen replacement therapy experienced nonsignificant decreases of <2.5% in bone density at both sites. Hergenroeder et al. investigated the effect of 12 mo of oral contraceptives, medroxy-progesterone, or placebo on bone density in 15 amenorrheic women aged 14–28 yr *(85)*. Four of the subjects had a current diagnosis of anorexia nervosa or bulimia, and one subject in each group did not exercise. The subjects randomized to oral contraceptives were younger than those randomized to medroxy-progesterone and placebo (18.8 ± 3.0, 20.3 ± 4.4, and 21.3 ± 5.2 respectively). Twelve months of oral contraceptive use led to a significant increase in bone density at the lumbar spine, but not the femoral neck (5.4 and 3.7%, respectively). The increase in lumbar spine bone density was independent of gain in body mass. After 12 mo, changes in bone density were not statistically significant for the medroxy-progesterone or placebo group (lumbar spine: –10.2 and –0.7%, respectively, and femoral neck: +4.2% and –3.4%, respectively). The results of these studies suggest that either estrogen replacement therapy or oral contraceptive use may be effective in increasing lumbar spine bone density and femoral neck bone density, although the latter may only be significant after at least 2 yr. Further studies are needed to confirm these results, since the sample sizes were small and, in the study by Hergenroeder et al. *(85)*, the subject sample was not homogenous (athletes and patients with eating disorders).

The above discussion highlights the negative effects of menstrual dysfunction on bone density. Therefore, attention should be paid to identifying athletes at risk of amenorrhea and then planning training loads and ensuring energy intakes are appropriate to expenditure to ensure normal menstrual function. It is recommended that athletes with amenorrhea be monitored for bone loss and early intervention be considered *(85,122)*.

THE OSTEOTROPHIC EFFECT OF EXERCISE DURING GROWTH

Childhood and adolescence are times when the skeleton undergoes rapid change owing to the processes of modeling and remodeling, which result in large gains in bone mass. The results of several studies have indicated that exercise training during growth may lead to large increases in bone density. These include large bilateral differences reported in the arms of young tennis and squash players *(124,125)*, higher bone density in athletes involved in high-impact sports during childhood and adolescence *(126,127)*, investigations that have reported a positive relationship between bone density and exercise during growth *(128–134)*, and the results of an exercise intervention study *(135)*. The reported increases in bone density in these studies ranged from 10 to 30%. If these benefits were maintained into adulthood, they would halve the risk of fracture.

Bone shape is also associated with bone strength *(2)*; however, there are no prevention strategies specifically targeted toward changing bone geometry to improve its biomechanical strength. The results of animal studies indicate that physical loading on immature bones altered bone shape and resulted in a stronger bone *(136–139)*. There are only limited retrospective data and no prospective data on the effect of exercise during growth on bone geometry in humans *(64,65,137)*. It is unknown whether exercise during growth has a role in the prevention of osteoporosis by changing bone geometry, but it is an issue that is currently being investigated. This section will review how exercise during growth may lead to increased peak bone density and greater bone strength.

The Osteotrophic Effects of Intense Training on the Immature Skeleton

The first studies to show that large increases in bone density may be achieved during growth were unilateral loading studies. The strength of these studies is that the nondominant limb controls for genetic determinants of bone density. That is, in unilateral sports, such as tennis, when the dominant and nondominant arms are compared in the same person, the "bilateral" differences that occur can be assumed to be environmental. Early studies using X-rays of the radius and humerus of tennis players revealed that men and women who had been involved in "lifetime tennis" had 28–35% greater cortical thickness and higher bone mass in their playing arm compared to the nonplaying arm *(64,65)*. More recently, Kannus et al. reported approx 9% greater bilateral differences (compared to controls) in the upper limbs of national level female tennis and squash players aged 27.7 ± 11.4 yr who had been training for 10 ± 6 yr *(125)*. After adjusting for height and age, the bilateral difference in bone mass was two to four times higher in those players who had started training before or at menarche (10–23%), compared to those who started more than 15 yr after menarche (2–9%) (Fig. 4). The results of these retrospective studies support the notion that training and playing tennis and squash before menarche may result in large increases in bone mass of the dominant arm. It is unknown whether the same increases occur at the femoral neck and lumbar spine with similar loading. The higher bone mass of elite prepubertal gymnasts suggests that this may be the case *(126,127)*.

Dyson et al. reported greater areal bone density at the femoral neck (8%) and trochanter (16%) in prepubertal gymnasts (aged 7–11 yr) who were training on average 18 h/wk *(127)*. Bone mineral apparent density was also higher in the gymnasts at the femoral neck (20%) and lumbar spine (8%). Volumetric bone density and bone cross-sectional areas were measured by QCT at the left distal radius. Volumetric bone density was greater at the distal radius: total (20%), cortical (16%), and trabecular (27%). There was a trend for the gymnasts to have a greater distal radial total bone cross-sectional area (unadjusted for the gymnasts shorter stature), but there were no differences in the proportion of trabecular or cortical bone distribution between the two groups. Bass et al. also reported that despite a smaller stature the bone density of elite prepubertal gymnasts was 10–30% higher than prepubertal controls matched for bone age *(126)*. Similar to the findings of Dyson et al. *(127)*, the greatest differences were found in the arms, a weight-bearing site in gymnastics. Further, the relative increase in areal bone density at the spine, femur, and arms was positively correlated with increasing years of training ($r = 0.3$–0.4, $p < 0.05$). The gymnasts also had higher volumetric bone mineral density at the lumbar spine and midfemoral shaft. The longitudinal data supported these cross-sectional observations. Over a 12-mo period, the areal bone density increased by 30–85% more in the prepubertal gymnasts compared to their age- and pubertal-matched controls (0.050 vs 0.027, 0.057 vs 0.043, and 0.020 vs 0.012 g/cm^2/yr: spine, legs, and arms for gymnasts and controls, respectively). Volumetric bone density also increased in the gymnasts and remained constant in the controls.

Selection bias is unlikely to explain a large proportion of the higher bone density reported in the gymnasts for several reasons. First, in both studies, the increase in bone density was site-specific to the loading patterns unique to gymnastics—the largest differences were found in the arms. Second, Bass et al. *(126)* reported that the surfeit in bone mass of the gymnasts increased with the increasing duration of training, with the

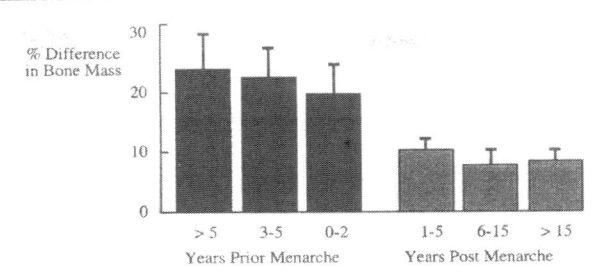

Fig. 4. The bilateral differences in bone mass at the humerus were two to four times higher in squash and tennis players who had started training before menarche than in those who had started up to 15 yr after menarche. Bars represent 95% CI's (adapted from ref. *125*).

regression line passing through zero. Third, the longitudinal data reported by Bass et al. *(126)* support the cross-sectional results, and finally, Dyson et al. *(127)* reported that there was no difference in bone density between the mothers of the gymnasts and controls.

Does Intense Training in Childhood Confer Benefits in Bone Density in Adulthood?

Although great osteotrophic gains may be made from intense exercise during growth, the clinical relevance lies in these benefits being maintained into adulthood and later life when osteoporotic fractures occur. To address this question accurately, a long-term exercise intervention study or a cohort study following active and nonactive children into adulthood is required. The long time interval between exposure and outcome makes these types of studies difficult to conduct. In the interim, researchers have looked toward retired athletes who began their training during childhood.

The osteotrophic benefits of intense exercise during childhood appear to be maintained into adulthood, as shown by the site-specific high bone density in retired gymnasts *(126)*. Despite reduced physical activity in retirement, bone density was 1–1.5 SD higher in the retired gymnasts at the weight-bearing sites, but normal at the nonweight-bearing sites compared to age-matched controls. Of particular interest is that the retired gymnasts (25.0 ± 0.9 yr) had a lower areal bone density (adjusted for age) compared to the active prepubertal gymnasts (bone aged 9.0 ± 0.2 yr) (Fig. 5) in the arms, but not the legs or spine. The reasons for this are uncertain, but may have been owing to one or a combination of factors. First, gymnastics training one to two decades ago was less intense, so the retired gymnasts may have attained a lower peak bone density compared to the current elite gymnasts. Second, the gymnasts may have experienced some bone loss early in retirement. This would have a greater effect on the arms than other weight-bearing sites, because the arms do not bear weight in everyday activities. This trend for retired athletes to have site-specific surfeits in bone density related to the unique loading patterns associated with training in childhood and adolescence has also been reported in tennis players *(64,65)*, gymnasts *(140,141)*, soccer players *(142)*, and weight lifters *(143,144)*.

Moderate Physical Activity and Bone Density in Active Nonathletic Children

The results of the aforementioned studies support the notion that long-term training during growth results in clinically important increases in bone density with benefits being preserved into adulthood. This provides a model of what is possible in competitive

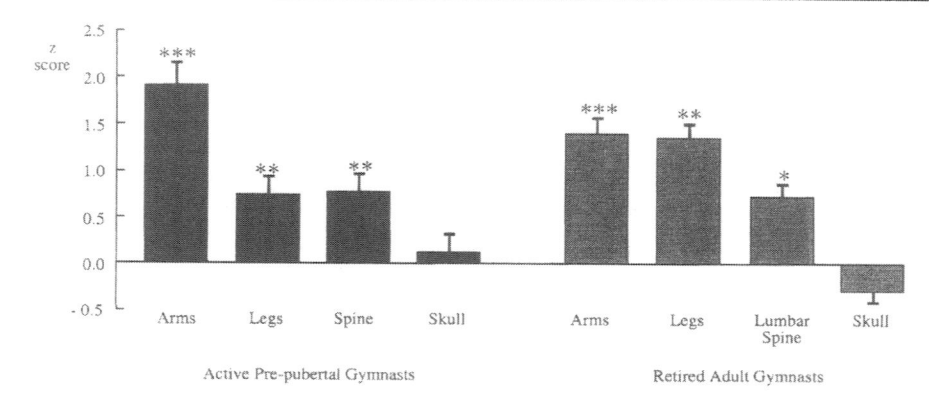

Fig. 5. Cross-sectional data showing regional areal bone density expressed as a standard deviation score (z score) in active prepubertal and retired adult gymnasts. The z scores were higher than zero (the predicted mean value in controls) at each site, except the skull. These site-specific surfeits in bone density are consistent with the loading patterns associated with gymnastic training. The lower surfeit in the arms of retired gymnasts (compared to the active prepubertal gymnasts) is likely to be the result of either a less vigorous training schedule and/or bone loss associated with retirement at a site that is not generally loaded in everyday living (adapted from ref. *126*). *$p < 0.05$, **$p < 0.01$, ***$p < 0.001$ compared to zero.

athletes and not what is probable in active nonathletic children. Nevertheless, the results of cross-sectional and cohort studies have reported a positive relationship between moderate exercise and bone density in active nonathletic children *(128–134)*.

Slemenda et al. reported that physical activity was a significant predictor of bone density at the femoral neck in prepubertal boys and girls, but not in either the peri- or postpubertal children *(132)*. Gunnes and Lehman reported similar results in forearm measurements in girls and boys (aged 8.5–17.0 yr) during 1 yr of observation *(130)*. They found weight-bearing exercise accounted for 5–16% of the variance in the change in bone density depending on the site, age, and gender. Exercise predicted the gain in bone density in prepubertal as well as adolescent boys, and was the best predictor of change in ultradistal radius bone density in girls younger than 11 yr. There was no detectable correlation found between exercise and bone density increments in adolescent girls. The mean gain in bone density was 14–128% higher in active compared to sedentary subjects. Of interest was that calcium intake was not correlated with change in bone density. However, exercise was a stronger predictor of the change in bone density when adjusted for calcium intake.

Several long-term cohort studies have investigated the associations between bone density in adulthood and lifestyle factors in childhood and adolescence. Welten et al. followed a group of males and females longitudinally for 15 yr from 13 yr of age *(134)*. In both genders, exercise was a predictor for adult bone density in the age periods of 13–17 yr, 13–21 yr, and the total period 13–27 yr. Cooper et al. also investigated the relationship between bone density in adulthood and lifestyle factors in late childhood and early adulthood *(128)*. Among the lifestyle factors, the strongest association was with exercise, and the effect was more apparent at the femoral neck than the lumbar spine, and stronger for bone density than for bone mass. Women in the highest activity category had 12% higher bone density at the femoral neck than women in the lowest activity category. Femoral neck bone density in the women in the moderate activity category was 7% higher than the least active group.

The results of these prospective and retrospective studies support the hypothesis that exercise during childhood increases bone density with benefits being maintained into adulthood. These results, however, may be biased, since children who have a larger musculoskeletal mass may be more likely to participate in physical activity. Intervention studies that are required to confirm this hypothesis are currently being conducted, but few have been published. Morris et al. conducted a 10-mo exercise program structured into the school curriculum for prepubertal girls (aged 9–10 yr). The bone density increased more in the exercise group compared with controls at the legs, arms, lumbar spine, and femoral neck *(135)*. There was an increase in volumetric bone density (BMAD) at the lumbar spine, but not at the femoral neck. Since there was a 13% increase in the femoral neck bone area, this suggests that the bone size and mass increased proportionally at this site in contrast to the lumbar spine, where there was either a disproportionately larger increase in bone mass compared with bone volume or an increase in bone mass of the spinous processes.

Is There a Stage of Growth When Exercise Will Result in the Greatest Osteotrophic Response?

It has been well documented that large osteotrophic benefits can be achieved through exercise during childhood and adolescence. It is unkown, however, if there is an "optimal" time during growth and maturation when exercise results in the greatest osteotrophic response. The investigation of this question is important for the development of pediatric exercise prescription programs for the prevention of osteoporosis later in life. This question is difficult to address for several reasons. First, the development of the skeleton is characterized by differing temporal patterns of growth in bone size and bone mass within a site, and between sites *(23)*. Further, unique biological phases that are linked to hormonal regulation divide the entire growth process into three additive and partly superimposed components: infancy, childhood, and puberty *(145)*. Growth hormone is responsible for growth during childhood (prepubertal growth, Tanner stage I), provided thyroid function is normal. However, growth during puberty (Tanner stage II to Tanner stage V) is related to growth hormone and sex steroids *(146–148)*. Therefore, before accurate comparisons can be made about the osteotrophic effects of exercise during growth, subjects must be matched by gender, ethnicity, age (bone and chronological age), stage of maturation, and growth velocity of the axial and appendicular skeleton.

Second, it is difficult to equate the relative mechanical load placed on skeletons of different sizes, such as that of an infant, child, or adolescent. Should the comparison incorporate a larger load on a larger skeleton? How should the relative increase in mass, length, or width be reported? A percentage increase is confounded by the different baseline measures. If measures are reported as areal densities, it will be impossible to distinguish whether the change was owing to an increase in mass or size. Further, how can a relative osteotrophic comparison be made with a 6-yr-old who grows on average five 5 cm/yr *(145,149)* and an 11-yr-old who may be growing up to 8–9 cm/yr *(149,150)*? This is made even more complex by the different temporal patterns of growth in bone size and bone mass at the axial and appendicular skeleton at different phases of growth *(23,150,151)*.

There are few data in the literature that address this complex question. Puberty is often reported to be the ideal time for exercise to result in the greatest osteotrophic response. The biological basis for this hypothesis is that puberty is the time in life of rapid skeletal growth and greatest mineral accrual—up to 50% in females (23,152). Bone turnover increases and reaches a lifetime peak, which coincides with the increasing secretions of sex steroids and growth hormone (23,148). It has been hypothesized that mechanical loading may enhance bone formation in a synergistic fashion in the presence of estrogen (124). As reported earlier (in the Osteotrophic Effects of Intense Training on the Immature Skeleton section), the bilateral difference in arm bone mass of tennis and squash players was two to four times higher in those players who had started training before or at menarche compared to those who started 15 yr after menarche (125). This group has also recently reported that the osteotrophic effect may be greatest during a relatively short period in puberty (124). Analysis of pre-, peri-, and postpubertal female tennis players (aged 7–17 yr) showed that bilateral differences in bone density of the arms of the players did not start to differ from controls until Tanner stage III. Haapasalo et al. (124) suggest that this demonstrates that the osteotrophic effect of exercise may be accentuated in the later stages of pubertal development. This observation is supported by bone physiology: the later stage of puberty is the only time in a female's life when bone is added in substantial amounts at the periosteal and endocortical surfaces (23,153). However, the players in these different phases of maturation were not matched for starting age of playing, number of training sessions per week, session length, years of training, or total training hours. Total training hours in the Tanner V group were more than fourfold greater than the Tanner I group (1131 vs 272 hours Tanner V and I, respectively), whereas the total training hours in the Tanner III group were 2.7-fold greater than the Tanner I group (744 vs 272 h Tanner III and I, respectively). Training intensity, the variable most likely to influence the osteotrophic response, was not reported. Haapasalo et al. (124) rationalize that these differences in training variables did not affect their interpretation of the results, because there was a large range in the training variables within every Tanner stage, but the correlation analysis was not significant between any training variable and bilateral differences in Tanner stages I or II. Also, there was a greater osteotrophic response in girls in Tanner III, IV, and V who had similar training histories to girls in Tanner I and II.

In another study, Khan et al. reported a significant correlation between hip bone density in retired ballet dancers (aged 51.4 yr) and the weekly hours of ballet training during the ages of 10–12 yr (154). This association persisted when the data were expressed as either absolute differences or as a standardized score. There was no detectable association between bone mass and weekly hours of ballet training at any other age younger or older than 10–12 yr. Surprisingly, there was no association between ballet training at each menarcheal age (years before or after menarche) and hip bone density. Khan et al. (154) suggest that there may be several reasons for this. First, there was a wide range of ages at menarche in the dancers (10–17 yr). Combining girls with similar menarcheal status would result in differences of up to 7 yr in chronological age, and therefore the hormone levels may not be comparable. Second, menarche is a late event in pubertal maturation and may not be as strongly associated with bone mass accrual (152) as earlier pubertal events, such as the early rise in estrogen (155), adrenarche, and peak growth hormone levels (156). Third, bone mass accrual at the femoral neck may not be as strongly influenced by maturation status as bone mass accrual at the lumbar spine (132).

In contrast, Bass et al. *(126)* hypothesized that the prepubertal years may be a uniquely opportune stage of growth during which the skeleton is responsive to exercise. There is also a sound biological basis for this hypothesis. First, growth is growth hormone-dependent and exercise is a potent stimulus for growth hormone secretion *(157,158)*; second, the prepubertal years are relatively sex hormone-independent. This may be an advantage, since the intensity of exercise needed to have an anabolic effect on bone mass may be similar to the intensity associated with interference with sex hormone cyclicity and a delay in pubertal maturation. Large increases in bone density have been reported in elite prepubertal gymnasts *(126,127)*, and positive associations with moderate exercise and bone density have been reported in prepubertal girls, but not pubertal girls *(130,132)*.

Comparing the relative responsiveness of the skeleton to physical loading during different stages of growth and maturation is difficult as has been highlighted by the conflicting results of the limited data available. Despite this conflict, it is generally accepted that large increases in bone density can be achieved from exercise in the pre- and peripubertal years, a time when the skeleton undergoes rapid change owing to the processes of modeling and remodeling. The results of studies conducted in postpubertal adolescents and young adults suggest that the osteotrophic response has already been tempered *(79,80,159)*.

The Effect of Physical Loading During Growth on Bone Geometry and Bone Strength

The majority of studies that have investigated the effect of exercise on bone strength and the risk of fracture have used bone density as the outcome measure. However, changes in bone geometric structure and internal architecture may significantly affect bone strength with or without significant changes in bone density *(160,161)*. Very little is known about the bone surface-specific effects of physical loading on bone geometry in humans. Further, it is unknown whether changes in bone geometry that occur during childhood are maintained into adulthood. The results of animal studies show that exercise during growth may alter bone geometry and result in a biomechanically stronger bone *(68,162–164)*. Mechanical loading in young rats during the growing period was associated with an increased cortical thickness and longitudinal curvature. In contrast, no consistent differences were detected from physical loading in mature animals *(163,164)*. Bone formation rate in rat tibia was also reported to be more responsive to exercise in the growing skeleton compared with the mature skeleton.

The limited data on the effects of physical loading on bone geometry in humans are from X-rays taken of the dominant arm in tennis players *(64,65)*. The pattern of humeral hypertrophy was different among the players. Some showed an increase in all cortical dimensions, as well as in the periosteal circumference. Others had a narrowed medullary cavity, but some had an enlarged periosteal and endocortical diameter. It has been hypothesized that the characteristics of the cortical dimensions—periosteal and endocortical diameters, and the cross-sectional bone shape—may have been determined by the time in life when the players began their training.

It has been suggested that mechanical loading increases bone apposition at the surfaces when there is a state of net formation. During childhood, there is net formation on the periosteal surface and net resorption on the endocortical surface. In contrast, from midpuberty to adulthood, the predominant site of apposition is at the endocortical surface. The periosteal surface undergoes minimal net formation *(23,153)*. Therefore, it is hypothesized that exercise during childhood and early in puberty will result in an increase in periosteal, but not endocortical apposition. Late in puberty and after menarche, however, the predominant effect of exercise may be an increase in endocortical apposition. This hypothesis of a differential response on the endocortical and periosteal surface to exercise has been based on one small retrospective study *(137)*. In support of this hypothesis, Margulies et al. reported that exercise resulted in endocortical apposition in young adults. Fourteen weeks of military training in 18- to 21-yr-old males resulted in an increase in areal bone density without a change in bone width *(165)*. Further, Dyson et al. reported that prepubertal gymnasts tended to have a larger cross-sectional area of the forearm despite a smaller stature *(127)*. In contrast, Bass et al. reported that prepubertal gymnasts increased their volumetric bone density at the midfemoral shaft owing to endocortical narrowing, not periosteal expansion as expected *(126)*.

The results from studies of animals also support the notion of maturity-dependent preferential change in cortical surfaces with mechanical loading *(138,163)*. Younger animals showed greater periosteal expansion, whereas older animals showed greater medullary cavity narrowing. Animal studies of reduced mechanical loading through limb immobilization or weightlessness also show preferential changes at the cortical surfaces. Younger animals show a greater periosteal response (inhibition of bone formation), whereas older animals showed a greater endocortical response (increased resorption) *(136–139)*.

Although these data support the concept of a maturity-dependent apposition on the periosteal and endocortical surfaces, the differing distribution of the load on the bone surface makes the analysis of this hypothesis more complex. For instance, a bone reacts differently when it is stretched (tensile strains) or compressed (compressive strains). When a bone is bent or curved, the concave side of the bone is subjected to compressive stresses, but the convex side to tensile stresses. At some point between the two surfaces, the strains are zero. This is referred to as the neutral axis *(166)*. Therefore, when a bone is loaded, the distribution of the load will be different depending on whether the surface is being subjected to tensile or compressive strains. The load placed on the periosteal surfaces will be greater than the loads placed on the endocortical surface because of the distance each surface is from the neutral point. The greatest stress will occur at the concave surface where there is the combination of the compressive stresses from axial loading and the compressive stresses from bending *(166)*.

There is a need for carefully planned longitudinal studies into the effects of exercise during growth, in particular, the surface-specific and geometric-specific effects of exercise during different stages of development. It is not known if the effect of mechanical loading on periosteal diameter may be more significant earlier in development. Greater gains in mechanical strength are achieved by periosteal expansion compared to endocortical contraction, since a greater periosteal diameter increases load-bearing capacity, because the moment of inertia increases as a function of the diameter to the power of 10^4. Other measures of bone strength that are also increased by a greater periosteal diameter and not by smaller endocortical diameter are the section modulus and the strength index *(166,167)*.

CONCLUSION

For exercise to have a role in the prevention of osteoporosis, the osteotrophic response must be large enough to be considered clinically important, and the surfeits gained from exercise must be maintained into adulthood and later in life when fractures occur. Large increases in bone density (up to 30%) have been reported in children and adolescents involved in exercise training. It is unknown whether these surfeits are maintained into adulthood, since there has been no long-term exercise intervention study following children or adolescents into adulthood. The site-specific higher bone density related to unique loading patterns reported in retired athletes supports the notion that large osteotrophic benefits from exercise training during childhood and adolescence can be maintained into adulthood, and are large enough to halve the risk of fracture. From a public health perspective, information is needed on what is probable in healthy nonathletic children rather than what is possible in an athlete. The results of many retrospective and limited prospective studies support the notion that moderate weight-bearing exercise in nonathletic children is associated with higher bone density in adulthood.

Exercise during the growing years may also reduce the risk of osteoporotic fracture by changing bone geometry and increasing the biomechanical strength of bone. It has been hypothesized that exercise during growth increases periosteal expansion, whereas the predominant response to exercise in the adult is increased endocortical contraction. Greater gains in mechanical strength are achieved by periosteal expansion (compared to endocortical contraction), because the load-bearing capacity of the bone increases as a function of the cross-sectional diameter to the power of 10^4. Longitudinal prospective studies are required to confirm this hypothesis.

To emphasize the importance of exercise during childhood and adolescence is not to deny its importance later in life. The former is concerned mainly with acquisition and the latter mainly with conservation of bone *(168)*. Exercise in premenopausal women is especially important considering that the adult skeleton is much more responsive to the adverse effects of unloading than to the beneficial effects of overloading *(168)*. Exercise may not always be beneficial, however, especially if it is associated with the development of amenorrhea or oligomenorrhea, which may lead to large deficits in bone density (up to 20%). Recent evidence has also shown that even long-term resumption of regular menses has failed to restore these deficits. The utility of exercise to offer protection or restore bone mass in amenorrheic athletes appears to be limited, and alternative measures for bone gain must be investigated and promoted.

In summary, exercise has an important role in increasing peak bone mass and bone strength during the growing years and maintaining bone mass in the premenopausal years. These findings support the development of public health campaigns that promote weight-bearing exercise in girls, teenagers, and young women, and highlight the importance of regular menstrual function.

REFERENCES

1. Seeman E. Osteoporosis: a public health problem. In: Marcus R, Feldman D, Kelsey J, eds. Osteoporos. Academic, California, 1996, pp. 25–40.
2. Marcus R. Clinical review 76: The nature of osteoporosis. J Clin Endocinol Metab 1996;81(1):1–5.
3. Melton LJI. Hip fractures: a worldwide problem today and tomorrow. Bone 1993;14(Suppl):1–8.
4. Mosekilde L, Mosekilde L, Danielsen CC. Biomechanical competence of vertebral trabecular bone in relation to ash density and age in normal individuals. Bone 1987;8:79–85.
5. Carter DR, Bouxsein ML, Marcus R. New approaches for interpreting projected bone densitometry data. J Bone Miner Res 1992;7:137–145.
6. Seeman E. Growth in bone mass and size: are racial and gender differences in bone density more apparent than real? J Clin Endocrinol Metab 1998;83:1–6.

7. Lu PW, Cowell CT, Lloyd-Jones SA, Broidy J, Howman-Giles R. Volumetric bone mineral density in normal subjects, aged 5–27 years. J Clin Endocrinol Metab 1996;81:1586–1590.
8. Cowell CT, Lu PW, Lloyd-Jones SA, Briody JN, Allen JR, Humphries JR, et al. Volumetric bone mineral density—a potential role in paediatrics. Acta Paediatr Suppl 1995;411:12–16.
9. Dunnill MS, Anderson JA, Whitehead R. Quantitative histological studies on age changes in bone. J Pathol Bacteriol 1967;94:275–291.
10. Kroger H, Kotaniemi A, Vainio P, Alhava E. Bone densitometry of the spine and femur in children by dual-energy X-ray absorptiometry. Bone Miner 1992;17:75–85.
11. Schonau E, Wentzlik U, Dietrich M, Scheidhauer K, Klein K. Is there an increase in bone density in children? Lancet 1993;342(September 11):689,690.
12. Trotter M, Hixon BB. Sequential changes in weight, density, and percentage ash weight of human skeletons from an early fetal period through old age. Anat Rec 1974;179:1–8.
13. Baron R. Anatomy and ultrastructure of bone. In: Favus MJ, eds. Primer on Metabolic Bone Diseases and Disorders of Mineral Metabolism, American Society for Bone and Mineral Research, California, 1990, pp. 3–7.
14. Burr D, Schaffler M, Yang KH, Lukoschek M, Sivaneri N, Biaha JD, et al. Skeletal change in response to altered strain environments: Is woven bone a response to elevated strain? Bone 1989;10:223–233.
15. Frost HM. Perspectives: the role of changes in mechanical usage set points in the pathogenesis of osteoporosis. J Bone Miner Res 1992;7:253–262.
16. Myers ER, Sebeny EA, Hecker AT, Corcoran TA, Hipp JA, Greenspan SL, et al. Correlations between photon absorbtion properties and failure load of the distal radius in vitro. Calcif Tissue Int 1991;49:292–297.
17. Garn S, Rohmannn C, Wagner B, Ascoli W. Continuing bone growth throughout life: a general phenomenon. Am J Phys Anthropol 1967;26:313–318.
18. Ruff C, Hayes W. Subperiosteal expansion and cortical remodeling of the human femur and tibia with aging. Science 1982;217:945–947.
19. Bouxsein ML, Myburgh KH, van der Meulen MCH, Lindenberger E, Marcus R. Age-related differences in cross-sectional geometry of the forearm bones in healthy women. Calcif Tissue Int 1994;54:113–118.
20. Garn SM, Wagner B. The Adolescent Growth of the Skeletal Mass and Its Implications to Mineral Requirements. Appleton-Century-Crofts, New York, 1969.
21. Mazess RB, Cameron JR. Skeletal growth in school children: Maturation and bone mass. Am J Phys Anthropol 1971;35:399–408.
22. Blimkie CJR, Chilibeck PD, Davison KS. Bone mineralization patterns: reproductive endocrine, calcium, and physical acivity influences during the life span. In: Perspectives in Exercise Science and Sports Medicine. Bar-Or D, Lamb D, Clarkson P, eds. Cooper Publishing Group, Carnel, IN, 1996; pp. 73–145.
23. Bass S, Delmas PD, Pearce G, Hendrich E, Tabensky A, Seeman E. The differing tempo of growth in size, mass and density in girls is region specific. J Clin Invest 1999;104:795–804.
24. Gordon C, Halton J, Atkinson S, Webber C. The contribution of growth and puberty to peak bone mass. Growth Dev Aging 1991;55:257–262.
25. Faulkner RA, Bailey DA, Drinkwater DT, Wilkinson AA, Houston CS, McKay HA. Regional and total body bone mineral content, bone mineral density, and total body tissue composition in children 8–16 years of age. Calcif Tissue Int 1993;53:7–12.
26. Bonjour JP, Theinz G, Buchs B, Slosman D, Rizzoli R. Critical years and stages of puberty for spinal and femoral bone mass accumulation during adolescence. J Clin Endocriol Metab 1991;73:555–563.
27. Geusens P, Cantatore F, Nijs J, Proesmans W, Emma F, Dequeker J. Heterogeneity of growth of bone in children at the spine, radius and total skeleton. Growth Dev Aging 1991;55:249–256.
28. Gilsanz V, Gibbens DT, Carlson M, Boechat MI, Cann CE, Schulz EE. Peak trabecular vertebral density: Comparison of adolescent and adult females. Calcif Tissue Int 1988;43:260–262.
29. Theintz G, Buchs B, Rizzoli R, Sloman D, Clavien H, Sizonenko P, et al. Longitudinal monitoring of bone mass accumulation in healthy adolescents: Evidence for a marked reduction after 16 years of age at the levels of the lumbar spine and femoral neck in female subjects. J Clin Endocrinol Metab 1992;75(4):1060–1065.
30. Teegarden D, Proulx WR, Martin BR, Zhao J, McCabe GP, Lyle RM, et al. Peak bone mass in young women. J Bone Miner Res 1995;10(5):711–715.

31. Matkovic V, Jelic T, Wardlaw GM, Ilich JZ, Goel PK, Wright JK, et al. Timing of peak bone mass in caucasian females and its implications for the prevention of osteoporosis. J Clin Invest 1994;93: 799–808.
32. Mazess RB, Barden HS. Bone density in premenopausal women: effects of age, dietary intake, physical activity, smoking, and birth-control pills. Am J Clin Nutr 1991;53:132–142.
33. Rodin A, Murby B, Smith MA, Caleffi M, Fentiman I, Chapman MC, et al. Premenopausal bone loss in the lumbar spine and neck of femur: a study of 225 Caucasian women. Bone 1990;211:1–5.
34. Recker RR, Davies K, Hinders SH, Heaney RP, Stegman MR, Kimmel DB. Bone gain in young adult women. JAMA 1992;268:2403–2408.
35. Parsons TJ, Prentice A, Smith EA, Cole TJ, Compston JE. Bone mineral mass consolidation in young british adults. J Bone Miner Res 1996;11(2):264–274.
36. Bennell KL, Malcolm SA, Khan KM, Thomas SA, Reid SJ, Brukner PD, et al. Bone mass and bone turnover in power athletes, endurance athletes, and controls: A 12-month longitudinal study. Bone 1997;20:477–484.
37. Micklesfield LK, Reyneke L, Fataar A, Myburgh KH. Long-term restoration of deficits in bone mineral density is inadequate in premenopausal women with prior menstrual irregularity. Clin J Sports Med, 1998;8:155–163.
38. Szejnfeld VL, Salomao CE, Baracat EC, Atra E, De Lima GR. Age and loss of bone density in premenopausal women. Revista. Paulista de Medicina 1993;111:289–293.
39. Peacock M. Vitamin D receptor alleles and osteoporosis: a contrasting view. J Bone Miner Res 1995;10:1294–1297.
40. Eisman JA. Vitamin D receptor gene alleles and osteoporosis: an affirmative view. J Bone Miner Res 1995;10:1289–1293.
41. Lutz J. Bone mineral, serum calcium, and dietary intakes of mother/daughter pairs. Am J Clin Nutr 1986;44:99–106.
42. Jouanny P, Guillemin F, Kuntz C, Jeandel C, Pourel J. Environmental and genetic factors affecting bone mass. Similarity of bone density among members of healthy families. Arthritis Rheum 1995;38(1):61–67.
43. Krall EA, Dawson-Hughes B. Heritable and life-style determinants of bone mineral density. J Bone Miner Res 1993;8(1):1–9.
44. Seeman E. Reduced bone density in women with fractures: contribution of low peak bone density and rapid bone loss. Osteoporos Int 1994;Suppl 1:S15–S25.
45. Armamento-Villareal R, Villareal DT, Aviolo LV, Civitelli R. Estrogen status and heredity are major determinants of premenopausal bone mass. J Clin Invest 1992;90:2464–2471.
46. Torgerson D, Campbell MK, Reid DM. Life-style, environmental and medical factors influencing peak bone mass in women. Br J Rheum 1995;34:620–624.
47. Seeman E, Hopper JL, Bach LA, Cooper ME, Parkinson E, McKay J, et al. Reduced bone mass in daughters of women with osteoporosis. N Eng J Med 1989;320(9):554–558.
48. Pocock NA, Eisman JA, Hopper JL, Yeates MG, Sambook PN, Eberl S. Genetic determinants of bone mass in adults: A twin study. J Clin Invest 1987;80:706–710.
49. Dequerker J, Nijs J, Verstraeten A, Guesens P, Gevers G. Genetic determinants of bone mineral content at the spine and radius: A twin study. Bone 1987;8:207–209.
50. Freenfield EM, Goldberg VM. Genetic determination of bone density. Lancet 1997;350: 1263,1264.
51. Gueguen R, Jouanny P, Guillemin F, Kuntz C, Pourel J, Siest G. Segregation analysis and variance components analysis and variance components analysis of bone mineral density in healthy families. J Bone Miner Res 1995;2:2017–2022.
52. Lutz J, Tesar R. Mother-daughter pairs: spinal and femoral bone densities and dietary intakes. Am J Clin Nutr 1990;52:872–877.
53. Ralston SH. The genetics of osteoporosis. Q J Med 1997;90:247–251.
54. Morrison NA, Qi JC, Tokita A, Kelly PJ, Crofts L, Nguyen TV, et al. Prediction of bone denisty from vitamin D receptor alleles. Nature 1994;367:284–287.
55. Houston LA, Grant SFA, Reid DM, Ralston SH. Vitamin D receptor polymorphism, bone mineral density, and osteoporotic vertebral fracture: studies in a UK population. Bone 1996;18:249–252.
56. Kobayashi S, Inoue S, Hosoi T, Ouchi Y, Shiraki M, Orimo H. Association of bone mineral density with polymorphism of the estrogen receptor gene. J Bone Miner Res 1996;11:306–311.

57. Lim SK, Park YS, Park JM, Song YD, Lee EJ, Kim KR, et al. Lack of association between vitamin D receptor genotypes and osteoporosis in koreans. J Clin Endocrinol Metab 1995;80(12):3677–3681.
58. Salamone LM, Ferrell R, Black DM, Palermo L, Epstein RS, Petro N, et al. The association between vitamin D receptor gene polymorphisms and bone mineral density at the spine, hip and whole-body in premenopausal women. Osteoporosis Int 1996;6:63–68.
59. Spotila LD, Caminis J, Devoto M, Shimoya K, Sereda L, Ott J, et al. Osteopenia in 37 members of seven families: analysis based on a model of dominant inheritance. Mol Med 1996;2:313–324.
60. Salamone LM, Glynne NW, Black DM, Ferrell RE, Palermo L, Epstein RS, et al. Determinants of premenopausal bone mineral density: the interplay of genetic and lifestyle factors. J Bone Miner Res 1996;11(10):1557–1565.
61. Parfitt AM. Genetic effects on bone mass and turnover-relevance to black/white differences. J Am Coll Nutr 1997;16(4):325–333.
62. Seeman E, Hopper JL. Genetic and environmental components of the population variance in bone density. Osteoporosis Int 1997;7(Suppl 3):S10–S16.
63. Montoye HJ, Smith EL, Fardon DF, Howley ET. Bone mineral in senior tennis players. Scand J Sports Sci 1980;2:26–32.
64. Jones HH, Priest JD, Hayes WC, Tichenor CC, Nagel DA. Humeral hypertrophy in response to exercise. J Bone Joint Surg 1977;59-A(2 March):204–208.
65. Huddleston A, Rockwell D, Kulund DN, Harrison B. Bone mass in lifetime tennis athletes. JAMA 1980;244(10):1107–1109.
66. Bouxsein ML, Marcus R. Overview of exercise and bone mass. Rheum Dis Clin North Am 1994;20 (3, August):787–802.
67. Drinkwater BL. Exercise in the prevention of osteoporosis. Osteoporos Int 1993;(Suppl 1):S169–S171.
68. Forwood M, Burr D. Physical activity and bone mass: exercises in futility? Bone Miner 1993;21:89–112.
69. Friedlander AL, Genant HK, Sadowsky S, Byl NN, Gluer C. A two-year program of aerobics and weight training enhances bone mineral density of young women. J Bone Miner Res 1995;10(4):574–585.
70. Glesson PB, Protas EJ, LeBlanc AD, Schneider VS, Evans HJ. Effects of weight lifting on bone mineral density in premenopausal women. J Bone Miner Res 1990;5(2):153–158.
71. Lohman T, Going S, Pamenter R, Hall M, Boyden T, Houtkooper L, et al. Effects of resistance training on regional and total bone mineral density in premenopausal women: a randomized prospective study. J Bone Miner Res 1995;10(7):1015–1024.
72. Rockwell JC, Sorensen AM, Baker S, Leahey D, Stock JL, Michaels J, et al. Weight training decreases vertebral bone density in premenopausal women: a prospective study. J Clin Endocrinol Metab 1990;71(4):988–992.
73. Snow-Harter C, Bouxsein JL, Lewis BT, Carter DR, Marcus R. Effects of resistance and endurance exercise on bone mineral status of young women: A randomized exercise intervention trial. J Bone Miner Res 1992;7(7):761–769.
74. Kerr DA, Morton A, Dick I, Prince RL. Exercise effects on bone mass in postmenopausal women are site specific and load-dependent. J Bone Miner Res 1996;11(2):218–225.
75. Bassey EJ, Ramsdale SJ. Increase in femoral bone density in young women following high-impact exercise. Osteoporosis Int 1994;4:72–75.
76. Dook JE, James C, Henderson NK, Price RI. Exercie and bone mineral density in mature female athletes. Med Sci Sports Exerc 1997;29(3):291–296.
77. Fehling PC, Alekel L, Clasey J, Rector A, Stillman RJ. A comparison of bone mineral densities among female athletes in impact loading and active loading sports. Bone 1995;17(3):205–210.
78. Risser WL, Lee EJ, Leblanc A, Poindexter GBW, Risser JMH, Schneider V. Bone density in eumenorrheic female college athletes. Med Sci Sports Exerc 1990;22(5):570–574.
79. Robinson TL, Snow-Harter C, Taaffee DR, Gills D, Shaw J, Marcus R. Gymnasts exhibit higher bone mass than runners espite similar prevalence of amenorrhea and oligomenorrhea. J Bone Miner Res 1995;10(1):26–35.
80. Taaffe DR, Robinson TL, Snow CM, Marcus R. High-Impact exercise promotes bone gain in well trained female athletes. J Bone Miner Res 1997;12(2):255–260.
81. Johnston GC, Slemenda CW, Melton LJ. Clinical use of bone densitometry. N Engl J Med 1991;324:1105–1109.

82. Cumming SR, Black DM, Nevitt MC, Browner W, Cauley J, Ensrud K, et al. Bone density at various sites for prediction of hip fracture. The study of osteoporotic fracture research group. Lancet 1993;341(April 10):962,963.
83. Vuori I, Heinonen A, Sievanen H, Kannus P, Pasanen M, Oja P. Effects of unilateral strength training and detraining on bone mineral density and content in young women: A study of mechanical loading and deloading on human bones. Calcif Tissue Int 1994;55:59–67.
84. Cann CE, Genant KH, Ettinger B, Gordan GS. Spinal mineral loss in oophorectomized women. JAMA 1981;244:2056–2059.
85. Hergenroeder AC, O'Brian Smith E, Shypailo R, Jones LA, Klish WJ, Ellis K. Bone mineral changes in young women with hypothalamic amenorrhea treated with oral contraceptives, medroxyprogesterone, or placebo over 12 months. Am J Obstet Gynecol 1997;176:1017–1025.
86. Bachrach LK, Guido D, Katzman D, Litt IF, Marcus R. Decreased bone density in adolescent girls with anorexia nervosa. Pediatrics 1990;86(3):440–447.
87. Seeman E, Szmukler G, Formica C, Tsalamandris C, Mestrovic R. Osteoporosis in anorexia nervosa: The influence of peak bone density, bone loss, oral contraception use, and exercise. J Bone Miner Res 1992;7:1467–1474.
88. Cann CE, Martin MC, Jaffe RB. Duration of amenorrhea effects rate of bone loss in women runners: Implication for therapy, abstracted. Med Sci Sports Exerc 1985;17:214.
89. Drinkwater B, Nilson K, Ott S, Chestnut CH III. Bone mineral density after resumption of menses in amenorrheic athletes. JAMA 1986;256(July 18):380–382.
90. Lindberg JS, Fears WB, Hunt MM. Exercise-induced ameorrhea and bone density. Ann Intern Med 1984;101:647,648.
91. Marcus R, Cann C, Madvig P, Minkoff J, Goddard M, Bayer M, et al. Menstrual function and bone mass in elite women distance runners: Endocrine metabolic features. Ann Intern Med 1985;102:158–163.
92. Rencken ML, Chestnut CH III, Drinkwater BL. Bone density at multiple skeletal sites in amenorrheic athletes. JAMA 1996;276(3):238–240.
93. Young N, Formica C, Szmukler G, Seeman E. Bone density at weight-bearing and nonweight-bearing sites in ballet dancers: The effects of exercise, hypogonadism, and body weight. J Clin Endocrinol Metab 1994;78:449–454.
94. Micklesfield LK, Lambert EV, Fataar AB, Noakes TD, Myburgh KH. Bone mineral density in mature, premenopausal, ultramarathon runners. Med Sci Sports Exerc 1995;27:688–696.
95. Rutherford OM. Spine and total body bone mineral density in amenorrheic endurance athletes. J Appl Physiol 1993;74:2904–2908.
96. Jonnavithula S, Warren MP, Fox RP, Lazaro MI. Bone density is compromised in amenorrheic women despite return of menses: a 2-year study. Obstet Gynecol 1993;81(5):669–674.
97. Halioua L, Anderson JJB. Lifetime calcium intake and physical activity habits: independent and combined effects on the radial bone of healthy premenopausal Caucasian women. Am J Clin Nutr 1989;49:534–541.
98. Warren MP, Brookes-Gunn J, Fox RP, Lancelot C, Newman D, Hamilton WG. Lack of bone accretion and amenorrhea: evidence for a relative osteopenia in weight-bearing bones. J Clin Endocrinol Metab 1991;72:847–853.
99. Cann CE, Martin MC, Genant HK, Jaffe RR. Decreased spinal mineral content in ameorrheic women. JAMA 1984;251:626–629.
100. Drinkwater B, Nilson K, Chestnut C, Bremner W, Shainholtz S, Southworth M. Bone mineral content of amenorrheic and eumenorrheic athletes. N Engl J Med 1984;311:277–281.
101. Linnell SI, Stager JM, Blue PW. Bone mineral content and menstrual regularity in female runners. Med Sci Sports Exerc 1984;16:343–348.
102. Otis CL. Exercise-associated amenorrhea. Clin Sports Med 1992;11(2):351–361.
103. Cook SD, Harding AF, Thomas KA, Morgan EL, Schnurpfeil KM, Haddad RJ. Trabecular bone density and menstrual function in women runners. Am J Sports Med 1987;15:503–507.
104. Lloyd T, Myers C, Buchanan JR, Demers LM. Collegiate women athletes with irregular menses during adolescence have decreased bone density. Obstet Gynecol 1988;72:639–642.
105. Drinkwater BL, Bruemner B, Chestnut CH III. Menstrual history as a determinant of current bone density in young athletes. JAMA 1990;263(4):545–548.
106. Grimston SK, Ensberg JR, Kloiber R. Menstrual, calcium, and training history: relationship to bone health in female runners. Clin Sports Med 1990;2:119–128.

107. Prior JC, Vigna YM, Schechter MT, Burgess AE. Spinal bone loss and ovulatory disturbances. N Engl J Med 1990;323(18):1221–1227.
108. Prior JC, Vigna YM, Barr SI, Rexworthy C, Lentle BC. Cyclic medroxyprogesterone treatment increases bone density: a controlled trial in active women with menstrual cycle disturbances. Am J Med 1994;96(June):521–530.
109. Waller K, Fenster L, Swann S, Windham G, Marcus R. Letters to the editor: An unsuccessful attempt to relate ovulatory disturbances to changes in bone density—authors response. JCE 1996; 81(11):4176–4179.
110. De Souza MJ, Miller BE, Sequenzia LC, Luciano AA, Ulreich S, Stier S, et al. Bone health is not affected by luteal phase abnormalities and decreased ovarian progesterone production in female runners. J Clin Endocrinol Metab 1997;82:2867–2876.
111. Rippon C, Noakes TD, Nash J. Abnormal eating attitudes—the best predictor of menstrual dysfunction in lean females. Int J Eating Disord 1988;7(5):617–624
112. Frisch RE, Gotz-Welbergen AV, McArthur JW, Albright T, Witschi J, Bullen B, et al. Delayed menarche and amenorrhea of college athletes in relation to age of onset of training. JAMA 1981;246(14):1559–1563.
113. Myburgh KH, Watkin VA, Noakes TD. Are risk factors for menstrual dysfunction cumulative? Phys Sports Med 1992;20:114–125.
114. Highet R. Athletic amenorrhea. An update on aetiology, complications and management. Sports Med 1989;7:82–108.
115. Lloyd T, Triantafyllou SJ, Baker ER, Houtes PS, Whiteside JA, Kalenak A, et al. Women athletes with menstrual irregularity have increased musculoskeletal injuries. Med Sci Sports Exerc 1986;18:374–379.
116. Mybugh KH, Hutchins J, Fataar AB, Hough SF, Noakes TD. Low bone density is an etiologic factor for stress fractures in athletes. Ann Int Med 1990;113:754–759.
117. Wilson JH, Wolman RL. Osteoporosis and fracture complications in an amenorrheic athlete: case study. Br J Rheumatol 1994;33:480,481.
118. Dugowson CE, Drinkwater BL, Clark JM. Nontraumatic femur fracture in an oligomenorrheic athlete. Med Sci Sports Exerc 1991;23(12):1323–1325.
119. Bennell KL, Malcolm SA, Thomas SA, Reid SJ, Brukner PD, Ebeling PR, et al. Risk factors for stress fractures in track and field athletes. Am J Sports Med 1996;24:810–817.
120. Pearce G, Bass S, Young N, Formica C, Seeman E. Does weight bearing exercise protect against the effects of exercise—induced oligomenorrhea on bone density? Osteoporosis Int 1996;6:448–452.
121. Slemenda C, Johnston C. High intensity activities in young women: site specific bone mass effects among female figure skaters. J Bone Miner 1993;20:125–132.
122. Keen AD, Drinkwater BL. Irreversible bone loss in former amenorrheic athletes. Osteoporosis Int 1997;7:311–315.
123. Cummings DC. Exercise-associated amenorrhea, low bone density, and estrogen replacement therapy. Arch Intern Med 1996;156:2193–2195.
124. Haapasalo H, Kannus P, Sievanen H, Pasanen M, Uusi-Rasi K, Heinonen A, et al. Effect of long-term unilateral activity on bone mineral density of female junior tennis players. J Bone Miner Res 1998;13(2):310–319.
125. Kannus P, Haapasalo H, Sankelo M, Sievanen H, Pasanen M, Heinonen A, et al. Effect of starting age of physical activity on bone mass in the dominant arm of tennis and squash players. Ann Intern Med 1995;123(1 July):27–31.
126. Bass S, Pearce G, Bradney M, Hendrick E, Delmas P, Harding A, et al. Exercise before puberty may confer residual benefits in bone density in adulthood: studies in active prepubertal and retired female gymnasts. J Bone Miner Res 1998;13(2):500–507.
127. Dyson K, Blimkie CJR, Davison S, Webber CE, Adachi JD. Gymnastic training and bone density in pre-adolescent females. Med Sci Sports Exerc 1997;29(4):443–450.
128. Cooper C, Cawley M, Bhalla A, Egger P, Ring F, Morton L, et al. Childhood growth, physical activity, and peak bone mass in women. J Bone Miner Res 1995;10(6):940–947.
129. Grimston SK, Willows ND, Hanley DA. Mechanical loading regime and its relationship to bone mineral density in children. Med Sci Sports Exerc 1993;25(11):1203–1210.
130. Gunnes M, Lehman EH. Physical activity and dietary constituents as predictors of forearm cortical and trabecular bone gain in healthy children and adolescents: a prosective study. Acta Paediatr 1996;85:19–25.

131. Slemenda CW, Miller JZ, Hui SL, Reister TK, Johnston CC. Role of physical activity in the development of skeletal mass in children. J Bone Miner Res 1991;6(11):1227–1333.
132. Slemenda CW, Reister TK, Hui SL, Miller JZ, Christian JC, Johnston CC. Influences of skeletal mineralization in children and adolescents: Evidence for varying effects of sexual maturation and physical activity. J Pediatr 1994;125(2):201–207.
133. Valimaki JM, Karkkainen M, Lamberg-Allardt C, Laitinen K, Alhava E, Heikkinen J, et al. Exercise, smoking, and calcium intake during adolescence and early adulthood as determinants of peak bone mass. Br Med J 1994;309:230–235.
134. Welten DC, Kemper HCG, Post GB, Van Mechelen W, Twisk J, Lips P, et al. Weight-bearing activity during youth is a more important factor for peak bone mass than calcium intake. J Bone Miner Res 1994;9(7):1089–1096.
135. Morris FL, Naughton GA, Gibbs JL, Carlson JS, Wark JD. Prospective ten-month exercise intervention in premenarchel girls: positive effects on bone and lean mass. J Bone Miner Res 1997;12(9):1453–1462.
136. Lanyon LE. Control of bone architecture by functional load bearing. J Bone Miner Res 1992;7(Suppl):S369–S375.
137. Ruff CB, Walker A, Trinkaus E. Postcranial robusticity in *Homo*. III: Ontogeny. Am J Phys Anthropol 1994;93:35–54.
138. Woo SLY, Kuei SC, Amiel D, Gomez MA, Hayes WC, White FC, et al. The effect of prolonged physical training on the properties of long bone: A study of Wolff's law. J Bone Joint Surg 1981;63A:780–787.
139. Wronski TJ, Morey ER. Effect of spaceflight on periosteal bone formation in rats. Am J Physiol (Regul Integrative Comp Physiol 13). 1983;244:R305–309.
140. Lindholm C, Hagenfeldt K, Ringertz H. Bone mineral content of young female former gymnasts. Acta Paediatr 1995;84:1109–1112.
141. Kirchner EM, Lewis RD, O'Connor P. Effect of past gymnastics participation on adult bone mass. J Appl Physiol 1996;80(1):226–232.
142. Duppe H, Gardsell P, Johnell O, Ornstein E. Bone mineral content in female junior, senior and former football players. Osteoporosis Int 1996;6:437–441.
143. Karlsson MK, Johnell O, Obrant KJ. Is bone mineral density advantage maintained long-term in previous weight lifters. Calcif Tissue Int 1995;57:325–328.
144. Karlsson MK, Hasserius R, Obrant KJ. Bone mineral density in athletes during and after career: a comparison between loaded and unloaded skeletal regions. Calcif Tissue Int. 1996;59:245–248.
145. Karlberg J. A biologically-oriented mathematical model (ICP) for human growth. Acta Paediatr 1989;Suppl 350:70–94.
146. Karlberg J. On the construction of the infancy-childhood-puberty growth standard. Acta Paediatr Scand 1989;Suppl 356:26–37.
147. Wollman HA, Ranke MB. GH treatment in neonates. Acta Paediatr 1996;85:398–400.
148. Bourguignon JP. Linear growth as a function of age at onset of puberty and sex steroid dosage: Therapeutic implications. Endocrinol Rev 1988;9(4):467–488.
149. Prader A. Pubertal growth. Acta Paediatr Jpn 1992;34:222–235.
150. Buckler JM. A Longitudinal Study of Adolescent Growth. Springer-Verlag, London, 1990.
151. Tanner JM. Growth at Adolescence, 2nd ed. Blackwell Scientific Publications and Springfield Thomas, London, 1962.
152. Bailey DA, Faulkner RA, McKay HA. Growth, physical activity and bone mineral acquisition. In: Holloszy JO, ed. Exercise and Sports Science Review. American College of Sports Medicine Series. Williams and Wilkins, Baltimore, 1996, pp. 233–266.
153. Garn S. The Earlier Gain and Later Loss of Cortical Bone. Charles C. Thomas, Spingfield, IL, 1970.
154. Khan KM, Bennell KL, Hopper JL, Flicker L, Nowson CA, Sherwin AJ, et al. Self-report ballet classes undertaken at age 10–12 years and hip bone mineral density in later life. Osteoporosis Int 1997;7:4–25.
155. Mauras N, Rogal AD, Veldhuis JD. Specific, time-dependent actions of low-dose ethinyl estradiol administration on the episodic release of GH, FSH and LH in prepubertal girls with Turner's syndrome. J Clin Endocrinol Metab 1989;69:1053–1058.
156. Malina RM, Bouchard C. Growth, Maturation and Physical Activity. Human Kinetics, Champaign, IL, 1991.

157. Borer KT. Exercise-Induced Facilitation of Pulsatile Growth Hormone (GH) Secretion and Somatic Growth. Serono Symposium from Raven Press Books Ltd., New York, 1989.
158. Eliakim A, Brasel JA, Mohan S, Barstow TJ, Berman N, Cooper DM. Physical fitness, endurance training, and the growth hormone-insulin like growth factor I system in adolescent females. J Clin Endocrinol Metab 1996;81(11):3986–3992.
159. Blimkie CJR, Rice S, Webber CE, Martin J, Levy D, Gordon CL. Effects of resistance training on bone mineral content and density in adolescent females. Can J Physiol Pharmacol 1996;74:1025–1033.
160. Smith EL, Gilligan C. Dose-response relationship between physical loading and mechanical competence of bone. Bone 1996;18(1):45S–50S.
161. Ammann P, Rizzoli R, Meyer JM, Bonjour JP. Bone density and shape as determinants of bone strength in IGF-I and/or Pamidronate-treated ovariectomized rats. Osteoporosis Int 1996;6:219–227.
162. Rubin CT. Suppression of the osteogenic response in the aging skeleton. Calcif Tissue Int 1992;50:305–313.
163. Steinberg ME, Trueta J. Effects of activity on bone growth and development in the rat. Clin Orthopaedics Rel Res 1981;156:52–60.
164. Lanyon LE. The influence of function on the development of bone curvature. An experimental study on the rat tibia. J Zool (Lond) 1980;192:457–466.
165. Margulies JY, Simkin A, Leichter I, Bivas A, Steinberg R, Giladi M, et al. Effect of intense physical activity on the bone-mineral content in the lower limbes of young adults. J Bone Jt Surg 1986;68-A (7, September):1090–1093.
166. Hayes WC, Gerhart TN. Biomechanics of bone: applications for assessment of bone strength. In: Peck WA, ed. Bone and Mineral Research. Elsevier Science Publishers, B.V., 1985, pp. 259–294.
167. Carter DR, van der Muelen CH, Beaupre GS. Skeletal development. Mechanical consequences of growth, aging and disease. In: Marcus R, Feldman D, Kelsey J, eds. Osteoporos. Academic, California, 1996, pp. 333–350.
168. Parfit M. The two faces of growth—benefits and risks to bone integrity. Osteoporosis Int 1994;4(6):382–398.

16 Interrelationships Between Acute and Chronic Exercise and the Immune and Endocrine Systems

Valéria M. Natale, MD
and Roy J. Shephard, MD, PhD, DPE

CONTENTS

> INTRODUCTION
> OVERVIEW OF THE IMMUNE SYSTEM
> THE IMMUNE SYSTEM AND ACUTE MUSCULAR EXERCISE
> PHYSICAL TRAINING
> CLINICAL APPLICATIONS
> CONCLUSIONS
> ACKNOWLEDGMENTS
> REFERENCES

INTRODUCTION

Exercise places a wide spectrum of demands on the body, depending on the form, intensity, and duration of the required effort, as superimposed on a background of physiological and psychological constraints peculiar to the host. Moreover, responses are modified by repetition of the exercise stimulus, giving rise to the typical training response.

Since 1893, when the first publication on exercise-induced leukocytosis was written by Schultz *(1)*, interrelationships between exercise and immune function have been widely studied and discussed. Several monographs now provide detailed reference sources *(2–4)*. An acute bout of exercise stimulates immune responses during the activity, but immune function is commonly subnormal for 2–24 h following a prolonged bout of endurance exercise. The ability of exercise to alter circulatory hemodynamics and thus homeostasis within the immune system is now well established *(5,6)*. Growing evidence also indicates that moderate exercise training can enhance resting immune responses, possibly decreasing susceptibility to viral infections of the respiratory tract *(7,8)*. In contrast, excessive training leads to immune suppression *(9–11)*, with an increased risk of illness.

From: *Contemporary Endocrinology: Sports Endocrinology*
Edited by: M. P. Warren and N. W. Constantini © Humana Press Inc., Totowa, NJ

Opinions vary regarding the mechanisms whereby exercise influences immune function. The current consensus is that exercise-induced immunomodulation is mediated by a complex interplay among hormones, cytokines, and neural and hematological factors. Possible underlying mechanisms include metabolic, physiological, and hormonal changes. Among potential metabolic and nutritional influences *(12)*, we may note the role of glutamine. The "glutamine hypothesis" *(13)* is grounded on two main facts: skeletal muscle provides an important reservoir of glutamine production and lymphocytes depend on glutamine for optimal growth. Thus, it has been hypothesized that plasma glutamine serves as a "metabolic link" between skeletal muscle and the immune system *(14)*. Plasma glutamine concentrations show a modest (15–20%) decline following sustained exercise *(15)*, particularly if it is pursued to the point of muscle glycogen depletion. It has therefore been suggested that during intense physical exercise, the demands on the muscle for glutamine exceed supply, so that the lymphoid system is forced into glutamine debt, with a temporary deterioration of its functional capacity *(14)*.

Vigorous exercise induces many physiological changes, including an increase of cardiac output and vascular shear forces and the secretion of stress hormones, but from the viewpoint of the immune system, the effects of the rise in core body temperature and local or general hypoxia may be of particular importance. A rise in body temperature also induces changes in circulating leukocyte counts that in many respects resemble those observed during exercise *(16–22)*. Acute hypoxia induces a recruitment of natural killer (NK) cells from reservoir sites to the circulating bloodstream *(23)*, possibly by increasing the secretion of catecholamines, and Kløkker et al. *(24)* have observed that the exercise-induced increases in NK cell activity is more pronounced during hypoxia than under normoxic conditions. Vigorous exercise does not induce a generalized decrease in arterial oxygen saturation, except in top-level athletes *(25)* and patients with chronic chest disease, but local hypoxia commonly arises from forceful contraction of muscles, obstructing local blood flow to the active limbs *(26)*.

Muscular exercise also increases the plasma concentrations of a number of stress hormones. Noradrenaline and adrenaline concentrations rise soon after the onset of exercise, and if the activity is sustained there are increases in cortisol, growth hormone, insulin, and β-endorphins. Associated microtrauma can increase plasma levels of prostaglandins, and these substances can have a substantial inhibitory influence on immune function.

The purpose of the present chapter is to discuss interrelationships among exercise, physical training, and the responses to these two stimuli observed in the neuroendocrine and immune systems. After making a brief survey of the immune system, we thus consider its responses to acute and chronic exercise, together with the contribution of hormonal factors to the observed changes. A concluding section discusses possible clinical applications of our current knowledge.

OVERVIEW OF THE IMMUNE SYSTEM

The immune system plays a major role in defending the integrity of the organism against foreign proteins and microorganisms, providing the essential basis of a discrimination between self and nonself or altered self. The immune system also makes a major contribution to homeostasis, and it provides important feedback loops running from the

Table 1
Cellular Components of the Immune System

Cells	Function
Innate	
NK cell (CD3⁻16⁺56⁺)	Lysis of virus-infected cells, tumor cells; antibody-dependent cellular cytotoxicity
Monocytes/macrophages	Phagocytosis; antigen presenting; cytokine secretion
Neutrophils	Phagocytosis; activation of bactericidal mechanisms
Eosinophils	Killing of antibody-coated parasites; inflammatory response
Basophils	Inflammatory response
Mast cells	Allergic response; inflammatory response
Adaptive	
T-cells (CD3⁺)	Antigen recognition; stimuli for B-cell growth and differentiation; macrophage and T-cytolytic activation
T-helper (CD4⁺)	by secreted cytokines; development of inflammation
T_{H1}	Macrophage activation; proinflammatory action; IL-1; IL-2, IFN-γ, and TNF-α secretion
T_{H2}	B-cell activation; anti-inflammatory action; IL-4, IL-5, IL-10 secretion
T-cytotoxic (CD8⁺)	Antibody-dependent cytotoxicity
T-suppressor (CD8⁺)	Downregulate the immune system
B-cells (CD19⁺)	Antibody production

[a]Cluster of differentiation (CD) markers are molecules of monoclonal antibodies (MAbs) that identify a given cell-surface molecule.
[b]Sources: refs. *28–30*.

working muscles to the secretory regions of the hypothalamus *(27)*. In this section, we offer a brief sketch of the immune system, its principal components, and its main functions.

The immune system comprises an intricate network of cells, hormones, and paracrine and autocrine mediators (*see* Tables 1 and 2). All of the cellular elements in the immune system arise initially from hematopoietic stem cells located in the bone marrow. These pluripotent cells divide to produce two more specialized types of stem cell: lymphoid stem cells (lymphoid progenitors, which give rise to T- and B-lymphocytes) and myeloid stem cells (myeloid progenitors, which give rise to the remaining categories of leukocyte). The T- and B-lymphocytes are distinguished by their site of differentiation; T-cells mature in the thymus, and B-cells in the bone marrow. They are also distinguished by their antigen receptors.

Leukocytes that are derived from the myeloid stem cells include the monocytes, and neutrophils, eosinophils, and basophils. The last three cell types are termed collectively polymorphonuclear leukocytes or granulocytes. The monocytes differentiate into macrophages; these are the main phagocytic cells of the immune system, which are to be found in muscle and other tissues. In contrast, neutrophils are the most important circulating phagocytic cells; they have functions similar to those of macrophages, but they

Table 2
Soluble Components of the Immune System

Components	Function[b]
Innate	
Major histocompatibility complex (MHC)	T-cells only recognize an antigen if bound to MHC
MHC class I	Present peptides to CD4+ cells
MHC class II	Present peptides to CD8+ cells
Complement	Opsonization, phagocytosis, cell lysis, and the removal of antibody/antigen complex
Lysozyme	Mechanism of defense against unencapsulated bacteria
Acute-phase proteins	Inflammatory response; complement activation; opsonization
Adhesion molecules	Role in margination of immune cells; facilitate interactions between cells and penetration of vascular endothelium
Adaptive	
Antibodies	Inflammatory response; immune memory
Cytokines[a]	Mediate natural immunity; regulate lymphocyte activation; regulate immune-mediated inflammation; stimulate the growth and differentiation of immature leukocytes

[a]Cytokines: interleukins, interferons, TNF, chemokines, hematopoietic growth factors.
[b]Sources: refs. *28–30*.

normally remain within the bloodstream. The eosinophils are blood-borne cells that are involved mainly in inflammation. Basophils are also found in the circulating blood; they are similar in some respects to mast cells, although they arise from a separate cell lineage. Mast cells also arise from precursor cells in bone marrow, but they complete their maturation within specific tissues; they are important to allergic responses.

There are two main classes of immune responses, innate or natural immunity and adaptive immunity. Innate or natural immunity is present from birth, and it includes numerous nonspecific defense mechanisms. Body surfaces, especially the skin, form the first line of defense against penetration by microorganisms. When these barriers are broken, the invading organisms encounter other elements of the innate immune system, cellular components (such as monocytes/macrophages, neutrophils, eosinophils, basophils, mast cells, and NK cells), along with soluble components (such as lysozyme, complement, acute-phase proteins, and α- and β-interferons).

The NK and lymphokine-activated killer (LAK) cells comprise a heterogeneous population of leukocytes that mediate the killing of a broad range of target cells. They are thought to play an important role in the first line of defense against acute and chronic virus infections and certain types of tumor cell, since they can exercise their functions without the intervention of major histocompatibility complex (MHC) class proteins. Nevertheless, their cytolytic activity is enhanced if T-cells are activated and plasma levels of interleukin 2 (IL-2) are increased.

If the innate immunity is overwhelmed, adaptive immune responses come into play, with the development of an inflammatory response. Adaptive responses are distinguished by a remarkable specificity against the offending agent and by a memory of previous responses to the same antigen. Mediators include cellular components (T- and B-lymphocytes) and soluble elements (antibodies and cytokines). Excessive inflammation can have serious negative consequences for health, either in its own right, or because of a secondary suppression of the immune system by counterregulatory cytokines. Clinical manifestations of excessive inflammation include bacterial penetration of the gut wall, sepsis, the respiratory distress syndrome, and the multiple-organ distress syndrome It is currently debated how far such reactions can account for the negative immunologic effects of prolonged and intense exercise *(31)*.

During an adaptive type of immune response, the antigen is initially taken up and processed by antigen-processing cells, primarily macrophages and related cells. Fragments of the ingested material become expressed as immunogenic epitopes, which are complexed on the surface of the antigen-presenting macrophage along with class II MHC molecules. The T-helper (T_H) cells bind with the macrophage through the action of certain adhesion molecules, recognizing characteristic features of both the epitope and the class II MHC molecule.

Activated T_H cells regulate the activities of other lymphocytes in a positive, cascade-like fashion through the secretion of soluble factors known collectively as lymphokines. One of these substances, IL-2, enhances the function of NK cells, and it also serves as an activating signal for a second class of T-cell, the T-cytotoxic (T_C) cell (which recognizes antigens expressed in the context of class I MHC molecules on the surface of target cells). Furthermore, the T_H cells furnish important growth and differentiation signals to B-cells, accelerating their proliferation and differentiation into antibody-secreting plasma cells.

The basis for memory in the immune response is the generation of antigen-specific T_H and B-cells following initial exposure to a given antigen. The memory cells have characteristic surface proteins, and they are prepared to make a more rapid and amplified response if they subsequently encounter the same antigen in a secondary, or anamnestic, response. T_C cells and antibodies use a variety of mechanisms to eliminate foreign antigens, some of which are integrally linked to the processes of inflammation and sepsis.

THE IMMUNE SYSTEM AND ACUTE MUSCULAR EXERCISE

Exercise induces an immediate leukocytosis, the magnitude of which is related to the intensity and duration of the activity that has been undertaken. The pattern of change in the leukocyte count postexercise is determined mainly by the time that has elapsed since the beginning of exercise, rather than by the intensity of effort or the total amount of work that has been performed.

The exercise-induced leukocytosis reflects increased numbers of circulating neutrophils, monocytes, and lymphocytes. The neutrophil count increases during exercise, and it continues to increase, sometimes for as long as several hours, following exercise *(6)*. During exercise, NK, T- and B-cells are all recruited to the circulating bloodstream, and there is an increase in the total lymphocyte count. However, the NK cell count increases more than the T-cell count, so that the CD3$^+$T cell percentage declines during exercise. The number of CD8$^+$ cells increase more than the number of CD4$^+$ cells, resulting in a decreased $CD4^+/CD8^+$ ratio *(32)*. Following long-duration exercise, the lymphocyte count decreases below its baseline level. The duration of this phase of immunosuppression depends on the intensity and duration of the exercise that has been undertaken *(33)*, but it generally seems of rather short duration to have any substantial clinical effect on resistance to either viral infections or tumor cells. The lymphocyte proliferative response per individual $CD4^+$ cell does not change substantially with exercise *(34)*.

Both the absolute cell count and the relative fraction of blood mononuclear cells (BMNC), which express characteristic NK cell-surface markers ($CD3 \cdot CD16^+CD56^+$) are markedly enhanced during physical exercise. The NK and LAK cell activities increase simultaneously, although there is at most only a small increase in lytic activity per fixed number of mononuclear cells. The intensity of exercise seems the prime determinant of the increase in NK cell count and activity during exercise, whereas the duration as well as the intensity of exercise determine if and to what extent a postexercise immunosuppression may occur *(35)*. NK and LAK cell activities are normally suppressed during the first few hours that follow a bout of intensive exercise, which lasts for 1 h or longer *(35)*.

The leukocytes carry receptors for various hormones, including catecholamines and cortisol. They are also capable of secreting hormones in their own right, as part of the feedback regulatory system. Catecholamine concentrations rise early during a bout of acute endurance exercise. Their secretion is associated with a mild leukocytosis, but a strong and rapid lymphocytosis. The lymphocytes are probably supplied from several storage sites, such as the spleen and the liver, together with the walls of high-endothelial venules *(36)*. The infusion of physiological doses of catecholamines can induce similar changes in cell counts to those seen during exercise *(37)*.

Cortisol concentrations increase in response to either high-intensity or prolonged submaximal exercise, particularly if the subject perceives the activity in question as stressful *(27)*. Cortisol can induce a leukocytosis. It promotes the entry of neutrophils into the circulation from bone marrow, while inhibiting the entry of lymphocytes and facilitating their egress to peripheral tissues and lymph nodes *(6,38,39)*. Thus, cortisol, which may remain elevated for at least 1.5 h following a prolonged period of endurance exercise *(38)*, reduces circulating lymphocyte numbers by encouraging their trafficking to peripheral tissues *(40)*. Cortisol also downregulates the IL-1 and IL-2 receptors on the T-cells. The immediate consequence of these actions is a reduction in both NK cell activity and the rate of B-cell proliferation *(41)*. In a more long-term perspective, a chronic elevation of cortisol levels increases the rate of catabolism, thus modifying the reserves of amino acids available for lymphocyte growth and proliferation *(14)*.

The effects of catecholamines probably predominate during and immediately following an acute bout of moderate exercise, explaining the large increase in number of circulating lymphocytes, but it is possible that cortisol plays a major role in maintaining a neutrophilia and lymphopenia following a prolonged period of intensive exercise.

Prostaglandin E_2 is secreted by macrophages in response to exercise-induced tissue injury. It depresses the proliferative response of peripheral blood mononuclear cells to mitogens, and decreases their IL-2 production *(42)*. The late suppression of NK cell activity following a bout of strenuous exercise can be largely abolished by administration of nonsteroidal anti-inflammatory drugs, such as indomethacin, which counter the effects of the prostaglandin *(43)*.

Table 3
Neuropeptides and Hormones That Influence Immune Function[a]

Neuropeptide or hormone	Effects on the immune system
Catecholamines	Via β-adrenoreceptors: induce leukocytosis
	May reduce endothelial adhesion of leukocytes to vessel walls
	Enhance the proliferation of $CD3^+$, $CD4^+$, and $CD8^+$ cells (by α-adrenergic stimulation)
	Inhibit the proliferation of $CD4^+$ and $CD8^+$ cells (by β-adrenergic stimulation)
	Inhibit the degranulation of mast cells and basophilic granulocytes
Cortisol	Enhance leukocyte liberation from bone marrow
	Mediate lymphocyte distribution
	Inhibit T-cell proliferation
	Inhibit IL-1, IL-2 production
	Enhance IL-4 production
β-Endorphin	Reduce phytohemagglutinin proliferation
	Promote NK cell activity
	Inhibit lymphocyte chemotactic factor
	May itself be a lymphocyte chemotactic factor
Growth Hormone	Promote T-cell generation

[a]Sources: Madden and Felten *(44)*, Shephard *(29)*, and Weicker and Werle *(45)*.

PHYSICAL TRAINING

Influence of Training on Immune and Endocrine Systems

There is a bilateral system of communication between the immune and neuroendocrine systems *(27)*. Hormones have significant effects on many aspects of immune function, including T-lymphocyte selection, splenic lymphocyte release, and the expression and secretion of intercellular mediators (*see* Table 3). Leukocytes also have both receptors for and the capacity to secrete a wide range of hormones *(44)*. Until now, around 20 different neuroendocrine peptides and/or their mRNAs have been identified in cells of the immune system. These peptides probably mediate autocrine and paracrine functions, and despite their rapid breakdown in vivo, it is possible that they have endocrine roles, regulating function elsewhere in both the immune and neuroendocrine systems. For example, T-lymphocytes can synthesize adrenocorticotrophic hormone (ACTH), endorphins, growth hormone, and others hormones *(46)*. Lymphocytes also have neural synapses *(47)*, and their function is modified by changes in sympathetic nerve activity *(48–50)*. Moreover, the various types of leukocyte all carry catecholamine receptors. Receptor densities are greater for B- and $CD8^+$ cells than for $CD4^+$ cells, and are still greater on NK cells *(36,51,52)*. However, the ranking of response to plasma-borne stimuli depends also on second messenger systems, which are poorly developed within the B-cells.

The immediate intercellular mediators between the various types of immune cell are called cytokines. These substances promote the regulation of immune and inflammatory responses, and they can exert a profound influence on neuroendocrine activity (*see*

Table 4
Effects of Cytokine Administration on the Concentrations
of Some Neuroendocrine Hormones in Blood[a]

Hormone	Cytokine	Blood	Author
ACTH	IL-1, IL-2, IL-6, TNF-α	∠ Concentration	Imura et al. (53), Turnbull and Rivier (54)
Corticosteroids	IL-1, IL-6, TNF-α	∠ Concentration	Turnbull and Rivier (54), Fantuzzi et al. (55)
Growth hormone	IL-1	∠ and) Concentration	Payne et al. (56), Wada et al. (57)
T_3 and T_4	IL-1, IL-6, TNF-α	) Concentration	Imura et al. (53)

[a] ∠ = increased,) = decreased.

Table 4). Cytokine receptors have been identified in neuroendocrine tissues, and they have been classified into three major families (58). The hematopoietic growth factor receptor family includes receptors for IL-6 and related cytokines. The tumor necrosis factor (TNF) receptor family includes receptors for both TNF-α and TNF-β. Finally, the immunoglobulin supergene family includes two identified IL-1 receptors, the 80-kDa type I receptor, which is found mainly on T-cells and fibroblasts, and the smaller 68-kDa type II receptor, which has been identified on B-cells and macrophages.

Interplay among the immune, endocrine, and nervous systems is most commonly associated with stressors that have a pronounced effect on the overall immune response. Any type of stress, including not only psychological and environmental challenges, but also vigorous physical activity, can initiate a hormonal stress response, with a potential for additive effects if there is exposure to more than one type of stress (59).

In the context of exercise, training, and immune responses, hormones that have attracted particular attention include components of the neurohormonal stress response and metabolic regulators (29), particularly catecholamines, cortisol, corticotropin-releasing hormone (CRH), adrenocorticotropic hormones, growth hormone, endorphins and enkephalins, insulin, thyroid hormones, prolactin, and prostaglandins. Unfortunately, the various studies that have examined the influence of physical training on the immune response differ widely from each other with respect to the type of subject recruited, the volume of training undertaken, and the immunological methodology employed. Moreover, when studies have involved athletes, it has been difficult to ensure adequate recovery from the effects of recent sessions of strenuous training. It is thus difficult to make reliable comparisons between studies.

The hypothalamic–pituitary–adrenal (HPA) axis is the key player in the stress response. The principal cell type involved within the HPA axis is the corticotroph. This cell produces, processes and stores peptides derived from a 31-kDa protein called propiomelanocortin (POMC). ACTH (corticotropin) and β-endorphin are products derived from POMC. During a typical stress response, cognitive recognition of stress by the higher centers of the central nervous system (CNS) causes the release of corticotropin-releasing hormone (CRH) from the hypothalamus. The CRH acts on the pituitary corticotrophs, causing a release of ACTH into the circulation. ACTH then acts on the adrenal gland, causing it in its turn to produce glucocorticoid hormone. Many of the physiological effects of stress are mediated by the glucocorticoids, which can modify both metabolism and immune function. These same substances also inhibit the synthesis and release of CRH and ACTH by a form of negative feedback.

β-endorphin is another substance released from the anterior pituitary in response to sustained and vigorous exercise. It elevates mood and may account for the occasional individual who becomes chemically dependent on regular bouts of prolonged exercise. The β-endorphin tends to suppress the formation of ACTH and cortisol, possibly by a feedback inhibition of CRH *(60)*. Although leukocytes carry receptors for the endorphins, the extent of their contribution to the immune response has yet to be clarified.

Activation of the sympathetic nervous system stimulates the release of catecholamines from the adrenal medulla and the sympathetic nerve terminals *(61)*. The response of the sympatheticoadrenomedullary system to exercise is more swift and more powerful than that of the HPA axis *(62)*. Sympathetic activation occurs within a few seconds of initiating physical activity, but the HPA response and secretion of glucocorticoids often do not begin until 20–30 min after commencing exercise *(63)*.

A period of physical training alters the response of most of the above hormones to exercise at any given power output, largely because the specified effort now represents a substantially smaller fraction of the individual's peak aerobic power. However, the response at a fixed fraction of peak aerobic power remains unchanged. Training also modulates the immediate resting concentrations of several stress hormones, particularly the catecholamines. Aerobic training decreases resting sympathetic β-adrenergic) activity, while increasing parasympathetic (vagal) tone *(64,65)*. Hack et al. *(66)* studied long-distance runners before and up to 24 h after they had performed a graded exercise test to exhaustion; the responses observed during periods of moderate and intensive training were compared with the responses seen in untrained (control) subjects. Probably because of incomplete recovery from previous training sessions, resting plasma adrenaline and noradrenaline levels were increased in subjects who were undertaking intensive training relative to controls or subjects who were performing only moderate training. However, the plasma catecholamine response at a given submaximal work rate was decreased following endurance training *(67,68)*.

Training programs may lead to a modification in the sensitivity and/or density of adrenergic receptors. Prolonged or habitual physical exercise tends to cause a downregulation of β-receptor density *(69)*, probably because of repeated exposure to high catecholamine levels. Butler et al. *(70)* observed an almost 60% decrease in the density of β-receptors on lymphocytes over 2 mo of intensive aerobic training. Because exercise training is so efficient in downregulating the sensitivity of the sympathetic nervous system (SNS), it has even been used as relaxation technique *(71)*. In support of the view that the mechanism of downregulation is the high catecholamine levels reached during training, Krawietz et al. *(72)* noted an inverse association between receptor density and circadian variations in catecholamine levels. However, Dorner et al. *(73)* found a higher β-receptor density on the granulocytes of subjects with a high level of aerobic fitness.

The magnitude of the neurohormonal response to any given physical task is augmented by associated emotional stress *(74)* and by any increase in core body temperature *(75,76)*. On the other hand, the secretion of endogenous opioids, such as β-endorphin *(77)*, and habituation to a given situation each reduce catecholamine secretion and the resultant physiologic and immunologic responses to exercise *(78)*.

When subjects have been compared at the same submaximal workrate, trained persons have generally had smaller increases in plasma cortisol levels than untrained persons (6,79).

Serum concentrations of several endogenous opiates or neuropeptides, including β-lipotropin, β-endorphin, and met-enkephalin, increase in response to exercise (80). Aerobic exercise was also found to augment β-endorphin release in seven women who participated in a rigorous 8-wk protocol consisting of conditioning exercises, cycling, and running (81). These results suggest that aerobically fit individuals who continue to exercise and maintain their aerobic fitness may release more endogenous opioids than their nonexercising, less-fit counterparts during exercise. This in turn would explain why they derive a sustained elevation of mood and perceived health from their exercise habit. It also seems reasonable to postulate that exercise training modifies psychological stress reactivity, and there is some empirical evidence of a reduced reaction to psychological stressors among those who are welltrained. LaPerriere has proposed a model in which exercise training reduces negative affective states by increasing the release of endogenous opiates, reducing HPAC activation, and enhancing immunity (27).

Cellular Responses to Training

Less information is available about the effects of training on the immune system than about acute exercise and immune responses (29). Several studies have made cross-sectional comparisons of the immune system between athletes and nonathletes (82–93). Others have followed sedentary individuals as they have initiated exercise programs, comparing pre- and postexercise training immune parameters relative to control groups (94–100). The majority of these studies have not demonstrated any important effects of regular exercise training on the circulating numbers of total leukocytes, lymphocytes, or their various subpopulations. However, several investigations of both humans and animal populations have shown significant increases in NK cell cytotoxic activity (NKCA) with exercise training (83,85,92,93,96,97,101,102). As yet, researchers disagree regarding whether the higher NKCA is owing to greater numbers of circulating NK cells or to an enhanced cytotoxic capacity per individual NK cell (92,93,97). With regard to lymphocyte proliferation, the data are conflicting; cross-sectional and prospective studies on both animals and humans have reported positive (97,100,103–105), neutral (34,84,87,97,106) or negative (91,103,107–109) effects of exercise training. We will now give brief consideration to some studies on the cellular component of immune responses to physical training.

Neutrophils—Numbers and Function

Resting Cell Counts. Analyzing studies that have compared sedentary and trained subjects, we found that resting neutrophil counts were higher in the trained group (110–113) when the intensity of training was moderate, but the opposite was true when training was intensive (93,97,114–116). Longitudinal studies have shown a similar picture (66,114,117–119). Thus, it is possible to conclude that moderate training is associated with a positive modulation of the resting neutrophil count, whereas intensive training seems to depress the numbers of circulating neutrophils, possibly because of a migration of these cells to injured muscles.

Exercise Cell Counts. During the first few minutes following an acute bout of exercise, there is a biphasic change in the neutrophil count (6). Studies comparing trained and untrained individuals have suggested that exercise produces a similar increase of neutrophil count in trained and untrained subjects *(86,110,120)*, or that the neutrophilia postexercise is substantially larger in trained subjects *(66,73,121)*. In contrast, Oshida et al. *(111)* found a smaller granulocytosis in trained than in untrained individuals. Longitudinal data, at this moment, are inconclusive.

Functional Activity. Some authors *(117,121,122)* have reported that neutrophils have a greater functional activity in trained individuals than in sedentary subjects. In contrast, Prasad et al. *(123)* suggested that heavy training causes a dysfunction of neutrophils.

Much of the available data suggest that conditioning programs induce little change of neutrophil function. In contrast, severe training may have a suppressant effect.

EOSINOPHILS AND BASOPHILS

Few studies have examined the influences of exercise and training on these cell categories. Nieman et al. *(124)* found higher resting eosinophil and lower resting basophil counts in marathoners than in control subjects. In contrast, Janssen et al. *(125)* observed no increase in resting eosinophil count and an increase in basophil count in subjects who had trained in preparation for a 15-km run.

MONOCYTES/MACROPHAGE COUNTS

Comparison between sedentary and trained subjects showed lower resting monocyte counts in the trained group *(86,124,126–128)*. Several authors have found little change in peripheral blood resting monocyte counts in response to training *(118,125,129)*. On the other hand, Ferry et al. *(130)* observed large increases in both resting and exercise counts after a period of vigorous training, and Ndon et al. *(118)* also noted a larger exercise-induced monocytosis in trained than untrained individuals.

T-CELL COUNTS

Sedentary and trained subjects commonly show little difference in resting $CD4^+$ counts *(97,126,131)*. However, some authors have noted substantially higher resting $CD8^+$ counts in active than in sedentary individuals *(130,132)*. Data on the $CD4^+/CD8^+$ ratio have been more consistent, with athletes showing low ratios in comparison with sedentary individuals *(93,97,126,130)*. The majority of longitudinal data have shown decreases in resting $CD4^+$ and $CD8^+$ *(93,129,132–134)* counts with training, but the influence of conditioning programs on $CD4^+/CD8^+$ ratio has varied from one study to another.

Cross-sectional data show little difference in exercise-induced changes in $CD4^+$ count between fit and unfit subjects *(111,130,132)*. However, exercise induced a larger increase in $CD8^+$ count in trained than in untrained individuals *(130,132)*. The exercise-induced changes in $CD4^+$ and $CD8^+$ counts and the $CD4^+/CD8^+$ ratio have been inconsistent in longitudinal training programs *(131,134,135)*.

B-CELL COUNTS

Cross-sectional comparisons of resting B-cell counts between trained and untrained subjects offer inconsistent results *(97,110,114)*. Studies of moderate training have shown a substantial increase *(97)*, no change *(114)*, or a decrease *(119)* in B-cell counts.

LYMPHOCYTE PROLIFERATION

Cross-sectional and prospective studies of animals and humans have reported positive *(97,100,103–105)*, neutral *(34,84,87,97,106)*, or negative *(91,103,107–109)* effects of exercise training on lymphocyte proliferation.

NK Cell Number and Function

Several studies have compared active and inactive groups. Cross-sectional data involving moderate training have sometimes shown substantially larger NK counts in trained individuals (92,93,111,112,126), but other studies have observed only small differences of resting NK cell count between active and trained groups (97,134). Liesen and Uhlenbruck (114) found very low resting NK counts in athletes who were undergoing rigorous training.

Different authors have found the resting NK cell count to increase (27,119,129,130) or to decrease (93,114,132) over the course of a training program. One explanation for a decrease in NK count may be incomplete recovery from recent training sessions.

Several investigations of both humans and animals have shown significant increases in NKCA with exercise training (83,85,92,93,96,97,101,102). Nevertheless, researchers still disagree on whether the higher NKCA is owing to a greater number of circulating NK cells or to an enhanced cytotoxic capacity per individual NK cell (92,93,97).

Cytokines

Cytokines and adhesion molecules comprise the main regulatory elements in the immune system. They govern the growth, differentiation, and functional activation of all cells in the immune system, and they are also responsible for the interaction of this system with somatic cellular systems.

Plasma levels of cytokines are often difficult to measure accurately, but they appear to change only slightly during exercise. However, an increased urinary excretion of several cytokines has been noted after intensive prolonged exercise, such as distance running or cross-country skiing (reviewed in *136*).

IL-6 is one of the easier substances to detect in the plasma. Sprenger et al. (*137*) noted an increased plasma IL-6 concentration and increases in the urinary excretion of IL-1, soluble IL-2 receptor (sIL-2r), IL-6, interferon (IFN), and TNF when male distance runners had covered a distance of 20 km. In general, moderate exercise causes little change in plasma or urinary excretion of cytokines. In contrast, strenuous exercise is associated with large increases in urinary excretion of most of the cytokines that have been measured to date (IL-1, sIL-2r, IL-6, IFN, TNF); the one possible exception is IL-2. There is also a decreased in vitro production of cytokines by cells isolated after exercise, with the exception of IFN (which appears to be produced in increased quantities *[136]*).

As yet, few studies have explored training-induced changes in cytokine secretion. Training may cause no change (*45*) in the level of IL-2, the cytokine responsible for initiating cell-mediated immune reactions. Rhind et al. (*119*) observed a small decrease in the plasma IL-2 level following 12 wk of moderate training. However, training has little influence on IL-1, IL-6, IFN, and TNF, the proinflammatory cytokines, unless the conditioning program is pushed to cause tissue injury and inflammation.

Other Soluble Factors

Moderate training tends to enhance both salivary and plasma levels of immunoglobulins. On the other hand, very heavy training can lead to a decrease in the concentrations of both secretory and circulating immunoglobulins (114,138).

There are few reports on complement levels. Concentrations may be lower in trained than in untrained individuals if the conditioning program is sufficiently intense to induce a chronic inflammatory reaction (88,139–141).

CLINICAL APPLICATIONS

Exercise and Upper Respiratory Tract Infections (URTI)

Many athletes develop upper respiratory infections, either following a single bout of prolonged exercise, such as a marathon run *(96)*, or in response to a period of heavy training as a major competition is approached *(114)*. Some authors have also reported that heavy training is associated with a reduction in immunoglobulin levels in serum, saliva, and nasal washings *(114,142)*. This has led to formulation of the so-called j-shaped hypothesis *(143)*, whereby moderate exercise exerts a protective effect, but heavy, stressful exercise suppresses immune function with negative consequences for defense mechanisms.

If immunoglobulin levels are reduced by a period of heavy training, then there would seem to be good grounds for suggesting an impairment of immune defenses. However, the evidence that a single bout of prolonged physical activity can cause a clinically significant depression of immune function is less convincing, since it is hard to envisage how the usual brief depression of immune response (2–24 h in duration) could have a sufficient impact on immune defenses to lower the resistance to infections for several weeks. The precise mechanism of any exercise-induced immunosuppression also continues to be a topic of discussion. Either the increase in total energy expenditure or the repair of tissue microinjuries could conceivably increase the formation of reactive species, with negative consequences for immune function. Given such a scenario, the athlete might be helped by administration of megadoses of antioxidant vitamins. However, the practical benefit from such therapy has been very limited among participants in the Comrades' marathon *(144)*. Alternatively, negative consequences might stem from microtraumata and an associated release of prostaglandin-E_2; if this were the *modus operandi*, it might be helpful to administer nonsteroidal anti-inflammatory drugs, such as indomethacin. Other hypotheses include hormone-induced changes in the trafficking of immune cells, the adverse influence of stress hormones (particularly cortisol) on lymphocyte function, and a depletion of the reserves of branch-chained amino acids needed for lymphocyte proliferation. Plainly, further research is needed to clarify which mechanisms underlie any changes in immune responses that develop with prolonged and intensive bouts of endurance exercise.

Several practical precautions may help athletes who are undergoing intensive training to reduce their risk of URTI. Guidelines include the adoption of a well-balanced diet *(145)*, ensuring adequate sleep *(146)*, spacing vigorous workouts and race events *(147)*, where possible avoiding contact with people who have viral infections *(148)*, keeping other life stresses to a minimum *(133)*, and having inoculations against influenza and other prevalent viruses. If immunoglobulin levels are low, it may also be helpful to administer immunoglobulin preparations, although this practice remains controversial.

Exercise and Cancer

In keeping with the discussion of interactions between exercise and susceptibility to acute viral infections, there is now a substantial volume of literature suggesting that regular moderate exercise has a helpful effect in reducing all-site cancer rates, together with susceptibility to cancers at specific sites, particularly the descending colon, but possibly also the lungs, the female reproductive tract and breast, and the prostate gland in men *(29)*. At some of these sites (for example, the female reproductive tract), benefit seems to arise from either a suppression of estrogen synthesis or an alteration of the pathway of estrogen metabolism in thinner individuals. There is also evidence that susceptibility varies with NK cell activity, so that the increases in NK function associated with moderate training may play some protective role. However, there is also animal and anecdotal human evidence that in a few instances excessive physical activity has predisposed to either the development of or the recurrence of a neoplasm *(149)*.

Exercise and Chronic Fatigue Syndrome

Excessive stress, whether induced through emotional shock alone, overvigorous training, or a combination of these two factors, can produce symptoms that merge with usual descriptions of chronic fatigue syndrome. It is important to monitor the condition of athletes closely to ensure that they do not reach such a level of stress, since treatment of chronic fatigue is prolonged and unsatisfactory. Unfortunately, few good markers of excessive training exist. Warning is provided by a deterioration in performance, despite rigorous training. Perhaps the simplest and often the most effective objective measure of overtraining is use of a simple psychological questionnaire, the Profile of Mood States (POMS) *(150)*; this usually shows a substantial deterioration of mood state in athletes who are training too hard.

Exercise and Aging

Human immune responses decline significantly with advancing age, and there is an associated increase in susceptibility to infectious diseases, inflammatory response-based disorders, and cancer, all of which are major health problems in older people. Aging leads to substantial changes in both the functional and phenotypic profiles of T-lymphocytes. Changes include a shift toward greater proportions of $CD4^+T$ cells of memory ($CD44^{hi}CD45RO^+$) phenotype and fewer cells of naive ($CD44^{lo}CD45RA^+$) phenotype *(151,152)*. In parallel with these modifications of phenotype, functional changes include a decreased proliferative response of T-cells to mitogens *(153)* and alterations in the profiles of cytokines, which are produced with T-cell activation *(154)*.

Few investigators have studied the influence of physical training on immune responses in the elderly. Xusheng et al. *(155)* found that the percentage of rosette forming (T) cells was lower in 24 elderly devotees of Taichiquan than in 24 age-matched controls. Nieman et al. *(97)* made both cross-sectional and 12-wk longitudinal assessments of the effects of training in women aged 67–85 yr. They found that the highly conditioned elderly women had greater NK and T-cell function than their sedentary counterparts, but that 12 wk of moderate exercise did not improve immune function in previously sedentary elderly women. Shinkai et al. (156) had similar findings in a cross-sectional study of trained and untrained elderly subjects. Rall et al. *(157)* compared the response of young and elderly individuals (65–80 yr) to high-intensity progressive resistance strength training; they concluded that 12 wk of training did not alter immune function in either group. Although the number of reports is small, there seems some support for the view that moderate exercise performed regularly throughout life may decrease the age-related decline in immune function, particularly if it is coupled with other positive lifestyle habits.

Exercise and Sepsis

Perhaps the most interesting aspect of the immune response to heavy exercise is the potential window it gives into human reactions to excessive inflammation and sepsis.

For ethical reasons, it is not possible to induce septic lesions by the deliberate infliction of injury on experimental subjects, but the study of cellular, hormonal, and cytokine responses in athletes who have produced tissue injury through excessive training can serve many of these same objectives *(29)*.

CONCLUSIONS

Physical training results in a variety of important biological changes. Particular interest attaches to interactions among the central nervous, endocrine, and immune systems, which result in modifications of the immune response. Moderate regular exercise appears to improve immune function, but in contrast, heavy physical training can suppress several immune parameters of the immune response. The exact mechanisms involved in both positive and negative reactions are not completely understood as yet. We may conclude that moderate physical training could be helpful in the prevention or treatment of diseases and conditions caused by or associated with a decline in immune function. However, further studies are needed to find the best way of attenuating those adverse immune changes that follow a period of very heavy exercise.

ACKNOWLEDGMENTS

V. M. Natale is grateful to the Fundação de Amparo à Pesquisa do Estado de São Paulo (São Paulo, SP, Brazil) (FAPESP) for support during her stay at the Defence and Civil Institute of Environmental Medicine, Toronto, Ontario, Canada. Shephard's research is supported by grants from the Defense & Civil Institute of Environmental Medicine and Canadian Tire Acceptance Limited.

REFERENCES

1. Schultz G. Experimentelle Untersuchungen über das Vorkommen und die diagnostische Bedeutung der Leukocytose (experimental research on the antecedents and diagnostic importance of leukocytosis). Dtsch Arch Klin Med 1893;51:234–281.
2. Hoffman-Goetz L, Husted J. Exercise, immunity and colon cancer. In: Hoffman-Goetz L, ed. Exercise and Immune Function. CRC, Boca Raton, FL, 1996, pp 179–197.
3. Mackinnon LT. Exercise and Immunology, 2nd ed. Human Kinetics, Champaign, IL, 1998.
4. Pedersen BK. Exercise Immunology, Landis, Austin, TX, 1997.
5. Keast D, Cameron K, Morton AR. Exercise and the immune response. Sports Med 1988;5:248–267.
6. McCarthy DA, Dale MM. The leucocytosis of exercise. A review and model. Sports Med 1988;6: 333–363.
7. Mackinnon LT. Exercise and Immunology. Current Issues in Exercise Science Series, Monograph No. 2, Human Kinetics, Champaign. IL, 1992, pp. 1–30.
8. Simon HB. Exercise and infection. Phys Sports Med 1987;15:135–141.
9. Kuipers H, Keizer HA. Overtraining in elite athletes. Review and directions for the future. Sports Med 1988;6:79–92.
10. Mackinnon LT, Tomasi TB. Immunology of exercise. Ann Sports Med 1986;3:1–4.
11. Roberts JA. Viral illness and sports performance. Sports Med 1986;3:296–303.
12. Shephard RJ, Shek PN. Heavy exercise, nutrition and immune function. Is there a connection? Int J Sports Med 1995;16:491–497.
13. Castell L, Newsholme E. Glutamine and the exhaustive exercise upon the immune response. Can J Physiol Pharmacol 1998;76:524–532.
14. Newsholme EA. Biochemical mechanisms to explain immunosuppression in well-trained and overtrained athletes. Int J Sports Med 1994;15:S142–147.
15. Keast D, Arstein D, Harper W, Fry RW, Morton AR. Depression of plasma glutamine concentration after exercise stress and its possible influence on the immune system. Med J Austr 1995;162:15–18.

16. Brenner IKM, Severs YD, Shek PN, Shephard RJ. Impact of heat exposure and moderate, intermittent exercise on cytolytic cells. Eur J Appl Physiol 1996;74:162–171.
17. Cross MC, Radomski MW, VanHelder WP, Rhind SG, Shephard RJ. Endurance exercise with and without a thermal clamp: effects on leukocytes and leukocyte subsets. J Appl Physiol 1996;81: 822–829.
18. Kappel M, Diamant M, Hansen MB, Kløkker M, Pedersen BK. Effects of in vitro hyperthermia on the proliferative response of blood mononuclear cells subsets, and detection of interleukins 1 and 6, tumour necrosis factor-alpha and interferon-gamma. Immunology 1991;73:304–308.
19. Kappel M, Stadeager C, Tvede N, Galbø H, Pedersen BK. Effects of in vivo hyperthermia on natural killer cell activity, in vitro proliferative responses and blood mononuclear cell subpopulations. Clin Exp Immunol 1991;84:175–180.
20. Kappel M, Tvede N, Hansen MB, Stadeager C, Pedersen BK. Cytokine production ex vivo: effect of raised body temperature. Int J Hyperthermia 1995;11:329–334.
21. Severs YD, Brenner IKM, Shek PN, Shephard RJ. Effects of heat and intermittent exercise on leukocyte and sub-population cell counts. Eur J Appl Physiol 1996;74:234–245.
22. Radomski M, Cross M, Buguet A. Exercise-induced hyperthermia and regulation of hormonal responses to exercise. Can J Physiol Pharmacol 1998;76:547–552.
23. Kløkker M, Kharazmi A, Galbø H, Bygbjerg I, Pedersen BK. Influence of in vivo hypobaric hypoxia on function of lymphocytes, neutrocytes, natural killer cells, and cytokines. J Appl Physiol 1993;74:1100–1106.
24. Kløkker M, Kjær M, Seche NH, Hanel B, Worm L, Kappel M, et al. Natural killer cell response to exercise in humans: effect of hypoxia and epidural anesthesia. J Appl Physiol 1995;78:709–716.
25. Dempsey JA. Is the lung built for exercise? Med Sci Sports Exerc 1986;18:143–155.
26. Kay C, Shephard RJ. On muscle strength and the threshold of anaerobic work. Int Z Angew Physiol 1969;27:311–328.
27. LaPerriere A, Ironson G, Antoni MA, Schneiderman N, Klimas N, Fletcher MA. Exercise and psychoneuroimmunology. Med Sci Sports Exerc 1994;26:182–190.
28. Abbas AK, Lichtman AH, Pober JS. Cellular and molecular immunology. Saunders Co., Philadelphia, PA, (1994)
29. Shephard RJ. Physical Activity, Training and the Immune Response. Cooper Publishing Group, Carmel, IN, 1997.
30. Stites DP, Terr AI. Basic and clinical immunology. Appleton & Lange, Prentice Hall, Englewood Cliffs, NJ, 1991
31. Shephard RJ, Shek PN. Physical exercise and immune changes: a potential model of subclinical inflammation and sepsis. Crit Rev Phys Rehabil Med 1996;8:153–181.
32. Pedersen BK. Influence of physical activity on the cellular immune system: mechanisms of action. Int J Sports Med 1991;2:S23–29.
33. Pedersen BK, Kappel M, Kløkker M, Nielsen HB, Secher NH. The immune system during exposure to extreme physiologic conditions. Int J Sports Med 1994;5:S116–121.
34. Tvede N, Pedersen BK, Bendix T, Christensen LD, Galbø H, Halkjær-Kristensen J. Effect of physical exercise on blood mononuclear cell subpopulations and in vitro proliferative responses. Scand J Immunol 1989;29:383–389.
35. Pedersen BK, Tvede N, Hansen FR, Andersen V, Bendix T, Bendixen G, et al. Modulation of natural killer cell activity in peripheral blood by physical exercise. Scand J Immunol 1988;27:673–678.
36. Crary B, Hauser SL, Borysenko M, et al. Epinephrine-induced changes in the distribution of lymphocyte subsets in peripheral blood of humans. J Immunol 1983;131:1178–1181.
37. Tvede N, Kappel M, Klarlund K, Duhn S, Halkjær-Kristensen J, Kjær M, et al. Evidence that the effect of bicycle exercise on mononuclear cell proliferative responses and subsets is mediated by epinephrine. Int J Sports Med 1994;15:100–104.
38. Nieman DC, Berk LS, Simpson-Westerberg M, et al. Effects of long endurance running on immune system parameters and lymphocyte function in experienced marathoners. Int J Sports Med 1989;10:317–323.
39. Robertson AJK, Ramesar KCRB, Potts RC, et al. The effect of strenuous physical exercise on circulating blood lymphocytes and serum cortisol levels. Clin Lab Immunol 1981;5:53–57.
40. Cupps TR, Fauci AS. Corticosteroid-mediated immunoregulation in man. Immunol Rev 1982;65: 133–155.

41. Beck LS, Nieman DC, Youngberg WS, Arabatzis K, Simpson-Westerberg M, Lee JW, et al. The effect of long endurance running on natural killer cells in marathoners. Med Sci Sports Exerc 1990; 22:207–212.
42. Shephard RJ, Rhind S, Shek PN. Response to exercise and training: NK cells, interleukin-1, interleukin-2 and receptor structures. Int J Sports Med 1994;15:S154–S166.
43. Kappel M, Tvede N, Galbø H, Haahr M, Kjær M, Linstouw M, et al. Evidence that the effect of physical exercise is mediated by adrenaline. J Appl Physiol 1991;70:2530–2534.
44. Madden KS, Felten DL. Experimental basis for neural-immune interactions. Physiol Rev 1995;75: 77–106.
45. Weicker H, Werle E. Interactions between hormones and the immune system. Int J Sports Med 1991;12(Suppl. 1):S30–S37.
46. Blalock JE. The syntax of immune-neuroendocrine communication. Immunol Today 1994;15: 504–511.
47. Ackerman KD, Bellinger DL, Felten SY. Ontogeny and senescence of noradrenergic innervation of the rodent spleen. In: Ader R, Felten DL, Cohen N, eds. Psychoneuroimmunology, vol. 2, Academic, San Diego, CA, (1991), pp 71–125.
48. Bachen EA, Manuck SB, Cohen S, Muldoon MF, Raibel R, Herbert TB, et al. Adrenergic blockage ameliorates cellular immune responses to mental stress in humans. Psychosom Med 1995;57:366–372.
49. Manuck SB, Cohen S, Rabin BS, Muldoon MF, Bachen EA. Individual differences in cellular immune response to stress. Psychol Sci 1991;2:111–115.
50. Rabin BS, Cunnick JE, Lysle DT. Stress-induced alteration of immune function. Progr Neuroendocrinol Immunol 1990;3:116.
51. Landmann R. Beta-adrenergic receptors in human leukocyte subpopulations. Eur J Clin Invest 1992;22(Suppl. 1):30–36.
52. Murray DR, Irwin M, Rearden CA, Ziegler M, Motulsky H, Maise AS. Sympathetic and immune interactions during dynamic exercise. Mediation via a beta-2-adrenergic dependent mechanism. Circulation 1992;86:203–213.
53. Imura H, Fukata J-I, Mori T. Cytokines and endocrine function: an interaction between the immune and neuroendocrine system. Clin Endocrinol 1991;35:107–115.
54. Turnbull AV, Rivier CL. Regulation of the HPA axis by cytokines. Brain Behav Immunol 1995;9: 253–275.
55. Fantuzzi G, Benigni F, Sironi M, Conni M, Carelli M, Cantonni L, et al. Ciliary neurotrophic factor (CNTF) induces serum amyloid A, hypoglycaemia and anorexia, and potentiates IL-1 induced corticosterone and IL-6 production in mice. Cytokine 1995;7:150–156.
56. Payne LC, Obal F, Poo MR, Krueger JM. Stimulation and inhibition of growth hormone secretion by interleukin-1β: the involvement of growth hormone-releasing hormone. Neuroendocrinology 1991;56:118–123.
57. Wada Y, Sato M, Niimi M, Tamaki M, Ishida T, Takahara J. Inhibitory effect of interleukin-1 on growth hormone secretion in conscious male rats. Endocrinology 1995;136:3936–3941.
58. Foxwell BMJ, Barret K, Feldmann M. Cytokine receptors: structure and signal transduction. Clin Exp Immunol 1992;12:1101–1114.
59. Shephard RJ. Immune changes induced by exercise in an adverse environment. Can J Physiol Pharmacol 1998;76:539–546.
60. Taylor C, Dluhy RG, Williams GH. Beta-endorphin suppresses adrenocorticotropin and cortisol levels in normal human subjects. J Clin Endocrinol Metab 1983;57:592–596.
61. Khansari DN, Murgo AJ, Faith RE. Effects of stress on the immune system. Immunol Today 1990;11:170–175.
62. Deuster PA, Chrousos GP, Luger A, DeBolt JE, Bernier LL, Trostman UH, et al. Hormonal and metabolic responses of untrained, moderately trained, and highly trained men to three exercise intensities. Metabolism 1989;38:141–148.
63. Rabin BS, Moyna NM, Kusnecov A, Zhou D, Shurin MS. Neuroendocrine effects on immunity. In: Hoffman-Goetz L, ed. Exercise and Immune Function. CRC, Boca Raton, FL, 1996, pp.21–37.
64. Frick M, Elovainio R, Somer T. The mechanism of bradycardia evoked by physical training. Cardiology 1967;51:46–54.
65. Moore R, Riedy M, Gollnick P. Effect of training on beta-adrenergic receptor number in rat heart. J Appl Physiol 1982;52:1133.

66. Hack V, Strobel G, Weiss M, Weicker H. PMN cell counts and phagocytic activity of highly trained athletes depend on training period. J Appl Physiol 1994;77:1731–1735.
67. Galbø H. Hormonal and Metabolic Adaptations to Exercise. Thieme Stratton, New York, 1983, pp. 2–27.
68. Winder M, Beattie MA, Holman RT. Endurance training attenuates stress hormone response to exercise in fasted rats. Am J Physiol 1982;243:R179–R184.
69. Opstad PK, Wiik P, Haugen A-H, Skrede KK. Adrenaline stimulated cyclic adenosine monophosphate response in leucocytes is reduced after prolonged physical activity combined with sleep and energy deprivation. Eur J Appl Physiol 1994;69:371–375.
70. Butler J, O'Brien M, O'Malley K, Kelly JG. Relationships of beta-adrenoreceptor density to fitness in athletes. Nature 1982;298:60–62.
71. Morgan WP, Horstman DH, Cymerman AR, Stokes JD. Exercise as a relaxation technique. Prim Cardiol 1980;6:48–57.
72. Krawietz W, Klein EM, Unterberg CH, Ackenheil M. Physical activity decreases the number of beta-adrenergic receptors on human lymphocytes. Klin Wschr 1985;63:73–78.
73. Dorner H, Heinhold D, Hilmer W. Exercise-induced leukocytosis—its dependence on physical capability. Int J Sports Med 1987;8:152.
74. Blimkie CJ, Cunningham DA, Leung FY. Urinary catecholamine excretion and lactate concentrations in competitive hockey players aged 11 to 23 years. In: Lavallée H. and Shephard RJ, eds. Frontiers of Activity and Child Health. Editions du Pélican, Québec City, 1977, pp. 313–321.
75. Melin B, Cure M, Pequignot JM, Bittel J. Body temperature and plasma prolactin and norepinephrine relationships during exercise in a warm environment: Effect of dehydration. Eur J Appl Physiol 1988;58:146–151.
76. Rowell LB. Hyperthermia: a hyperadrenergic state. Hypertension 1990;15:505–507.
77. Angelopoulos TJ, Denys BG, Weikart C, Dasilva SG, Michael TJ, Robertson RJ. Endogenous opioids may modulate catecholamine secretion during high intensity exercise. Eur J App Physiol 1995;70:195–199.
78. Leavitt JA, Turner AK, Battinelli NJ, Coats MH, Falk RH. Reproducibility of the catecholamine response to serial exercise testing in normals. Am J Med Sci 1992;303:160–164.
79. Galbø H Endocrinology and metabolism in exercise. Int Sports Med 1981;2:203–211.
80. Harber VJ, Sutton JR. Endorphins and exercise. Sports Med 1984;1:154–171.
81. Carr DB, Bullen BA, Skrinar GS, Arnold MA, Rosenblatt M, Beitins IZ, et al. Physical conditioning facilitates the exercise induced secretion of beta-endorphin and beta-lipotropin in women. N Engl J Med 1981;305:560–563.
82. Brahmi Z, Thomas JE, Park M, Dowdeswell IAG. The effect of acute exercise on natural killer-cell activity of trained and sedentary human subjects. J Clin Immunol 1985;5:321–328.
83. Crist DM, Mackinnon LT, Thompson RF, Atterbom HA, Egan PA. Physical exercise increases natural cellular-mediated tumor cytotoxicity in elderly women. Gerontology 1989;35:66–71.
84. Green RL, Kaplan SS, Rabin BS, Stanitsk CL, Zdziarski U. Immune function in marathon runners. Ann Allergy 1981;47:73–75.
85. Kusaka Y, Kondou H, Morimoto K. Healthy lifestyles are associated with higher natural killer cell activity. Prev Med 1992;21:602–615.
86. Lewicki R, Tchórzewski H, Denys A, Kowalska M, Golinska A. Effect of physical exercise on some parameters of immunity in conditioned sportsmen. Int J Sports Med 1987;8:309–314.
87. MacNeil B, Hoffman-Goetz L, Kendall A, Houston AM, Arumugam Y. Lymphocyte proliferation responses after exercise in men: fitness, intensity, and duration effects. J Appl Physiol 1991;70:179–185.
88. Nieman DC, Tan SA, Lee JW, Berk LS. Complement and immunoglobulin levels in athletes and sedentary controls. Int J Sports Med 1989;10:124–128.
90. Nieman DC, Henson DA, Sampson C, Herring JL, Suttles J, Conley M, et al. Natural killer cell cytotoxic activity weight lifters and sedentary controls. J Strength Cond Res 1994;8:251–254.
91. Papa S, Vitale M, Mazzoti G, Neri LM, Monti G, Manzoli FA. Impaired lymphocyte stimulation induced by long-term training. Immunol Let 1989;22:29–33.
92. Pedersen BK, Tvede N, Christensen LD, Klarlund K, Kragbak S, Halkjær-Kristensen J. Natural killer cell activity in peripheral blood of highly trained and untrained persons. Int J Sports Med 1989;10:129–131.
93. Tvede N, Steensberg J, Baslund B, Halkjær-Kristensen J, Pedersen BK. Cellular immunity in highly-trained elite racing cyclists and controls during periods of training with high and low intensity. Scand J Sports Med 1991;1:163–166.

94. Blaslund B, Lyngberg K, Andersen V, Dristensen JH, Hansen M, Kløkker N, et al. Effect of 8 wk of bicycle training on the immune system of patients with rheumatoid arthritis. J Appl Physiol 1993;75:1691–1695.
95. Nehlsen-Cannarella SL, Nieman DC, Balk-Lamberton AJ, Markoff PA, Chritton DBW, Gusewitch G, et al. The effects of moderate exercise training on immune response. Med Sci Sports Exerc 1991; 23:64–70.
96. Nieman DC, Nehlsen-Cannarella SL, Markoff PA, Balk-Lamberton AJ, Yang H, Chritton DBW, et al. The effects of moderate training on natural killer cells and acute upper respiratory tract infections. Int J Sports Med 1990;11:467–473.
97. Nieman DC, Henson DA, Gusewitch G, Warren BJ, Dotson RC, Butterworth DE, et al. Physical activity and immune function in elderly women. Med Sci Sports Exerc 1993;25:823–831.
98. Nieman DC, Cook VD, Henson DA, Suttles J, Rejeski WJ. Moderate exercise training and natural killer cell cytotoxic activity in breast cancer patients. Int J Sports Med 1995;6:334–337.
99. Soppi E, Varjo A, Eskola J, Laitinen LA. Effect of strenuous physical stress on circulatin lymphocyte number and function before and after training. J Clin Lab Immunol 1982;8:43–46.
100. Watson RR, Moriguchi S, Jackson JC, Werner L, Wilmore JH, Freund BJ. Modification of cellular immune functions in humans by endurance exercise training during β-adrenergic blockade with atenolol or propranolol. Med Sci Sports Exerc 1986;18:95–100.
101. MacNeil B, Hoffman-Goetz L. Chronic exercise enhances in vivo and in vitro cytotoxic mechanisms of natural immunity in mice. J Appl Physiol 1993;74:388–395.
102. Simpson JR, Hoffman-Goetz L. Exercise stress and murine natural killer cell function. Proc Soc Exp Biol Med 1990;195:129–135.
103. Nasrullah I, Mazzeo RS. Age-related immunosenescence in Fischer 344 rats: influence of exercise training. J Appl Physiol 1992;73:1928–1932.
104. Peters BA, Sothmann M, Wehrenberg WB. Blood leukocyte and spleen lymphocyte immune responses in chronically physically active and sedentary hamsters. Life Sci 1989;45:2239–2245.
105. Tharp GC, Preuss TL. Mitogenic response of T-lymphocytes to exercise training and stress. J Appl Physiol 1991;70: 535–2538.
106. Jensen M. The influence of regular physical activity on the cell-mediated immunity in pigs. Acta Vet Scand 1989;30:19–26.
107. Ferry A, Rieu P, Laziri F, Guezennec CA, Elhabazi A, Le Page C, et al. Immunomodulation of thymocytes and splenocytes in trained rats. J Appl Physiol 1991;71: 815–820.
108. Lin YS, Jan MS, Chen HI. The effect of chronic and acute exercise on immunity in rats. Int J Sports Med 1993;14:86–92.
109. Pahlavani MA, Cheung TH, Chesky JA, Richardson A. Influence of exercise on the immune function of rats of various ages. J Appl Physiol 1988;64:1997–2001.
110. Boas SR, Joswiak ML, Bufalino K, O'Connor MJ, Nixon PA, Orenstein DM, et al. Effects of anaerobic exercise on the immune system in 8 to 17 year old trained and untrained males. Med Sci Sports Exerc 1995;27:S175 (Abstract).
111. Oshida Y, Yamanouchi K, Hayamizu S, Sato Y. Effect of acute physical exercise on lymphocyte sub-populations in trained and untrained subjects. Int J Sports Med 1988;9:137–140.
112. Rhind S, Shek PN, Shinkai S, Shephard RJ. Differential expression of interleukin-2 receptor alpha and beta chains in relation to natural killer subsets and aerobic fitness. Int J Sports Med 1994;15: 911–918.
113. Seneczko F. White blood cell count and adherence in sportsmen and non-training subjects. Acta Physiol Pol 1983;34:601–610.
114. Liesen H, Uhlenbruck G. Sports Immunology. Sport Sci Rev 1992;1:94–116.
115. Nieman DC, Buckley KS, Henson DA, Warren BJ, Suttles J, Ahle A, et al. Immune function in marathon runners versus sedentary controls. Med Sci Sports Exerc 1995;27:986–992.
116. Pyne DB, Baker MS, Fricker PA, McDonald WA, Telford RD, Weidemann MJ. Effects of intensive 12-week training program by elite swimmers on neutrophil oxidative activity. Med Sci Sports Exerc 1995;27:536–542.
117. Benoni G, Bellavite P, Adami A, Chirumbolo S, Lippi G, Giulini GM, et al. Changes in several neutrophil functions in basketball players, before during and after sports season. Int J Sports Med 1995;16:34–37.
118. Ndon JA, Snyder AC, Foster C, Wehrenber WB. Effects of chronic intense exercise training on the leukocyte response to exercise. Int J Sports Med 1992;13:176–182.

119. Rhind S, Shek PN, Shinkai S, Shephard RJ. Effects of moderate endurance exercise and training on lymphocyte activation: in vitro lymphocyte proliferative response, IL-2 production, and IL-2 receptor expression. Eur J Appl Physiol 1996;74:348–360.
120. Hack V, Strobel G, Rau JP, Weicker H. The effect of maximal exercise on the activity of neutrophil granulocytes in highly trained athletes in am moderate training period. Eur J Appl Physiol 1992;65:520–524.
121. Benoni G, Bellavite P, Adami A, Chirumbolo S, Lippi G, Cuzzolini L. Effect of acute exercise on some hematological parameters and neutrophil functions in active and inactive subjects. Eur J Appl Physiol 1995;70:187–191.
122. Ortega E, Barriga C, De la Fuente M. Study of the phagocytic process of the neutrophils from elite sportswomen. Eur J Appl Physiol 1993;66:60–64.
123. Prasad K, Chaudhary AK, Kalra J. Oxygen derived free radical producing activity and survival of activated polymorphonuclear leukocytes. Mol Cell Biol 1991;103:51–62.
124. Nieman DC, Brendle DA, Henson DA, Suttles J, Cook VD, Warren BJ, et al. Immune function in athletes versus non-athletes. Int J Sports Med 1995;16:329–333.
125. Janssen GM, van Wersch JWJ, Kaiser V, Does R. White cell system changes associated with a training period of 18–20 months: a transverse and a longitudinal approach. Int J Sports Med 1989;10:S176–S180.
126. Baum M, Bialluch S, Liesen H. Die Wirkung eines sechswöchigen moderaten Ausdauertrainings auf immunologische Parameteren (The effect of 6 weeks moderate training on immunologic parameters). In: Kindermann W and Schwarz L, eds. Bewegung und Sport—eine Herausforderung für die Medizin (Movement and Sport—A Challenge for Medicine). CIBA-Geigy, Wehr, 1995, p. 144 (Abstract).
127. Davidson RJ, Robertson JD, Maughan RJ. Hematological changes associated with marathon running. Int J Sports Med 1987;8:19–25.
128. Gabriel H, Schwarz L, Urhausen A, Kindermann W. Leukocytes and lymphocyte subpopulations in peripheral blood of female and male athletes under resting conditions. Dtsch Z Sportmed 1992;43:196–210.
129. Pizza FX, Flynn MG, Sawyer T, Brolison PG, Starling RD, Andres FF. Run training versus cross-training: effect of increased training on circulation leukocyte subsets. Med Sci Sports Exerc 1995;27:363–370.
130. Ferry A, Picard F, Duvallet A, Weill B, Rieu M. Changes in blood leucocyte populations induced by acute maximal and chronic submaximal exercise. Eur J Appl Physiol 1990;59:435–442.
131. Hoffman-Goetz L, Simpson JR, Cipp N, Arumagam Y, Houston ME. Lymphocyte subset response to repeated submaximal exercise in men. J. Appl Physiol 1990;68:1069–1074.
132. Baj Z, Kantorski J, Majewska E, Zeman K, Pokoca I, Fornalczk E, et al. Immunological status of competitive cyclists before and after the training season. Int J Sports Med 1994;15:319–324.
132. Kendall A, Hoffman-Goetz L, Houston M, MacNeil B, Arumagam Y. Exercise and blood lymphocyte subset responses: intensity, duration and subject fitness effects. J App Physiol 1990;69:251–260.
133. Hoffman-Goetz L, Pedersen BK. Exercise and the immune system: a model for the stress response? Immunol Today 1994;15:382–387.
134. Neisler HM, Bean MH, Thompson WR, Hall M. Alteration of lymphocyte subsets during a competitive swim training session. In: MacLaren D, Reilly T, and Lee A, eds. Biomechanics and Medicine in Swimming. Swimming Science VI. E & F N Spon, London, 1990, pp.333–336.
135. Verde T, Thomas S, Moore RW, Shek PN, Shephard RJ. Immune responses and increased training of the athlete. J Appl Physiol 1992;73:1494–1499.
136. Northoff H, Weinstock C, Berg A. The cytokine response to strenuous exercise. Int J Sports Med 1994;15:S167–171.
137. Sprenger H, Jacobs C, Main M, Gressner AM, Prinz H, Wesemann W, et al. Enhanced release of cytokines, interleukin 2 receptors, and neopterin after long distance running. Clin Immunol Immunopathol 1992;63:188–194.
138. Mackinnon LT. Exercise and immunoglobulins. Exerc Immunol Rev 1996;2:1–34.
139. Eberhardt A. Influence of motor activity on some serologic mechanisms of nonspecific immunity. II. Effect of strenuous physical effort. Acta Physiol Polonica 1971;22:185–194.
140. Smith JA, Telford RD, Mason IB, Weidemann MJ. Exercise training and neutrophil microbicidal activity. Int J Sports Med 1990;11:179–187.

141. Thomsen BS, Rodgaard A, Tvede N, Hansen FR, Steensberg J, Halkjær-Kristensen J, et al. Levels of complement receptor type one (CR1, CD35) on erythrocytes, circulating immune complexes and complement C3 split products C3d and C3c are not changed by short-term physical exercise or training. Int. J. Sports Med. 1992;13:172–175.
142. Mackinnon LT, Ginn E, Seymour G. Temporal relationship between exercise-induced decreases in salivary IgA concentration and subsequent appearance of upper respiratory illness in elite athletes. Med Sci Sports Exerc 1991;23:S45 (Abstract).
143. Nieman DC. Exercise and resistance to infection. Can J Physiol Pharmacol 1998;76:573–580.
144. Peters-Futre E. Vitamin C, neutrophil function, and upper respiratory tract infection risk in distance runners: The missing link. Ex Immunol Rev 1997;3:32–52.
145. Chandra RK. McCollom Award Lecture. Nutrition and Immunity: lessons from the past and new insights into the future. Am J Clin Nutr 1990;53:1087–1101.
146. Irwin M, Smith TL, Gillin JC. Electroencephalographic sleep and natural killer activity in depressed patients and control subjects. Psychosom Med 1992;54:10–21.
147. Nieman DC. Exercise, upper respiratory tract infection, and the immune system. Med Sci Sports Exerc 1994;26:128–139.
148. Jackson GG, Dowling HF, Anderson TO, Riff L, Saporta J, Turck M. Susceptibility and immunity to common upper respiratory viral infections—the common cold. Ann Intern Med 1960;53:719–738.
149. Shephard RJ, Shek PN. The risk of cancer in the international athlete. Acta Acad Olymp Est 1996; 4:5–24.
150. Verde T, Thomas S, Shephard RJ. Potential markers of heavy training in highly trained distance runners. Br J Sports Med 1992;26:167–175.
151. Lerner A, Yamada T, Miller RA. Pgp-1^{hi} T lymphocytes accumulate with age in mice and respond poorly to concanavalin A. Eur J Immunol 1989;19:977–982.
152. Gabriel H, Schmitt B, Kindermann W. Age-related increase of CD45RO$^+$ lymphocytes in physically active adults. Eur J Immunol 1993;23:2704–2706.
153. Song L, Kim YH, Choppra RK, Proust JJ, Nagel JE, Nordin AA, et al. Age-related effects in T cell activation and proliferation. Exp Gerontol 1993;28:313–321.
154. Hobb VM, Weigle WO, Noonan DJ, Torbett BE, McEvilly, RJ, Koch RJ, et al. Patterns of cytokine gene expression by CD4$^+$ T cells from young and old mice. J Immunol 1993;150:3602–3614.
155. Xusheng S, Yugi XX, Ronggang Z. Detection of AC rosette-forming lymphocytes in the healthy aged with Taichiquando (88 style) exercise. J Sports Med Phys Fitness 1990;30:401–405.
156. Shinkai S, Khono H, Kimura K, Komura T, Asai H, Inai R, et al. Physical activity and immune senescence in men. Med Sci Sports Exerc 1995;27:1516–1526.
157. Rall LC, Roubenoff R, Cannon JG, Abad LW, Dinarello CA, Meydani SN. Effects of progressive resistance training on immune response in aging and chronic inflammation. Med Sci Sports Exerc 1996;28:1356–1365.

17 Exercise and the Developing Child
Endocrine Considerations

*Sita M. Sundaresan, BA,
James N. Roemmich, PhD,
and Alan D. Rogol, MD, PhD*

Contents

    Introduction
    Pubertal Growth and the Growth Hormone–Insulin-Like
        Growth Factor/Hypothalamic–Pituitary–Gonadal
        (GH–IGF/HPG) Axes
    The Effects of Acute Exercise on Hormone Release
    Exercise Training and Hormonal Alterations
        in the Neuroendocrine Axes
    Effects of Training for Sport on Growth and Puberty
    Confounding Factors and Their Influence
        on Growth and Pubertal Development
    Conclusions
    References

INTRODUCTION

With increasing numbers of children training for and competing in sports, questions arise about the effects of daily, physically intense exercise regimens on somatic growth and maturational processes. The search to identify and nurture the talented athlete has extended to younger and younger children, raising concern about potential negative influences of intensive exercise on their physical and psychological well-being.

In normal children and adolescents, physical activity is an important aspect of a healthy lifestyle. As for adults, exercise and the developing child produces many physiologic benefits, including increased strength, improved blood lipid levels (*1*), and psychological benefits, such as learning a sense of competence and control, increased confidence and self-esteem, and social development (*2*). However, children who participate in organized sports often are involved in physical activity at higher levels of intensity and for

From: *Contemporary Endocrinology: Sports Endocrinology*
Edited by: M. P. Warren and N. W. Constantini © Humana Press Inc., Totowa, NJ

longer periods of time than recreational participants. The influence of frequent bouts of intense physical training on growth and maturation has been debated in recent years *(3–6)*. The lack of consensus is owing, in part, to multiple confounding factors, such as genetics, nutrition, socioeconomic status, and nonstandardized experimental methodology. The principal topic addressed in this chapter is the effect of exercise on growth and maturation. The effects of acute and chronic exercise on the neuroendocrine axes controlling growth and maturation of children will also be described.

PUBERTAL GROWTH AND THE GROWTH HORMONE–INSULIN-LIKE GROWTH FACTOR/HYPOTHALAMIC–PITUITARY–GONADAL (GH–IGF/HPG) AXES

Overview

The pubertal growth spurt is one of the most dynamic periods of physiologic and somatic change in physique, sexual maturation, and body composition. With pubertal growth comes improvement in sports performance, associated with increases in body size, muscle strength and power, and skill level. These physiologic changes are controlled, in large part, by the GH–IGF and HPG axes.

GH is the primary hormone responsible for somatic growth, having, in addition, potent actions on protein, carbohydrate, and lipid metabolism. Many of the effects of GH are indirectly mediated through IGFs, primarily IGF-1, which can be locally synthesized by target tissues or by the liver, the predominant locus of circulating IGF-1. GH has direct end-organ effects as well, initiating complex cellular processes that result in cell differentiation and proliferation. At the growth plate, IGF-1-induced epiphyseal cartilage proliferation and differentiation of stem cell chondrocytes increase the formation of cartilage and elongation of bone *(7)*.

The neuroendocrine regulation of GH production and pulsatile GH release is subject to various influences as a child's biological age advances to reproductive maturity *(8,9)*. Prepubertally, resting GH secretion is modulated primarily through GH-releasing hormone (GHRH) originating from the arcuate nucleus of the hypothalamus, and through somatostatin released from the preoptic and paraventricular nuclei. Genetic determinants and environmental influences, such as diet, nutrition, or chronic disease, may influence GH release and growth potential from infancy to childhood.

At the onset of puberty, a marked acceleration in growth velocity results from a complex network of interactions between the GH–IGF and HPG axes. Total GH secretion increases two- to threefold, modulated through increased amplitude of secretory bursts, independent of pulse frequency *(10)*. Increases in circulating IGF-1 and insulin-like growth factor binding protein 3 (IGF-BP3) parallel the augmented GH secretion *(11)*.

Increases in the mass and rate of GH released per secretory burst during puberty may be modulated by the increasing concentrations of sex steroid hormones. Once believed to be primarily androgen-dependent *(10,12,13)*, the activation of the HPG and GH/IGF axes are now thought to be controlled by rising estrogen concentrations. Data suggest that estrogen may control feedback amplification of GH secretion during puberty, even in the male *(14,15)*. Ultrasensitive measurements demonstrate the pattern of rising estrogen concentrations in boys during their progress through puberty *(16)*. The first measured rise in estrogen concentrations occurs at the time of peak growth velocity. Thus, estrogen in girls, or aromatization of testosterone to estrogen in boys, may likely be the initial trigger of amplified GH secretion in puberty *(17)*. Estrogen may act synergistically with increasing testosterone and GH concentrations to mediate skeletal growth in boys and girls at low concentrations, while at higher concentrations, inducing epiphyseal fusion in both sexes. Recently, osteoporosis, unfused epiphyses, and continuing linear growth in adulthood was described in a man with an estrogen-receptor mutation rendering him unresponsive to estrogens. Previously thought to be lethal, the estrogen receptor mutation in a living human provides valuable clinical evidence supporting the hypothesis that estrogen may be responsible for normal male and female skeletal growth and development *(18)*. Identification of aromatase deficiency in a man revealed a similar clinical presentation to that of mutated estrogen receptor phenotype. Epiphyseal closure occurred only after estrogen (not androgen) therapy *(19)*. In addition, boys with androgen insensitivity have female characteristics in timing and duration of pubertal growth if there is no therapeutic response to androgen administration *(20)*. These findings and other supporting studies *(21)* are contrary to previous hypotheses that pubertal growth is mediated by an androgen-dependent process.

In summary, the complex interrelationship of the GH/IGF axis and HPG axis governs normal growth and puberty. Recent advances have further characterized the neuroendocrine alterations controlling GH secretion at puberty. Our greater understanding of the physiology of pubertal growth will soon lead to improved therapeutic options in pathologic conditions, and will heighten awareness of potential positive and negative influences from additional factors, such as exercise.

Leptin

Leptin, the protein product of the obesity *(ob)* gene, has been the focus of many recent studies in humans *(22–24)*. Secreted from adipocytes into the bloodstream, leptin may be an important link between peripheral fat mass and the brain's central control of metabolism (Fig. 1) *(24)*. Extensively studied in *ob/ob* mice, leptin deficiency is associated with a decreased metabolic rate, increased appetite, decreased energy expenditure, obesity, and infertility. These abnormalities are reversed after leptin administration *(23)*. Leptin treatment also accelerates pubertal onset in *ob/ob* mice *(25)*. The mechanisms by which leptin regulates body weight and integrates adiposity with other neuroendocrine axes remain unclear *(24)*. Congenital leptin deficiency has been reported in two severely obese children, both of whom had a markedly increased fat mass but low serum leptin concentration *(26)*. These findings support the hypothesis that leptin is an important regulator of energy balance in humans and may be the first genetic evidence that leptin deficiency can cause obesity in humans.

Leptin may affect the timing and tempo of puberty, since it is involved in energy balance and reproduction in small laboratory animals, although this has not yet been shown in humans *(25)*. Leptin may be one of the factors through which exercise training and reduced adiposity affects the neuroendocrine axes *(8)*. In effect, leptin may be a molecular signal linking nutritional status to the activation of the HPG axis *(22)*. Leptin has been hypothesized to be a possible trigger for the onset of puberty because leptin concentrations rise (approximately twofold) prior to the pubertal increase in testosterone in males *(27)* and prior to activation of the HPG axis in females *(28)*. However, the physiologic mechanisms for the leptin surge remain unknown. Others have also reported increases in leptin concentrations in the prepubertal to pubertal transition of girls and boys and then pubertal reductions in leptin concentrations in boys *(29,30)*.

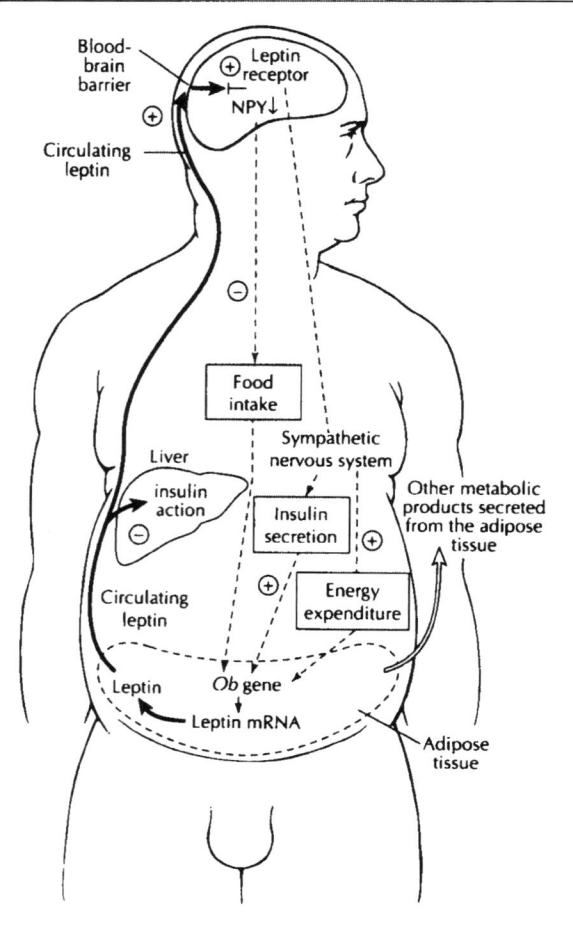

Fig. 1. Leptin, secreted from adipocytes, may represent a link between peripheral fat mass and central control mechanisms of metabolism in the brain. The binding of leptin to receptors in the hypothalamus decreases neuropeptide Y (NPY) secretion, causing appetite suppression and sympathetic nervous system-mediated increases in insulin secretion and energy expenditure. Other hormonal systems may also be involved. (From ref. 24, with permission.)

The relationship among gender, leptin concentration, and body fat mass accumulation during puberty remains unclear. Recently, Roemmich et al. *(31)* described that the gender difference in leptin concentration of boys and girls was related to differences in the amount of subcutaneous fat and greater androgen concentrations of boys. Leptin concentrations were more highly related to the subcutaneous fat than the total fat mass as measured by a criterion four-compartment model. The gender differences in leptin concentration remained after correcting for the amount of subcutaneous fat or total fat mass. Although previously hypothesized to increase energy expenditure and physical activity by others *(32)*, serum leptin concentrations were inversely related to the total energy expenditure (measured by $^2H_2^{18}O$ dilution) when adjusted for the amount of fat-free mass. Energy expenditure may reduce leptin concentrations by reducing the subcutaneous fat and total fat mass *(31)*. Nagy et al. *(33)* also found that body fat distribution (subcutaneous and intra-abdominal adipose tissue measured by computed tomography) could account for gender differences in serum leptin concentrations.

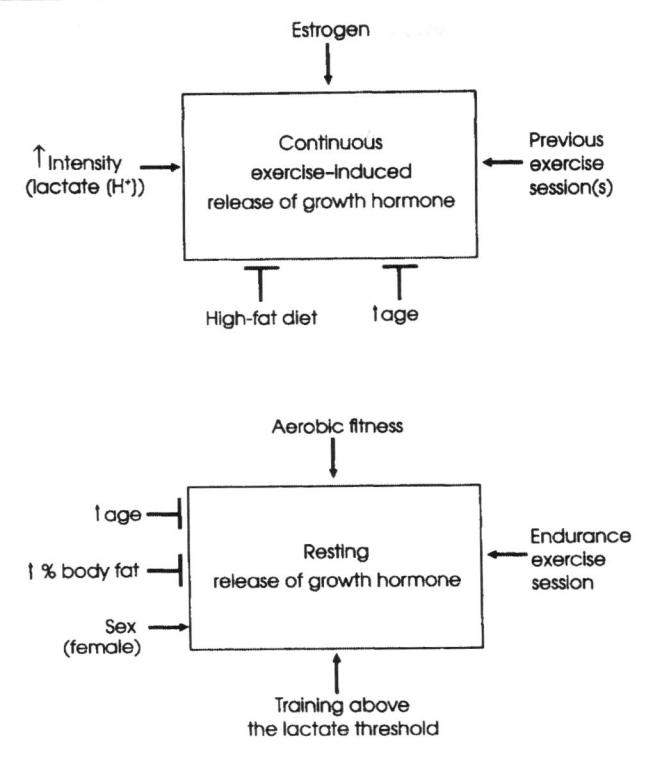

Fig. 2. Factors that influence the continuous exercise-induced release of GH (top box) and the resting release of GH in endurance exercise-trained people (bottom box). (From ref. *40*, with permission.)

Other investigators have found significant gender effects on leptin concentrations in children after correcting for the adiposity with noncriterion estimates of body composition *(30,34,35)*. Thus, gender differences in leptin concentration may be owing to differences in leptin synthesis, bioactivity, clearance rates, and other biokinetic properties *(35)*. Pubertal increases in testosterone concentration may also reduce the leptin concentration in adolescent males *(30,36,37)*. Testosterone enanthate therapy reduces leptin concentrations in adolescent boys with delayed puberty *(38)*. The fat mass also decreased in subjects; however, the authors did not report the effects of testosterone treatment on leptin concentrations independent of the change in fat mass. More studies in children and adolescents are needed in order to elucidate the role of leptin in pubertal development and to define further the relationship among gender, sex steroids, body composition, body fat distribution, energy expenditure, and leptin.

THE EFFECTS OF ACUTE EXERCISE ON HORMONE RELEASE

GH–IGF-1 Axis and Acute Exercise

Acute bouts of exercise increase the plasma concentration of GH in children and adolescents *(39)*. Stimulation of GH release during acute exercise is influenced by several factors, including sex steroid hormones, blood lactate concentration, macronutrient composition, age, and previous exercise sessions (Fig. 2) *(40)*. Pubertal development influences the response of the GH–IGF-1 axis to acute exercise *(41,42)*. The peak

GH response to treadmill exercise and arginine-insulin stimulation increases in both boys and girls as the pubertal stage advances. The peak GH response is similar in boys and girls at the same pubertal stage. Sex steroids play a major role in enhancing exercise-induced GH release during puberty. Estrogen priming of prepubertal subjects increases the peak GH response to exercise, arginine, or insulin to pubertal levels *(42)*. Increased aerobic fitness, reduced adiposity, younger age, greater training intensities and female gender enhance the basal (resting) GH release in adults *(40)*. These same factors may modulate resting GH release in children, but few data are available to support such a claim.

Acute Exercise and the Male HPG Axis

Alterations have also been described in the male HPG axis as a result of acute exercise. Studies have shown that the testosterone concentration rises after the onset of short-term exercise activity and increase in proportion to the exercise intensity *(43)*. Similarly, testosterone concentration increases after the onset of a prolonged exercise bout (>60 min), but decline substantially as exercise is maintained, finally returning to baseline after a recovery period. Luteinizing hormone (LH) concentrations also increase in response to maximal and submaximal exercise bouts, whereas follicle-stimulating hormone (FSH) concentrations remain relatively unaffected. These findings have been reported in many different modalities of exercise, including running, weight lifting, rowing, swimming, and high intensity sprinting *(43)*. A recent study by Elias et al. *(44)* reported contradictory findings in normal male subjects exercised to exhaustion. Sampling at baseline and immediately after a single bout of exercise showed no significant increases in LH and FSH up to 180 min after cessation of exercise. Testosterone concentration was not measured in this study. Others have also reported that light to moderate exercise did not influence testosterone or LH concentrations, but higher exercise intensity and longer duration increased the testosterone concentration despite the low LH concentration *(45)*. The impact of acute exercise on the immature and developing male reproductive system has not been well studied.

Acute Exercise and the Female HPG Axis

Hormonal alterations in adult female athletes during acute exercise have been the focus of much research in the last 25 years owing to the prevalence of menstrual disturbances observed in these women. Exercise-induced sympathoadrenal secretion of catecholamines stimulates endocrine secretion of secondary hormones and impairs production of gonadotropins *(46)*. Subsequent luteal-phase deficiency and anovulation are commonly reported in this population *(47)*. Several possible mechanisms for the decline in gonadotropin secretion with exercise have been proposed *(48,49)*, but conclusive evidence is still lacking.

To investigate the hypothesis that exercise-related hypoestrogenemia results from norepinephrine-mediated disruption of gonadotropin pulsatility, investigators evaluated the effects of acute exercise on estrogen, catecholestrogens, and catecholamine concentrations *(50)*. Resting, submaximal intensity, and maximal intensity determinations of plasma estrogen, catecholestrogens, and catecholamine responses were made during exercise (cycle ergometer) in both the follicular and luteal phase of nine previously untrained women. Increased circulating estrogen and catecholamines concentrations were reported in response to acute exercise were reported, but only a minor effect on catecholestrogen concentration was observed. More detailed discussions of these issues have previously been published *(46–49,50)*.

Acute Exercise and Leptin

Little information is available about the influence of acute exercise on the serum leptin concentration. Not surprisingly, the data on children and adolescents are even more limited. Apparently a single bout of exercise does not significantly affect the leptin concentration in humans. Perusse et al. *(52)* determined that serum leptin concentrations were not affected by an acute maximal bout of exercise in sedentary men and women. Other investigators reported plasma leptin concentrations sampled simultaneously from the venous (drainage from subcutaneous adipose tissue) and arterial circulation did not change during moderate intensity exercise (cycle ergometer) for 60 min *(53)*. Leptin concentrations appear not to be significantly altered in highly trained individuals after a prolonged (20 mile) exercise bout *(54)*. Thus, in both sedentary and trained subjects, serum leptin concentrations are not significantly influenced by single bouts of exercise.

EXERCISE TRAINING AND HORMONAL ALTERATIONS IN THE NEUROENDOCRINE AXES

Exercise Training and the GH–IGF-1 Axis

In women, 1 yr of endurance training increases 24-hr mean serum GH concentrations *(55)*. Intensity of exercise may be a crucial factor in the stimulation of the GH–IGF-1 axis with the requirement being a training intensity above the lactate threshold. A much shorter (2 wk) training study of 10 healthy, young, nonobese men showed increased GH release through increased plasma IGF-1 concentrations *(56)*. Growth hormone binding protein (GHBP), the extracellular domain of the receptor, concentrations rose significantly after the exercise training, representing a possible upregulation of the GH receptor. Fitness level and athletic training may also modulate the GH–IGF-1 axis in children and adolescents *(40)*. Eliakim et al. *(57)* reported that fitness, as measured by peak oxygen uptake, was directly related to serum IGF-1 concentrations in adolescent females. However, the effects of endurance exercise training on the GH–IGF-1 axis of children and young adults cannot be characterized owing to a lack of well-controlled exercise training studies.

Gymnastics training does not appear to enhance GH release as readily as distance running. No significant differences in serum IGF-1 concentrations were observed in collegiate female gymnasts compared to control women before or after the sport season *(58)*. In trained adolescent female gymnasts, circulating IGF-1 concentrations decreased after 3 d of intensive exercise *(59)*. In both studies, poor nutritional status may have altered the adaptation of the GH–IGF-1 axis to training, a potentially common occurrence in these athletes who often self-impose dietary restrictions in an effort to maintain a slim body physique.

Wrestling training and the associated dietary restriction temporarily lead to negative energy balance, decreased lean tissue, and reduced protein nutrition over a sports season, but do not appear to affect skeletal growth and maturation adversely *(60,61)*. Adolescent wrestlers were assessed for growth, maturation, hormonal concentrations, and nutrition before and after their sports season and compared to recreationally active controls matched for chronologic age, biological age, and sexual maturation. As a result of reduced energy intake and high-energy expenditures by the wrestlers, the body weight decreased primarily owing to a significant reduction in fat, but not fat-free, mass during the season. However, a subsequent postseason catch-up growth in fat-free mass by wrestlers suggests the normal pubertal accrual of lean tissue was slowed during the season. Resting hormonal analyses at late season revealed reductions in free and total testosterone, IGF-1, IGF-BP3, and GHBP concentrations, but normal LH and increased GH concentrations. Reductions in IGF-1 in the presence of elevated GH concentrations suggest a sports seasonal GH resistance. This adaptation may be mediated through reduced numbers of GH receptors (as indexed by concentrations of GHBP). Analysis performed 4 mo after the end of the season showed compensatory reversal of these hormonal alterations. However, separation of training effects from undernutrition requires study of a group of wrestlers who train daily without weight loss.

Exercise Training and the HPG Axis

Many studies have examined the effects of exercise training on the HPG axis of adults *(43,51,62)*, but fewer data are available in children and adolescents *(46)*. Implications about the influences of exercise on the HPG axis of children must be extended from adult data.

Disruption of the normal menstrual cycle in women who participate in high amounts of exercise and drain the body's energy stores is referred to as "athletic amenorrhea" *(63)*. Altered neuroendocrine regulation of gonadotropin secretion in these women likely results from decreased activity of the hypothalamic gonadotropin-releasing hormone (GnRH) pulse generator *(64)* and, thus, lowered pituitary secretion of FSH and LH. The pathophysiologic mechanism(s) causing the reversible hypoestrogenism has not yet been elucidated. Proposed mechanisms for the observed hypothalamic inhibition include increased activation of the HPA axis and energy drain *(62,65)*. There are numerous implications on women's health issues resulting from athletic amenorrhea, including reduced bone density, osteoporosis, scoliosis, and cardiovascular risks *(47)*. Bullen et al. *(66)* reported suppression of the LH surge, follicular and luteal development, and ovulation within the first month of an acutely very intensive exercise training program, and increased incidence of menstrual irregularities in the second month.

However, some studies have not found an effect of exercise training on the menstrual cycle of adult women. A prospective, longitudinal study had previously untrained adult women run at and above their lactate threshold 3 d/wk for 12–14 mo *(55)*. No significant effects on menstrual cycle length, follicular- and luteal-phase lengths, LH pulsatility, and integrated serum progesterone or estradiol concentrations were found. Loucks et al. *(67)* reported endurance exercise-trained women had a reduced LH pulse frequency, increased LH pulse amplitude, and reduced FSH responsiveness to GnRH. Despite the alterations in the HPG axis, the trained women maintained their menstrual cycles, demonstrating the plasticity of the HPG axis *(67)*. Stress and psychological factors may be partly responsible for the inconsistencies among the studies.

Women who initiate training closer to age of menarche may be more susceptible to menstrual cycle disruption *(65,68,69)*. In girls, the timing of release of gonadotropins, the activation of the gonadal axis, and the tempo of puberty may be disrupted by athletic training *(7,47,65,70–72)*. However, social influences also affect menarche in athletes *(73,74)* making the hypothesis that exercise training alone causes delayed menarche debatable *(65)*.

Mode of exercise training may be an important consideration when determining whether exercise training induces alterations in the HPG axis. Menstrual dysfunction in adolescent competitive swimmers may result from physiologic mechanisms different from inhibition of the hypothalamic GnRH pulse generator observed in dancing and long distance running, modes of exercise typically associated with low body mass *(75)*. More intensive investigations of the influence of exercise mode are required to determine the effects of exercise training on the neuroendocrine axes of children and adolescents.

The impact of endurance exercise training on the male reproductive system has been less extensively studied. Mild abnormalities in the HPG axis, primarily a normal LH concentration but reduced testosterone concentration, suggest a central HPG impairment in adult endurance-trained men, but many conflicting findings have been reported *(43)*. Single blood samples of the resting hormonal profiles of adult trained men show reduced free and total testosterone concentrations, but no significant change in LH concentration *(76–79)*. Prospective exercise studies report both reductions *(80–82)* and no significant changes *(83,84)* in the resting concentrations of testosterone, LH, and FSH in endurance-trained adult males. Studies utilizing serial blood sampling to allow for detection of LH pulse frequency and amplitude reported contradictory results as well *(43)*. Lucia et al. *(85)* found no adverse effects on the LH and testosterone concentrations of professional cyclists, elite triathletes, and recreational marathon runners who were studied prospectively over their sports seasons. Semen characteristics also were normal and unchanged by training.

Few studies have examined the effects of endurance exercise training on the HPT axis of prepubertal or pubertal male athletes. Rowland et al. *(86)* studied previously trained adolescent male runners and found no significant changes in total and free testosterone concentrations. These data suggest that endurance training does not disturb the male adolescent HPG axis. However, the intensity of the exercise training and the duration of the season may not have been great enough to impact this neuroendocrine axis significantly.

Exercise Training and Leptin

Since leptin may be an important signal between the body fat mass and the neuroendocrine regulation of nutrient metabolism and energy expenditure, exercise training may modulate leptin synthesis and/or release. Few studies have evaluated the effects of exercise training on resting leptin concentrations in humans *(52,54,87,88)*. The current data suggest that there are no independent effects of chronic exercise on resting leptin concentration, apart from those related to changes in fat mass during the training. However, some recent data show decreases in leptin concentration after adjusting for changes in fat mass *(87,89)*. Hickey et al. *(89)* have proposed that exercise training affects the leptin concentration independent of changes in fat mass and more so in females than males. Serum leptin concentrations decreased in nine females after 12 wk of aerobic exercise training, but not in nine males matched for aerobic capacity. Exercise training produced improvements in aerobic capacity, but no significant alterations in fat mass. Pasman et al. *(87)* also found that exercise training decreased plasma leptin concentrations independently from percent body fat and plasma insulin levels. Fifteen obese adult males underwent 4 mo of dietary restriction and endurance exercise training (swimming, cycling, and running), followed by either 12 mo of continued endurance exercise training (trained group) or resumption of minimal physical activity (nontrained group). The trained group had significantly lowered leptin concentrations, after correction for changes in insulin and body fat percentage, compared to the nontrained group. Additionally, the hours of moderate-intensity exercise per week in the trained group were inversely correlated with changes in leptin concentrations. The long duration of exercise training may have been an important factor in this study. More prospective studies in adults and children are needed to determine the effects of exercise training on serum leptin concentration.

EFFECTS OF TRAINING FOR SPORT ON GROWTH AND PUBERTY

Data from several longitudinal studies of female dancers, swimmers, and gymnasts imply that intensive exercise negatively affects growth and/or pubertal development *(4,70–72,90–93)*. Age at menarche has been accepted as a marker of pubertal onset, although initially girls can have cyclical changes in hormone concentrations without menstrual bleeding. Merzenich et al. *(94)* concluded that increased time spent in training was associated with a delay in menarche. Warren *(72)* noted a late age of menarche in ballet dancers with slim body physiques. Thientz et al. *(93)* prospectively evaluated height, sitting height, leg length, weight, body fat, and pubertal stage of adolescent female gymnasts training 22 h/wk, and swimmers who trained 8 h/wk. Their pubertal development revealed a discordance between thelarche (GnRH and therefore central gonadotropin dependent) and gonadarche (adrecarche, perhaps dependent on a central adrenal androgen-stimulating factor). Without the presence of estrogen to mature (and fuse) the epiphyseal plates of the long bones, these young women grew to an adult height greater than that predicted at a younger age. Over time, the gymnasts had a lower growth velocity and decreased predicted height compared to swimmers. They concluded intensive gymnastics training initiated before and maintained throughout puberty may significantly decrease growth rate and final adult height, although genetics, selection bias, and nutrition probably also influenced the results.

Pigeon et al. *(92)* reported a 5-yr longitudinal study of the growth and maturation of female dancers followed to adult height. Diminished growth velocity and pubertal delay were reported in the dancers compared to recreationally active controls. Decreased pubertal growth velocity was observed in 16% of the dancers who were also leaner and had poorer dietary habits compared to the rest of the dancers. No differences in chronologic age, time spent in training, age of initiation of ballet training, height at age 6, maternal menarcheal age, or mean parental height were found in the dancer subgroups. Mean age of menarche was delayed by 1.5 yr in the dancers (13.5 yr) compared to controls (12 yr). As expected, reduced energy and nutritional intake were more evident in the subset of dancers who experienced delayed growth and puberty.

Another 5-yr longitudinal study also reported delayed growth and pubertal development in competitive adolescent gymnastics who had a delayed age of menarche, slower growth rate, but also less body fat (from skinfold thickness) and smaller body physiques (height and weight) compared to nontraining, age-matched controls and normal population means *(70)*. The development of anorexia nervosa was reported in two gymnasts, but specific analyses of nutritional intake, dietary practices, and energy balance were not performed. Genetics for linear growth (predicted height), but not pubertal development (maternal age at menarche) were assessed, and the adult height was found to be less than predicted in 6 of the 22 (27%) gymnasts. These findings support the hypothesis that intensive gymnastics training may produce negative effects on pubertal development and linear growth, in conjunction with other factors, such as body physique and nutritional factors

CONFOUNDING FACTORS AND THEIR INFLUENCE ON GROWTH AND PUBERTAL DEVELOPMENT

Often, confounding factors are not considered in research studies that conclude that exercise has adverse effects on the growing child and adolescent. Environmental factors influence the linear growth and pubertal development of a child, and can delay or prevent a child from reaching his or her adult height or reproductive maturity. Additionally, hereditary determinants of stature as well as timing and tempo of maturational processes can also play a key role in determining whether a healthy child will be able to grow and mature in a normal pattern.

Nutrition is a major environmental factor influencing growth and pubertal development *(95,96)*. Malnutrition stunts growth and delays maturation, as is tragically evident in underdeveloped countries *(97)*. When food intake is inadequate, the limited energy resources are utilized for sustaining basic life processes, and not for growth and development. Energy balance can be difficult to maintain in some sports *(98)*, such as gymnastics and wrestling, given the pressures exerted by coaches, peers, or the child to maintain a low body weight and/or ideal body physique, which is thought to enhance performance *(99–101)*. Young female athletes have a higher incidence of eating disorders and preoccupation with body weight *(96,102)*. Thus, the dietary habits and nutritional status of exercising youth are important considerations when interpreting growth and maturation data. If not measured, it makes it difficult to implicate the exercise regimen itself as a negative influence on a child's linear growth and progression into adolescence.

Psychological factors also influence the growth and pubertal development of exercising youth. In encouraging and grooming these young athletes for competition and athletic success, coaches, parents, and peers may expose the child to external pressures to perform and participate in training regimens *(103)*. The media may also contribute to the psychological stress that athletes experience. Though not extensively studied, psychological pressures can produce mental stress in an athlete. These psychological disturbances may be manifested as physical symptomatology, including disorders of growth, eating disorders, and derangements of the timing and tempo of puberty *(9,73)*.

There is no consensus on whether exercise training *per se* in children and adolescents can alter growth and biological maturation. For the majority of young athletes, intensive training for a sport itself may not exert negative effects on these processes; rather, associated environmental and genetic factors, or the interaction of exercise with these factors is more likely the cause of altered growth and puberty of these young athletes *(73,103)*. A cause–effect sequence between training and the biological processes of growth and sexual maturation may not be inferred from strong associations *(103)*. Ultimately, it may be impossible for one to conclude that exercise alone causes deleterious effects on a child's height or reproductive maturity. Delayed growth and maturation of athletes may actually be more a result of preselection of individuals who display desirable characteristics for the sport *(65,73,103)*. Sports selection for linearity of physique, for example, is associated with later maturation in both sexes *(103)*. In an extensive review of growth and maturation data in team and individual youth sport, Malina *(103)* summarized the many data that have been presented that are pertinent to this topic. Preselection for sport, genetic determinants of growth and maturation, diet and nutrition, coaching practices, and associated adverse emotional and psychological pressures were often overlooked in these studies. Prior to their sports selection, gymnasts measured shorter than average at a young age, even as young as 2 yr old, and linear growth patterns in young female swimmers and track/rowing athletes as well as gymnasts showed no change in statural growth as a result of exercise activity *(103)*. The swimmers and track athletes were already taller than average during childhood, and maintained their position relative to reference data for nonathletes during adolescence. The female gymnasts were already shorter than average prior to their participation in sports. Thus, preselection for a sport creates a nonrandom population that may skew the data about patterns of growth and maturation.

Another factor that is not consistently normalized in growth studies is the skeletal maturation of the subject *(103,104)*. Inconsistencies in skeletal age prior to exercise training may then be mistaken as resulting from athletic activity. No differences exist between the pubertal development of active and nonactive boys and girls, based on several retrospective longitudinal studies *(103,105)*. Additional familial factors, such as the age of menarche in female relatives, often do not receive ample consideration. Mothers and sisters of university athletes and gymnasts have a delayed age of menarche, and a greater number of children in a family increases the age of menarche *(103)*. However, some investigators have evaluated the effects of genetic factors on age of menarche in dancers *(106)* and swimmers *(107)*. Maternal puberty alone did not predict age of menarche in the athletes. The amount and intensity of physical training also influenced menarcheal age in the athletes.

Exercise may have no significant effects on the physical growth of children. Obert et al. *(108)* compared prepubertal girls participating in swimming 10–12 h/wk for a period of 40 mo to a control group of recreationally active girls. No significant differences in growth were observed, suggesting that intense swimming training early in life has no immediate influences on the physical growth of children. As expected, physiologic differences were observed in the two groups, with an increased peak oxygen uptake found in the exercising group. Similarly, high-intensity resistance training in children may have little effect on somatic growth (height or weight) and body composition *(109)*.

Exercise may be necessary for stimulation of normal linear growth *(106)*. A recent study in preschool children (ages 24–48 mo) recovering from protein-energy malnutrition demonstrated that active children (stimulated to play more physically demanding games) grew more in length and lean body mass as compared to less active children over a 6 wk period *(110)*.

CONCLUSIONS

Although athletic training and exercise can be associated with later menarche and delayed growth, there are many interactions and multiple confounding factors that do not permit the isolation of a specific effect of training *per se* on growth and maturation. Valid assessments of the effects of exercise on growth must consider the energy balance of the child and include measurements of energy intake and energy expenditure. There are marked effects of acute exercise and exercise training on the neuroendocrine axes controlling the growth and maturation of adults, but further research is needed to characterize fully if similar alterations occur in the immature hormonal axes of children. Long-term implications of intense training for sports on later health remain unclear, and further investigation is warranted. Future studies should account for as many confounding factors as possible.

REFERENCES

1. Zauner CW, Maksud MG, Melichna J. Physiological considerations in training young athletes. Sports Med 1989;8:15–31.
2. Hughson R. Children in competitive sports—a multi-disciplinary approach. Canad J Appl Sport Sci 1986;11:162–172.
3. Malina RM. Physical activity and training: effects on stature and the adolescent growth spurt. Med Sci Sports Exer 1994;26:759–766.
4. Theintz G, et al. The child, growth and high-level sports. Schweizerische Zeitschrift für Medizin und Traumatologie 1994;3:7–15.
5. Beunen GP, Malina RM, Renson R, Simons J, Ostyn M, Lefevre J. Physical activity and growth, maturation and performance: a longitudinal study. Med Sci Sports Exerc 1992;24:576–585.
6. Mansfield MJ, Emans SJ. Growth in female gymnasts: should training decrease during puberty? J Pediatr 1993;122:237–240.
7. Roemmich JN, Rogol AR. Physiology of growth and development: Its relationship to performance in the young athlete. Clin Sports Med 1995;14:483–502.
8. Rogol AD. Growth and development: editorial overview. Curr Opinion Endocrinol 1995;2:79–82.
9. Westphal O. Normal growth and growth disorders in children. Acta Odontol Scand 1995;53:174–178.
10. Kerrigan JR, Veldhuis JD, Rogol AD. Androgen-receptor blockade enhances pulsatile luteinizing hormone production in late pubertal males: evidence for a hypothalamic site of physiologic androgen feedback action. Pediatr Res 1994;35:102–106.
11. Loche S, Casini MR, Faedda A. The GH/IGF-1 axis in puberty. Br J Clin Pract—Symp Suppl 1996;85:1–4.
12. Ulloa-Aguirre A, Blizzard RM, Garcia-Rubi E, Rogol AD, Link K, Christie CM, et al. Testosterone and oxandrolone, a nonaromatizable androgen, specifically amplify the mass and rate of growth hormone (GH) secreted per burst without altering GH secretory burst, duration or frequency or the GH half-life. J Clin Endocrinol Metab 1990;71:846–854.
13. Link K, Blizzard RM, Evans WS, Kaiser DL, Parker MW, Rogol AD. The effect of androgens on the pulsatile release and the twenty-four-hour mean concentration of growth hormone in peripubertal males. J Clin Endocrinol Metab 1986;62:159–164.
14. Mauras N, Rogol AD, Haymond MW, Veldhuis JD. Sex steroids, growth hormone, insulin-like growth factor-I: Neuroendocrine and metabolic regulation in puberty. Horm Res 1996;45:74–80.
15. Smith EP, Korach KS. Oestrogen receptor deficiency: consequences for growth. Acta Paediatr Suppl 1996;417:39–43.
16. Klein KO, Martha PM Jr, Blizzard RM, Herbst T, Rogol AD. A longitudinal assessment of hormonal and physical alterations during normal puberty in boys. II. Estrogen levels as determined by an ultrasensitive bioassay. J Clin Endocrinol Metab 1996;81:3203–3207.
17. Veldhuis JD, Metzger DL, Martha PM Jr, Mauras N, Kerrigan JR, Keenan B, et al. Estrogen and testosterone, but not a nonaromatizable androgen, direct network integration of the hypothalamo-somatotrope (growth hormone)-insulin-like growth factor I axis in the human: evidence from pubertal pathophysiology and sex-steroid hormone replacement. J Clin Endocrinol Metab 1997;82:3414–3420.
18. Smith EP, Boyd J, Frank GR, Takahasi H, Cohen RM, Specker B, et al. Estrogen resistance caused by a mutation in the estrogen-receptor gene in a man. N Engl J Med 1994;331:1056–1061.
19. Carani C, Qin K, Simoni M, Faustini-Fustini M, Serpente S, Boyd J, et al. Effect of testosterone and estradiol in a man with aromatase deficiency. N Engl J Med 1997;337:91–95.
20. Ritzen EM. Pubertal growth in genetic disorders of sex hormone action and secretion. Acta Paediatr 1992;383(Suppl):S22–S25.
21. Zachmann M, Prader A, Sobel EH, Crigler JF Jr, Ritzen EM, Atares M, et al. Pubertal growth in patients with androgen insensitivity: indirect evidence for the importance of estrogens in pubertal growth of girls. J Pediatr 1986;108:694–697.

22. Apter D. Leptin in puberty. Clin Endocrinol 1997;47:175–176.
23. Dryden S, Williams G. Leptin as a neuromodulator of feeding and energy balance. Curr Opinion Endocrinol 1997;4:124–129.
24. Lonnqvist F, Schalling M. Role of leptin and its receptor in human obesity. Curr Opinion Endocrinol 1997;4:164–171.
25. Cameron JL. Search for the signal that conveys metabolic status to the reproductive axis. Curr Opinion Endocrinol 1997;4:158–163.
26. Montague CT, Farooqi IS, Whitehead JP, Soos MA, Rau H, Wareham NJ, et al. Congenital leptin deficiency is associated with severe early-onset obesity in humans. Nature 1997;387:903–908.
27. Mantzoros CS, Flier JS, Rogol AD. A longitudinal assessment of hormonal and physical alterations during normal puberty in boys. V. Rising leptin levels may signal the onset of puberty. J Clin Endocrinol Metab 1997;82:1066–1070.
28. Garcia-Mayor RV, Andrade MA, Rios M, Lage M, Dieguez C, Casanueva FF. Serum leptin levels in normal children: relationship to age, gender, body mass index, pituitary-gonadal hormones, and pubertal stage. J Clin Endocrinol Metab. 1997;82:2849–2855.
29. Clayton PE, Gill MS, Hall CM, Tillmann V, Whatmore AJ, Price DA. Serum leptin through childhood and adolescence. Clin Endocrinol 1997;46:727–733.
30. Blum WF, Englaro P, Hanitsch S, Juul A, Hertel NT, Muller J, et al. Plasma leptin levels in healthy children and adolescents: dependence on body mass index, body fat mass, gender, pubertal stage, and testosterone. J Clin Endocrinol Metab 1997;82:2904–2910.
31. Roemmich JN, Clark PA, Bern SS, et al. Alterations in growth and body composition during puberty. II Gender differences in leptin levels during puberty are related to the subcutaenous fat depot and sex steroids. Am J Physiol 1998;275:E543–E551.
32. Salbe AD, Nicolson M, Ravussin E. Total energy expenditure and the level of physical activity correlate with plasma leptin concentrations in five-year old children. J Clin Investig 1997;99:592–595.
33. Nagy TR, Gower BA, Trowbridge CA, Dezenberg C, Shewchuk RM, Goran MI. Effects of gender, ethnicity, body composition, and fat distribution on serum leptin concentrations in children. J Clin Endocrinol Metab 1997;82:2148–2152.
34. Caprio S, Tamborlane WV, Silver D, Robinson C, Leibel R, McCarthy S, et al. Hyperleptinemia: an early sign of juvenile diabetes. Relations to body fat depots and insulin concentrations. Am J Physiol 1996;271:E626–E630.
35. Ellis KJ, Nicolson M. Leptin levels and body fatness in children: effects of gender, ethnicity, and sexual development. Pediatr Res 1997;42:484–488.
36. Wabitsch M, Blum WF, Muche R, Braun M, Hube F, Rascher W, et al. Contribution of androgens to the gender differences in leptin production in obese children and adolescents. J Clin Invest 1997;100:108–113.
37. Lahlou N, Landais P, De Boissieu D, Bougneres PF. Circulating leptin in normal children and during the dynamic phase of juvenile obesity: relation to body fatness, energy metabolism, caloric intake, and sexual dimorphism. Diabetes 1997;46:989–993.
38. Arslanian S, Suprasongsin C. Testosterone treatment in adolescents with delayed puberty: changes in body composition, protein, fat, and glucose metabolism. J Clin Endocrinol Metab 1997;82:3213–3220.
39. Ghigo E, Bellone J, Aimaretti G, Bellone S, Loche S, Cappa M, et al. Reliability of provocative tests to assess growth hormone secretory status. Study in 472 normally growing children. J Clin Endocrinol Metab 1996;81:3323–3327.
40. Roemmich JN, Rogol AD. Exercise and growth hormone: does one affect the other? J Pediatr 1997;131:S75–S80.
41. Bouix O, Brun JF, Fedou C, Raynaud E, Kerdelhue B, Lenoir V, et al. Plasma beta-endorphin, corticotrophin and growth hormone responses to exercise in pubertal and prepubertal children. Horm Metab Res 1994;26:195–199.
42. Marin G, Domene HM, Barnes KM, Blackwell BJ, Cassorla FG, Cutler GB Jr. The effects of estrogen priming and puberty on the growth hormone response to standardized treadmill exercise and arginine-insulin in normal girls and boys. J Clin Endocrinol Metab 1994;79:537–541.
43. Hackney AC. The male reproductive system and endurance exercise. Med Sci Sports Exerc 1996;28:180–189.

44. Elias AN, Wilson AF, Naqvi S, Pandian MR. Effects of blood pH and blood lactate on growth hormone, prolactin, and gonadotropin release after acute exercise in male volunteers. Proc Soc Exp Biol Med 1997;214:156–160.
45. Duclos M, Corcuff JB, Rashedi M, Fougere V, Manier G. Does functional alteration of the gonadotropic axis occur in endurance trained athletes during and after exercise? Eur J Appl Physiol Occupat Physiol 1996;73:427–433.
46. Bunt JC. Hormonal alterations due to exercise. Sports Med 1986;3:331–345.
47. Constantini NW, Warren MP. Special problems of the female athlete. Baillieres Clin Rheum 1994;8:199–219.
48. Bergendahl M, Evans WS, Veldhuis JD. Current concepts on ultradian rhythms of luteinizing hormone secretion in the human. Hum Repro Update 1996;2:507–518.
49. Elias AN, Wilson AF. Exercise and gonadal function. Hum Reprod 1993;8:1747–1761.
50. Decree C, Ball P, Seidlitz B, Van Kranenburg G, Geurten P, Keizer HA. Plasma 2-hydroxycatecholestrogen responses to acute submaximal and maximal exercise in untrained women. J Appl Physiol 1997;82:364–370.
51. Arena B, Maffuli N, Maffuli F, Morleo MA. Reproductive hormones and menstrual changes with exercise in female athletes. Sports Med 1995;19:278–287.
52. Perusse L, Collier G, Gagnon J, Leon AS, Rao DC, Skinner JS, et al. Acute and chronic effects of exercise on leptin levels in humans. J Appl Physiol 1997;83:5–10.
53. Racette SB, Coppack SW, Landt M, Klein S. Leptin production during moderate-intensity aerobic exercise. J Clin Endocrinol Metab 1997;82:2275–2277.
54. Hickey MS, Considine RV, Israel RG, Mahar TL, McCammon MR, Tyndall GL, et al. Leptin is related to body fat content in male distance runners. Am J Physiol 1996;271:(Endocrinol Metabol 34):E938–E940.
55. Rogol AD, Weltman JY, Evans WS, Veldhuis JD, Weltman AL. Long-term endurance training alters the hypothalamic-pituitary axes for gonadotropins and growth hormone. Endocrinol Metabol Clin North Am 1992;21:817–832.
56. Roelen CA, de Vries WR, Koppeschaar HP, Vervoorn C, Thijssen JH, Blankenstein MA. Plasma insulin-like growth factor-I and high affinity growth hormone-binding protein levels after two weeks of strenuous physical training. Internat J Sports Med 1997;18:238–241.
57. Eliakim A, Brasel JA, Mohan S, Barstow T, Berman N, Cooper D. Physical fitness, endurance training, and the growth hormone-insulin-like growth factor I system in adolescent females. J Clin Endocrinol Metab 1996;81:3986–3992.
58. Nichols DL, Sanborn CF, Bonnick SL, Ben-Ezra V, Gench B, DiMarco NM. The effects of gymnastics training on bone and mineral density. Med Sci Sports Exerc 1994;26:1220–1225.
59. Jahreis G, Kauf E, Frohner G, Schmidt HE. Influence of intensive exercise on insulin-like growth factor I, thyroid and steroid hormones in female gymnasts. Growth Regul 1991;1:95–99.
60. Roemmich JN, Sinning WE. Weight loss and wrestling training: effects on nutrition, growth, maturation, body composition, and strength. J Appl Physiol 1997;82:1751–1759.
61. Roemmich JN. Weight loss effects on growth, maturation, growth-related hormones, protein nutrition markers and body composition of adolescent wrestlers. Dissertation, Kent State University, 1994.
62. Loucks AB. Effects of exercise training on the menstrual cycle: existence and mechanisms. Med Sci Sports Exerc 1990;22:275–280.
63. Loucks AB, Horvath SM. Athletic amenorrhea: a review. Med Sci Sports Exerc 1985;17:56–72.
64. Veldhuis JD, Evans WS, Demers LM, Thorner MO, Wakat D, Rogol AD. Altered neuroendocrine regulation of gonadotropin secretion in women distance runners. J Clin Endocrinol Metab 1985;61:557–563.
65. Loucks AB, Vaitukaitis J, Cameron JL, Rogol AD, Skrinar G, Warren MP, et al. The reproductive system and exercise in women. Med Sci Sports Exerc 1992;24:S288–S293.
66. Bullen BA, Skrinar GS, Beitins IZ, Von Mering G, Turnbull BA, MacArthur JW. Induction of menstrual disorders by strenuous exercise in untrained women. N Engl J Med 1985;312:1349–1353.
67. Loucks AB, Mortola JF, Girton L, Yen SSC. Alterations in the hypothalamic–pituitary–ovarian and the hypothalamic–pituitary–adrenal axes in athletic women. J Clin Endocrinol Metab 1989;68:402–411.
68. Lindholm C, Hagenfeldt K, Ringertz B. Bone mineral content of young female former gymnasts. Acta Paediatr 1995;84:1109–1112.
69. Lutter JM, Cushman S. Menstrual patterns in female runners. Physician Sports Med 1982;10:60.

70. Lindholm C, Hagenfeldt K, Ringertz B. Pubertal development in elite juvenile gymnasts: effects of physical training. Acta Obstet Gynecol Scand 1994;73:269–273.
71. Frisch RE, Gotz-Welbergen AB, McArthur JW, Albright T, Witschi J, et al. Delayed menarche and amenorrhea of college athletes in relation to age of onset of training. JAMA 1981;246:1559–1563.
72. Warren MP. The effects of exercise on pubertal progression and reproductive function in girls. J Clin Endocrinol Metab 1980;51:1150–1157.
73. Malina RM. Growth and Maturation of Female Gymnasts. Spotlight on Youth Sports 1996;19:1–3.
74. Malina RM. Menarche in athletes: a synthesis and hypothesis. Ann Hum Biol 1983;10:1–24.
75. Constantini NW and Warren MP. Menstrual dysfunction in swimmers: a distinct entity. J Clin Endocrinol Metab 1995;80:2740–2744.
76. Hackney AC, Dolny DG, Ness RJ. Comparison of resting reproductive hormonal profiles in select athletic groups. Biol Sport 1988;4:200–204.
77. Hackney AC, Sinning WE, Brout BC. Reproductive hormonal profiles of endurance-trained and untrained males. Med Sci Sport Exerc 1988;20:60–65.
78. Ayers JWT, Komesu V, Romani T, Ansbacher R. Anthropomorphic, hormonal, and psychologic correlates of semen quality in endurance-trained male athletes. Fertil Steril 1985;43:917–921.
79. Wheeler GD, Wall SR, Belcastro AN, Cumming DC. Reduced serum testosterone and prolactin levels in male distance runners. JAMA 1984;252:514–516.
80. Busso T, Hakkinen K, Parkarinen A, Kauhanen H, Komi PV, Lacour JR. Hormonal adaptations and modeling responses in elite weightlifters during 6 weeks of training. Eur J Appl Physiol 1992;64:381–386.
81. Wheeler GC, Singh M, Pierce WD, Epling WF, Cumming DC. Endurance training decreases serum testosterone levels in men without change in luteinizing hormone pulsation release. J Clin Endocrinol Metab 1991;72:422–425.
82. Hakkinen K, Pakarinen A, Alen M, Kauhanen H, Komi PV. Relationships between training volume, physical performance capacity, and serum hormone concentrations during prolonged training in elite weightlifters. Int J Sports Med 1987;8(S):61–65.
83. Hackney A.C, Sharp RJ, Runyan WS, Ness RJ. Relationship of resting prolactin and testosterone in males during intensive training. Br J Sports Med 1989;23:194.
84. Fellman N, Coudert J, Jarrige F, Dedu M, Denis C. Effects of endurance training on the androgenic response to exercise in man. Int J Sports Med 1985;6:215–219.
85. Lucia A, Chicharro JL, Perez M, Serratosa L, Bandres F, Legido JC. Reproductive function in male endurance athletes: sperm analysis and hormonal profile. J Appl Physiol 1996;81:2627–2636.
86. Rowland TW, Morris AH, Kelleher JF, Haag BL, Reiter EO. Serum testosterone response to training in adolescent runners. Amer J Dis Child 1987;141:881–883.
87. Pasman WJ, Westerterp-Plantenga MS, Saris WHM. The effect of exercise training on leptin levels in obese males. Am J Physiol 1998;274:(Endocrinol Metab 37):E280–E286.
88. Kohrt WM, Landt M, Birge SJ Jr. Serum leptin levels are reduced in response to exercise training, but not hormone replacement therapy, in older women. J Clin Endocrinol Metab 1996;81:3980–3985.
89. Hickey MS, Houmard JA, Considine RV, Tyndall GL, Midgette JB, Gavigan KE, et al. Gender-dependent effects of exercise training on serum leptin levels in humans. Am J Physiol 1997;272:E562–E566.
90. Casey MJ, Jones EC, Foster F, Pollock ML. Effect of the onset and intensity of training on menarchal age and menstrual irregularity among elite speedskaters in: Sport and Elite Performers. Landers DM, ed., Human Kinetics, Champaign, IL, 1986, pp. 33–44.
91. Hamilton LH, Brooks-Gunn J, Warren MP, Hamilton WG. The role of selectivity in the pathogenesis of eating problems in ballet dancers. Med Sci Sports Exerc 1988;20:560–565.
92. Pigeon P, Oliver I, Charlet JP, Rochiccioli P. Intensive dance practice. Repercussions on growth and puberty. Am J Sports Med 1997;25:243–247.
93. Thientz GE, Howald H, Weiss U, Sizonenko PC. Evidence for a reduction of growth potential in adolescent female gymnasts. J. Pediatr 1993;122:306–313.
94. Merzenich H, Boeing H, Wahrendorf J. Dietary fat and sports activity as determinants for age at menarche. Am J Epidemiol 1993;138:217–224.
95. Pirke KM, Schweiger U, Lemmel W, et al. The influence of dieting on the menstrual cycle of healthy young women. J Clin Endocrinol Metab 1985;60:1174–1179.
96. Warren MP. Effects of undernutrition on reproductive function in the human. Endocr Rev 1983;4:363–377.

Chapter 17 / Exercise and the Developing Child

97. Delemarre-van de Waal HA. Environmental factors influencing growth and pubertal development. Environ Health Perspect 1993;101(Suppl 2):39–44.
98. Warren MP, Brooks-Gunn J. Delayed menarche in athletes: The role of low energy intake and eating disorders and their relation to bone density in: Hormones and Sport. Laron Z, Rogol AD, eds. Raven, New York, NY, 1989, pp. 41–53.
99. Roemmich JN, Sinning WE. Sport-seasonal changes in body composition, growth, power, and strength of adolescent wrestlers. Int J Sports Med 1996;17:92–99.
100. Roemmich JN, Sinning WE. Weight loss and wrestling training: effects on nutrition, growth, maturation, body composition, and strength. J Appl Physiol 1997;82:1751–1759.
101. Moore DC. Body image and eating behavior in adolescents. J Amer Coll Nutr 1993;12:505–510.
102. Van de Loo DA, Johnson MD. The young female athlete. Clin Sports Med 1995;14:687–707.
103. Malina RM. Physical growth and biological maturation of young athletes. Exerc Sports Sci Rev 1994;22:389–433.
104. Borer KT. The effects of exercise on growth. Sports Med 1995;20:375–397.
105. Malina RM, Bielicki T. Retrospective longitudinal growth study of boys and girls active in sport. Acta Paediat 1996;85:570–576.
106. Brooks-Gunn J, Warren MP. Mother-daughter differences in menarcheal age in adolescent dances and nondancers. Ann Hum Biol 1988;15:435–438.
107. Stager JM, Hatler LK. Menarche in athletes: the influence of genetics and prepubertal training. Med Sci Sports Exerc 1988;20:369–373.
108. Obert P, Courteix D, Lecoq AM, Guenon P. Effect of long-term intense swimming training on the upper body peak oxygen uptake of prepubertal girls. Euro J Appl Physiol Occup Physiol 1996; 73:136–143.
109. Blimkie CJ. Resistance training during preadolescence. Issues and controversies. Sports Med 1993;15:389–407.
110. Torun B, Viteri FE. Influence of exercise on linear growth. Eur J Clin Nutr 1994;48(Suppl 1): S186–S190.

18 Exercise and the Female Reproductive System
The Effect of Hormonal Status on Performance

David M. Quadagno, PhD

CONTENTS
  INTRODUCTION
  PHYSIOLOGICAL RESPONSES TO AEROBIC EXERCISE
    DURING THE MENSTRUAL CYCLE
  EFFECTS ON STRENGTH AND ENDURANCE
  INFLUENCE OF THE MENSTRUAL CYCLE ON ATHLETIC PERFORMANCE
  OCs AND PERFORMANCE
  AREAS OF FUTURE RESEARCH
  ACKNOWLEDGMENTS
  REFERENCES

INTRODUCTION

This chapter assesses studies dealing with the effect of the menstrual cycle on various parameters of exercise performance, including athletic performance. Past studies are divided into three categories: selected physiological responses to exercise during sustained aerobic performance, including ventilation, cardiovascular responses, and thermoregulation; the effect of the cycle on strength performance; and the influence of the cycle on athletic performance as measured by changes in performance in a particular sporting event over the course of the cycle.

To date, only four studies have actually monitored the menstrual cycles of athletes prospectively and compared the results to their athletic performance, and none of these confirmed cycle phase with hormone assays. The most common approach taken by researchers interested in this problem involves studies measuring the responses of physiological parameters, such as oxygen uptake, heart rate, time to exhaustion, and thermoregulation to exercise under laboratory conditions, e.g., on a treadmill or cycle ergometer, during different cycle phases.

Determining the influence of the menstrual cycle on exercise parameters, like oxygen uptake or performance in athletic events, is not easy because of the methodological

From: *Contemporary Endocrinology: Sports Endocrinology*
Edited by: M. P. Warren and N. W. Constantini © Humana Press Inc., Totowa, NJ

problems involved and lack of comparability among studies. Much of the research examining the effect of cycle phase on performance recalls the cliché "comparing apples to oranges." One problematic area is the determination of menstrual cycle phase *(1)*. Throughout this chapter, the methods used to determine cycle phase will be stated, since this key area has often created difficulties in comparing studies. Methods have ranged from menstrual cycle charting (the least precise) to monitoring of hormones for cycle phase and confirmation of ovulation (the most precise).

Very few studies have monitored the actual levels of ovarian steroids for an accurate determination of cycle phase and the presence of ovulatory cycles. As a result, we must assume that ovulatory and anovulatory cycles were "lumped" together. The results of Pivarnik et al. *(2)* reveal the enormous consequences this lumping can have for interpretation of data, especially in view of the small sample sizes employed in many studies. They studied temperature regulation in nine eumenorrheic women performing endurance exercise during different phases of the cycle. One woman did not ovulate (had shown no increase in progesterone 1 wk after predicted ovulation), and this woman exhibited responses markedly different from those of the remaining subjects *(2)*. The study by Pivarnik et al. also illustrates another frequent problem in this field of research: small sample sizes. A comprehensive review article established that the mean sample size for published work was 9.9, the medium 8.5, and the range 4–21 subjects *(3)*.

Another problem is that some researchers used highly trained athletes, whereas others recruited subjects who engaged in only light to moderate exercise, creating problems with comparison of studies using women of different levels of physical fitness *(4)* and mental preparedness *(1,5)*. Trained and untrained women have been shown to differ in exercise performance, suggesting that some aspects of exercise performance can be voluntarily altered by training *(4,5)*. For example, trained women may show higher thresholds of perceived exertion, i.e., will exercise longer before indicating exertion. Trained athletes may also have fewer negative perceptions about the menstrual cycle and performance.

Another confounding factor is changes induced in the menstrual cycle by exercise *(6,7)*. For example, levels of the steroid hormone testosterone rise in response to exercise in both trained and untrained women during the follicular and luteal phases *(8)*, and Kraemer et al. *(7)* found that low-volume resistance exercise in untrained women elevated estradiol, growth hormone, and the androgen androstenedione. The effects on performance of these elevated levels of hormones, whether between individuals in resting endogenous levels or within individuals as a result of exercise, are unknown. Despite these limitations, many conclusions can still be drawn, provided the reasons for discrepancies between studies are taken into account.

Cyclic variations in physiological and hormonal variables are well documented in the eumenorrheic menstrual cycle. The ovulatory cycle shows large and consistent variations in ovarian steroid hormones. The principal estrogen, estradiol, rises during the first half of the cycle and peaks shortly before ovulation. Estradiol levels then fall, but rise again and show a broader secondary peak during the midluteal phase *(9)*. Therefore, during the first half of the cycle, the follicular phase (the time between the ending of menses and ovulation, also called the estrogenic phase), estradiol is the dominant hormone. Progesterone, the dominant progestin, remains low during the follicular phase, begins to increase at the time of ovulation, and reaches a peak during the second half of the cycle, the luteal phase (the time between ovulation and the onset of the next menses, also called the progestational phase). Therefore, progesterone is the dominant hormone during the luteal phase. The luteal phase is characterized by an increase in basal body temperature (BBT) owing to the thermogenic effects of progesterone *(10)*, and this rise in BBT, although not always reliable *(11,12)*, is often used to confirm that ovulation has occurred.

PHYSIOLOGICAL RESPONSES TO AEROBIC EXERCISE DURING THE MENSTRUAL CYCLE

This section examines the influence of the menstrual cycle on selected physiological responses to aerobic exercise. The list of responses is not exhaustive, but includes those that are clearly linked to athletic performance *(1)*. For earlier comprehensive reviews of this topic, see Lebrun *(1,3)*.

Thermoregulation

During extended exercise, the ability to maintain a relatively constant temperature near 37°C (98.6°F) is essential for optimum function. The increase of approx 0.5°C in BBT during the luteal phase, associated with increased concentrations of progesterone from the corpus luteum *(9)*, means that during that phase, the exercising female begins with a higher BBT than at other times. Does this higher BBT have consequences for the exercising female?

It has been proposed that the "set point" of central neuronal structures of the thermoregulatory system is higher during the luteal phase *(10)*. If so, one might hypothesize that all thermoregulatory responses should be activated at higher threshold temperatures during the luteal phase than at other times, including responses designed to reduce BBT (*see* Table 1). In the well-done study of Pivarnik et al. *(2)*, temperature regulation during exercise during two different cycle phases was monitored in nine eumenorrheic women who were trained and heat-acclimatized to ambient outdoor temperatures. The investigators confirmed cycle phase from the luteinizing hormone (LH) surge in the urine that indicates ovulation, followed by progesterone assays from serum. The women were required to perform two continuous 60-min rides on a cycle ergometer at 65–70% of their peak VO_2 at 22°C and 60% relative humidity (ambient temperature and humidity for that time of the year). One ride was performed during the midfollicular phase (approx 7 d before ovulation as determined by LH surge) and the other during the midluteal phase (approx 7 d after ovulation as determined by LH surge).

Rectal temperature reached a plateau at 38.3°C midway through the exercise bout during the follicular phase, but rose to 38.9°C during the lutealphase bout and had not reached a plateau by the time the bout ended *(2)*. Skin temperatures were not influenced by cycle phase; they reached plateaus in both exercise bouts at approx 20 min. Perceived exertion by the subjects was also greater during the luteal than during the follicular phase. Interestingly, perceived exertion was similar during the two phases until the latter half of the exercise bout. The difference in perceived exertion arose soon after rectal temperatures during the luteal phase rose above those in the follicular phase *(2)*.

The basic findings of Pivarnik et al. *(2)* replicate those of Hessemer and Bruck *(10)*. In their subjects, the thresholds for chest sweating and cutaneous vasodilation, both responses designed to reduce BBT, were higher during the luteal phase than during the follicular phase *(10)*. Hessemer and Bruck *(10)* used 10 subjects and monitored menstrual

Table 1
Effect of Cycle Phase on Thermoregulation[a]

Reference	No. of subjects	Trained/ untrained	Cycle phase determination	Results
Pivarnik et al. (2)	9	Trained	LH, P	Higher rectal temperatures recorded during luteal phase compared to follicular phase in response to exercise
Hessemer and Bruck (10)	10	9 Untrained, 1 trained	BBT, P	Higher thresholds for sweating and cutaneous vasodilation higher in luteal phase compared to follicular phase; no difference between cycle phase and onset of sweating or total sweat loss
Carpenter and Nunneley (13)	7	Not stated	BBT, E, P, LH, FSH	No difference between cycle phase in threshold for onset of sweating or total sweat loss
Frye and Kamon (15)	4	Untrained	BBT	No difference between cycle phase in threshold for onset of sweating or total sweat loss
Sargent and Weinman (14)	12	Untrained	Charting	No difference between cycle phase in threshold for onset of sweating or total sweat loss

[a]Abbreviations: BBT = basal body temperature, E = estradiol, P = progesterone, LH = luteinizing hormone, FSH = follicle-stimulating hormone.

cycle phase by rectal BBT, verified by progesterone assays in venous blood. They also documented greater heat loss (chest sweat rate) during the luteal than during the follicular phase.

Carpenter and Nunneley (13) used BBT plus multiple measurements of the hormones estradiol-17b, progesterone, LH, and follicle-stimulating hormone to determine cycle phase in a group of seven normally cycling women. Their experimental design involved an acclimation phase during which each subject pedaled a cycle ergometer in a dry heat chamber for 2 h at 30% of her VO_2max during the menstrual flow, ovulation, and luteal phases of the cycle. The exercise bouts continued daily until each subject achieved a steady state during the second hour of exercise for two consecutive days. Steady state was defined as a change in rectal temperature of $\leq 0.1°C$ and a variation in heart rate of <10 beats/min. At the completion of this phase, each subject was tested during the same three phases of the menstrual cycle.

Rectal and skin temperatures were always significantly higher during the luteal phase than during the other two phases, both at rest and during the exercise bout, but hormonal status had no significant effect on total sweat loss (13). Carpenter and Nunneley concluded that the luteal phase is associated with a stable, but small, increase in BBT and that, although temperature changes were not caused by changes in sweat production, they may have been the result of phase-related differences in the threshold for the onset of sweating. Carpenter and Nunneley did not test perceived exertion, nor did they indicate whether subjects reached a plateau in temperature during the luteal phase. Their results show that both BBT and skin temperature were still rising at the end of the ride during the luteal phase, but were declining during the menstrual phase.

Not all researchers have found differences in thermoregulatory responses during different cycle phases. Carpenter and Nunneley *(13)*, Sargent and Weinman *(14)*, and Frye and Kamon *(15)* found no differences between cycle phases in threshold for onset of sweating or for total sweat loss. Frye and Kamon used BBT, and Sargent and Weinman used charting (counting of days from the onset of menses) to determine cycle phase.

In summary, the hypothesis that the thresholds of responses designed to reduce BBT will be higher during the luteal than during other phases appears to have support. These results have potential negative implications for prolonged athletic activity at high ambient temperatures during the luteal phase, but could have potential positive implications for athletic activities, such as aquatic or winter sports, in which heat conservation could be a factor. Although there is evidence that thermoregulation is influenced by cycle phase, few data exist to indicate that cycle phase influences heart rate, perceived exertion, or aerobic capacity *(4,16–18)*.

Heart Rate and Perceived Exertion

The effect of the menstrual cycle on heart rate and perceived exertion (time to fatigue) has been studied under a variety of conditions. Pivarnik et al. *(2)* used a design in which trained women exercised on a cycle ergometer while self-rating their perceived exertion on a 15-point Borg scale *(19)* (*see* Table 2). Heart rate was monitored by telemetry from a pulse monitor attached to each subject's chest. The subjects were instructed to state their levels of perceived exertion throughout the 60-min exercise bout at 65–70% of peak oxygen uptake (VO_2).

Pivarnik et al. *(2)* found that heart rate was lower during exercise performed in the follicular phase than during that in the luteal phase, and heart rate differences remained constant throughout the exercise bouts. Perceived exertion was found to be similar during the two cycle phases until 50 min into the bout, when perceived exertion was reported to be greater during the luteal phase. Hessemer and Bruck *(10)* also found heart rate to be elevated during the luteal phase when subjects were exposed to thermoneutral conditions. Higgs and Robertson *(20)*, using charting to monitor cycle phase, showed that perceived exertion was greater during the premenstrual and menstrual phases than at midcycle when 12 untrained subjects were tested at 90 and 100% VO_2max on a treadmill.

The majority of findings do not support the results of Pivarnik et al. *(2)*. Bemben et al. *(21)*, using five untrained women performing a maximal treadmill exercise test, found no differences between menstrual cycle phases in heart rate, as monitored by telemetry, or voluntary termination of the test at exhaustion. Cycle phase was determined by BBT and serum progesterone assays. Bryner et al. *(22)* also found no differences between cycle phases in volitional fatigue on a maximal treadmill test. The authors used 10 untrained subjects and monitored cycle phase by transabdominal ultrasound, used to confirm ovulation. Higgs and Robertson *(20)* found no change in heart rate over the cycle, a finding confirmed by Lebrun et al. *(18)*, who also found no change in perceived exertion (*see* Aerobic Capacity, *below* for details of experimental design).

Table 2
Effect of Cycle Phase on Heart Rate and Perceived Exertion[a]

Reference	No. of subjects	Trained/ untrained	Cycle phase determination	Results
Pivarnik et al. (2)	9	Trained	LH, P	Heart rate lower in follicular phase compared to luteal phase in response to exercise; perceived exertion greater in luteal phase
Hessemer and Bruck (10)	10	9 Untrained, 1 trained	BBT, P	Heart rate lower in follicular phase compared to luteal phase in response to exercise; perceived exertion not recorded
Higgs and Robertson (20)	12	Untrained	Charting	Perceived exertion greater in luteal phase compared to follicular phase in response to exercise; no change in heart rate during any cycle phase in response to exercise
Bemben et al. (21)	5	Untrained	BBT, P	No change in heart rate or perceived exertion between cycle phase in response to exercise
Lebrun et al. (20)	16	Trained	E, P	No change in maximal heart rate or perceived exertion between cycle phases in response to exercise
Bryner et al. (22)	10	Untrained	Ultrasound to confirm ovulation	No differences in perceived exertion between cycle phase in response to exercise

[a] Abbreviations: BBT = basal body temperature, E = estradiol, P = progesterone, LH = luteinizing hormone, FSH = follicle-stimulating hormone.

Aerobic Capacity

Many studies have sought to determine whether aerobic capacity, as measured by oxygen uptake, changes with menstrual cycle phase. Oxygen uptake (VO_2), the amount of oxygen consumed by the body in L/min, is usually measured by collection of expired air over a period of 1–5 min.

Maximal oxygen uptake (VO_2max) is generally thought to be the best single indicator of the cardiovascular-respiratory component of fitness and maximal aerobic power (23). Many other factors, including strength, contribute to overall fitness, but VO_2max is an excellent indicator of superior fitness because of the strong relationship between VO_2max and total work output and the good estimate it provides of cardiovascular system potential and endurance capacity (24).

Studies that examined maximal or submaximal cardiorespiratory responses at different phases of the menstrual cycle and used hormone assays to confirm cycle phase have produced few definitive findings *(2,4,16,17)*. Lebrun et al. *(18)*, using a sample of 16 moderately trained subjects and monitoring cycle phase by means of serum estradiol and progesterone levels, did find a higher absolute VO$_2$max during the follicular phase than during the luteal phase, but not a higher relative VO$_2$max. They did not find differences between cycle phases in highest recorded minute ventilation, maximal heart rate, or maximum respiratory exchange ratio.

EFFECTS ON STRENGTH AND ENDURANCE

Isometric muscular strength refers to the force or tension that can be generated by a muscle or muscle group during one maximal effort, and muscular endurance is the ability to perform many repetitions at submaximal loads.

It has been hypothesized that increasing or elevated levels of estrogen will be associated with increased muscle strength and endurance. The rationale for this hypothesis is taken from the findings of Phillips et al. *(25)*, who found that the maximum voluntary force exerted by the adductor pollicis muscle (a muscle in the hand that brings the thumb closer to the palm) relative to its cross-sectional area was 28% lower in old than in young individuals and that in women the decline occurs at the time of menopause. Further, this decline could be reversed in postmenopausal women by hormone-replacement therapy using preparations containing estrogen *(25)* (*see* Table 3). Using:

1. Athletically trained and untrained women who did not use oral contraceptives;
2. An athletically trained group using oral contraceptives; and,
3. Male controls.

Phillips and coworkers found a significant increase in the maximal voluntary force of the adductor pollicis muscle during the follicular (estrogenic) phase of the cycle *(26)*. This increase was seen in both the trained and the untrained groups that were not using oral contraceptives, but not in the trained group using oral contraceptives or in the male control group.

The athletically trained subjects in the Phillips et al. study *(26)* were members of rowing clubs (10 women, 17–39 yr of age) who trained 6 d/wk; the untrained subjects (12 women, 17–39 yr of age; 6 men, 23–35 yr of age) were not engaged in any regular athletic training. Phillips et al. *(26)* monitored cycle phases by means of BBT and measurements of both LH and 17-B estradiol.

The results of Phillips et al. *(26)* confirm those of Sarwar et al. *(27)*, who found a higher maximal hand grip during the first half of the menstrual cycle than during the second half. Using 10 untrained subjects, Sarwar et al. *(27)* also found that the large quadriceps muscle group showed an 11% increase in isometric force between the 1st and 14th d of the cycle. Cycle phases were estimated by charting.

Reis et al. *(28)* found clear evidence of an increase in strength of the quadriceps femoris muscle group with increasing levels of estrogen. The maximal strength of the muscle group was registered during leg extension by means of an isokinetic leg press with hydraulic regulation. Maximal extension (both strength and repetitions) occurred during the late follicular and early luteal phases, when subjects were documented to have high levels of estradiol. The authors used seven untrained women, and cycle phase was monitored by BBT supplemented by urinary assay of LH and serum assays of ovarian steroids.

Table 3
Effect of Cycle Phase on Strength and Endurance[a]

Reference	No. of subjects	Trained/ untrained	Cycle phase determination	Results
Phillips et al. (26)	26 12	Trained Untrained	BBT, LH, E	Increase in strength during follicular phase compared to luteal phase
Sarwar et al. (27)	10	Untrained	Charting	Increase in strength during follicular phase compared to luteal phase
Reis et al. (28)	7	Untrained	BBT, LH, E, P	Increase in strength during times of high estrogen (late follicular and early luteal phases)
Lebrun et al. (18)	6	Trained	BBT, E, P	No influence of cycle phase on strength
Petrofsky et al. (29)	7	Untrained 4 Cycling 3 Using OCs	BBT	No influence of cycle phase on strength
Higgs and Robertson (20)	12	"Active" was used to describe sample	Charting	No influence of cycle phase on strength
Dibrezzo et al. (30)	21	Untrained	Charting	No influence of cycle phase on strength or endurance
Davies et al. (5)	12	Untrained	Charting	No influence of cycle phase on strength
Quadagno et al. (31)	12	Trained	Charting	No influence of cycle phase on strength or endurance
Wirth and Lohman (32)	10 7 9	Non-OC users OC users OC users plus taking vitamin B-6	Charting	No influence of cycle phase on strength, but increase in endurance during luteal phase

[a]Abbreviations: BBT = basal body temperature, E = estradiol, P = progesterone, LH = luteinizing hormone.

In a carefully controlled study, Lebrun et al. (18) found no influence of cycle phase on isokinetic strength as measured by peak torque generated by maximal knee flexion and extension. The six trained subjects were 18–40 yr old, had regular menstrual cycles, and had not taken oral contraceptives for the past 6 mo. The cycles were monitored by BBT and serum hormone measurements. Subjects were tested during the early follicular phase (between d 3 and 8 before estrogen increase) and midluteal phase (between d 4 and 9 after ovulation; estrogen levels were higher than in early follicular phase). It is interesting to note that estrogen levels are lower in the follicular phase than in the luteal phase in this study. Perhaps at the time of a follicular-phase estrogen peak, an increase in strength might have been observed. These results confirm those of Petrofsky et al. (29), who used BBT to monitor cycle phase.

Higgs and Robertson *(20)*, Dibrezzo et al. *(30)*, Davies et al. *(5)*, Quadagno et al. *(31)*, and Wirth and Lohman *(32)* failed to identify changes in strength with menstrual cycle phase. In all of these studies, cycle phase was monitored by charting.

Fewer studies have looked at muscular endurance. Quadagno et al. *(31)* examined the mean number of times 12 moderately trained women could lift 70% of the maximum weight they could lift in the bench and leg presses and found no significant differences between cycle phases. Dibrezzo et al. *(30)* also found no effect of cycle phase in 26 untrained women on repetitions using the muscles of knee flexion and extension on a Cybex II isokinetic dynamometer. Wirth and Lohman *(32)* found that their 10 untrained subjects showed an increase during the luteal phase in the length of time they could maintain 50% of their maximum grip strength on a hand-grip device.

In summary, good data exist to indicate that increasing or elevated levels of estrogen are associated with increased muscle strength. Increasing levels of estrogen do not appear to increase muscle endurance as measured by repetitions or latency to maintain a set muscle exertion.

INFLUENCE OF THE MENSTRUAL CYCLE ON ATHLETIC PERFORMANCE

Examination of the influence of menstrual cycle phase on performance in sporting events "in the field" brings into play many confounding factors that are eliminated in laboratory experiments. Only limited research has addressed this problem *(1,31)*. Brooks-Gunn et al. *(33)* speculated that little research has been done because belief in menstrual cycle-related performance decrements is so pervasive.

In the early 1960s, Erdelyi *(34)* questioned more than 500 female athletes about their athletic performance during different phases of their menstrual cycles. Approximately 31% reported performance decrements during either the premenstrual or menstrual phases, whereas about 15% stated that performance improved during the menstrual phase. From these retrospective self-reports, Erdelyi concluded that athletic performance was negatively affected during the premenstrual period and the first 2 d of the menses.

Erdelyi found, however, that the women's self-perceptions about the cycle's effect on performance differed with the sports in which they participated. For example, rowers reported poor performance during the menses, but sprint swimmers reported less influence of the cycle on their performance. From his findings, Erdelyi hypothesized that athletic events requiring relatively more and longer effort would be more influenced by the cycle.

Athletic Events of Long Duration

In an investigation of 164 women (18–22 yr of age) who participated in cross-country ski events of long duration (5 and 12.5 km), Fomin et al. *(35)* reported that performance did change over the course of the cycle. Specifically, poorer performance was reported during the premenstrual and menstrual phases than during other phases of the cycle. The authors did not record performance times or apply statistical tests to the findings. Cycle phase was monitored by BBT and cyclic cervical mucus changes.

A prospective study of 15 highly trained postadolescent university varsity swimmers found no significant differences in performance in the 200-m freestyle event during any cycle phase *(31)*. Although the 200-m event is not nearly as long as a cross-country skiing race, it is the longest athletic event for which we have prospective data. The women performed repeated time trials, which were averaged. Cycle phase was monitored by charting, confirmed by the onset of menstrual flow. The women were tested during the premenstrual (3–5 d before menses), menstrual (d 1–3 of flow), and postmenstrual (10–12 d after onset of menses) phases. Although the difference was not significant, the slowest times were recorded during the menstrual phase, the fastest during the premenstrual phase (late luteal), and intermediate times during the postmenstrual phase (late follicular or early luteal depending on cycle length).

Thus, in two studies of athletic events of relatively long duration, the menstrual phase was associated with poorer performance. Neither of the two studies confirmed cycle phase with hormonal determinations.

Athletic Events of Short Duration

In a prospective study of four trained adolescent swimmers, the fastest swimming times for both the 100-yd freestyle and the 100-yd event of the swimmer's choice occurred during the menses and the slowest during the premenstrual phase *(36)*. These findings conflicted with those of another prospective study of 20 trained adolescent sprint swimmers, in which faster times were recorded during the postmenstrual phase than during the premenstrual and menstrual phases *(37)*. A later prospective study of 15 highly trained postadolescent university varsity swimmers found no differences in performance in the 100-m freestyle event during any phase of the cycle *(31)*. None of the women in any of the studies was using oral contraceptives (OCs).

OCs AND PERFORMANCE

Numerous hormonal preparations intended to prevent pregnancy are on the market. They range from OCs containing estrogen and progesterone or progesterone alone to injectable progestins and implants containing progesterone. The OCs come in two basic formulations: single phase (delivering the same amounts of estrogen and progesterone on every day of the cycle) and triphasic (delivering different amounts of both estrogen and progesterone at different phases of the cycle to mimic the "natural" cycle) *(38)*. The doses of estrogen and progesterone vary with pill preparation and may also produce different levels of suppression of endogenous estrogen in different individuals *(39)*.

All hormonal methods of contraception act to suppress the surge of LH at midcycle, and, hence, ovulation. All hormonal preparations also prevent, to varying degrees, the cyclic release of endogenous estrogen and progesterone from the ovaries and thus provide a situation in which the effect of this supression on performance can be studied. Depending on the formulation, the levels of the steroid hormones tend to remain fairly constant while the contraceptives are taken *(39)*. A problem with interpretation of research results is that many authors combine results from women on different OC regimens.

One might hypothesize that women on hormonal contraceptives will not show changes in performance with cycle phase, because the "natural" cyclic release of ovarian steroids is inhibited to varying degees. Only studies comparing women taking and not taking OCs and in which an effect of cycle phase was found are addressed in this section. In almost all such cases, women on OCs did not show changes in performance with cycle phase. Wirth and Lohman *(32)* found significant differences in endurance and force ouput in grip strength between cycle phases in women not taking OCs, but found no such differences in women taking OCs. The authors state that 8 different OC regimens were used by the 16 subjects taking OCs, but no other specifics were given. Sarwar et al. *(27)* found significantly higher quadriceps and handgrip strength at midcycle (highest estrogen levels) than during early follicular and luteal phases in women not taking OCs. They found no such differences in women using single-phase OCs. Phillips et al. *(26)* found similar results for strength of the adductor pollicis muscle; OC use reduced the differences between cycle phases in strength. These authors did not indicate the type of OCs employed in their study. In summary, it appears that hormonal contraceptives reduce any influences of the cycle on performance.

AREAS OF FUTURE RESEARCH

One of the greatest problems facing researchers in this field is the confirmation of cycle phase and determination of whether ovulation has occurred. With the advent of noninvasive methods for assaying ovarian steroids in saliva *(40)*, it should be more feasible to document cycle phase and to monitor the effects of the menstrual cycle on selected aspects of performance, including studies of athletic performance "in the field."

Small sample sizes have also been a problem, in part because of the difficulty of using invasive methods, such as venipuncture, to secure plasma for hormone assays. Subjects are reluctant to have blood drawn, and multiple samples compound the problem. A study using saliva samples could include many subjects, each of whom would have only to place a saliva sample in a small plastic vial each day for the duration of two to three cycles. Cycle phase and ovulation could be confirmed by assay of all of the steroid hormones produced by the ovaries. Particularly convenient features of saliva samples are that they can be stored for days at room temperature before analysis with little effect on steroid levels *(41)*, that their noninvasive nature allows frequent and repeated testing for very close monitoring of hormonal status, and that they would even permit sampling both before and after a single exercise bout or actual field event.

More difficult to resolve is the problem of comparison of results from trained and untrained subjects. Although untrained subjects are more readily available to some researchers, those working on college or university campuses should be able to work with women varsity athletes.

ACKNOWLEDGMENTS

Thanks are due to Suzanne Walter-Geissler for helpful comments on the manuscript and to Anne B. Thistle for critical comments and editorial help.

REFERENCES

1. Lebrun C. The effect of the phase of the menstrual cycle and birth control pill on athletic performance. The Athletic Woman 1994;13:419–441.
2. Pivarnik J, Marichal C, Spillman T, Morrow J. Menstrual cycle phase affects temperature regulation during endurance exercise. J Appl Physiol 1992;72:543–548.
3. Lebrun C. Effect of different phases of the menstrual cycle and oral contraceptives on athletic performance. Sports Med 1993;16:400–430.
4. Schoene R, Robertson H, Pierson D, Peterson R. Respiratory drives and exercise in menstrual cycles of athletic and nonathletic women. J Appl Physiol 1981;50:1300–1305.

5. Davies B, Elford J, Jamieson K. Variations in performance in simple muscle tests at different phases of the menstrual cycle. J Sports Med Phys Fitness 1991;31:532–537.
6. Arena B, Maffulli N, Maffulli F, Morleo A. Reproductive hormones and menstrual cycle changes with exercise in female athletes. Sports Med 1995;19:278–287.
7. Kraemer R, Heleniak R, Tryniecki J, Kraemer G, Okazaki N, Castracane D. Follicular and luteal phase hormonal responses to low-volume resistive exercise. Med Sci Sports Exerc 1995;27:809–817.
8. Keizer H, Poortman J, Bunnik G. Influence of physical exercise on sex hormone metabolism. J Appl Physiol 1980;48:765–769.
9. Wood J. Dynamics of Human Reproduction. Aldine De Gruyter, New York, NY, 1994.
10. Hessemer V, Bruck K. Influence of menstrual cycle on shivering, skin blood flow, and sweating responses measured at night. J Appl Physiol 1985;59:1902–1910.
11. Bauman J. Basal body temperature: unreliable method of ovulation detection. Fertil Steril 1981;36:429–433.
12. Hilgers T, Bailey A. Natural family planning, II: Basal body temperature and estimated time of ovulation. Obstet Gynecol 1980;55:333–339.
13. Carpenter A, Nunneley S. Endogenous hormones subtly alter women's response to heat stress. J Appl Physiol 1988;63:2313–2317.
14. Sargent F, Weinman K. Eccrine sweat gland activity during the menstrual cycle. J Appl Physiol 1966;21:1685–1687.
15. Frye A, Kamon E. Responses to dry heat of men and women with similar aerobic capacities. J Appl Physiol 1981;50:65–70.
16. De Souza M, Maguire M, Rubin K, Maresh C. Effects of menstrual cycle phase and amenorrhea on exercise performance in runners. Med Sci Sports Exerc 1990;22:575–580.
17. Dombovy M, Bonekat H, Williams T, Staats B. Exercise performance and ventilatory response in the menstrual cycle. Med Sci Sports Exerc 1987;19:111–117.
18. Lebrun C, McKenzie D, Prior J, Taunton J. Effects of menstrual cycle phase on athletic performance. Med Sci Sports Exerc 1995;27:437–444.
19. Borg G. Perceived exertion as an indicator of somatic stress. Scand J Rehabil Med 1970;2:92–98.
20. Higgs S, Robertson L. Cyclic variations in perceived exertion and physical work capacity in females. Can J Appl Sports Sci 1981;6:191–196.
21. Bemben D, Salm P, Salm J. Ventilatory and blood lactate responses to maximal treadmill exercise during the menstrual cycle. J Sports Med Phys Fitness 1995;35:257–262.
22. Bryner R, Toffle R, Ullrich I, Yeater R. Effect of low dose oral contraceptives on exercise performance. Br J Sports Med 1996;30:36–40.
23. Wells CL. Women, Sport and Performance. Human Kinetics Books, Champaign, IL, 1991.
24. O'Toole M, Douglas P. Fitness: definition and development. In: Shangold M, Mirkin G, eds. Women and Exercise: Physiology and Sports Medicine. FA Davis Co., Philadelphia, PA, 1988, pp. 3–22.
25. Phillips S, Rook K, Siddle N, Bruce S, Woledge R. Muscle weakness in women occurs at an earlier age than in men, but strength is preserved by hormone replacement therapy. Clin Sci 1993;84:95–98.
26. Phillips S, Sanderson A, Birch K, Bruce S, Woledge R. Changes in maximal voluntary force of human adductor pollicis muscle during the menstrual cycle. J Physiol 1996;496:551–557.
27. Sarwar R, Beltran N, Rutherford O. The effect of the menstrual cycle on the human quadriceps strength, contractile properties and fatiguability. J Physiol 1995;483:128P.
28. Reis E, Frick D, Schmidtbleicher D. Frequency variations of strength training sessions triggered by the phases of the cycle. Int J Sports Med 1995;16:545–550.
29. Petrofsky JS, Ledonne DM, Rinehart JS, Lind AR. Isometric strength and endurance during the menstrual cycle. Eur J Appl Physiol 1976;35:1–10.
30. Dibrezzo R, Fort IM, Brown B. Relationships among strength, endurance, weight and body fat during three phases of the menstrual cycle. J Sports Med Fitness 1991;31:89–94.
31. Quadagno D, Faquin L, Lim G, Kuminka W, Moffatt R. The menstrual cycle: does it affect athletic performance. Physician Sports Med 1991;19:121–124.
32. Wirth J, Lohman T. The relationship of static muscle function to use of oral contraceptives. Med Sci Sports Exerc 1982;14:16–20.
33. BrooksGunn J, Gargiulo J, Warren M. The menstrual cycle and athletic performance. In: Puhl J, Brown C, eds. The Menstrual Cycle and Physical Activity. Human Kinetics, Champaign, IL, 1986, pp. 13–28.
34. Erdelyi GJ. Gynecological survey of female athletes. J Sports Med 1962;2:174–179.

35. Fomin S, Pivovarova V, Vorovova V. Changes in the special working capacity and mental stability of well-trained woman skiers at various phases of the biological cycle. Sports Training Med Rehabil 1989;1:89–92.
36. Brooks-Gunn J, Gargiulo J, Warren M. The effect of cycle phase on the performance of adolescent swimmers. Physician Sports Med 1986;14:182–192.
37. Bale P, Nelson G. The effects of menstruation on performance of swimmers. Aust J Sci Med Sport, 1985;March:19–22.
38. Winikoff B, Wymelenberg S. Contraception. John Henry Press (National Academy Press), Washington, DC. 1997.
39. Hatcher R, Trussell J, Stewart F, Stewart G, Kowal D, Guest F, et al. Contraceptive Technology. Irvington, NY, 1994.
40. Dabbs J. Salivary testosterone measurements in behavioral studies. Ann NY Acad Sci 1993;694: 177–183.
41. Dabbs J. Salivary testosterone measurements: reliability across hours, days and weeks. Physiol Behav 1990;48:83–86.

19 Exercise and Pregnancy
Hormonal Considerations

Fred K. Lotgering, MD, PhD

CONTENTS
INTRODUCTION
MATERNAL RESPONSES
FETAL RESPONSES
SUMMARY
REFERENCES

INTRODUCTION

Forty-two percent of US women perform physical exercises during pregnancy, and half of them continue to exercise for more than 6 mo *(1)*. It is apparently safe to do so, despite the potentially conflicting large energy demands of both the exercising muscles and the growing fetus. Healthy women, as well as females of other species, meet the increased demands through effective metabolic and circulatory adaptations even under the most strenuous circumstances, i.e., during heavy exercise in the third trimester *(2,3)*. More specifically, in healthy women, pregnancy does not affect the maximal aerobic capacity ($\dot{V}O_2$max) *(4)*, and maximal exercise does not elicit hypoxic stress in the fetus *(5,6)*. A recent study suggests that even if placental reserve is compromised, as in fetal growth retardation, moderately strenuous exercise to a maternal heart rate of 150 beats/min is not harmful *(7)*.

The study of exercise in pregnancy is intriguing, but complex: intriguing because the heavy burden of the combined demands of pregnancy and exercise stresses physiologic adaptation mechanisms to their limits, and complex because many variables are involved. Therefore, results of studies on exercise in pregnancy must be interpreted with care. The two major determinants of physiologic responses to exercise are the shape of the individual and the burden of exercise. Shape is markedly affected by the baseline variables gestational age, body mass and its distribution, and physical condition, or $\dot{V}O_2$max. The physiological burden is highly affected by the type, intensity, and duration of work, in addition to environmental conditions. Comparative studies are bound to be misleading if experimental conditions have not been rigorously controlled for these variables. This

From: *Contemporary Endocrinology: Sports Endocrinology*
Edited by: M. P. Warren and N. W. Constantini © Humana Press Inc., Totowa, NJ

chapter will explore the question of to what extent endocrine mechanisms are involved in the remarkably effective metabolic and circulatory adaptations to the combined demands of exercise and pregnancy.

MATERNAL RESPONSES

Metabolism

The energy requirements of the body are met predominantly by metabolism of carbohydrates and fats; protein metabolism is quantitatively unimportant. Most studies on exercise in pregnancy have been limited to measurements of blood concentrations of substrates and hormones. Such blood concentrations are acutely affected by the exercise-induced hemoconcentration of up to 14% *(2)*. More importantly, however, blood concentrations of substrates poorly reflect their utilization, which is the difference between uptake and production on the one hand and output and breakdown on the other hand. In addition, blood concentrations of hormones do not adequately reveal if exercise affects the hormone receptors.

The second half of pregnancy is a diabetogenic period, because peripheral tissues, including muscle and fat, become relatively resistant to insulin *(8)*. Various hormones are produced in large quantities during pregnancy and affect insulin resistance. These include, in order of progressive potency, estradiol, prolactin, human placental lactogen, progesterone, and cortisol *(8)*. From a teleological point of view, the pregnancy-induced insulin resistance would seem to benefit the fetus, because more glucose is available for diffusion across the placenta to the fetus when maternal glucose utilization is reduced and the concentration of glucose in the blood is higher. In contrast, exercise would seem to reduce fetal glucose availability as a result of competitively increased muscular glucose uptake.

Notwithstanding the potential fuel competition between muscles and fetus, maximal power and oxygen uptake are unaffected by pregnancy and fetal outcome in physically active women is good *(4–6)*. Although outcome is generally reported as good, some authors have suggested that exercise negatively affects fat mass through fuel competition in a dose–response manner *(9,10)*. Selection bias, however, may have affected the results, and others have found no negative effects of exercise on birthweight or the incidence of low-birthweight infants *(11–13)*.

INSULIN AND GLUCAGON

Glucose metabolism is regulated primarily by insulin, which lowers the blood glucose concentration, and by glucagon, which increases it. Several authors have reported on the acute blood glucose and insulin responses to exercise in pregnancy. The responses vary with the stress of exercise. Mild exercise, of <50% VO$_2$max, hardly affects the circulating concentrations of glucose *(14–17)*, insulin *(15)*, or glucagon *(16)*, in healthy women and in class-B diabetic patients *(16)*. More pronounced changes occur at higher exercise intensities. In pregnant and nonpregnant women who performed moderately strenuous exercise, by cycling for 30 min at an average heart rate (HR) of 140 beats/min, the mean blood concentration of glucose in nonpregnant controls at rest was 3.9 ± 0.3 mmol/L, and that of insulin 150 ± 14 pmol/L *(18)*. In pregnancy, the control values at rest were not different except in the third trimester, when the glucose and insulin concentrations increased by 20 and 56%, respectively. During exercise, the glucose and insulin concentrations decreased by 15 and 37% in the nonpregnant state, by 25 and 44% in the second trimester, and by 35 and 47% in the third trimester, respectively. In the third trimester, but not in the second trimester, the reduction in insulin concentration during exercise was significantly more pronounced than in the nonpregnant state. Nonetheless, the glucose-to-insulin ratio remained significantly higher throughout gestation *(18)*. Following exercise, the insulin concentration was below its resting control value for more than 30 min, whereas the glucose concentration returned to control within 15 min. Subsequent studies have shown similar responses, although with a somewhat slower recovery of the glucose concentration *(19–21)*. One might speculate that the more pronounced reduction in blood glucose level during exercise in pregnant than in nonpregnant women *(18,21)* could be associated with a faster shift toward fat metabolism, the so-called accelerated starvation response *(22)*. However, one might also speculate that pregnancy could change the insulin sensitivity of the muscles in a way that would vary with the intensity and duration of exercise. One study might suggest that this is the case *(23)*. In that study, 75 women were studied before and after, but not during 20 min of either treadmill or aerobic exercise at a heart rate comparable to that of the woman's daily exercise routine. The intensity of the exercise performance was classified as <60, 60–69, 70–79, and 80% $\dot{V}O_2$max. The exercise-induced change in glucose concentration in the nonpregnant state was described as Δ glucose = –2.02 mmol/L + 0.042 * % $\dot{V}O_2$max. During pregnancy, the slope of the relationship decreased with gestational age to 0.034, 0.027, and 0.010 at 8, 15, and 23 wk, respectively, and was ~0 after 30 wk of gestation *(23)*. Thus, the postexercise glycemic response reportedly varied with gestational age and exercise intensity. The insulin concentrations following exercise in this study were 50–60% lower than at rest, in both pregnant and nonpregnant women, but they were not reported in relation to exercise intensity. Reversal of the nonpregnant, hyperglycemic response in the third trimester is more pronounced in heavy endurance exercise than in progressive maximal testing of short duration *(24)*. The mechanism behind the change in glycemic response to strenuous exercise in pregnancy cannot be derived from the study of blood concentrations alone.

Blood concentrations reflect the balance among absorption, gluconeogenesis, and utilization *(25)*. Experiments in horses have shown that exercise conditioning may increase glucose uptake by 50% in the absence of a significant change in blood glucose concentration *(25)*. Despite lower blood concentrations of glucose and insulin of 40 and 14%, respectively, in pregnant and nonpregnant rats, muscle glucose uptake following glucose loading is 75–110% higher in pregnancy *(26)*. When pregnant rats are exercised, the glucose uptake following glucose loading increases further by 40 and 240% in red and white gastrocnemius muscles, respectively, despite insignificant changes in insulin concentration *(26)*. This shows that the pregnancy-induced muscle insulin resistance is reversible, and that blood concentrations of glucose and insulin are indeed not very informative. One study has reported on glucose kinetics during exercise in pregnant women *(27)*. Five women were studied with the use of stable isotopes before, during, and after mild exercise, 30 min of cycling at an HR of 135 beats/min, about 6 wk before and after delivery. The glucose turnover rate at rest in pregnancy was not significantly different from postpartum, with values of 8 ± 3 and 6 ± 4 µmol/kg/min, respectively. During exercise, the turnover rate increased threefold, without significant differences between pregnant and nonpregnant women, in the absence of significant changes in the blood concentrations of glucose and insulin *(27)*. Further studies are needed to determine the extent to which pregnancy affects the glucose turnover rate and insulin response to strenuous exercise.

Physical training increases the cellular responsiveness to insulin *(28)* and, therefore, should lower the average blood glucose concentration. This mechanism is of potential use in the treatment of gestational diabetic women. A controlled study of 19 women with gestational diabetes, 10 of whom performed moderately strenuous exercise regularly, reported a positive effect of such exercise on glycemic control *(29)*. The exercise consisted of arm ergometer training, 20 min/d for 6 wk at 70% HR_{max}, in addition to dietary treatment. It reduced the fasting glucose concentration by 30% and the concentration 1 h after a 50-g oral glucose load by 54%. The reductions were significantly greater than those of control women treated with diet alone, in which the fasting glucose concentration decreased by 10% and the concentration after loading by 17% *(29)*. A positive effect of exercise on glycemic control was also noted in a study of 41 insulin-requiring gestational diabetic patients, randomized between diet plus exercise and diet plus insulin *(30)*. Cycling 3 × 15 min/day 3 times/wk for 6 wk at 50% $\dot{V}O_2max$ reduced the fasting glucose concentration by an average 0.4 mmol/L, which was not significantly less than the 0.9 mmol/L reduction in the insulin-treated controls *(30)*. No positive effect of exercise on glycemic control, however, was reported in another study of 33 women with gestational diabetes who performed dynamic exercise for 30 min/d 3 times/wk for 4–8 wk at 70% HR_{max} *(31)*. Hemoglobin A_1C levels as well as fasting and postprandial glucose concentrations were not different between trained women and nontrained controls on diet alone. The Third International Workshop on Gestational Diabetes reportedly endorsed the prescription of exercise as an additional treatment in gestational diabetic patients, since it is apparently safe *(32)*. The efficacy of regular exercise as additional treatment in gestational diabetic patients, however, requires further proof.

HUMAN PLACENTAL LACTOGEN (HPL)

HPL, also named human chorionic somatomammotropin, has growth hormone-like properties, is present in high concentrations in the blood during pregnancy, and contributes to the diabetogenic effect of pregnancy *(8)*. Twenty minutes of mild to moderate cycling, 10 min at 50 W, followed by 10 min at 75 W did not significantly affect the blood concentrations of HPL or glucose *(33)*. Other studies reported that strenuous cycling, for more than 30 min at an HR of 160 beats/min *(34)* and 25 min of aerobic exercises at an HR of 150 beats/min *(19)* did not affect plasma HPL levels. The limited data available suggest no major role of HPL in the regulation of exercise metabolism in pregnancy.

CORTISOL

Cortisol has been indicated as the most potent diabetogenic hormone, and its concentration increases during pregnancy *(8)*, with mean values of 400–550 nmol/L during gestation, as compared to 165 nmol/L postpartum *(35)*. In one study, mild exercise, 15 min walking on a treadmill at 2 mph at an HR of 104 beats/min, was found not to affect the serum cortisol concentration in pregnant women *(15)*. Also, no effect on the serum cortisol concentration was observed with more strenuous exercise, 10 min cycling at an HR of 157 beats/min *(36)* or 40 min of aerobic dancing at an HR of 135 beats/per *(20)*. Surprisingly, in the latter study, the cortisol concentration was reported to increase 25% in response to walking for 40 min at the same HR of 135 beats/min *(20)*.

Cycle exercise in the water, for 20 min at 60% predicted HR_{max}, showed no significant change from control cortisol values during immersion, which were lower than on land *(35)*. Although cortisol concentrations have not been measured under strenuous circumstances in pregnancy, there is little reason to believe that pregnancy affects the normal role of cortisol in exercise metabolism.

PROGESTERONE AND ESTROGENS

Progesterone and estrogens are produced in large quantities by the ovaries and the placenta, and they are likely to contribute to the pregnancy-induced insulin resistance. In trained rats that run on a treadmill at 28 m/min for 1 h/d throughout pregnancy, serum progesterone levels at rest were not different from those in sedentary control animals, with mean values of 335 and 300 nmol/L, respectively *(37)*. In third trimester pregnant women, cycling for 10 min at an HR of 157 beats/min significantly increased the concentration of estriol by 8%, but not those of progesterone and estradiol during exercise *(36)*. During recovery from exercise, the concentrations of the three hormones were reported to decrease and to reach a significantly lower level at 60 min after exercise, with reductions of 12 and 8% for progesterone and estrogens, respectively *(36)*. In contrast, no significant changes in progesterone and estriol concentrations were observed after 45 min of recovery from 25 min of aerobic exercises at an HR of 150 beats/min *(19)*. The limited data on progesterone and estrogens suggest that their role in exercise metabolism in pregnancy is negligible.

PROLACTIN

It has been suggested that maternal exercise could negatively affect breast milk production. Early this century, it had been observed that lactating rats exercise little *(38)*. A more recent study also showed that mice perform less voluntary exercise during lactation *(39)*. This could be interpreted as saving fuel for lactation. In contrast, however, milk yield was 10% better in mice that were allowed to exercise voluntarily on a treadwheel than in confined control animals *(39)*. In cows, forced walking, 8 km/d for 5 d/wk for 8 wk, did not affect milk production or composition *(40)*. In women, the volume and composition of breast milk were studied in relation to moderate training, 45 min/d for 5 d/wk for 12 wk at 65% HR reserve *(41,42)*. Energy expenditure in the exercising women was higher than in sedentary controls by 1675 kJ/d, but this was compensated for a higher caloric intake. There were no significant differences between the two groups with respect to the volume or composition of the breast milk *(42)*. Also in a recent experiment in which treadmill exercise >75% $\dot{V}O_2max$ was strenuous enough to increase the blood lactate concentration to 10 mmol/L and the breast milk concentration to 1 mmol/L, pH and milk volume were unaffected *(43)*.

When the volume and composition of breast milk are little affected by exercise, one would expect little change in hormonal control. One study in pregnant women reported that the plasma concentration of prolactin did not change during aerobic exercise at 60% $\dot{V}O_2max$, but that it increased temporarily by 45% during recovery from exercise *(36)*. In contrast, in lactating postpartum women, the prolactin concentration was reported to decrease by 23% during exercise in the water at 60% $\dot{V}O_2max$ as compared to immersion alone *(44)*. Despite possible small acute changes in prolactin concentrations, basal concentrations are unaffected by regular exercise. In one study, prolactin concentrations, measured at the onset of labor, were similar in women who in the third trimester had cycled for 30 min 3 times/wk at 65 HR_{max} and in untrained controls *(45)*. Another study showed that plasma prolactin concentrations before and after sucking were not different between trained women and sedentary controls *(42)*. A third study reported that resting plasma concentrations of cortisol, free T_3, and insulin in lactating women who trained for 45 min/d for 5 d/wk at 70% $\dot{V}O_2max$, were not different from those in sedentary lactating women *(41)*. Thus, exercise does not affect basal plasma levels of prolactin, or lactation performance.

Circulation

The major circulatory changes that occur during pregnancy are likely to be controlled by the fetal–placental–maternal endocrine system *(46)*. Among the most pronounced changes are an increase in uteroplacental blood flow equal to 25% of cardiac output, a 30% reduction in systemic vascular resistance, and a 50% increase in cardiac output, whereas blood pressure is only slightly affected. The reduced vascular resistance and increased venous capacitance are associated with a 40% larger blood volume, through a 50% increase in plasma volume and a 25% increase in red cell mass *(46,47)*. These circulatory changes start to develop early in pregnancy, continue to increase in the first two trimesters, and level off in the third trimester. Although one might expect the profound circulatory changes to affect endocrine control, for example, through the increase in plasma volume or the concomitant reduction in protein concentration, there is little evidence to suggest that endocrine responses to exercise are indeed markedly affected by these changes. This stresses both the need for adequate control measurements of hormonal responses to exercise in pregnancy and the fact that circulating hormone concentrations poorly reflect their biological effect.

Circulatory adaptation is required to supply adequate amounts of fuel and oxygen to the muscles during exercise. The sympathetic nervous system is actively involved in the circulatory adaptation to exercise, through an increase in cardiac output and blood flow redistribution. Circulating concentrations of catecholamines provide only a crude estimate of sympathetic nervous activity, since they are the result of release from the nerve endings minus local reuptake and elimination from the circulation.

CATECHOLAMINES

Pregnancy does not markedly affect the resting control values of circulating catecholamines *(24,48,49)*. The physiologic response to an exercise load varies notably with exercise intensity and duration, muscle mass, and physical condition. Because plasma catecholamine concentrations reflect the physiological stress of exercise, they vary to some extent with heart rate. Sheep experiments have shown that the circulatory responses to a fixed load of 45 min of treadmill exercise at 2.5 mph 0° grade vary highly *(50)*. They divided the animals in two groups, a severe response group with a mean HR of 227 beats/min and a moderate response group with a mean HR of 148 beats/min, and observed that norepinephrine (NE) increased 4.8- and 2.7-fold, epinephrine (E) 7.3- and 1.2-fold, and dopamine (D) 3.1- and 3.3-fold, respectively. Pygmy goats exercising strenuously at an HR of 209 beats/min showed similar results *(51)*. Also in humans, catecholamine responses vary with exercise intensity. Pregnant women who performed mild exercise and increased their HR to 103–130 beats/min showed increases in NE and E of up to 40 and 20%, respectively, comparable to postpartum increases *(52,53)*. In third trimester women who performed more strenuous exercise, 10 min of cycling at a mean HR of

157 beats/min, NE increased 1.4-fold and E 1.5-fold *(36)*. Much more pronounced increases in circulating catecholamines are seen at maximal effort, and these responses are not significantly different between third trimester women and postpartum controls *(24,49)*. During progressive maximal cycling, concentrations of NE increased eightfold, E eightfold, and D threefold, both at 32 wk pregnancy and postpartum *(24)*. Also during endurance exercise, 40 min of cycling at 75% $\dot{V}O_2$max with an HR of 175 beats/min, plasma catecholamine concentrations increased equally in pregnant and postpartum women *(24)*. Although the response to dynamic exercise is apparently unaffected by pregnancy, one study has suggested that the catecholamine response to isometric exercise may be slightly blunted by pregnancy. Two minutes of 50% maximal handgrip exercise that increased HR to 120 beats/min, increased the concentrations of NE and E 2.3- and 1.6-fold in pregnancy and 4.4- and 2.3-fold postpartum, respectively *(48)*. It seems safe, however, to conclude that pregnancy does not appear to have a marked effect on the catecholamine response to exercise, as reflected by their concentrations in the circulation.

PLASMA RENIN ACTIVITY

The sympathetic nervous system may express itself during exercise not only through catecholamine release, but also through activation of the renin-angiotensin system. Plasma renin activity (PRA) at rest increases early in gestation, remains elevated throughout pregnancy, and returns to nonpregnant values within hours after delivery *(54)*. Despite eightfold higher levels of PRA, however, blood pressure is not increased in normal pregnancy *(49)* because of reduced angiotensin sensitivity. In one study, progressive strenuous cycling to an HR > 170 beats/min was found not to increase PRA during pregnancy, in contrast to a 2.3-fold increase postpartum, whereas blood pressure increased more during pregnancy than it did postpartum *(49)*. During isometric exercise, consisting of 2 min of 50% maximal handgrip, PRA reportedly increased in both pregnant and postpartum women *(48)*. Without information on angiotensin sensitivity, measured values of PRA are clearly not informative of physiologic responses.

Miscellaneous

RELAXIN

Joint laxity is considered to increase in pregnancy despite absence of firm experimental evidence. Relaxin could be related to joint laxity as it is also increased during pregnancy and has a connective tissue softening effect. In one study, relaxin concentrations were studied in relation to laxity *(55)*. Serum relaxin levels in pregnancy were 9- to 17-fold higher in pregnancy than postpartum, whereas laxity of the knee joint increased during gestation and remained elevated for 6 wk after delivery. There appeared to be no relationship between relaxin concentrations and knee joint laxity.

β-ENDORPHIN

The physiological role of β-endorphin is not well understood, but strenuous muscular exercise and labor contractions are known to increase endogenous opioid secretion. Only one study has addressed the question if pregnancy affects the acute β-endorphin response to exercise in pregnancy. That study took place in the water *(56)*. β-endorphin concentrations at rest were elevated during pregnancy and decreased with gestational age, with values of 43, 21, and 15 pmol/L at 15, 25, and 35 wk, respectively, compared to 6 pmol/L postpartum. Immersion in 30°C water had no consistent effect, but β-endorphin levels increased with exercise, which consisted of 20 min of cycling in the water at 60% maximal capacity. The exercise-induced increase in β-endorphin concentration was most pronounced in early pregnancy, when resting values were the highest, and decreased with advancing gestation, with mean changes of 13, 11, 5, and ~0 pmol/L at 15, 25, and 35 wk pregnancy and postpartum, respectively *(56)*. Although the authors recommended additional studies to clarify the β-endorphin response to exercise in pregnancy, no such studies have been published. Any further studies should preferably be undertaken on land under strenuous circumstances.

Physical training may enhance the exercise-induced β-endorphin response. One study has reported on the effect of physical training, 30 min of cycling 3 times/wk at 65% HR_{max}, on plasma β-endorphin concentrations measured at the onset and end of labor *(45)*. β-endorphin levels were slightly higher in the trained group than in the untrained group of women, with mean values of 35 and 28 pg/mL, respectively, at the onset of labor and increased to a similar extent in both groups during labor. Obviously, however, onset of labor does not represent the true resting state, and labor is not a standard exercise trial. It remains to be determined if pregnancy modifies the effect of training on the exercise-induced endorphin response.

FETAL RESPONSES

Metabolism

Glucose and lactate are the two most important substrates for the fetus. Because both substrates cross the placenta by diffusion, the fetal concentrations are highly affected by those of the mother, and they are not very informative of actual substrate utilization. Since fetal endocrine autonomy is well developed in the second half of pregnancy *(57)*, fetal glucose metabolism is affected by fetal insulin and glucagon concentrations, which will vary in response to trans-placental glucose supply. In sheep, moderately strenuous exercise induces an increase in fetal glucose concentration of 86%, from 0.86 ± 0.06 mmol/L, in conjunction with a 72% increase in maternal concentration and a 68% increase in uterine glucose extraction *(58)*. Increased fetal glucose uptake accounts for about 20 and 60% of the increase in total uterine uptake in fed and underfed sheep, respectively *(57)*. One study has reported on the hormonal responses to maternal exercise in the sheep fetus (55). In these experiments, near the end of 60 min moderate exercise on a treadmill at 2.5 km/h up a 10° slope, the fetal concentrations of insulin and glucagon were unaffected, whereas the fetal concentrations of glucose and lactate were increased by 30 and 90%, respectively. This suggests a blunted fetal endocrine response to the exercise-induced glucose load. Also, acute experiments in rats showed that the fetal concentrations of insulin and glucagon after exercise of the mother were not different from those in sedentary controls, when the glucose concentration was also unaffected *(60,61)*. Another acute study in rats showed that fetal rat glucose uptake after maternal glucose loading was 40% lower in fetuses from exercised mothers compared to those of control mothers, even though the maternal blood glucose concentration was slightly higher in the exercised animals *(26)*. This stresses the point that blood concentrations provide little information on uptake or control mechanisms. Further studies are needed to explore the question why the fetal endocrine response to an exercise-induced maternal glucose load appears to be blunted.

Circulation

One might expect a relationship between fetal heart rate and catecholamine concentrations during exercise, but this is not clearly the case. In one sheep study, the fetal NE and D concentrations increased by 79% in strenuously exercised mothers with an HR of 212 beats/min as well as in those with an HR of only 150 beats/min, whereas the fetal heart rate increased by 20% in the severe response group only *(50)*. In another sheep study, the fetal NE concentration tended to increase with exercise intensity to a twofold higher value at maternal exhaustion, without reaching statistical significance, despite no change in fetal heart rate *(5)*. Absence of changes in fetal blood pressure *(5)*, cardiac output *(5)*, cardiac output distribution *(5)*, and cord blood erythropoietin concentration *(62)* confirms the absence of marked catecholamine release or hypoxemia in the fetus during maternal exercise.

SUMMARY

The pronounced hormonal changes that occur in pregnancy appear not to affect markedly the physiologic mechanisms underlying the metabolic and circulatory adaptations to exercise, except for reversal of the normal hyperglycemic response to strenuous exercise. This may reflect so-called accelerated starvation, which is attributed to a faster shift toward fat metabolism or altered insulin sensitivity of the muscles. The acute and marked metabolic and circulatory changes that occur during exercise do not seem to have a major impact on the maternal endocrine system. The fetus is so well protected by the effective maternal adaptations that there appears to be little need for autonomous fetal endocrine regulation in response to maternal exercise.

REFERENCES

1. Zhang J, Savitz DA. Exercise during pregnancy among US women. Ann Epidemiol 1996;6:53–59.
2. Lotgering FK, Gilbert RD, Longo LD. Maternal and fetal responses to exercise during pregnancy. Physiol Rev 1985;65:1–36.
3. Van Doorn MB, Lotgering FK, Wallenburg HCS. Physiology and practical implications of dynamic exercise in pregnancy. Fetal Med Rev 1991;3:11–28.
4. Lotgering FK, Van Doorn MB, Struijk PC, Pool J, Wallenburg HCS. Maximal aerobic exercise in pregnant women: heart rate, O_2 consumption, CO_2 production, and ventilation. J Appl Physiol 1991;70:1016–1023.
5. Lotgering FK, Gilbert RD, Longo LD. Exercise responses in pregnant sheep: blood gases, temperatures, and fetal cardiovascular system. J Appl Physiol 1983;55:842–850.
6. Van Doorn MB, Lotgering FK, Struijk PC, Pool J, Wallenburg HCS. Maternal and fetal cardiovascular responses to strenuous bicycle exercise. Am J Obstet Gynecol 1992;166:854–859.
7. Nabeshima Y, Sasaki J, Mesaki N, Sohda S, Kubo T. Effect of maternal exercise on fetal umbilical artery waveforms: the comparison of IUGR and AFD fetuses. J Obstet Gynaecol Res 1997;23:255–259.
8. Jovanovic-Peterson L, Peterso CM. Review of gestational diabetes mellitus and low-calorie diet and physical exercise as therapy. Diabetes Metab Rev 1996;12:287–308.
9. Clapp JF, Capeless EL. Neonatal morphometry after endurance exercise during pregnancy. Am J Obstet Gynecol 1990;163:1805–1811.
10. Bell RJ, Palma SM, Lunley JM. The effect of vigorous exercise during pregnancy on birth-weight. Aust NZ J Obstet Gynaecol 1995;35:46–51.
11. Hatch MC, Shu XO, McLean DE, Levin B, Begg M, Reuss L, et al. Maternal exercise during pregnancy, physical fitness, and growth. Am J Epidemiol 1993;173:1105–1114.
12. Schramm WF, Stockbauer JW, Hoffman HJ. Exercise, employment, other daily activities, and adverse pregnancy outcomes. Am J Epidemiol 1996;143:211–218.

13. Sternfield B. Physical activity and pregnancy outcome. Review and recommendations. Sports Med 1997;23:33–47.
14. Berg A, Mroß F, Hillemans HG, Keul J. Die Belastbarkeit der Frau in der Schwangerschaft. Med Welt 1977;28:1267–1269.
15. Artal R, Platt LD, Sperling M, Kammula RK, Jilek J, Nakamura R. Exercise in pregnancy I. Maternal cardiovascular and metabolic responses in normal pregnancy. Am J Obstet Gynecol 1981;140: 123–127.
16. Artal R, Wiswell R, Romem Y. Hormonal responses to exercise in diabetic and nondiabetic pregnant patients. Diabetes 1985;34(Suppl.2):78–80.
17. Artal R, Rutherford S, Romem Y, Kammula RK, Dorey FJ, Wiswell RA. Fetal heart rate responses to maternal exercise. Am J Obstet Gynecol 1986;155:729–733.
18. Bonen A, Campagna P, Gilchrist L, Young DC, Beresford P. Substrate and endocrine responses during exercise at selected stages of pregnancy. J Appl Physiol 1992;73:134–142.
19. Bonen A, Campagna PD, Gilchrist L, Beresford P. Substrate and hormonal responses during exercise classes at selected stages of pregnancy. Can J Appl Physiol 1995;20:440–451.
20. McMurray RG, Hackney AC, Guion WK, Katz VL. Metabolic and hormonal responses to low-impact aerobic dance during pregnancy. Med Sci Sports Exerc 1996;28:41–46.
21. Soultanakis HN, Artal RA, Wiswell R. Prolonged exercise in pregnancy: glucose homeostasis, ventilatory and cardiovascular responses. Semin Perinatol 1996;20:315–327.
22. Freinkel N, Dooley SL, Metzger BE. Care of the pregnant woman with insulin-dependent diabetes mellitus. N Engl J Med 1985;313:96–101.
23. Clapp JF III. The changing glycemic response to exercise during pregnancy. Am J Obstet Gynecol 1991;165:1678–1683.
24. Lotgering FK, Spinnewijn WEM, Struijk PC, Boomsma F, Wallenburg HCS. Respiratory and metabolic responses to endurance cycle exercise in pregnant and postpartum women. Int J Sport Med 1998;19:1–16, in press.
25. Evans JW. Effect of fasting, gestation, lactation and exercise on glucose turnover in horses. J Anim Sci 1971;33:1001–1004.
26. Treadway JL, Young JC. Decreased glucose uptake in the fetus after maternal exercise. Med Sci Sports Exerc 1989;21:140–145.
27. Cowett RM, Carpenter MW, Carr S, Kalhan S, Maguire C, Sady B, et al. Glucose and lactate kinetics during a short bout in pregnancy. Metabolism 1996;45:753–758.
28. Craig BW, Treadway J. Glucose uptake and oxidation in fat cells of trained and sedentary pregnant rats. J Appl Physiol 1986;60:1704–1709.
29. Jovanovic-Peterson L, Durak EP, Peterson CM. Randomized trial of diet versus diet plus cardiovascular conditioning on glucose levels in gestational diabetes. Am J Obstet Gynecol 1989;161:415–419.
30. Bung P, Artal R, Khodiguian N. Regelmäßige Bewegungstherapie bei Kohlehydratstoffwechselstörungen in der Schwangerschaft—Ergebnisse einer prospectiven, randomisierten Longitudinalstudie. Geburtsh Frauenheilk 1993;53:188–193.
31. Avery MD, Leon AS, Kopher RA. Effects of a partially home-based exercise program for women with gestational diabetes. Obstet Gynecol 1997;89:10–15.
32. Artal R. Exercise and pregnancy. Clin Sports Med 1992;11:363–377.
33. Pavlou C, Chard T, Landon J, Letchworth AT. Circulating levels of human placental lactogen in late pregnancy: the effect of glucose loading, smoking and exercise. Eur J Obstet Gynecol Reprod Biol 1973;3:45–49.
34. Lindberg BS, Nilsson BA. Variations in maternal plasma levels of human placental lactogen (HPL) in normal pregnancy and labour. J Obstet Gynaecol Br Commonw 1973;80:619–626.
35. McMurray RG, Katz VL, Berry MJ, Cefalo RC. The effect of pregnancy on metabolic responses during rest, immersion, and aerobic exercise in the water. Am J Obstet Gynecol 1988;158:481–486.
36. Rauramo I, Andersson B, Laatikainen T. Stress hormones and placental steroids in physical exercise during pregnancy. Br J Obstet Gynecol 1982;89:921–925.
37. Garris DR, Kasperek GJ, Overton SV, Alligood GR. Effects of exercise on fetal-placental growth and uteroplacental blood flow in the rat. Biol Neonate 1985;47:223–229.
38. Wang GH. The relation between "spontaneous activity" and oestrus cycle in the white rat. Comp Psychol Monogr 1923;2:1–27.
39. Karasawa K, Suwa J, Kimura S. Voluntary exercise during pregnancy and lactation and its effect on lactational performance in mice. J Nutr Sci Vitaminol 1981;27:333–339.

40. Lamb RC, Anderson MJ, Walters JL. Forced walking prepartum for dairy cows of different ages. J Dairy Sci 1981;64:2017–2024.
41. Lovelady CA, Lonnerdal B, Dewey KG. Lactation performance of exercising women. Am J Clin Nutr 1990;52:103–109.
42. Dewey KG, Lovelady CA, Nommsen-Rivers LA, McCrory MA, Lönnerdal B. A randomized study of the effects of aerobic exercise by lactating women on breast-milk volume and composition. N Engl J Med 1994;330:449–453.
43. Carey GB, Quinn TJ, Goodwin SE. Breast milk composition after exercise of different intensities. J Hum Lact 1997;13:115–120.
44. Katz VL, McMurray R, Turnbull CD, Berry M, Bowman C, Cefalo RC. The effects of immersion and exercise on prolactin during pregnancy. Eur J Appl Physiol 1989;60:191–193.
45. Varrassi G, Bazzano C, Edwards TW. Effects of physical activity on maternal plasma β-endorphin levels and perception of labor pain. Am J Obstet Gynecol 1989;160:707–712.
46. Longo LD. Maternal blood volume and cardiac output during pregnancy; a hypothesis of endocrinologic control. Am J Physiol 1983;245:R720–R729.
47. Clark SL, Cotton DB, Pivarnik JM, Lee W, Hankins, GDV, Benedetti THJ, et al. Position change and central hemodynamic profile during normal third-trimester pregnancy and post partum. Am J Obstet Gynecol 1991;164:883–887.
48. Barron WM, Mujais SK, Zinaman M, Bravo EL, Lindheimer MD. Plasma catecholamine responses to physiologic stimuli in normal human pregnancy. Am J Obstet Gynecol 1986;154:80–84.
49. Eneroth-Grimfors E, Bevegård S, Nilsson BA, Sätterström G. Effect of exercise on catecholamines and plasma renin activity in pregnant women. Acta Obstet Gynecol Scand 1988;67:519–523.
50. Palmer SM, Oakes GK, Champion JA, Fisher DA, Hobel CK. Catecholamine physiology in the ovine fetus: III. Maternal and fetal response to acute maternal exercise. Am J Obstet Gynecol 1984; 149:426–434.
51. Hohimer AG, Bissonnette JM, Metcalfe J, McKean TA. Effect of exercise on uterine blood flow in the pregnant Pygmy goat. Am J Physiol 1984;246:H207–H212.
52. Platt LD, Artal R, Semel J, Sipos L, Kammula RK. Exercise in pregnancy: II. Fetal responses. Am J Obstet Gynecol 1983;147:487–491.
53. Cooper KA, Hunyor SN, Boyce ES, O'Neill ME, Frewin DB. Fetal heart rate and maternal cardiovascular and catecholamine responses to dynamic exercise. Aust NZ J Obstet Gynecol 1984;27:220–223.
54. Broughton Pipkin F, Symonds EM. The renin-angiotensin system in the maternal and fetal circulation in pregnancy hypertension. Clin Obstet Gynaecol 1977;4:651–664.
55. Schauberger CW, Rooney BL, Goldsmith L, Shenton D, Silva PD, Schaper A. Peripheral joint laxity increases in pregnancy but does not correlate with serum relaxin levels. Am J Obstet Gynecol 1996;174:667–671.
56. McMurray RG, Berry MJ, Katz V. The beta-endorphin responses of pregnant women during aerobic exercise in the water. Med Sci Sports Exerc 1990;22:298–303.
57. Bell AW, Bassett JM, Chandler KD, Boston RC. Fetal and maternal endocrine responses to exercise in the pregnant ewe. J Develop Physiol 1983;5:129–141.
58. Chandler KD, Bell AW. Effects of maternal exercise on fetal and maternal respiration and nutrient metabolism in the pregnant ewe. J Dev Physiol 1981;3:161–176.
59. Chandler KD, Leury BJ, Bird AR, Bell AW. Effects of undernutrition and exercise during late pregnancy on uterine, fetal and uteroplacental metabolism in the ewe. Br J Nutr 1985;53:625–635.
60. Levitsky LL, Kimber A, Marchichow JA, Uehara J. Metabolic response to fasting in experimental intrauterine growth retardation induced by surgical and nonsurgical maternal stress. Biol Neonate 1977;31:311–315.
61. Carlson KI, Yang HT, Bradshaw WS, Conlee RK, Winder WW. Effect of maternal exercise on fetal liver glycogen late in gestation in the rat. J Appl Physiol 1986;60(4):1254–1258.
62. Clapp JF, Little KD, Appleby-Wineberg SK, Widness JA. The effect of regular maternal exercise on erythropoietin in cord blood and amniotic fluid. Am J Obstet Gynecol 1995;172:1445–1451.

20 The Endocrine System in Overtraining

*Axel Urhausen, MD, PhD
and Wilfried Kindermann, MD, PhD*

CONTENTS

SUMMARY
THE OVERTRAINING SYNDROME
ADRENALINE (EPINEPHRINE) AND NORADRENALINE (NOREPINEPHRINE)
TESTOSTERONE AND CORTISOL
PITUITARY HORMONES
OTHER HORMONES
PATHOPHYSIOLOGICAL CONSIDERATIONS
PERSPECTIVES
REFERENCES

SUMMARY

An imbalance between physical exercise and other stressors superimposed on individual tolerance induces an overreaching or overtraining (OT) syndrome. This syndrome is characterized by a diminished sport-specific physical performance, an accelerated fatigability, and (inconstant) vegetative symptoms. Although the OT syndrome represents the most frequent and feared dysfunction of the athlete, there are still no single objective parameters suitable for its diagnosis.

Endogenous hormones are essential for physiological reactions and adaptations during physical work and influence the regeneration phase by modulating anabolic and catabolic processes. The OT syndrome is characterized by a central—probably (supra)hypothalamic—hormonal dysregulation involving corticotropin-releasing hormone, prolactin, and/or β-endorphin. In overtrained athlete studies, a disturbed stress response occurs showing an intraindividually decreased maximum exercise-induced response of pituitary hormones (adrenocorticotropic hormone [ACTH], growth hormone), cortisol, and insulin. The blood testosterone/cortisol ratio, indicator of the so-called anabolic/catabolic balance, decreases during periods of intense training or repetitive competitions and can be reversed by regenerative measures. However, the testosterone/cortisol ratio indicates rather the actual physiological strain in training than an OT syndrome.

From: *Contemporary Endocrinology: Sports Endocrinology*
Edited by: M. P. Warren and N. W. Constantini © Humana Press Inc., Totowa, NJ

The sympatho-adrenergic system may be involved in the pathogenesis of OT. Its chronic form typically shows a diminished maximal secretion of catecholamines and impaired mobilization of anaerobic lactic reserves. In particular, workloads exceeding the individual anaerobic threshold and psychic stress during competitive events are characterized by a dysproportional increase of catecholamines. Thus, the frequency of training sessions with higher anaerobic lactic demands or competitions should be limited in order to prevent an OT.

Individual reference values of hormonal concentrations for "normal" exercise tolerance as well as easier and less expensive laboratory methods are still lacking. External factors influencing the hormonal blood concentrations require well-standardized sampling conditions that are often difficult to realize in training practice. However, hormonal disorders may precede the appearance of OT symptoms, suggesting that further investigation is needed to characterize hormonal monitoring of training.

THE OVERTRAINING SYNDROME

The efficiency of physical training essentially depends on intensity, volume, and periodization of training stimuli. An optimal training program also requires an adequate assessment of the current individual tolerance of stress, including training and competitions, as well as other external stressors, including physical disease and social problems. For practical use, this concept is what is called the "stress barrel," which can be filled by stressors of different origins (Fig. 1).

An imbalance between the strain during training and the individual tolerance of stress leads to short-term OT, called overreaching, with unexpected reduction of performance, which can be reversed by a prolonged period of regeneration of several days up to approx 2 wk. It has to be differentiated from short-term (lasting maximally 1–2 d) fatigue after overload training. The further training stress will induce an OT syndrome or "staleness," which can no longer be reversed by a prolonged regenerative period *(1–3)*. The sympathicotonic form of the OT syndrome is easier to recognize because of more pronounced vegetative complaints, whereas the more advanced chronic parasympathicotonic ("addisonoid") typically is associated with less obvious symptoms *(4,5)*. Generally the OT is characterized by a decreased sports performance capacity and with the training load maintained or increased, an enhanced fatiguability and more or less pronounced vegetative complaints *(4,5)*. The diagnosis of OT remains a clinical diagnosis of exclusion because other (organic) diseases must be excluded.

Even today, the frequent occurrence of this feared "disease" of the athlete (the term "malfunction" or "dysregulation" would be more suitable) is in contrast with the lack of available diagnostic tools. The data on overtraining are frequently based on experience or individual observations rather than on experimental findings.

The evaluation of the decrease in performance, the cardinal symptom during OT, often causes difficulties. It requires a specific and standardized test methodology. An impairment of speed endurance or short-term endurance with limited anaerobic lactic capacity has been reported *(5–10)*, and is primarily recognized when reaching the limit of physical performance.

Endogenous hormones are essentially involved in exercise-induced acute or chronic adaptations and influence the regeneration phase through the modulation of anabolic and catabolic processes after exercise. Thus, apart from routine measurements of sub-

Chapter 20 / Overtraining   349

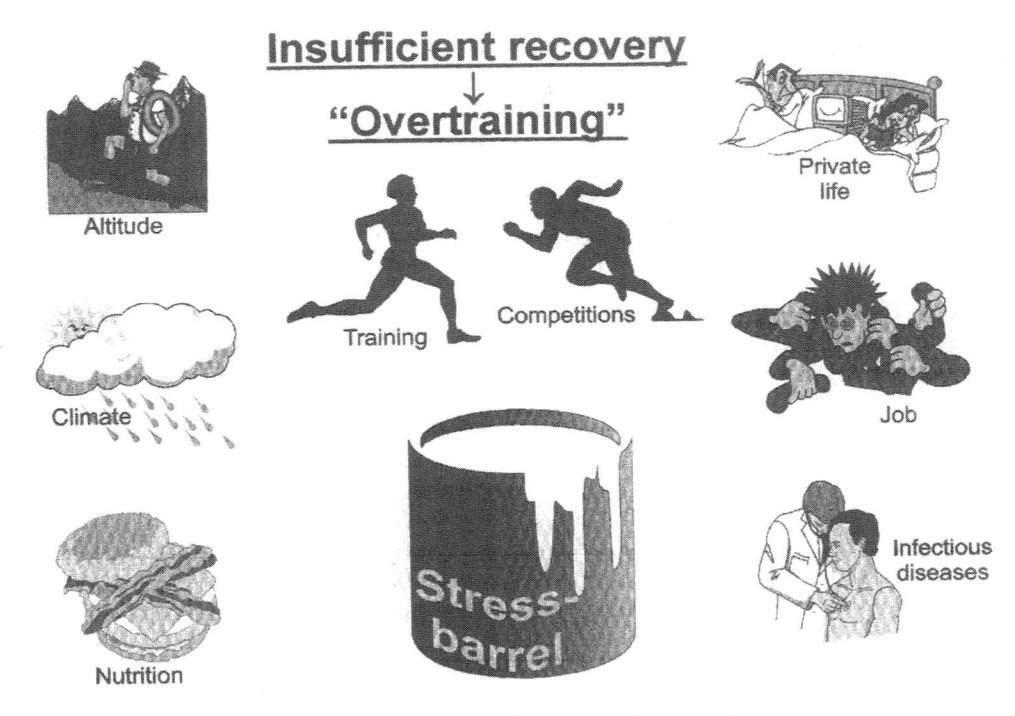

Fig. 1. Multifactorial genesis of overtraining syndrome.

strates (lactate, ammonia, urea, and so forth) or enzyme activity (creatine kinase) in blood, in the last few years, attention has focused on an objective monitoring of exercise intensity and training by determinations of hormones ("hormonal monitoring of training") *(11–13)*.

Table 1 provides a summary survey of studies published in connection with athletes claiming OT syndrome (some cases are questionable). A longer period of observation (as in refs. *9,14*) has the advantage of including other stressful factors in addition to training in generating an OT. These factors—typically infectious diseases, frequent competitions, and psychic social distress (examinations, business, family life)—are an essential part of the multifactorial genesis of the OT (Fig. 1).

Studies involving endurance athletes *(5,7,15)* suggest an essential role for the intensity of physical exercise in the genesis of an OT. During prolonged exercises at intensities above the individual anaerobic threshold, without a lactate steady state, the metabolic and psychic demands increase considerably with an overproportional increase in free plasma catecholamines *(16)*. Other authors, however, report an OT achieved solely by a very drastic increase in training volume *(17,18)*, or partly owing to a combination of a limited intake of carbohydrate causing reduced muscular glycogen stores associated with training *(17)*. Few prospective studies have been done with athletes with OT induced by resistance training. In their excellent review, Fry and Kraemer *(12)* point out different neuroendocrine responses to high-intensity and high-volume resistive exercise OT, the latter being similar to OT resulting from aerobic activities.

Table 1
Studies Involving Blood Hormone Levels of Athletes in a State
of Overtraining/Overreaching Syndrome (OT) over a Period of at least 1 wk.[a]

Reference	Number of overtrained athletes	Observation period	Overtraining	Objective indicators of overtraining	Subjective indicators of overtraining	Hormonal parameters
Barron et al. (58)	4 M marathon runners	4 mo	Intensive training, frequent races during 8–14 wk	Racing and training performance ↓	Emotional and behavioral symptoms	Cortisol-, ACTH-, STH-, and PRL-response to insulin-induced hypoglycemia ↓; normal response of LH, TSH, and PRL to LHRH
Häkkinen et al. (126)	21 M physically active subjects (2 groups)	36 wk	3 strength training sessions/wk (2 protocols) during 24 wk	Maximal strength during the first 20 wk ↑, followed by a 4-wk plateau phase (OT?)	?	During training phase: cortisol ↓ and testosterone shortly ↑ in one experimental group (n = 11); during the plateau and the following regeneration phase testosterone/cortisol and testosterone/SHBG correlate to the changes of maximum strength; LH, FSH, STH, and SHBG unchanged
Adlercreutz et al. (11)	M long-distance runners		"Very intensive training programme during 1 week"	?	?	Free testosterone/ cortisol <70% or <0.35 × 10⁻³
Kindermann (5)	M/F mid-distance runners		Case reports	Maximal anaerobic lactic performance on treadmill (stepwise increasing and speed endurance tests ↓	Vegetative complaints (sympathetic or parasympathetic form of OT)	Maximal exercise-induced rise of free epinephrine and norepinephrine in parasympathicotonic OT ↓
Häkkinen et al. (41)	11 M weightlifters	1 yr, including 6 wk of preparation for main competition	11% increase of training volume during 2 wk	No significant changes in competitive results (OT?)	?	After intensive training: testosterone ↓ LH ↑; after the following normal and reduced training: testosterone unchanged; cortisol and LH ↓; the changes of testosterone/SHBG correlate with those of the competitive results

350

Kirwan et al. (49)	12 M swimmers, 4 in OT	24 d	110% increase in training distance at 94% VO$_2$max for 10 d	Swimming tests, training speed ↓	Subjective rating of training effort ↑	Cortisol at rest after maximal incremental treadmil test ↑; ACTH and β-endorphin after exercise ↓
Kraemer et al. (15)	7 M/F physically active subjects	10 wk	3 longer sprint intervals and 3 maximal 30 min runs/wk	VO$_2$max ↑ (!) (OT?)	?	Testosterone, SHBG, cortisol, LH, FSH unchanged
Fry et al. (7)	5 M elite soldiers	15 d	2 intensive interval running sessions/d on treadmill during 10 d	Time to exhaustion on treadmill at 18 km/h/1% gradient ↓	Subjective complaints	Nocturnal catecholamine excretion ↓, submaximal free norepinephrine ↑; epinephrine (↑); cortisol at rest (↑), after exercise ↓; (free) testosterone, insulin, STH, C-peptide, prolactin, LH, FSH, thyroid hormones, aldosterone, free catecholamines at rest and after exercise unchanged
Lehmann et al. (18)	8 M mid- and long-distance runners	5 wk	Training volume approx +100% over 3 wk	Treadmill running speed at 4 mmol/L lactate unchanged, total running distance in incremental test ↓	Daily rating of "well-being" ↓	
Hooper et al. (29)	14 M/F swimmers, 3 in OT	6 mo	Training volume approx +10% during tapering for 2–3 wk before trials	Competitive results ↓	Level of fatigue >5 (scale from 1–7) over 7 d without illness	Resting norepinephrine before trials ↑; epinephrine, cortisol unchanged
Flynn et al. (42b)	5 M swimmers	21 wk	Training volume +88% with approx the same percentage of high intensive training over 2 wk	Performance in swimming tests ↓	Global mood state impaired	(Free) testosterone ↓; cortisol unchanged
Urhausen et al. (14)	15 M cyclists and triathletes	19 mo	Time of intensive training +180% over at least 2 wk in addition to individual stressors (competitions, short recovery after illness, social pressure)	Competitive/training performance ↓	Impaired mood profile and subjective rating of effort, vegetative complaints	Maximal exercise-induced rise of ACTH, STH, insulin ↓, cortisol (↓), submaximal norepinephrine (↑); all hormones including testosterone, SHBG, LH, FSH (at rest), β-endorphin, and free epinephrine/norepinephrine (at rest and maximal) unchanged

(continued)

Table 1
Studies Involving Blood Hormone Levels of Athletes in a State
of Overtraining/Overreaching Syndrome (OT) over a Period of at least 1 wk.[a] (continued)

Reference	Number of overtrained athletes	Observation period	Overtraining	Objective indicators of overtraining	Subjective indicators of overtraining	Hormonal parameters
Snyder et al. (64)	8 M cyclists	4 wk	Training volume +4%, time >90% VO$_2$max +200%	Wmax ↓	Daily questionnaires, RPE during ex. tests ↑	Cortisol ↓ in 6/8 subjects
Mackinnon et al. (30)	8 M/F swimmers	4 wk	Training volume +37%, dry land resistance ex. +22%	200-m-time ↓ by 1.2–6.5%	Fatigue rating in log book, sleep disturbances	Urinary norepinephrine excretion ↓; no changes in plasma norepinephrine, cortisol, testosterone
O'Connor et al. (63)	14 F college swimmers, 3 in OT	5.5 mo	Training volume +600% over 3 wk	Performance ↓ by 3–10% for at least 2 wk	POMS depression scores ↑, also after 4 wk of progressive training reduction	Saliva cortisol ↑
Gabriel et al. (28) Urhausen et al. (8)	12 M cyclists and triathletes	14 wk	Periods of intensive (total volume +38%, intensive training +260%), normal and regenerative training	Cycle ergometer performance in 1-min-anaerobic test ↓, time to exhaustion at 110% of individual anaerobic threshold	Impaired mood profile and subjective rating of effort, vegetative complaints	Maximal exercise-induced rise of ACTH, STH, cortisol, (nor)epinephrine ↓; no changes in resting levels including testosterone, LH and FSH. (Hyper) normalization after 2 wk of regenerative training

[a] m = male, f = female, ( ) = tendencial statistical significance

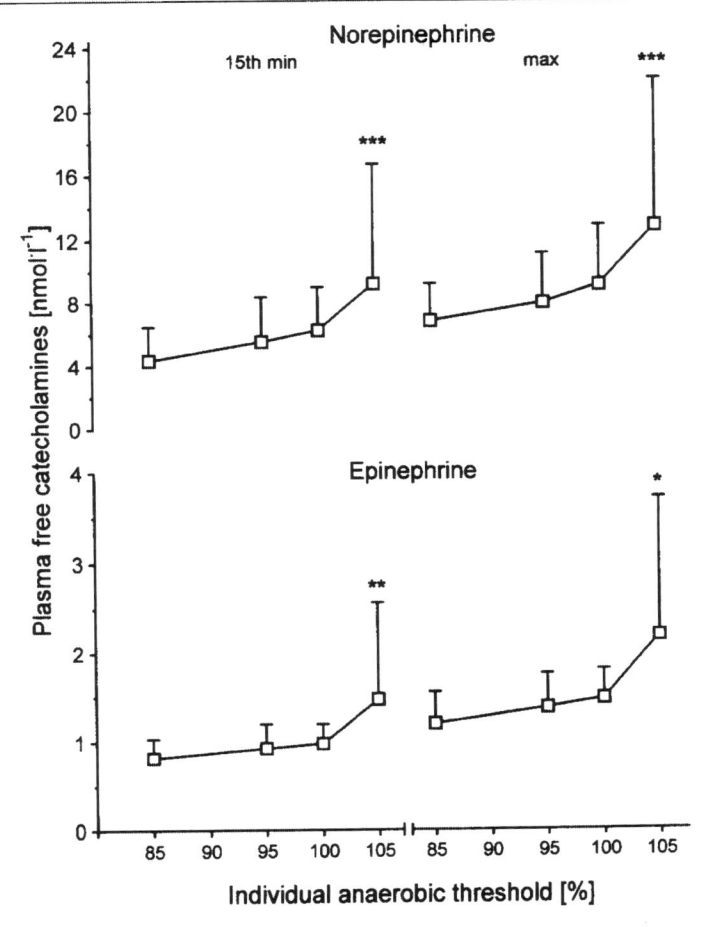

Fig. 2. Free plasma adrenaline and noradrenaline during 45-min lasting endurance runnings on treadmill in relation to the intensity of the individual anaerobic threshold (IAT). Means ± SD; $n = 14$ endurance trained male runners, $*p < 0.05$; $**p < 0.01$; $***p < 0.001$. From ref. *16*.

ADRENALINE (EPINEPHRINE) AND NORADRENALINE (NOREPINEPHRINE)

Free catecholamines measured in plasma reflect sympatho-adrenergic activation associated with exercise *(19,20)*. Catecholamines play an important role in many metabolic and cardiocirculatory reactions and adaptations to physical and psychic work. During incremental graded physical work, free adrenaline and noradrenaline correlate with the exponential increase in lactate *(21)*. During prolonged exercise with intensities below the individual anaerobic threshold, the catecholamines increase in a time-dependent manner, although the blood lactate concentration remains constant or even decreases *(16)*. If the exercise intensity exceeds the individual anaerobic threshold by 5% or more, the lactate concentration exceeds the maximal steady state, which eventually leads to progressive acidosis *(22)*. At the same time, there is a dysproportional time- and intensity-dependent rise in adrenaline and noradrenaline as a sign of an increased sympatho-adrenergic activation (Fig. 2). This suggests that in accordance with the concept of

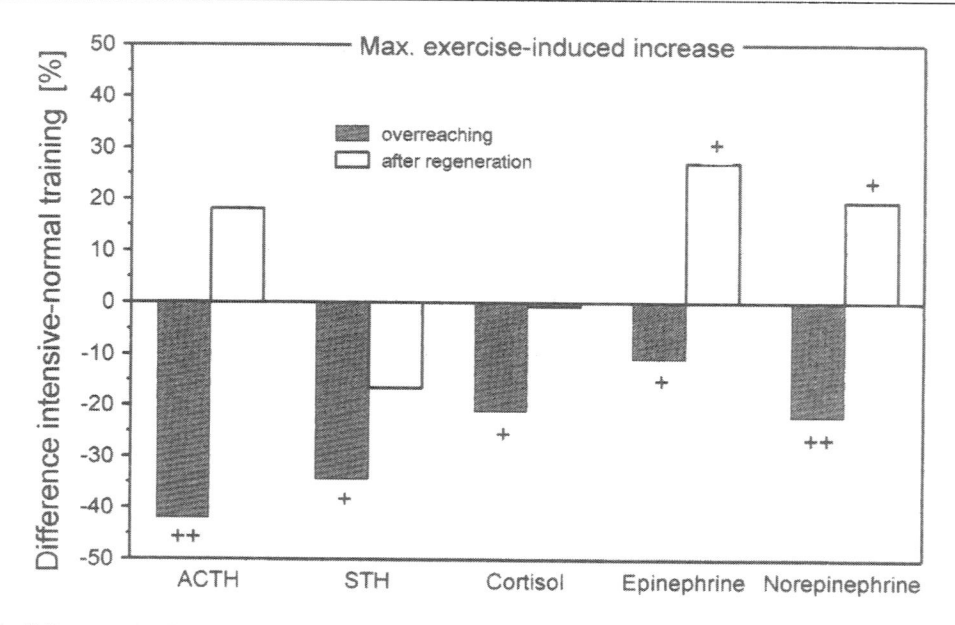

Fig. 3. Percentage changes of ACTH, STH, cortisol, epinephrine, and norepinephrine after an exhaustive bicycle endurance test at 110% of the individual anaerobic threshold after 4 wk of overreaching and 2 wk of regenerative training. Means ± SD; $n = 12$ endurance trained male triathletes and cyclists, $+ p < 0.05$, $++ p < 0.01$. From ref. 9.

"aerob-anaerobic transition" (23) a physiological breakpoint occurs, which corresponds to the range for the individual anaerobic threshold. Shorter high-intensive (anaerobic lactic) exercises are characterized by a higher catecholamine secretion and a higher adrenaline/noradrenaline ratio in comparison to aerobic work (24,25). During prolonged exercise at 85–100% of the individual anaerobic threshold, the concentrations of adrenaline or noradrenaline demonstrate only discrete differences (16). A positive training effect is characterized by lower catecholamine concentrations at the same relative submaximal workload (26). Apart from thermoregulatory demands, the increase in catecholamine concentrations in the course of the prolonged exercise is attributed to a reduced intramuscular glycogen availability during training (27).

In some studies involving overtrained endurance athletes, a disturbed glycolytic energy mobilization with reduced maximal blood lactate concentrations had been described (5,9,28). This is accompanied by lowered plasma values of free adrenaline and noradrenaline after maximal treadmill and cycle ergometric tests lasting 30 s to approx 20 min. However, after 2 wk of regenerative training, the exercise-induced catecholamine (and lactate) responses had returned to (supra)normal levels in previously overreached cyclists and triathletes (9) (Fig. 3). In another study, during submaximal exercise, increased noradrenaline values were measured in runners overtrained by volume overload (18). Despite their limited validity, resting noradrenaline values are also occasionally reported to be increased in a retrospective evaluation of three swimmers during early OT (29), but could not be confirmed by our examinations (5,9,28). The form of the OT probably plays an important role: it has been hypothesized that the initial stage (sympathicotonic form) of OT is characterized by increased exercise-induced catecholamine levels and downregulated skeletal muscle β-receptors (12) and progresses to a chronic (parasympathicotonic) form of OT with decreased exercise-induced concentrations. The 40–70% decrease of nocturnal urinary catecholamine excretion is similar to patients with autonomic sympathetic insufficiency *(3)*. It is interesting to note that neuroendocrine disorders may precede the symptoms of OT and thus constitute early markers of OT: a decreased urinary noradrenaline excretion is induced by rising swimming training volume as well as an increased exercise-induced catecholamine response by high-intensity resistance training, even before the performance declines *(12,30)*.

A counterregulatory decrease in the sensitivity and density of the β-adrenoreceptors during OT owing to chronically increased catecholamine levels in stressful training *(3)* can be speculated to be similar to that reported following long-term stimulation by isoproterenol *(31)*. This would explain the reduced maximal heart rate response during OT *(9)*. A modified neuronal activity possibly plays a role through muscle receptors *(18)*, and metabolites in active muscles may stimulate the adrenergous activity via afferent fibres during exercise *(32)*. However, catecholamines may be less important to glycolysis and glycogenolysis during physical exercise than generally assumed *(3)*; a blood lactate level of about 8 mmol/L can still be measured at low exercise intensities in patients with defect sympathetic regulation (Shy-Drager Syndrome).

In the future, the application of measurements of catecholamines as an assessment of sympatho-adrenergic activity could be used in different training regimens as well as in competition. Exercise regimens with high nervous stress components are probably more susceptible to inducing an OT, especially if the adequate periods of regeneration are neglected. Blood lactate concentrations may less helpful. During competition badminton, players showed similar adrenaline and noradrenaline values in comparison to highly intensive training, whereas lactate was clearly (about three times) lower *(33)*. This is most likely a reflection of the pronounced psychic stress specific to competition.

TESTOSTERONE AND CORTISOL

Testosterone

Serum testosterone shows a biphasic behavior with physical exercise: after exercises of shorter duration, testosterone increases in relation to intensity, volume, and the muscle mass involved. This is because of a decreased hepatic and extrahepatic clearance or sympathetic stimulation of β-receptors in the testis *(34,35)*. Following exercise of more than approx 3 h, the values decrease *(34,35)*. During the following regeneration phase, lowered concentrations at rest were observed for hours to days, e.g., after a triathlon competition *(36)*, but also after repeated anaerobic exercises *(37)*. The chronic training effect on testosterone levels is controversial, with most studies involving longer training programs showing unchanged concentrations *(12)*. Endurance athletes, when compared with untrained subjects, are reported to have lower blood testosterone concentrations. These studies have been criticized as retrospective and cross-sectional, with wide differences among the subjects. The subjects were not controlled for training and other variables, such as diet, age, differences of the time of blood sampling, and genetic influences *(38)*.

Secretion of hormones with anabolic or catabolic properties, such as testosterone and cortisol, depends on the intensity and duration of preceding physical work. These hormones show quantitative changes signaling a catabolic state, which can be reversed by appropriate regenerative measures *(13,26,39,40)*. For the diagnosis of OT, Adlercreutz et al. *(11)* proposed a decrease in the ratio of (measured) free testosterone/cortisol >30% or <$0.35/10^{-3}$. The respective advantages of directly measuring or calculating the biologically active free testosterone fraction (by using the blood concentration of sexual hormone binding globulin = SHBG) is controversial. Häkkinen et al. *(41)* observed a parallel development between the testosterone/cortisol ratio and the training-induced changes in strength in power athletes and also during a plateau phase of performance interpreted as OT. An increase in strength, however, is not necessarily connected with a simultaneous increase in the testosterone/cortisol ratio. Sensitivity to androgens was enhanced by a rapid increase in the number of receptors in exercised muscles *(42a)*. During resistive training, in which OT was induced by volume overload, resting total, and especially free testosterone decrease, but not following increased training intensity (*see* review in ref. *12*).

There exist only a few studies relating changes in free testosterone or the testosterone/cortisol ratio to objective parameters of performance in endurance athletes *(13)*. Flynn et al. *(42b)* observed a decrease in (free) testosterone associated with reduced swimming times and altered mood state after the training volume was increased by 80% for 2 wk. Female athletes are also reported to present lower testosterone values in comparison to untrained women *(43)*. With respect to the low physiological testosterone concentration (about 7–10% of the male values), negative correlation to the training intensity was seen in female rowers *(44,45)* or speed skaters *(46)*. These studies are hampered by the small number of subjects.

Recent prospective studies with overreached or overtrained endurance athletes, however, show no essential changes in concentrations at rest with regard to testosterone, cortisol, and SHBG *(8,14)*. The testosterone/cortisol ratio is occasionally also overinterpreted. Although significantly reduced ratios were related to a decline in the performance during competition *(44,47)*, even a decrease in (free) testosterone/cortisol >30% during intensive training or competition phases *(12,45,48)* does not necessarily indicate an OT. It is probable that the behavior of (free) testosterone and cortisol is more likely a physiological indicator of current training load *(13,44,46,49,50)*.

The significance of changes in carrier protein SHBG is unclear. An SHBG increase in response to a decrease in testosterone may suggest an OT *(11)*. An increased concentration of the carrier protein somewhat protects the testosterone pool from a sudden metabolic turnover, but leads to a further decrease in the biologically active testosterone fraction, which could be interpreted as unfavorable. In contrast to that, low SHBG values are regarded as being a sign of an "insufficient adaptation" to training loads based on empiric observation *(51)*. There is also an influence of diet on the SHBG concentration, with increased values during fasting, and correspondingly decreased free testosterone fraction *(52,53)*. In most of the studies, SHBG showed no changes during OT.

There are several hypotheses concerning the pathomechanism responsible for the decreased testosterone concentrations incurred by endurance training or during OT *(13)*. These include a transient suppressive effect on testicular luteinizing hormone (LH) receptors as a result of the exercise-induced increase in adrenocorticotropin (=ACTH) and cortisol, a direct influence on the testicular testosterone secretion (through the inhibition of an enzymatic step or a decreased sensitivity of the Leydig cells to stimulating hormones), a catecholamine-induced increase in the testicular vascular resistance, a desensitizing effect on LH receptors through reduced prolactin levels, or an increased metabolic rate of testosterone. Many reports, however, suggest these may be a central mechanism in the sense of a (supra) hypothalamo–pituitary dysregulation with disturbed gonadotropin-releasing hormone (GnRH) release and LH pulsatility *(13,38,54)*.

To what extent decreased testosterone levels influence the energy-supplying processes cannot be definitely answered. Testosterone plays an important role in muscle metabolism during the regeneration phase after physical exercise in that its anabolic effect not only encourages protein synthesis, but also seems to increase the ability of the muscle to refill its glycogen storage through an increased activity of the muscle glycogen synthetase *(55)*. This is important for adequate regeneration after prolonged exercise and during intensive training periods. Although transitory decreased testosterone levels are of only of minor importance, significant effects in target cells are noted with testosterone levels that decreased for a prolonged period of time *(39)*. Anabolic deficits occur characterized by a decreased counterregulation to the catabolic effect of cortisol *(56)*. Androgen pathways significantly influence the exercise-induced muscle hypertrophy. In animal experiments, an increased protein catabolism occurs as the result of the activation of intracellular nonlysosomal proteinases after the administration of glucocorticoids *(40)*. Exhausting prolonged exercises can have effects comparable to glucocorticoids. In experiments on isolated rat muscle, these effects could be reversed or prevented *(40,57)* through the administration of anabolic steroids or testosterone.

Cortisol

The exercise-induced cortisol increase depends on the duration and intensity of physical exercise *(13,24,26,47)*. A significant increase in the blood cortisol concentration usually requires a duration of exercise of more than 20 min with at least 60% of the maximal oxygen uptake and is primarily the consequence of a higher secretion rate. During the postexercise phase, cortisol usually decreases quickly and, within hours, reaches the initial value again *(36,37)*. Apart from physical strain and psychic factors (e.g., mental stress before starting the effort), diet may also influence cortisol levels through a modification of metabolic clearance *(53)*.

The maximal exercise-induced cortisol response during OT seems to be lowered *(8,14,18,58)* (Figs. 3 and 4). Decreased submaximal cortisol concentrations together with sustained fatigue are also reported in distance runners *(60)*. An increased cortisol response with exercise is described as training effect in an induced adaptation *(61,62)*. Nevertheless, it can be assumed that different training forms (aerobic or anaerobic) can also lead to different hormonal adaptations *(15)*.

Repeated determinations of cortisol have been suggested as a possible important tool in the diagnosis of OT. The data on resting cortisol levels are conflicting. Increased concentrations during OT *(15,49,58,63)* are reported in some, but not all reports *(8,14,29,42b)*. Some report decreasing concentrations *(18,40,64)* or, in spite of training reduction, "unexpected" cortisol increases *(65)*. Higher cortisol concentrations are also interpreted as a long-term adaptation to training in oligo-amenorrhoic female skiers, suggesting a chronic catabolic state *(66)*. During several weeks of overload training in female rowers, we observed significant correlations between changes of resting capillary cortisol and mood state, without a drop in performance *(48)*. Interestingly, in patients with psychological depression, higher blood cortisol concentrations are reported as well *(67)*.

When the exercise duration is prolonged, the cortisol increase is important for the energy supply, since cortisol prevents the re-esterfication of fatty acids released by

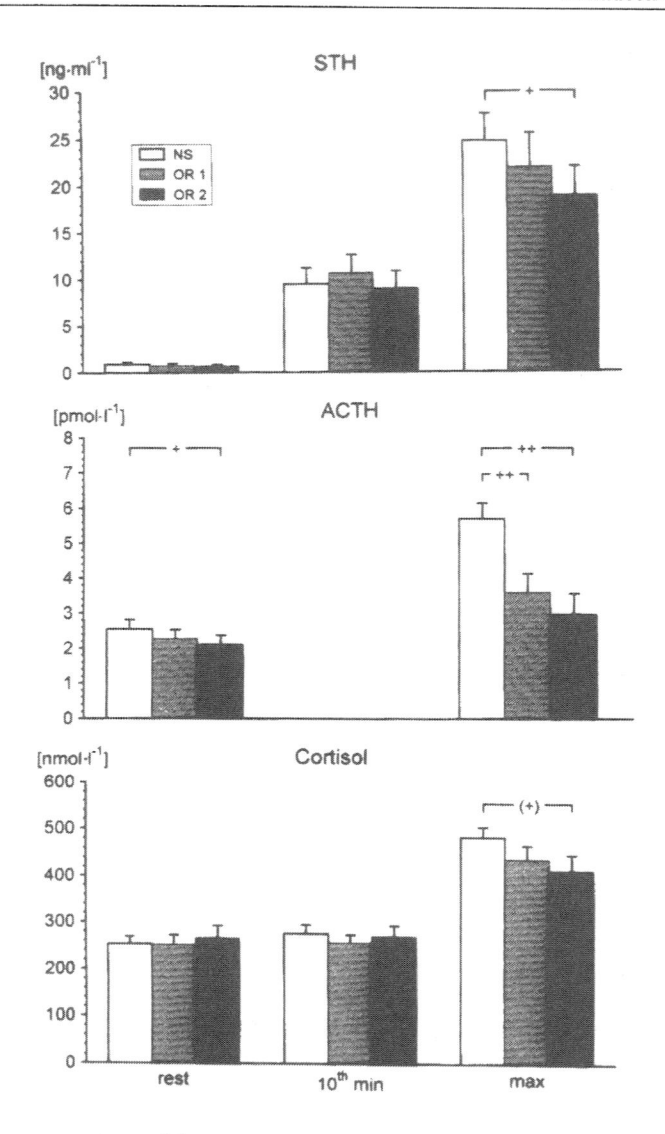

Fig. 4. Serum concentrations of STH, ACTH, and cortisol before, during (10th min), and after an exhaustive bicycle endurance test at 110% of the individual anaerobic threshold. Means ± SE; $n = 17$ endurance trained male triathletes and cyclists, (+) $p = 0.06$, + $p < 0.05$, ++ $p < 0.01$; NS = normal state, OR1 = overreaching, OR2 = severe overreaching/OT syndrome. From ref. *14*.

the catecholamine-induced lipolysis *(26)*. During the postexercise phase, cortisol may participate in the muscular glycogen resynthesis *(68)*. A transfer of glycogen depots to the liver at the expense of the muscle stores is also reported. Through the decrease in glucoplastic amino acids with increased gluconeogenesis, however, cortisol has a protein-catabolic effect on the skeletal muscle *(69)*, which is probably of importance during recovery.

PITUITARY HORMONES

Gonadotrophins

After acute physical exercise, LH usually decreases and the LH response to GnRH is not changed *(58,70)*. During very intensive training phases, a reduced pulsatile LH secretion and response to GnRH was found in marathon runners and other athletes *(71–73)*. However, this may be owing to insufficient energy intake on pulsatile LH release *(74)*, suggesting a possible impaired hypothalamic–pituitary mechanism in OT. Single measurements of hormonal concentrations in peripheral blood are not sensitive enough to investigate these complex pulsatile mechanisms, however. In fact, decreased testosterone levels after a 6-mo training or in high-mileage runners were not connected with an impaired LH secretion *(75,76)*.

Female athletes experience menstrual cycle irregularities, especially if stressful training is combined with an insufficient energy balance, possibly induced by eating disorders. In amenorrheic athletes, a partly irreversible loss of bone density increases the risk of stress fractures (*see* Chapters 9 and 14). Some authors even claim that training-induced amenorrhoea may be one manifestation of OT in female athletes *(77)*. Suppressed LH and follicle-stimulating hormone (FSH) pulsations may result from augmented corticotropin-releasing hormone (CRH) secretion or another metabolic signal and subsequent hypothalamic downregulation of GnRH, possibly through increased endogenous opioids *(78)*. Findings in overstrained (eumenorrhoeic) female athletes include significantly reduced pulsatile GnRH release (which depends on regulation by neurotransmitters, such as β-endorphin and dopamine) and LH secretion. In amenorrhoeic athletes, decreased and disordered LH pulses and increased responsiveness to GnRH were shown *(79)*. This suggests a central, perhaps (supra)hypothalamic alteration, which may relate to the genesis of an OT.

In men, the biologic effects of training or OT-induced decreased testosterone concentrations are unknown. In runners, the training mileage has been found to correlate with sperm motility and density. At the same time, total and free testosterone were significantly lower in high-mileage runners *(75)*. However, both the sperm quality and the testosterone and LH concentrations of the high-mileage runners were still measured within the (low) normal range. In some cases, decreased testosterone values together with a subjective feeling of tiredness, a slightly impaired spermatogenesis ($n = 5$), and a decreased libido are reported after an endurance training of only 14 d *(80)*. In another case, a very low testosterone level is discussed as the reason for an osteoporotic fracture in one walker *(81)* and for recurrent muscular injuries in a soccer player *(82)*.

Adrenocorticotropic Hormone (ACTH)

ACTH secretion depends on the intensity and duration of the exercise. It is stimulated by different stressors, especially by decreasing concentrations of blood glucose *(26,69)*. It primarily occurs as a response to the CRH, but is also influenced by catecholamines. Higher ACTH levels were found in trained as compared with untrained women during exercise, which is rated as an indication of possibly increased pituitary or hypothalamic sensitivity by the investigators *(83)*.

Despite speculations on an essential participation of hypothalamo–pituitary hormonal changes in the pathogenesis of OT, only few results in athletes in a state of OT are available. Two prospective studies involving overtrained and overreached athletes showed an impaired exercise-induced increase in ACTH, somatotropic hormone (STH), cortisol, and insulin after an exhausting short-endurance test *(8,14)*. These exercises were performed at the intensity of 110% of the individual anaerobic threshold (approx 80% of VO_2max) *(8,14,28)* (Figs. 3 and 4). Barron et al. *(58)* were able to prove a reduced increase in ACTH, growth hormone, prolactin, and cortisol in response to an insulin-induced hypoglycemia in four overtrained marathon runners, with an adequate response of the pituitary hormones after the administration of the LH-releasing hormone (LHRH). Thus a "central depression" of hypothalamic dysfunction is suggested with OT. In animal experiments *(84)*, a transient impaired pituitary function with lower ACTH values after repetitive stimulation by electrical shocks occurs, and may represent self-protection of the organism *(40)*, possibly by a negative feedback of cortisol or a depletion of the pituitary ACTH pool.

In other studies that described lowered ACTH values after a 3-mo endurance training *(85)*, peripheral mechanisms are speculated to be involved, such as a change in the intracellular homeostasis influenced by chemoreceptors *(86)*. The feeling of heavy legs is one typical complaint in OT and occurs despite low lactate values *(9,87)*. It could be connected to a modified sensitivity of chemoreceptors. In athletes during OT, Kraemer et al. *(15)* also reported an impaired exercise-induced rise in ACTH. However, they measured increased cortisol values. The sensitivity of the adrenal cortex to ACTH was sometimes found reduced in overtrained horses *(88)*, but could not be confirmed by others *(3,14)*.

Growth Hormone (STH)

STH exerts its metabolic effects by somatomedins. Somatomedins as well as insulin growth factor (IGF) binding-protein-3 are reported to correlate with maximal aerobic capacity and isometric force *(89)*. STH release is controlled by a hypothalamic pulsatile mechanism with numerous sleep-induced secretions. The secretion of hypothalamic hormones (growth hormone-releasing and inhibiting hormone) is influenced by neurotransmitters (including catecholamines), hormones (including adrenal hormones and endogenous opioids), amino acids, as well as physiological stimuli (stress, exercise, hypoglycemia, sleep, and so forth) *(69,90)*. The exercise-induced increase occurs in relation to the duration and intensity of the physical exercise *(24,26,37,91,92)* and is also pronounced especially after repeated anaerobic exercise *(91)*.

Training enhances the basal pulsatile STH release as well as the response to an acute exercise stimulus *(92–94)*. In overtrained athletes, however, an impairment of the maximal exercise-induced STH response occurs *(8,14)* (Figs. 3 and 4). Other authors found depressed levels of somatomedine C after excessive physical exercise with negative energetic balance *(95)*. Athletes overreached by increased volumes of resistance training also showed lower resting and acute responses of STH *(12)*. It is interesting to note that the spontaneous nocturnal secretion of the growth hormone during highly intensive training phases was impaired *(96)*, but increased in normally trained athletes *(97)*.

β-Endorphins

As for endurance exercises at an intensity in the range of the individual anaerobic threshold, the duration of exercise usually has to exceed 60 min before significantly increasing blood concentrations of β-endorphin occur *(98)* (*see also* Chapter 2 in this volume). Findings in literature suggest a relationship between the increase of β-endorphin and the extent of anaerobic lactic energy supply (or acidosis tolerance) as well as an enhancement of hormone secretion by training *(61,98)*. Following administration of naloxone, an opioid antagonist, the catecholamine secretion during high-intensive exercise is increased, suggesting an opioid-mediated modulation of the catecholamine response during severe stress to prevent excessive activity *(99)*. Endogenous opioids also inhibit the GnRH release *(70)*. However, in overtrained athletes *(15,100)*, a decreased β-endorphin response after physical exercise and stimulation test is observed. Those runners with "psychological exhaustion" after an ultraendurance race showed significantly lowered β-endorphin, norepinephrine, and ACTH concentrations *(101)*.

Prolactin

The response of prolactin (PRL) to exercise reveals large interindividual differences. It depends partly on the intracellular glucose availability *(26,85)*. The exercise-induced rise in PRL only seems to be significant in better-trained subjects *(26,61)* or at higher exercise intensities (>90% VO_2max in untrained subjects). As a result of training, the release of PRL is reported to be enhanced or starts at lower exercise intensities *(85,102)*, but this could not be confirmed in all studies *(86)*. The exercise response may be associated with anaerobic lactic contribution *(103)*, which would be interesting in view of the hypothesis of anaerobic lactic exercise forms being one important trigger mechanism for inducing an OT. An OT induced by an excessive increase in training volume did not lead to any changes of resting and exercise-induced PRL values *(18)*, which was also true for those in high-mileage runners *(75)*. After a strenuous 5-d ranger training combined with sleep deprivation and caloric deficit *(104)*, however, the concentrations at rest were reduced (as well as testosterone and estradiol). Elevated PRL values can inhibit the GnRH release through an enhanced dopaminergic tone *(105)*.

OTHER HORMONES

Insulin

Little data exist with respect to athletes in intensive training periods or even in a state of OT for the other hormones. We found a significantly reduced maximal exercise-induced concentration of insulin without altered blood glucose or correlation to the duration of exercise *(14)*. One review reports athletes with parasympathicotonic OT and a hypoglycemic state with physical exercise *(2)*. During prolonged physical work the insulin level decreases, because the catecholamine increase inhibits the insulin secretion *(24,26,92)*. This pattern is favorable to the glucose homeostasis with increased glucose availability for the central nervous system. At the onset of exercise, the adrenergic inhibition of the insulin secretion disappears: the blood glucose concentration leads to the increase in insulin, which enhances the muscular glycogen repletion during the postexercise phase. In addition, insulin accelerates the muscular growth both by means of somatomedines and insulin receptors, probably through decreased proteolysis *(106)*. Training has been shown to increase the insulin response after exhausting endurance exercise *(92)*.

The hypothesis of an impaired (supra) hypothalamo–pituitary axis in OT is supported by Elias and Wilson *(70)*, who reported an enhanced hypothalamic opioid tone as a result of low insulin levels *(107)*. These changes can result in a depressed GnRH pulsatility and subsequent gonatotropin secretion, as seen in insulino-deficient patients *(108)*. High insulin concentrations attenuate the central increase in neuropeptides *(109)*.

Thyroid Hormones

Measurements of the blood concentrations of thyroid hormones or thyroid-stimulating hormone (TSH) do not appear to have an application in the monitoring of training or diagnosis of OT. After a stressful combat course of 5 d, the secretion of thyroxine and triiodothyroxine decreased, but TSH was depressed *(104)*. An imbalance between dietary intake and energy expenditure also seems to play an important role in the induction of low-T3 syndrome *(53,110)*.

PATHOPHYSIOLOGICAL CONSIDERATIONS

Multiple studies suggest that exposure to repetitive stress leads to an altered neuroendocrine regulation and possibly inhibits the pulsatile hypothalamic release of GnRH through the CRH and/or opioid pathways (Fig. 5). This could be interpreted as a mechanism of self-protection. Elevations of central CRH or peripheral cortisol levels inhibit the GnRH, LH, and growth hormone (GH) release *(70,74)*. In animal experiments, the stress-induced impaired LH pulsatility is blocked by administration of CRH antagonists *(111)*.

At present, there are only few findings concerning the role of anabolic and catabolic hormones during the regeneration phase after physical exercise. The impaired secretion of centrally or peripherally acting hormones during OT contrasts with the usually increased hormonal concentrations induced by training *(59)*. A decreased exercise-induced rise in pituitary hormones, as well as cortisol and insulin, and lower resting concentrations of testosterone possibly affect the resynthesis of protein and glycogen during the regeneration phase after physical exercise *(26,40,55)*. The lower respiratory quotient repeatedly described in OT *(9,112)* probably indicates a shift of the energy-supplying processes in favor of increased fat utilization associated with a decreased carbohydrate supply. In hypophysectomized rats, the replenishing of muscular glycogen decreased during the first 4 h after exhausting exercise, but after 24–48 h, no essential differences could be seen *(113)*.

It is possible that during OT, peripheral and central mechanisms have a synergetic effect (Fig. 5). The (supra) hypothalamo–pituitary–adrenal axis can also be influenced by peripheral stimuli, e.g., the accumulation of lactic acid, changes in pH, or activation of muscular chemoreceptors *(70)*. The repeated exposure to stress hormones (particularly cortisol), which increase during prolonged intensive exercises, may lead to a suppression of the hypothalamo–pituitary axis with subsequent impaired release of ACTH and consecutively cortisol *(40,114)*. In chronically stressed rats, a restricted muscular Na,K-ATPase activity is associated with reduced cortisol levels, suggesting the importance of an intact pituitary–adrenal axis for an adequate function of the muscular Na,K-pump *(40)*. The Na,K-pump is useful for maintaining the membrane potential

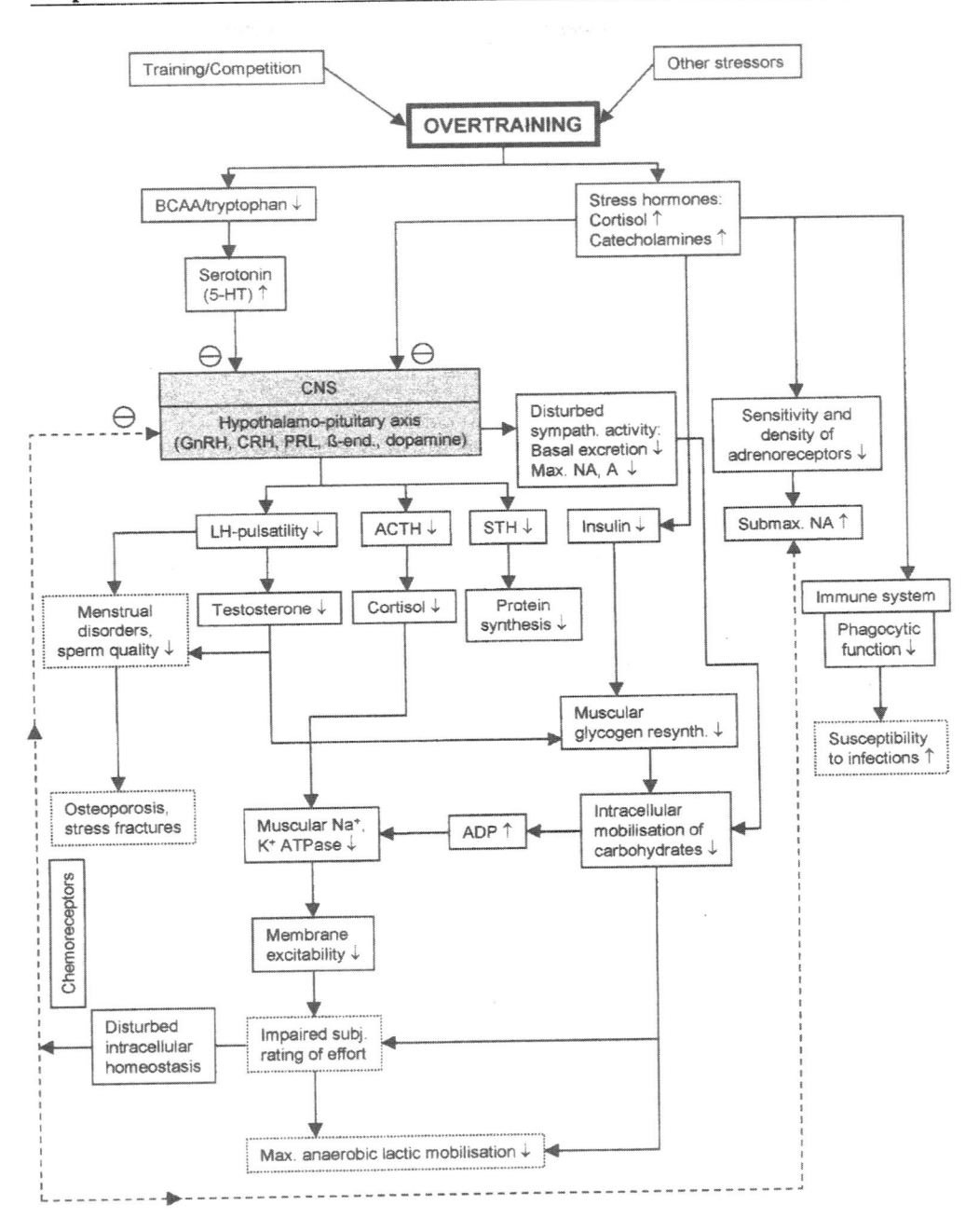

Fig. 5. Postulated neuroendocrine mechanisms in overtraining.

and counteracts the loss of potential caused by the extracellular potassium increase associated with decreased excitability. Training enhances the activity of the Na,K-pump *(115,116)* and increases the membrane potential in animals and humans *(116,117)*. The Na,K-pump is primarily, but not exclusively, activated by β_2-receptors *(118,119)*. An ion shift with increased extracellular potassium concentration is also suggested as a possible cause for the occurrence of complaints during exercise under β-blockade similar to those observed in OT (119). Muscular fatigue may be at least partly caused by such a mechanism (120,121), and this could be an explanation for some of the muscular complaints in OT. Lower testosterone concentrations may also have negative effects on neural regulation of skeletal muscle activity (12).

One result of the reduced muscular glycogen availability in OT is a higher blood concentration of tryptophan compared to branched chain amino acids (122). This is owing to a higher muscular utilization of branched chain amino acids and/or a shifted binding of tryptophan to albumin with the increased occurrence of free fatty acids. The subsequent enhanced uptake and transformation to the neurotransmitter 5-hydroxytryptamin (5-HT) in the brain may be the cause of central fatigue. Differences in the run time of rats actually could be attributed to changes in the brain 5-HT activity, perhaps in interaction with subsequent modifications of the brain dopamine concentration (123). Increased muscle and liver glycogen contents also occured compared to controls, which is in keeping with our hypothesis of an impaired intramuscular glycolytic mobilization in overtrained athletes (13). However, an enhanced 5-HT activity has been found to elevate the plasma concentrations of hormones resulting from the hypothalamo-pituitary–adrenocortical axis and sympathoadrenal system (124). Furthermore, data from prolonged exercise in rats cannot be simply transferred to chronically overtrained athletes, where reduced maximal concentrations of pituitary hormones and free catecholamines exist. Some studies find unchanged plasma levels of tryptophan and branched chain amino acids after 40% increases of training over 2 wk leading to elevated fatigue scores as judged by a profile of mood state in runners (125).

PERSPECTIVES

Future basic research should include studies of the (supra) hypothalamic level, e.g, by considering releasing hormones, as well as the changes of CRH, prolactin, β-endorphin, and leptin. A more exact recording of the activity of the hypothalamic–pituitary axis, however, requires serial determinations of pulsatile secreted hormones. Assessments of the activity of the central nervous system could be possible by using electroencephalography during exercise and transcranial magnetic stimulation. The peripheral regulation of hormonal action at the receptor level also remains relatively unexplored, since it may modulate the effect of the measured blood concentrations.

Descriptions of the OT syndrome are only possible through research involving a sufficient number of athletes actually in this state, and at a minimum in the state of overreaching. Transferring results obtained during intensive phases of (overload) training is not suitable. Unfortunately, the induction of an OT often requires the addition of other stressors, which are difficult to plan in a prospective study design.

Although of essential importance, the regeneration period after OT has not yet been investigated systematically. In our own study (8,28), following 4 wk of overload training, we observed a normalization of both the impaired performance and the exercise-induced maximal response of pituitary hormones and catecholamines after 2 wk of regenerative training.

The systematic use of hormonal measurements in the monitoring of training is currently somewhat restricted by the rather high intra- and interassay variability of the laboratory methods. Determinations of hormones remain problematical because of their dependence on circadian and/or pulsatile rhythms, different half-lives, feedback mechanisms, and psychological factors. Also, the influence of a disturbed energy balance has to be taken into account. This requires carefully standardized sampling conditions as well as individual comparative data. At present, there are no standard values that indicate when the regeneration is complete and the next training stimulus can be restarted, or when there is an insufficient recovery with the danger of overreaching. The development of micromethods allowing hormonal measurements from capillary blood samples are promising. Hormone measurements in blood will, in future, represent an essential link in the concept of psycho-neuroendocrine regulation of metabolic as well as immunological reactions and adaptations to physical exercise, including OT.

REFERENCES

1. Fry RW, Morton AR, Keast D. Overtraining in athletes. An update. Sports Med 1991;12:32–65.
2. Kuipers H, Keizer HA. Overtraining in elite athletes. Review and directions for the future. Sports Med 1988;6:79–92.
3. Lehmann M, Foster C, Keul J. Overtraining in endurance athletes: a brief review. Med Sci Sports Exerc 1993;25:854–862.
4. Israel S. Die Erscheinungsformen des Übertrainings. Sportmed 1958;9:207–209.
5. Kindermann W. Overtraining—expression of a disturbed autonomic regulation [in German]. Dtsch Z Sportmed 1986;37:238–245.
6. Callister R, Callister RJ, Fleck SJ, Dudley GA. Physiological and performance responses to overtraining in elite judo athletes. Med Sci Sports Exerc 1990;22:816–824.
7. Fry RW, Morton AR, Garcia Webb P, Crawford GP, Keast D. Biological responses to overload training in endurance sports. Eur J Appl Physiol 1992;64:335–344.
8. Urhausen A, Gabriel HHW, Brückner F, Kindermann W. Effects of two training phases of different intensities on the exercise-induced hormonal response and psychological parameters in endurance athletes. Int J Sports Med 1998;19(Suppl 1):S43,S44.
9. Urhausen A, Gabriel HHW, Weiler B, Kindermann W. Ergometric and psychological findings during overtraining: a prospective long-term follow-up study in endurance athletes. Int J Sports Med 1998;19:114–120.
10. Warren BJ, Stone MH, Kearney JT, Fleck SJ, Johnson RL, Wilson GD, et al. Performance measures, blood lactate and plasma ammonia as indicators of overwork in elite junior weightlifters. Int J Sports Med 1992;13:372–376.
11. Adlercreutz H, Härkönen M, Kuoppasalmi K, Näveri H, Huhtaniemi I, Tikkanen H, et al. Effect of training on plasma anabolic and catabolic steroid hormones and their response during physical exercise. Int J Sports Med 1986;7(Suppl 1):27–28.
12. Fry AC, Kraemer WJ. Resistance exercise overtraining and overreaching. Sports Med 1997;23:106–129.
13. Urhausen A, Gabriel H, Kindermann W. Blood hormones as markers of training stress and overtraining. Sports Med 1995;20:251–276.
14. Urhausen A, Gabriel HHW, Kindermann W. Impaired pituitary hormonal response to exhaustive exercise in overtrained endurance athletes. Med Sci Sports Exerc 1998;30:407–414.
15. Kraemer WJ, Fleck SJ, Callister R, Shealy M, Dudley GA, Maresh CM, et al. Training responses of plasma beta-endorphin, adrenocorticotropin, and cortisol. Med Sci Sports Exerc 1989;21:146–153.
16. Urhausen A, Weiler B, Coen B, Kindermann W. Plasma catecholamines during endurance exercise of different intensities as related to the individual anaerobic threshold. Eur J Appl Physiol 1994;69:16–20.
17. Costill DL, Flynn MG, Kirwan JP, Houmard JA, Mitchell JB, Thomas R, et al. Effects of repeated days of intensified training on muscle glycogen and swimming performance. Med Sci Sports Exerc 1988;20:249–254.
18. Lehmann M, Gastmann U, Petersen KG, Bachl N, Seidel A, Khalaf AN, Fischer S, et al. Training-overtraining: performance, and hormone levels, after a defined increase in training volume versus intensity in experienced middle- and long-distance runners. Br J Sports Med 1992;26:233–242.
19. Christensen NJ, Galbo H. Sympathetic nervous activity during exercise. Annu Rev Physiol 1983;45:139–153.

20. Yamaguchi N, de Champlain J, Nadeau R. Correlation between the response of the heart to sympathetic stimulation and the release of endogenous catecholamines into the coronary sinus of the dog. Circ Res 1975;36:662–668.
21. Mazzeo RS, Marshall P. Influence of plasma catecholamines on the lactate threshold during graded exercise. J Appl Physiol 1989;67:1319–1322.
22. Urhausen A, Coen B, Weiler B, Kindermann W. Individual anaerobic threshold and maximum lactate steady state. Int J Sports Med 1993;14:134–139.
23. Kindermann W, Simon G, Keul J. The significance of the aerobic-anaerobic transition for the determination of work load intensities during endurance training. Eur J Appl Physiol 1979;42:25–34.
24. Kindermann W, Schnabel A, Schmitt WM, Biro G, Cassens J, Weber F. Catecholamines, growth hormone, cortisol, insulin, and sex-hormones in anaerobic and aerobic exercise. Eur J Appl Physiol 1982;49:389–399.
25. Kjær M. Epinephrine and some other hormonal responses to exercise in man: with special reference to physical training. Int J Sports Med 1989;10:2–15.
26. Galbo H. Hormonal and metabolic adaption to exercise. Thieme, Stuttgart, New York, 1983.
27. Pequignot JM, Peyrin L, Peres G. Catecholamine-fuel interrelationships during exercise in fasting men. J Appl Physiol 1980;48:109–113.
28. Gabriel HHW, Urhausen A, Schwarz S, Weiler B, Kindermann W. Cycle ergometric performance capacity, lactate and respiratory parameters during an intensive training period of endurance athletes. Int J Sports Med 1998;19(Suppl 1):S24.
29. Hooper SL, MacKinnon LT, Gordon RD, Bachmann AW. Hormonal responses of elite swimmers to overtraining. Med Sci Sports Exerc 1993;25:741–747.
30. Mackinnon LT, Hooper SL, Jones S, Gordon RD, Bachmann AW. Hormonal, immunological, and hematological responses to intensified training in elite swimmers. Med Sci Sports Exerc 1997; 29:1637–1645.
31. Tomeh JF, Cryer PE. Biphasic adrenergic modulation of β-adrenergic receptors in man. J Clin Invest 1980;65:836–840.
32. Kniffki KD, Mense S, Schmidt RF. Muscle receptors with fine afferent fibers which may evoke circulatory reflexes. Circ Res 1981;48(Suppl 1):25–31.
33. Weiler B, Urhausen A, Coen B, Weiler S, Huber G, Kindermann W. Sports medical performance diagnostic (basic endurance and sprinting ability) and determination of stress hormone concentrations in competition of badminton players of national and international top level [in German]. Sportorthopädie-Sporttraumatologie 1997;13:5–12.
34. Cadoux-Hudson TA, Few JD, Imms FJ. The effect of exercise on the production and clearance of testosterone in well trained young men. Eur J Appl Physiol 1985;54:321–325.
35. Kindermann W, Schmitt WM, Schnabel A, Berg A, Biro G. Behavior of testosterone in blood serum during physical exertion of differing duration and intensity [in German]. Dtsch Z Sportmed 1985;36:99–104.
36. Urhausen A, Kindermann W. Behavior of testosterone, sex hormone binding globulin (SHBG) and cortisol before and after a triathlon competition. Int J Sports Med 1987;8:305–308.
37. Kuoppasalmi K, Näveri H, Rehunen S, Härkönen M, Adlercreutz H. Effect of strenuous anaerobic running exercise on plasma growth hormone, cortisol, luteinizing hormone, testosterone, androstenedione, estrone and estradiol. J Steroid Biochem 1976;7:823–829.
38. Hackney AC. Endurance training and testosterone levels. Sports Med 1989;8:117–127.
39. Kuoppasalmi K, Adlercreutz H. Interaction between catabolic and anabolic steroid hormones in muscular exercise. In: Fotherby K, Pal S, eds. Exercise Endocrinology. De Gruyter W & Co, Berlin, New York, NY, 1985, pp. 65–98.
40. Viru A. Hormones in muscular activity. CRC Press, Boca Raton, 1985.
41. Häkkinen K, Pakarinen A, Alèn M, Kauhanen H, Komi PV. Relationships between training volume, physical performance capacity, and serum hormone concentrations during prolonged training in elite weight lifters. Int J Sports Med 1987;8(Suppl 1):61–65.
42a. Inoue K, Yamasaki S, Fushiki T, Kano T, Moritani T, Itoh K, et al. Rapid increase in the number of androgen receptors following electrical stimulation of the rat muscle. Eur J Appl Physiol 1993;66:134–140.
42b. Flynn MG, Pizza FX, Boone JB Jr, Andres FF, Michaud TA, Rodriguez Zayas JR. Indices of training stress during competitive running and swimming seasons. Int J Sports Med 1994;15:21–26.
43. Marx K, Kische B, Hoffmann P. Die Gonadotropine und Sexualsteroide während des Menstruationszyklus bei jungen sporttreibenden Frauen Med Sport 1986;26:51–54.

44. Urhausen A, Kullmer T, Kindermann W. A 7-week follow-up study of the behaviour of testosterone and cortisol during the competition period in rowers. Eur J Appl Physiol 1987;56:528–533.
45. Vervoorn C, Vermulst LJ, Boelens Quist AM, Koppeschaar HP, Erich WB, Thijssen, JH, et al. Seasonal changes in performance and free testosterone: cortisol ratio of elite female rowers. Eur J Appl Physiol 1992;64:14–21.
46. Banfi G, Marinelli M, Roi GS, Agape V. Usefulness of free testosterone/cortisol ratio during a season of elite speed skating athletes. Int J Sports Med 1993;14:373–379.
47. Dessypris A, Kuoppasalmi K, Adlercreutz H. Plasma cortisol, testosterone, androstenedione and luteinizing hormone (LH) in a non-competitive marathon run. J Ster Biochem 1976;7:33–37.
48. Urhausen A, Coen B, Weiler B, Werremeier S, Kindermann W. Hormonal and biochemical parameters, psychovegetative profile, and ergometric performance during training in rowing. Med Sci Sports Exerc 1998;30(Suppl):S174.
49. Kirwan JP, Costill DL, Flynn MG, Mitchell JB, Fink WJ, Neufer PD, et al. Physiological responses to successive days of intense training in competitive swimmers. Med Sci Sports Exerc 1988;20:255–259.
50. Vervoorn C, Quist AM, Vermulst LJ, Erich WB, de Vries WR, Thijssen, JH. The behaviour of the plasma free testosterone/cortisol ratio during a season of elite rowing training. Int J Sports Med 1991;12:257–263.
51. Sattler R, Rademacher G, Appelt D, Hotz G. Die Beeinflussung des SHBGC sex-hormone-binding globulin) durch physische Belastung. In: Häcker R, de Marées H, eds. Hormonelle Regulation und psychophysische Belastung im Leistungssport. Deutscher Ärzteverlag, Köln, 1991, pp. 32–38.
52. Adlercreutz H. Western diet and Western diseases: some hormonal and biochemical mechanisms and associations. Scand J Clin Lab Invest 1990;50(Suppl 201):3–23.
53. Tegelman R, Lindeskog P, Carlstrom K, Pousette A, Blomstrand R. Peripheral hormone levels in healthy subjects during controlled fasting. Acta Endocrinol Copenh 1986;113:457–462.
54. Cumming DC, Wheeler GD, McColl EM. The effects of exercise on reproductive function in men. Sports Med 1989;7:1–17.
55. Gillespie CA, Edgerton VR. The role of testosterone in exercise-induced glycogen supercompensation. Horm Metab Res 1970;2:364–366.
56. Mayer M, Rosen F. Interaction of anabolic steroids with glucocorticoid receptor sites in rat muscle cytosol. Am J Physiol 1975;229:1381–1386.
57. Dahlmann B, Widjaja A, Reinauer H. Antagonistic effects of endurance training and testosterone on alkaline proteolytic activity in rat skeletal muscles. Eur J Appl Physiol 1981;46:229–235.
58. Barron JL, Noakes TD, Levy W, Smith C, Millar RP. Hypothalamic dysfunction in overtrained athletes. J Clin Endocrinol Metab 1985;60:803–806.
59. Borer KT. Neurohumoral mediation of exercise-induced growth. Med Sci Sports Exerc 1994;26:741–754.
60. Verde T, Thomas S, Shephard RJ. Potential markers of heavy training in highly trained distance runners. Br J Sports Med 1992;26:167–175.
61. Bullen BA, Skrinar GS, Beitins IZ, Carr DB, Reppert SM, Dotson CO, et al. Endurance training effects on plasma hormonal responsiveness and sex hormone excretion. J Appl Physiol 1984;56:1453–1463.
62. Fellmann N, Coudert J, Jarrige JF, Bedu M, Denis C, Boucher D, et al. Effects of endurance training on the androgenic response to exercise in man. Int J Sports Med 1985;6:215–219.
63. O'Connor PJ, Morgan WP, Raglin JS, Barksdale CM, Kalin NH. Mood state and salivary cortisol levels following overtraining in female swimmers. Psychoneuroendocrinology 1989;14:303–310.
64. Snyder AC, Kuipers H, Cheng B, Servais R, Fransen E. Overtraining following intensified training with normal muscle glycogen. Med Sci Sports Exerc 1995;27:1063–1070.
65. Häkkinen K, Keskinen KL, Alèn M, Komi PV, Kauhanen H. Serum hormone concentrations during prolonged training in elite endurance-trained and strength-trained athletes. Eur J Appl Physiol 1989;59:233–238.
66. Tegelman R, Johansson C, Hemmingsson P, Eklof R, Carlstrom K, Pousette A. Endogenous anabolic and catabolic steroid hormones in male and female athletes during off season. Int J Sports Med 1990;11:103–106.
67. Kalin NH, Dawson GW. Neuroendocrine dysfunction in depression: hypothalamic anterior pituitary systems. Trends Neurosci 1986;9:261–266.
68. Poland JL, Myers TD, Witorsch RJ, Brandt RB. Plasma corticosterone and cardiac glycogen levels in rats after exercise. Proc Soc Exp Biol Med 1975;150:148–150.

69. Siegenthaler W. Klinische Pathophysiologie. Thieme, Stuttgart, 1987.
70. Elias AN, Wilson AF. Exercise and gonadal function. Hum. Reprod. 1993;8:1747–1761.
71. Hackney AC, Sinning WE, Bruot BC. Hypothalamic-pituitary-testicular axis function in endurance-trained males. Int J Sports Med 1990;11:298–303.
72. MacConnie SE, Barkan A, Lampman RM, Schork MA, Beitins IZ. Decreased hypothalamic gonadotropin-releasing hormone secretion in male marathon runners. N Engl J Med 1986;315:411–417.
73. Ronkainen H. Depressed follicle-stimulating hormone, luteinizing hormone, and prolactin responses to the luteinizing hormone-releasing hormone, thyrotropin-releasing hormone, and metoclopramide test in endurance runners in the hard-training season. Fertil Steril 1985;44:755–759.
74. Loucks AB, Mortola JF, Girton L, Yen SSC. Alterations in the hypothalamic-pituitary-ovarian and the hypothalamic–pituitary–adrenal axes in athletic women. J Clin Endocrinol Metab 1989;68:402–411.
75. De Souza MJ, Arce JC, Pescatello LS, Scherzer HS, Luciano AA. Gonadal hormones and semen quality in male runners. A volume threshold effect of endurance training. Int J Sports Med 1994;15:383–391.
76. Wheeler GD, Singh M, Pierce WD, Epling WF, Cumming DC. Endurance training decreases serum testosterone levels in men without change in luteinizing hormone pulsatile release. J Clin Endocrinol Metab 1991;72:422–425.
77. Keizer HA, Rogol A.D. Physical exercise and menstrual cycle alterations. Sports Med 1990;10:218–235.
78. Ruffin MT IV, Hunter RE, Arendt E. Exercise and secondary amenorrhoea linked through endogenous opioids. Sports Med 1990;10:65–71.
79. Reame NE, Sauder SE, Case GD, Kelch RP, Marshall JC. Pulsatile gonadotropin secretion in women with hypothalamic amenorrhea: evidence that reduced frequency of gonadotropin-releasing hormone secretion is the mechanism of persistent anovulation. J Clin Endocrinol Metab 1985;61:851–858.
80. Griffith RB, Dressendorfer RH, Fullbright CD. Effects of overwork on testosterone, sperm count and libido. Med Sci Sports Exerc 1988;20(Suppl):S39.
81. Kuntz JL, Caillard C, Werle CL, Bloch JG, Simonasch L. Ostéoporose avec déficit androgénique chez un marcheur. Rev Rhum 1990;57:5–7.
82. Naessens G, De Slypere JP, Dijs H, Driessens M. Hypogonadism as a cause of recurrent muscle injury in a high level soccer player. A case report. Int J Sports Med 1995;16:413–417.
83. Keizer HA, Kuipers H, de Haan J, Beckers E, Habets L. Multiple hormonal responses to physical exercise in eumenorrheic trained and untrained women. Int J Sports Med 1987;8(Suppl 3):139–150.
84. Rivier C, Vale W. Diminished responsiveness of the hypothalamic–pituitary–adrenal axis of the rat during exposure to prolonged stress: a pituitary-mediated mechanism. Endocrinology 1987;121:1320–1328.
85. Keizer HA, Kuipers H, de Haan J, Janssen GM, Beckers E, Habets L, et al. Effect of a 3-month endurance training program on metabolic and multiple hormonal responses to exercise. Int J Sports Med 1987;8(Suppl 3):154–160.
86. Buono MJ, Yeager JE, Sucec AA. Effect of aerobic training on the plasma ACTH response to exercise. J Appl Physiol 1987;63:2499–2501.
87. Snyder AC, Jeukendrup AE, Hesselink MK, Kuipers H, Foster C. A physiological/psychological indicator of over-reaching during intensive training. Int J Sports Med 1993;14:29–32.
88. Persson SG, Larsson M, Lindholm A. Effects of training on adreno-cortical function and red-cell volume in trotters. Zentralbl Veterinarmed 1980;27:261–268.
89. Brun JF, Blachon C, Micallef JP, Fédou C, Charpiat A, Bouix O, et al. Protéines porteuses des somatomédines et force isométrique de préhension dans un groupe de gymnastes adolescents soumis à un entraînement intensif. Sci Sports 1996;11:157–165.
90. Macintyre JG. Growth hormone and athletes. Sports Med 1987;4:129–142.
91. Dulac S, Brisson GR, Péronnet F, Decarufel D, Quirion A. Réponses hormonales à une répétition d'exercises anaérobiques lactacides chez des sujets masculins. Can J Appl Sport Sci 1986;11:178–185.
92. Hartley LH, Mason JW, Hogan RP, Jones LG, Kotchen TA, Mougey EH, et al. Multiple hormonal responses to prolonged exercise in relation to physical training. J Appl Physiol 1972;33:607–610.
93. Borer KT. The effects of exercise on growth. Sports Med 1995;20:375–397.
94. Weltman A, Weltman JY, Schurrer R, Evans WS, Veldhuis JD, Rogol AD. Endurance training amplifies the pulsatile release of growth hormone: effects of training intensity. J Appl Physiol 1992;72:2188–2196.

95. Smith AT, Clemmons DR, Underwood LE, BenEzra V, McMurray R. The role of exercise on plasma somatomedin C/insulin-like growth factor I concentrations. Metabolism 1987;36:533–539.
96. Beyer P, Witt D, Knuppen S, Zehendner R, Ball P, Brack C, et al. Änderung spontaner nächtlicher Hormonsekretion während eines Trainingsjahres. In: Bernett P, Jeschke D, eds. Sport und Medizin—Pro und Contra. Zuckschwerdt, München, 1991, pp. 511–513.
97. Walsh BT, Puig Antich J, Goetz R, Gladis M, Novacenko H, Glassman AH. Sleep and growth hormone secretion in women athletes. Electroencephalogr Clin Neurophysiol 1984;57:528–531.
98. Schwarz L, Kindermann W. Changes in beta-endorphin levels in response to aerobic and anaerobic exercise. Sports Med 1992;13:25–36.
99. Angelopoulos TJ, Denys BG, Weikart C, Dasilva SG, Michael TJ, Robertson RJ. Endogenous opioids may modulate catecholamine secretion during high intensity exercise. Eur J Appl Physiol 1995;70:195–199.
100. Keizer HA, Platen P, Koppeschaar H, De Vries WR, Vervoorn C, Geurten P, et al. Blunted β-endorphin responses to corticotropin releasing hormone and exercise after exhaustive training. Int J Sports Med 1991;12:97.
101. Odagiri Y, Shimomitsu T, Iwane H, Katsumura T. Relationships between exhaustive mood state and changes in stress hormones following an ultraendurance race. Int J Sports Med 1996;17:325–331.
102. Boyden TW, Pamenter RW, Grosso D, Stanforth P, Rotkis T, Wilmore JH. Prolactin responses, menstrual cycles, and body composition of women runners. J Clin Endocrinol Metab 1982;54: 711–714.
103. De Meirleir KL, Baeyens L, L'Hermite-Baleriaux M, L'Hermite M, Hollmann W. Exercise-induced prolactin release is related to anaerobiosis. J Clin Endocrinol Metab 1985;60:1250–1252.
104. Aakvaag A, Sand T, Opstad PK, Fonnum F. Hormonal changes in serum in young men during prolonged physical strain. Eur J Appl Physiol 1978;39:283–291.
105. Ojeda SR, McCann SM. Control of LH and FSH release by LHRH: influence of putative neurotransmitters. Clin Obstet Gynaecol 1978;5:283–303.
106. Florini JR. Hormonal control of muscle cell growth. J Anim Sci 1985;61:21–37.
107. Morley JE. Appetite regulation by gut peptides. Annu Rev Nutr 1990;10:383–395.
108. South SA, Asplin CM, Carlsen EC, Booth RA Jr, Weltman JY, Johnson ML, et al. Alterations in luteinizing hormone secretory activity in women with insulin-dependent diabetes mellitus and secondary amenorrhea. J Clin Endocrinol Metab 1993;76:1048–1053.
109. Malabu UH, McCarthy HD, McKibbin PE, Williams G. Peripheral insulin administration attenuates the increase in neuropeptide Y concentrations in the hypothalamic arcuate nucleus of fasted rats. Peptides 1992;13:1097–1102.
110. Loucks A, Heath EM. Induction of low-T3 syndrome in exercising women occurs at a threshold of energy availability. Am J Physiol 1994;266:R817–R823.
111. Rivier C, Rivier J, Vale W. Stress-induced inhibition of reproductive functions: role of endogenous corticotropin-releasing factor. Science 1986;231:607–609.
112. Costill DL, Bowers R, Branam G, Sparks K. Muscle glycogen utilization during prolonged exercise on successive days. J Appl Physiol 1971;31:834–838.
113. Kochan RC, Lawrence DR, Kochan BMJ, Lamb DR. Hypophysectomie and skeletal muscle glykogen replenishment after exercise. Med Sci Sports Exerc 1978;10:44–48.
114. Dallman MF, Jones MT, Vernikos Danellis J, Ganong WF. Corticosteroid feedback control of ACTH secretion: rapid effects of bilateral adrenalectomy on plasma ACTH in the rat. Endocrinology 1972;91:961–968.
115. Kjeldsen K, Richter EA, Galbo H, Lortie G, Clausen T. Training increases the concentration of [3H]ouabain-binding sites in rat skeletal muscle. Biochim Biophys Acta 1986;860:708–712.
116. Knochel JP, Blachley JD, Johnson JH, Carter NW. Muscle cell electrical hyperpolarization and reduced exercise hyperkalemia in physically conditioned dogs. J Clin Invest 1985;75:740–745.
117. Moss RF, Raven PB, Knochel JP, Peckham JR, Blachley JD. The effect of training on resting muscle membrane potentials. Int Ser Sports Sci 1983;13:806–811.
118. Clausen T, Flatman JA. Beta 2-adrenoceptors mediate the stimulating effect of adrenaline on active electrogenic Na-K-transport in rat soleus muscle. Br J Pharmacol 1980;68:749–755.
119. Kullmer T, Kindermann W. Physical performance and serum potassium under chronic beta-blockade. Eur J Appl Physiol 1985;54:350–354.
120. Jones DA. Muscle fatigue due to changes beyond the neuromuscular junction. Ciba Found Symp 1981;82:178–196.

121. Juel C. The effect of beta 2-adrenoceptor activation on ion-shifts and fatigue in mouse soleus muscles stimulated in vitro. Acta Physiol Scand 1988;134:209–216.
122. Newsholme EA, Blomstrand E, McAndrew N, Parry-Billings M. Biochemical causes of fatigue and overtraining. In: Shepard RJ, Astrand PO, eds. Endurance in Sport. Blackwell Scientific Publications, Oxford, 1992, pp. 351–364.
123. Bailey SP, Davis JM, Ahlborn EN. Neuroendocrine and substrate responses to altered brain 5-HT activity during prolonged exercise to fatigue. J Appl Physiol 1993;74:3006–3012.
124. Bagdy G, Calogero AE, Murphy DL, Szemeredi K. Serotonin agonists cause parallel activation of the sympathoadrenomedullary system and the hypothalamo–pituitary–adrenocortical axis in conscious rats. Endocrinology 1989;125:2664–2669.
125. Tanaka H, West KA, Duncan GE, Bassett DR Jr. Changes in plasma tryptophan/branched chain amino acid ratio in responses to training volume variation. Int J Sports Med 1997;18:270–275.
126. Hökkinen K, Pakarinen A, Alèn M, Komi PV. Serum hormones during prolonged training of neuromuscular performance. Eur J Appl Physiol 1985;53:287–293.

21 The Effects of Altitude on the Hormonal Responses to Exercise

Roland J. M. Favier, Dr. es Sci.

CONTENTS

INTRODUCTION
ACUTE HIGH-ALTITUDE EXPOSURE
CHRONIC HIGH-ALTITUDE EXPOSURE
ACKNOWLEDGMENTS
REFERENCES

INTRODUCTION

Changes in plasma concentration of hormones with physical activity have been thoroughly examined during the last 30 years and have been shown to play a key role in ventilatory, circulatory, and metabolic adaptations to the increase in metabolism with exercise *(1,2)*. Plasma concentration of hormones reflects a balance among synthesis, release, and clearance of the substance, and only for very few hormones have turnover studies been performed. A variety of factors, including environmental conditions, have been found to be susceptible to influence the hormonal response to exercise *(1)*.

In addition to the effects of intrinsic characteristics of the exercise stimulus (i.e, intensity and/or duration of exercise, physical fitness of individuals *[3,4]*), other environmental factors (e.g., oxygen availability, hydration, nutrition, low temperature, and so forth) can modify the hormonal response to exercise *(1)*. In this respect, reduced availability of oxygen owing to low barometric pressure is the basic problem associated with high altitude as Paul Bert's experiments showed conclusively *(5)*. However, hypohydration and undernutrition are also environmental hazards that face living organisms at high altitudes *(6,7)*. As a consequence, some of the hormonal responses to exercise at altitude, originally attributed to reduced oxygen availability, could, in fact, be linked to some alterations in nutritional and/or body fluid homeostasis *(8,9)*.

From: *Contemporary Endocrinology: Sports Endocrinology*
Edited by: M. P. Warren and N. W. Constantini © Humana Press Inc., Totowa, NJ

ACUTE HIGH-ALTITUDE EXPOSURE

Sympathoadrenergic Activity

Even though peripheral venous concentrations of catecholamines can be an imprecise index of sympathetic nervous activity, the best means of assessing the functional state of the sympathoadrenal system relies mostly on determination of the main chemical transmitters in this system, i.e., epinephrine (E), norepinephrine (NE), and dopamine (DA). The major source of E is derived from the adrenals, whereas NE levels represent a spillover of the neurotransmitter from sympathetic nerve endings. Thus far, the origin of plasma DA is unclear, and adrenal glands, sympathetic neurons, chromaffin paraganglia, or specific dopaminergic neurons have been suggested as putative sources (10).

At sea level, an increase in the concentration of these amines in plasma has been reported in humans during dynamic as well as during static exercise (1,2). The plasma concentration of catecholamines for a given type of exercise increases exponentially with work intensity when it is expressed on a relative basis (i.e, as a percentage of individual maximal oxygen uptake, VO_2max) (3,11). Furthermore, the duration of exercise is the determinant in the sympathoadrenergic response to exercise; thus, at a given VO_2, plasma NE and E levels increase progressively during prolonged exercise to reach a maximum at exhaustion. In addition, if a certain work intensity is achieved by small muscle groups (e.g, arms), the increase in plasma catecholamine concentration above resting value is higher than if the same VO_2 is obtained with large muscle groups (i.e, legs) (12).

Although hypoxia is known as a potent activator of the sympathetic nervous system by stimulating arterial chemoreceptors, Rostrup (13) underlined that most studies on the effects of acute hypoxia on catecholamines failed to show any changes in resting plasma or urinary NE. In contrast, more than 90% of the studies on subjects staying for more than 1 wk at high altitude reported an increased sympathoadrenergic activity, suggesting that the duration of hypoxic exposure is one of the major determinants of the sympathoadrenergic response (14).

There are several reports concerning the acute effects of hypoxic exposure on the catecholamine response to exercise (15–20). With mild exercise (40% VO_2max), Bubb et al. (16) found that plasma levels of E and NE are not affected by inhaling gas mixtures containing 19 to 13% O_2 (equivalent to an altitude ranging from 700 to 3700 m above sea level). Subsequently, hypoxemia was found to result in significant increments in plasma E and NE levels when exercising at intensities higher than 50% of VO_2max (17). As previously shown in normoxia, the plasma catecholamine response to short-duration exercise under hypoxia is closely related to the relative workload (15,18), i.e, when the reduction of VO_2max that occurs under acute hypoxia is taken into account (21). In a series of comprehensive studies, Mazzeo and his colleagues (19,22–26) examined the arterial catecholamine response during exercise under acute high-altitude exposure. They provided evidence for a differential adaptive response between sympathetic neural activity and that of the adrenal medulla during exposure to 4300-m altitude. Indeed, within 4 h of arrival at high altitude, arterial concentrations of E are significantly increased both at rest and during prolonged low-intensity exercise (50% VO_2max). In contrast, resting arterial NE on arrival at high altitude decreased compared with sea level and increased during 45 min of constant submaximal exercise to values similar to those encountered at sea level (19).

Since skeletal muscles represent a large percentage of body mass, an increase in sympathetic activity from the muscular vascular bed is expected to make a significant contribution to NE spillover in the blood during exercise at altitude. Indeed, plasma NE levels correlate to resting muscle sympathetic nerve activity (MSNA) *(27)* and there is a close relationship between plasma NE level and MSNA during graded arm exercise *(28)*. The relative increase in MSNA is approximately two- to fourfold greater than the corresponding increase in plasma NE.

At rest, hypoxemia raises muscle sympathetic activity without increasing venous plasma concentrations of E and NE *(29)*. When submaximal rhythmic exercise is superimposed on hypoxia, MSNA is enhanced in nonactive skeletal muscles *(30)*. According to Seals et al. *(30)*, MSNA potentiation with hypoxemia is linked to a greater stimulation of chemosensitive afferents by some yet unknown metabolic stimulus (pH, lactic acid, byproducts of prostaglandin metabolism). Saito et al. *(31)* suggested that the responsiveness of MSNA is increased dominantly by peripheral chemoreflex activation under moderate hypoxia, while being modulated by central nervous mechanisms under severe hypoxia (~6000 m).

Even though circulating catecholamines originate, in humans, mainly from sympathetic nerve endings of working and nonworking muscles, it should be kept in mind that they could also come from the myocardium or from splanchnic and renal vascular beds *(32)*. Furthermore, in some species (e.g, dog), plasma catecholamines are also of adrenomedullary origin *(33–35)*. Because hypoxia increases myocardial turnover of NE *(36)*, one can thus hypothesize that the heart might play an endocrine role when exercising in hypoxia *(37,38)*.

That sympathoadrenergic response to exercise is affected by oxygen availability is also corroborated by the reduction in exercise-induced changes in plasma catecholamines when breathing 100% O_2 *(39)*. Nevertheless, hyperoxia lowers efferent sympathetic activity to skeletal muscle under resting conditions without altering plasma NE concentrations, but has no obvious modulatory effect on the nonactive MSNA to rhythmic handgrip exercise *(40)*. It is likely that the magnitude of the sympathetic activation evoked during exercise in humans is partly determined by the size of the active muscle mass *(41)*.

INFLUENCE OF HYPOHYDRATION AND UNDERNUTRITION ON THE SYMPATHOADRENERGIC RESPONSE TO EXERCISE

As mentioned earlier, there is ample evidence of a major disturbance of fluid homeostasis during exposure to high altitude linked to an immediate decrease in water intake and increase in water losses *(7,42,43)*. Two mechanisms are responsible for increased water losses from the body. First, the partial pressure of water vapor and water concentration decrease in ambient air as a result of decreased temperature at increasing altitudes. In air breathers, the passage of air with low water content over the moist surfaces of the airways, coupled with hypoxic hyperventilation, considerably increases evaporation from the respiratory tract, particularly during muscular activity *(44)*. The second mechanism responsible for increased water losses at high altitude relates to the increase in the diffusion coefficient of water vapor, which, as for any gas, is inversely proportional to the barometric pressure. Thus, at an altitude of 5500 m, one would, theoretically, expect water losses through permeable surfaces to be exactly twice as great as at sea level. Therefore, the rarefied and arid conditions of the atmosphere at altitude would favor dehydration of organisms in the absence of either structural or behavioral special adaptation. Hypoxia may also act independently in reducing thirst, at least in rats, the mechanisms of the hypodipsic effects of hypoxia remaining to be clarified *(7)*.

To compensate for increased water losses and decreased water intake, there is an immediate decrease in urinary output *(7)*. The influence of the hypoxic environment on water and electrolyte balance has been the focus of extensive research for many years *(45)*, and the question arises regarding which hormones might be affected by exercise under altitude exposure for controlling body fluid homeostasis *(46)*. By comparison with heat exposure, which also results in hypohydration *(47)*, it can be expected that the cascade of endocrinological and physiological adjustments necessary to meet cardiovascular, metabolic, and thermoregulatory demands during exercise in hypoxia should be increased. Most of the studies on hormones affecting fluid regulation during exercise at high altitude concentrated on the renin–angiotensin–aldosterone system *(48–50)*. However, it has been recently shown that acute hypovolemia in the dog is a sufficient stimulus to intensify the sympathoadrenal response to moderate exercise *(9)*, suggesting that the sympathoadrenergic stimulation during exercise at altitude *(19,25)* could be, in some circumstances, linked to the hypoxia-induced state of hypohydration.

On the other hand, inadequate nutrition is a condition tied to high altitude *(6,51)*. In newcomers to highland areas, but also in those exposed to hypobaric hypoxia in a low-pressure chamber, anorexia and hypophagia are known to be most pronounced during the acute phase of hypoxic exposure. Underlying mechanisms are still poorly understood, but reduced food intake is thought to be responsible for loss in body weight, and negative water and nitrogen balances in adults *(6,51)*. Unfortunately, only few studies have allowed these effects to be evaluated, and to be distinguished from those of hypoxia *(52)*. Recently, it was found that dietary restriction appears to result in increased circulating levels of catecholamines during the early stages of undernutrition *(53)*. The impact of hypoxia-induced states of undernutrition and hypohydration on the catecholamine response to exercise remains to be explored.

PHYSIOLOGICAL SIGNIFICANCE OF THE SYMPATHOADRENERGIC ACTIVATION DURING EXERCISE AT HIGH ALTITUDE

The sympathoadrenal system plays a critical role in regulating a number of key physiological (heart rate, stroke volume, vascular resistance, blood pressure) and metabolic (substrates mobilization and use) functions necessary to adjust to the stress imposed either by exercise or/and by altitude exposure. Indeed, the catecholamines, by binding to α- and β-adrenergic receptors, can exert a powerful vasomotor effect on vascular smooth muscle *(54)*.

In acute hypoxia, cardiac output increases by about 20% both at rest and during submaximal exercise *(55)*. However, maximal cardiac output and heart rate cannot increase, and the reduction in oxygen content in arterial blood decreases the potential for oxygen extraction so that VO_2max is decreased by about 25% at 4000 m altitude *(55)*. Although an increase in cardiac output may be considered appropriate for a short-term solution to the problem of hypoxia, a sustained increase in cardiac output is costly in terms of cardiac work. Therefore, with prolonged exposure to altitude, the organism appears to elect a less costly mode of delivering oxygen during submaximal exercise by increasing oxygen extraction rather than elevating blood flow *(56)*. On the other hand, acute hypoxia causes essentially no change in the mean systemic arterial blood pressure in humans *(26)*. This is in contrast to the dog, where acute hypoxia results in a rise in mean arterial pressure *(57)*. Even though sympathetic stimulation is expected to play a significant role in these cardiovascular adaptations to exercise in hypoxia, Wolfel et al. *(58)* have shown that increased O_2 extraction, and not preserved cardiac output, is responsible for the maintenance of oxygen uptake during sub-maximal exercise in the presence of nonselective β-adrenergic blockade.

Another striking cardiovascular change at high altitude is the occurrence of pulmonary hypertension caused by an increase in pulmonary vascular resistance, which is seen in healthy subjects during hypoxic breathing at sea level and in lowlanders exposed acutely to high altitude *(59)*. The pulmonary hypertension of acute hypoxia is alleviated by oxygen breathing. It has been hypothesized that catecholamines help to set the background tone that is necessary for the pulmonary vascular smooth muscle to respond to the vasoconstricting effects of hypoxia *(60)*. Recently, it was shown that healthy subjects had minimal changes in pulmonary vascular pressures with heavy exercise at sea level, but developed pulmonary hypertension at 3810-m altitude *(61)*. Similarly, we found that chronic administration of almitrine, a piperazine derivative acting selectively on arterial chemoreceptors like hypoxia, did not modify pulmonary arterial pressure at rest *(62)*. Nevertheless, when exercise was superimposed on almitrine medication, pulmonary arterial pressure remained elevated throughout the exercise bout, an effect that could be possibly related to enhanced plasma E levels *(62)*.

In addition to their role in cardiovascular adjustments to exercise in hypoxia, strong correlations have been reported between catecholamines and glucose/lactate turnovers *(19,22,63,64)*. Thus, circulating NE concentration correlates with the glucose rate of appearance *(63)*, allowing an increased use of blood glucose during exercise under acute exposure to hypoxia. However, on the basis of an enhanced glucose use during exercise at altitude after nonselective β-adrenergic blockade, Roberts et al. *(64)* concluded that E is not a major factor in regulating hepatic glucose production. On the other hand, Mazzeo et al. *(19)* reported a high correlation between blood lactate and E concentrations consistent with a causal relationship existing between the two. Such a causal relationship is further supported by the influence of nonselective β-adrenergic blockade, which reduces blood lactate concentration by ~50% on acute exposure to hypoxia *(64)*.

The impact of oxygen availability is not restricted to the sympathoadrenal system, but can also affect other glucoregulatory hormones (insulin, glucagon), the hypothalamic–pituitary–adrenal axis, and hormones that play a role in the regulation of fluid and electrolyte balance *(43,65)*.

Hormones of the Islets of Langerhans

Plasma concentration of insulin decreases during exercise in an intensity-dependent fashion *(66)*, the minimal work intensity required for decreasing plasma insulin level (~50% VO_2max) being similar to that necessary to influence sympathoadrenal activity *(1)*. The decrease in insulin release during exercise is probably owing to inhibition of $α_2$-adrenergic receptors of the β-pancreatic cells *(67)*.

Initially, Sutton *(65)* suggested that serum insulin level decreases during exercise to a greater extent under hypoxic conditions and displays a greater rebound in the postexercise period. However, Roberts et al. *(64)* have recently re-evaluated the influence of hypoxia on carbohydrate metabolism during submaximal exercise and found that acute exposure to 4300-m altitude causes an increased dependence on glucose as a fuel compared with sea level at rest and during exercise at the same absolute submaximal workload, this effect being enhanced by β-adrenergic blockade. However, arterial insulin concentration decreased during exercise under all conditions, but did not differ between control and β-blocked subjects. Because large changes in glucose rate of disappearance and net leg glucose uptake were accomplished with essentially the same arterial insulin levels, Roberts et al. *(64)* concluded that exercise and acute hypoxia resulted in a large increase in apparent insulin action. This conclusion contrasts, however, with a recent study by Larsen et al. *(68)* showing a markedly reduced insulin action after 2 d of altitude hypoxia, which has been attributed to an increase in plasma cortisol.

In humans, plasma glucagon concentration decreases during brief, intense exercise, and a significant increase above resting levels is not found until several hours of prolonged submaximal exercise *(1)*. In humans, in contrast to other species (rat, dog), the autonomic nervous system is not of major importance for the increase in plasma glucagon during prolonged exercise *(1)*, and during high-intensity exercise, it has been proposed that α-adrenergic activity inhibits the glucagon response to exercise *(2)*.

Plasma glucagon decreased to a similar extent in acute hypoxia and normoxia when exercising at the same relative workload (85% VO_2max) *(18)*. Subsequently, Roberts et al. *(64)* found that at sea level, plasma glucagon increased significantly during 45 min of exercise at ~50% of sea level VO_2max and the response was not affected either by acute exposure to high altitude or by β-adrenergic blockade. The finding that during exercise under different conditions, the plasma glucagon response is closely related to plasma glucose level has given rise to the proposal that instead of autonomic nervous control of glucagon secretion, glucose availability is the major determinant of the glucagon response to exercise *(1)*. This hypothesis is somewhat supported by the blunting of the exercise-induced response of glucagon when glucose is ingested prior to or during exercise *(69)*.

RENIN–ANGIOTENSIN–ALDOSTERONE SYSTEM

Acute exposure to altitude increases sodium and water diuresis, bringing about a shift of fluid out of the intravascular space into the interstitial and/or intracellular space *(45)*, which results in a relative increase in hematocrit to counterbalance the reduced supply of oxygen to peripheral tissues. Most of the studies in which renin and aldosterone levels have been simultaneously determined reported a decrease in aldosterone to renin ratio associated with hypoxia *(43,70)*. A similar dissociation between aldosterone and plasma renin activity response was reported during prolonged exercise at the same relative intensity under hypoxia *(48,50)*. This dissociation of renin and aldosterone reponse during exercise under acute hypoxia has been attributed to an inhibition of the angiotensin-converting enzyme *(59)*. However, several studies measuring angiotensin II failed to confirm this inhibition in vivo *(14)*. An alternative explanation for the uncoupling aldosterone from renin control during exercise in hypoxia might be linked to variations in plasma potassium level. However, Bouissou et al. *(49)* found that variations in plasma K^+ had no effect on aldosterone level during exercise in normoxic or hypoxic conditions. Other investigators have tried to correlate the dissociation of renin and aldosterone with the possible role of atrial natriuretic peptide (ANP) in the response to exercise in hypoxia *(71)*. This conclusion was, however, recently refuted by Vuolteenaho et al. *(72)*, who found a blunted ANP response to maximal exercise in acute hypobaric exposure. Apart from the fact that this latter study was performed in hypobaric conditions during maximal exercise, a possible factor that could explain the conflicting results with those of Lawrence and Shenker *(71)* could be related to the fact that these authors examined untrained subjects, whereas the study of Vuolteenaho et al. *(72)* involved well-trained individuals. These data suggest that aldosterone and ANP response to exercise are more or less totally independent in hypoxia and that other influences could explain the apparent dissociation of renin and aldosterone reported in these conditions. A more likely explanation is that aldosterone secretion is controlled differently at altitude, thus allowing ANP to exert a greater inhibitory influence compared with that at sea level *(50)*.

Arginine Vasopressin (AVP)

The neurohypophyseal hormone AVP increases during exercise *(73)*. Of note is that AVP response to exercise is variable between subjects, but remarkably reproducible within an individual *(74)*. In response to an increasing workload, plasma AVP concentrations display a threshold response at ~70% of VO_2max. It is also well documented that at a similar workload (e.g, 65% of VO_2max) short-term exercise fails to increase significantly plasma AVP, whereas after 2 h, AVP increases by 88% *(73)*. Thus, the response of AVP to exercise is modulated by intensity and duration of exercise.

Initially, short-term exposure (20 min) to mild hypoxia (equivalent to ~3400-m altitude) was found to result in a significant reduction in plasma AVP, which returns toward sea level values with more severe hypoxia (~5000 m) *(75)*. Actually, it is believed that diuresis, at least partly allowed by a decrease or lack of increase in AVP, is a normal response to hypoxia as long as altitude is tolerated. As soon as hypoxia begins to become intolerable (nausea, headache, respiratory distress), AVP is increased, antidiuresis ensues, and edema worsens *(14)*. Water restriction, which increases AVP by itself by increasing osmolality and decreasing plasma volume, augments the AVP response to acute hypoxemia in rats *(76)*. However, no interaction for AVP response was found between hypoxia and prolonged mild exercise *(77)*.

Adrenocorticotrophic Hormone (ACTH) and Adrenal Glucocorticoids

The ACTH response to hypoxia has long been of interest because of its possible involvement in high-altitude acclimatization *(78)*. Its secretion is mostly evaluated from estimates of adrenal glucocorticoid production, i.e, from determination of cortisol level in humans and corticosterone in the rat. Whereas acute exposure to moderate altitude (<5000 m) does not appear to increase plasma glucocorticoid levels, more severe hypoxia does result in an increase in ACTH and corticosteroids in various species *(14)*. During physical exercise, the cortisol response was found to be unchanged *(71)*, augmented *(65)*, or decreased *(79)* under moderate hypoxia. However, some of these studies *(65)* examined the cortisol response at the same absolute intensity of exercise, although it is assumed that the cortisol response relies rather on the relative than the absolute workload *(18)*. In addition, the cortisol response to exercise is correlated with ACTH in normoxic, but not under hypoxic conditions *(79)*, suggesting a decreased adrenal sensitivity to ACTH when exercising in hypoxia. However, cortisol release from adrenal cells in vitro is not affected by changes in oxygenation or blood flow to the adrenals *(14)*. Because chronic carotid body chemodenervation attenuates the ACTH and cortisol response to acute hypoxia *(14)*, it can be hypothesized that peripheral arterial chemoreceptors are essential to the hypothalamic–pituitary–adrenocortical response to exercise under acute hypoxia.

Hormones from the Anterior Pituitary

Physical exercise is regarded as a physiological stimulant of growth hormone (GH) and prolactin (PRL) release *(1)* from the anterior pituitary. A delay in plasma GH changes with exercise has been thoroughly described, but the progressive course of the increase in plasma GH during incremental exercise suggests that GH secretion is directly influenced by intensity and duration of exercise. However, Hartley et al. *(3,4)* have reported lower plasma GH levels during maximal than during submaximal exercise. This could be owing either to the characteristic pulsatile secretion of GH, to inhibition of GH secretion by high cortisol levels *(3,4)* or to a decreasing secretion rate of GH when steady state is not achieved during exercise *(1)*.

Initially, a large increase in plasma GH levels was found during exercise at altitude, whereas at the same absolute workload (750 kpm/min), serum growth hormone displayed only minor changes when performed at sea level *(65)*. Subsequently, Raynaud et al. *(80)* demonstrated a shorter delay in exercise-induced GH increase during acute exposure to hypoxia with no difference in peak plasma GH. On the basis of a close association between GH secretion and the oxygen demand/availability ratio over a wide range of exercise in both untrained and trained subjects and under both normoxic and hypoxic conditions, VanHelder et al. *(81)* suggested that imbalance between oxygen demand and supply is an important regulator at the muscle site of GH secretion during exercise.

In addition to GH secreting cells, other acidophil cells in the human anterior pituitary gland secrete PRL. Both GH and PRL share a marked structural homology. Like GH, plasma PRL level has been shown to increase during intense exercise, but to a lower extent. Furthermore, PRL may increase during the postexercise period when a steady state is not reached during exercise *(82)*. In a recent study, Struder et al. *(83)* reported that during exercise, PRL increased drastically with oxygen breathing, but did not change in normoxia. This effect was attributed to an inhibition of the dopaminergic system by some unknown mechanisms. Compatible with the view that secretion of PRL is influenced by oxygen availability, an inhibition of exercise-induced blood PRL response is observed following acute exposure to hypoxia *(84)*. From experiments in which glucose and insulin levels are artificially raised during exercise *(1)*, it appears that glucose availability might play a role in the PRL response to exercise at altitude.

CHRONIC HIGH-ALTITUDE EXPOSURE

Sympathoadrenergic Activity

From a theoretical point of view, the synthesis of plasma catecholamines should be decreased by chronic exposure to hypoxia. Indeed, the rate-limiting enzyme of catecholamine biosynthesis, tyrosine hydroxylase (TH), requires molecular oxygen as a substrate *(84)*. However, elevated plasma and urinary catecholamine levels were reported after 17 d at ~4500 m *(85)*. Whereas comparison of data from different studies is sometimes difficult because various methods have been used for the dosage of plasma catecholamines, hyperactivity of the sympathoadrenergic system with altitude exposure was confirmed recently with the use of high-performance liquid chromatography *(19,24,25)*.

These authors also provided evidence for a dissociation between the two limbs of the sympathoadrenergic system, namely the activity of sympathetic nerves and the adrenal medullary activity. Thus, with altitude acclimatization, arterial E concentration during submaximal exercise returned to sea level values, but a progressive increase in plasma NE level was reported whether at rest or during exercise *(19,24,25,86)*. It should be mentioned that during the conduct of Operation Everest II, Young et al. *(86)* examined the effect of gradual ascent over the course of 40 d to an altitude equivalent to Mount Everest (8848 m) and reported a blunted catecholamine response to exercise in severe hypoxia (SaO_2 = 39%). Earlier literature indicating normal values for plasma and urine NE levels in newcomers residing at altitude for several months *(87)* suggests that the hypoxia-induced sympathoadrenergic activation may not persist with longer residence at altitude. Indeed, we found that high-altitude natives do not display any sign of a greater sympathoadrenergic activation during chronic hypoxia and the exercise-induced hormonal changes remained unaffected by acute inhalation of a normoxic gas mixture *(88)*.

It is well documented that plasma catecholamine response to exercise is closely related to relative and not absolute work intensity *(1)*. Because maximal oxygen uptake is similarly decreased by acute and chronic hypoxia *(21)*, it was suggested that acclimatization in adrenal medullary responsiveness during chronic hypoxia is linked to improved oxygenation ventilatory acclimatization and erythropoiesis *(19)*. Indeed, a strong inverse relationship ($r = 0.94$) between arterial saturation and circulating E was reported both at rest and during exercise. The sympathetic nerve stimulation and NE response to chronic hypoxia are more complex with relatively little information being known. It is doubtful that hypoxemia is responsible for the pattern of the NE response because plasma NE level increases over time, while arterial oxygen saturation is increasing. On the basis of a high correlation between the drop in plasma volume and the rise in norepinephrine during altitude acclimatization, Mazzeo et al. *(19)* suggested that net increase in sympathetic nerve stimulation with chronic hypoxia could serve to redistribute blood to vital organs for ensuring adequate oxygenation. However, Sawka et al. *(89)* reported that plasma volume decreased from sea level by ~10% after 10–14 h after arrival at 4300 m with no additional changes from the 1st to the 9th d of altitude exposure. These data contrast with several other studies showing a progressive plasma volume loss during chronic exposure to hypoxia (*see* ref. 89 for additional references). The absence of change in plasma volume during altitude acclimatization in the study from Sawka et al. *(89)* could be attributed to the high level of physical activity performed by the subjects. Indeed, Hoyt and Honig *(45)* have proposed that physical exercise, by increasing extracellular osmolality, may influence the effects of hypoxia on total body water and body fluid distribution.

In a recent study *(90)*, muscle sympathetic activity was found to be significantly elevated both at rest and during exercise with altitude acclimatization, and the authors concluded that muscle is a major contributor to the increase in plasma NE levels observed after 3 wk at 4300 m *(19)*. The functional significance of the enhanced muscle sympathetic activity with altitude acclimatization is reflected by a number of ventilatory, circulatory, and metabolic adjustments.

First, hypoxia causes progressive accumulation of tyrosine hydroxylase, the rate-limiting enzyme in catecholamine synthesis both in peripheral chemoreceptors *(91)* and in the caudal region of the solitary complex where carotid sinus afferents project *(92)*. The stimulatory influence of hypoxia on tyrosine hydroxylase activity in these peripheral and central structures is correlated with ventilatory acclimatization to hypoxia, and some studies have shown that carotid body excision impairs ventilatory acclimatization *(93)*. Second, systemic hypertension at high altitude is found to be related to sympathoadrenal activity both at rest and during submaximal exercise *(26,94)*, suggesting that heightened sympathetic neural activity, probably acting primarily via NE, is responsible for the increase in vascular resistances observed in subjects residing for days to weeks at altitude. However, mean arterial pressure and vascular resistance do not return to normoxic values after acute inhalation of 35% O_2 in subjects after 3 wk of residence at high altitude *(95)*, and on return to sea level, an elevation of blood pressure is still present despite a normalization of urinary catecholamines *(87)*. These data suggest that sympathoadrenergic activity is not the only factor involved in the persistence of systemic hypertension at high altitude. Third, acclimatization to high altitude was found to result in an increased dependence on blood glucose both at rest and during sustained exercise conditions *(63)*. Indeed, a significant correlation between glucose rate of appearance and blood NE concentration was observed after 3 wk at 4300 m, suggesting a primary role for muscle sympathetic nerve activity in determining fuel utilization during exercise in chronic hypoxia. Fourth, blood lactate concentration for a given exercise workload falls after acclimatization to high altitude compared with acute hypoxia *(63)* with a similar pattern to that found for E *(19)*, suggesting that a relationship exits between activation of β-adrenergic pathways and lactate production. As a consequence, it was hypothesized that a fall in β-adrenergic stimulus with altitude acclimatization should result in reduced lactate release. However, reduction in β-adrenergic activity with altitude acclimatization (lowered circulating E) accounts for only a part of the fall in exercise lactate during chronic hypoxia *(22,23)*.

Whereas the increased activity of the β-adrenergic limb of the sympathetic systems results in tachycardia during the initial phase of hypoxia, maximal exercise heart rate decreases as exposure to hypoxia is prolonged *(55)*. The decrease in maximal heart rate during altitude acclimatization in spite of continued increased sympathetic activity could involve several mechanisms.

First, the sustained elevated adrenergic activity may induce an uncoupling of the β-receptor/adenylate cyclase complex (desensitization) and/or a decrease in the number of active myocardial β-adrenergic receptors (downregulation) *(96)*. Indeed, blunted increases in heart rate have been reported during β-adrenergic stimulation *(97)*, and β-adrenergic blockade produces smaller decreases in heart rate both at rest and during exercise up to maximum *(98)*. The altered responsiveness seems to be related to the magnitude and duration of altitude exposure *(99)*.

Second, adenosine released in the extracellular space by the hypoxic myocardium would appear to modulate the response of β-receptor to adrenergic stimulation by stimulating adenosinergic (A_1) receptor and altering the adenylate cyclase complex *(100)*. Thus, altered neurotransmission seems to contribute to the reduced chronotropic response to hypoxia.

Another mechanism that could account for the observed reduction in maximal heart rate in chronic hypoxia is a central reduction in sympathetic activation. It may be that the sympathetic system is not activated centrally because of a reduced chemoreflex feedback from exercising muscles during maximal exercise at lower workload in chronic hypoxia *(99)*. On the basis of higher heart rate, and plasma lactate levels during one-leg compared with two-leg exercise after 2–3 mo at altitudes between 5250 and 8700 m, these authors suggest that signals from contracting muscles, perhaps through group III and IV afferents, may be important for setting the upper limit for heart rate during exercise at very high altitude, as well as for determining the level of sympathetic stimulation of the system. Alternatively, alterations in the interaction between sympathetic neural responses and the brain–renin–angiotensin–AVP systems have been proposed *(99)*.

Hormones of the Islets of Langerhans

In response to hypoxia, fasting plasma glucose and insulin concentration are transiently increased during the first 48–72 h and then return to normoxic value after altitude acclimatization *(63,86)*. It seems therefore that the acute decrease in insulin action during the first days of altitude is quickly reversed with more prolonged exposure to hypoxia *(63,68)*. However, at higher altitude (from 5450 to 7615 m), it was found that both pre- and postexercise plasma insulin concentrations are increased by approximately twofold as compared to sea level *(86)*. On the other hand, in lowlanders acclimatized to high altitude for several months and in high-altitude natives, it was suggested that long-term elevation of GH limits glucose transport into the cells and produces insulino-resistance *(101)*. Nevertheless, in lifelong highland residents from South America, insulin displays a gradual decrease during incremental exercise, which is not affected by acute exposure to normoxia *(88)*.

In humans, there is much evidence to indicate that the autonomic nervous system is not of major importance for the exercise-induced increase in plasma glucagon concentrations *(1)*. However, after 3 wk at 4300 m, Roberts et al. *(64)* reported that circulating glucagon levels are significantly greater than those measured at sea level or during acute altitude exposure whether at rest or during submaximal exercise. Furthermore, arterial glucagon values tended to be higher following β-adrenergic blockade at rest, but were significantly elevated during exercise compared with control values. Nevertheless, in high-altitude natives, we found that plasma glucagon remained unchanged during incremental exercise when exercising in hypoxia, but increased progressively when inhaling a normoxic gas mixture *(88)*. During exercise eliciting an increase in glucagon concentration, the decrease in plasma glucose concentration is often very small, suggesting an increased sensitivity of the α-cells during exercise compared to rest *(102)*. Thus, it is likely that the slight increase in circulating glucagon in highlanders during exercise in normoxia was linked to a slightly lower plasma glucose *(88)*.

Renin–Angiotensin–Aldosterone System

Raff et al. *(70)* provided evidence for a significant reduction by hypoxia of aldosterone release from bovine adrenocortical cells in vitro, but a number of in vivo studies yielded conflicting results with respect to the effects of altitude hypoxia on plasma renin activity (PRA) and aldosterone secretion *(see ref. 14)*.

One of the first determinations of PRA-aldosterone dynamics during exercise at high altitude *103)* reported that the reduction in aldosterone secretion during graded exercise with acute exposure to hypoxia was partially restored when altitude exposure was extended to 11 d. Milledge et al. *(104)* studied the time-course of the effect of altitude over a 6-wk stay at 4500 m and above, and found that the initial suppression of aldosterone secretion was restored to sea level value after 12–20 d of hypoxia. The time-course of changes in the renin–angiotensin–aldosterone system during hypoxic exposure might differ according to species. Thus, Martin et al. *(105)* found that aldosterone remained elevated in rats exposed to a simulated altitude of 4400 m for 10 wk, but returned to baseline level only after 7 mo at 5500 m *(106)*.

Exercise stimulates renin release via activation of the adreno-sympathetic system, this effect being inhibited by administration of β-adrenergic blockers *(1)*. Whereas during acute exposure to high altitude, resting level and response to exercise of renin are lower than at sea level, under chronic altitude, the inhibitory influence of hypoxia on plasma renin activity at rest and during exercise is canceled *(50,103)*.

Arginine Vasopressin (AVP)

In the absence of pulmonary edema, plasma AVP does not appear to increase significantly during exposure to chronic hypoxia in humans *(14)*, sheep, or rats *(76)*. Recently, Bärtsch et al. *(107)* examined plasma levels of AVP in subjects before and during a sojourn of 3–4 d at 4559 m both at rest and during 30 min of exercise on a cycle ergometer. No significant changes in AVP occur at rest under exposure to altitude for 4 d, whether the subjects are susceptible or not to acute mountain sickness (AMS). During the exercise test, performed at a level comparable to the efforts of mountaineering, a significantly greater increase in AVP was observed in subjects developing AMS compared to those who stayed without symptoms during the 4-d sojourn at 4500 m. In the same study, a significantly higher level of ANP was found in resting conditions, irrespective of the susceptibility of the subjects to AMS *(107)*. However, the ANP response to exercise was similar in subjects without and with AMS and comparable to the exercise response at sea level. It seems, nonetheless, that if exposure to hypoxia is extended over a 2-wk period, the ANP response to exercise is blunted *(50)*. The reduced ANP response to exercise with altitude acclimatization might be related to a decrease in mechanical stretch of atria owing to a decrease in stroke volume. More research is needed to confirm that chronic hypoxia decreases the response of ANP to exercise and to explore the mechanism by which this effect occurs.

ACTH and Adrenal Glucocorticoids

There is some evidence for an increase in pituitary ACTH content and an increased number of corticotrophic cells of the adenohypophysis in rats chronically exposed to hypoxia, suggesting a chronic activation of the hypothalamo–pituitary–adrenal axis *(14)*. Indeed, pituitary and adrenal hypertrophy have been demonstrated in rats exposed to 5500 m simulated altitude *(108)*. In humans, plasma and urinary cortisol increases both with the time and the level of exposure to altitude and/or to the development of AMS (*see* ref. *14*). Little information is available concerning the effects of lifelong exposure to hypoxia on cortisol concentration. Maresh et al. *(109)* reported a greater cortisol response to a simulated altitude of 4760 m in lowlanders as compared to moderate-altitude natives (1830–2200 m), suggesting some adaptation of the system to chronic hypoxia. However, the cortisol response to maximal exercise was similar in both groups whether tested at their respective residence altitude or in hypobaric chamber, suggesting that the stimulus provided by exercise alone, and not the hypoxic environment is responsible for an increased cortisol level after exercise *(110)*.

Hormones from the Anterior Pituitary

In animals exposed to hypobaric hypoxia in a low-pressure chamber, anorexia and hypophagia are most pronounced during the early phase of hypoxic exposure *(52)*. The reduced food intake may be responsible for loss of body weight and may be associated with depressed growth in immature animals. Indeed, Nelson and Cons *(111)* have shown that female rats exposed from birth to 40 d of age to simulated altitude of 3800 m display striking growth impairment associated with a significantly reduced content of GH in pituitary gland, whereas plasma GH did not differ from control values.

In high-altitude natives, concentration of immunoreactive human GH was found to be significantly higher than in sea level natives *(80)*. Furthermore, the GH response to exercise under hypoxia is characterized by a sudden rise at the beginning of exercise and a sharp decrease as soon as exercise has stopped. It has been hypothesized that faster GH changes in hypoxia were linked either to a relatively lower hepatic blood flow or to acid–base alterations at onset of exercise. However, these hypotheses remain unproven, and Raynaud et al. *(80)* suggested that the magnitude of GH release depends not only on secretion and catabolism of the hormone, but also on the state of repletion of the pituitary gland, which in turn could depend on factors not directly related to muscular exercise.

In a recent study, it was reported that in humans acclimatized to an altitude of 3500 m for periods ranging from 3 to 12 mo as well as in high-altitude natives resident at 3300–3700 m, plasma prolactin level is similar to sea level values *(112)*. One study in women reported a decrease in basal prolactin related to the degree of hypoxemia *(113)*. These data are consistent with the low-serum prolactin levels measured in native high-altitude women *(114)*. Low-serum prolactin level observed at high altitude could be owing to a high dopaminergic activity and could explain the low prevalence of menstrual abnormalities associated with hyperprolactinemia in female highlanders *(114)*. Whereas in men with hypoxemic chronic lung disease prolactin responses to hypoglycemia and thyrotrophin-releasing hormone administration are normal *(14)*, it is possible that prolactin secretion in women might be inhibited at rest, but not during exercise at moderate altitude *(113)*.

Thyroid Hormones

The frequency of goiter in mountainous areas is well known and is mainly due to low iodine content of the soil *(59)*. From a theoretical point of view, a relative hypothyroidism might be expected when exposed to hypoxia to reduce the needs for oxygen. In the pituitary gland, the number of thyrotrophic cells is reduced, suggesting a reduced output of thyroid-stimulating hormone (TSH) *(14)*. In humans, however, thyroid activity is increased in lowlanders acclimatized to high altitude and in high-altitude natives *(115)*. Thyroxine (T4) and triiodothyronine (T3) plasma levels increase after a few hours of exposure to hypoxia without an increase in hormone binding proteins. Plasma TSH did not show any appreciable change at moderate altitude (3700 m), but decreased at extreme altitude (5000–6300 m) *(115)*. Moderate exercise increases T3 and T4, and the changes were enhanced after a 3-wk sojourn at 3650 m *(116)*. The fact that these increases occurred so rapidly without any corresponding change in TSH levels suggests that increases in plasma thyroid hormones are probably owing to a shift from extrathyroidal tissue compartments to the extracellular compartment. Changes in plasma levels of thyroid hormones are found to be correlated with plasma free fatty acid (FFA) levels *(25)*. The physiological significance of the relationship between circulating thyroid hormones and plasma FFA changes is not immediately obvious, but could be linked to the increased sympathetic activity reported after 3 wk at high altitude *(19)*.

Erythropoietin (EPO)

To adapt red cell mass to oxygen demand of the organism, the glycoprotein hormone erythropoietin (EPO) is produced by kidney in inverse correlation with the oxygen content of the arterial blood *(117)*. Following acute hypoxia, an increase in renal EPO mRNA has been demonstrated after 1–2 h to reach maximal values after 6–24 h in rodents and within 48 h in humans. Despite continued hypoxia, serum EPO levels decline before an increase in blood oxygen-carrying capacity *(117)*. The decline in serum EPO is accompanied by a marked reduction of renal EPO mRNA content, which provides evidence for a reduction in EPO production rather than an enhanced hormone clearance or consumption *(118)*.

During very heavy exercise, oxygen demand may exceed supply and lead to tissue hypoxia, which was hypothesized to stimulate EPO production *(117)*. This hypothesis seems to be supported by peripheral reticulocyte counts, which have been shown to increase within a few days following different types of exercise *(119)*. Recently, Schmidt et al. *(120)* reported that EPO is not directly influenced by a short period of maximal or a long period of submaximal exercise under normoxia, whereas higher EPO levels were found 24–48 h after submaximal exercise in hypoxia. The increased number of reticulocytes observed within days after exercising in hypoxia and after maximal exercise in normoxia suggests a higher erythrocyte production rate, probably under hormonal influence. However, EPO is likely not the only hormonal system responsible for the delayed exercise-induced reticulocytosis. Indeed, other factors influenced by exercise at high altitude, such as GH and insulin-like growth factor *(121)*, may play a significant role in regulation of EPO.

In high-altitude natives, the mean resting plasma EPO level does not differ from that of sea level residents *(122)*, but is higher than one would expect from the relationship between EPO and hematocrit at sea level. Exercise under chronic hypoxia in high-altitude natives does not appear to stimulate EPO production, as previously reported for lowlanders after exercising under acute hypoxic conditions. The apparent inhibition of EPO production during exercise might be related to more efficient O_2 transport in chronically adapted subjects *(123)*.

ACKNOWLEDGMENTS

To avoid a cumbersome bibliography, review articles and books have sometimes been cited instead of original papers. We apologize to all contributors not directly quoted.

The author would like to thank Brigitte Sempore for technical assistance, C. Gharib, and J. M. Pequignot for suggestions and comments, and John Carew for help in preparing the English version of the manuscript.

REFERENCES

1. Galbo H (ed.) Hormonal and Metabolic Adaptation to Exercise. Georg Thieme Verlag, New York, NY, 1983.
2. Kjær M. Regulation of hormonal and metabolic responses during exercise in humans. Exerc Sport Sci Rev 1992;20:161–84.
3. Hartley LH, Mason JW, Hogan RP, Jones LG, Kotchen TA, Mougey EH, et al. Multiple hormonal responses to graded exercise in relation to physical training. J Appl Physiol 1972;33:602–606.
4. Hartley LH, Mason JW, Hogan RP, Jones LG, Kotchen TA, Mougey EH, et al. Multiple hormonal responses to prolonged exercise in relation to physical training. J Appl Physiol 1972;33:607–610.

5. Bert P (ed.) La Pression Barométrique, recherches de physiologie expérimentale. Centre National de la Recherche Scientifique, Paris, 1979.
6. Rose MS, Houston CS, Fulco CS, Coates G, Sutton JR, Cymerman A. Operation Everest. II: Nutrition and body composition. J Appl Physiol 1988;65:2545–2551.
7. Tenney SM, Jones RM. Water balance and lung fluids in rats at high altitude. Respir Physiol 1992;87:397–406.
8. Gonzalez-Alonso J, Mora-Rodriguez R, Below PR, Coyle EF. Dehydration reduces cardiac output and increases systemic and cutaneous vascular resistance during exercise. J Appl Physiol 1995; 79:1487–1496.
9. Turlejska E, Falecka-Wieczorek I, Titow-Stupnicka E, Uscilko HK. Hypohydration increases the plasma catecholamine response to moderate exercise in the dog (Canis). Comp Biochem Physiol C 1993;106:463–465.
10. Esler M, Jennings G, Lambert G, Meredith I, Horne M, Eisenhofer G. Overflow of catecholamine neurotransmitters to the circulation: source, fate, and functions. Physiol Rev 1990;70:963–985.
11. Banister EW, Griffiths J. Blood levels of adrenergic amines during exercise. J Appl Physiol 1972;33:674–676.
12. Davies CT, Few J, Foster KG, Sargeant AJ. Plasma catecholamine concentration during dynamic exercise involving different muscle groups. Eur J Appl Physiol 1974;32:195–206.
13. Rostrup M. Catecholamines, hypoxia and high altitude. Acta Physiol Scand 1998;162:389–399.
14. Raff H. Endocrine adaptation to hypoxia. In: Fregly MJ, Blatteis CM, eds. Handbook of Physiology: Environmental Physiology. Oxford University Press, New York, NY, 1996, pp. 1259–1275.
15. Bouissou P, Peronnet F, Brisson G, Helie R, Ledoux M. Metabolic and endocrine responses to graded exercise under acute hypoxia. Eur J Appl Physiol 1986;55:290–294.
16. Bubb WJ, Howley ET, Cox RH. Effects of various levels of hypoxia on plasma catecholamines at rest and during exercise. Aviat Space Environ Med 1983;54:637–640.
17. Escourrou P, Johnson DG, Rowell LB. Hypoxemia increases plasma catecholamine concentrations in exercising humans. J Appl Physiol 1984;57:1507–1511.
18. Kjær M, Bangsbo J, Lortie G, Galbo H. Hormonal response to exercise in humans: influence of hypoxia and physical training. Am J Physiol 1988;254:R197–R203.
19. Mazzeo RS, Bender PR, Brooks GA, Butterfield GE, Groves BM, Sutton JR, et al. Arterial catecholamine responses during exercise with acute and chronic high-altitude exposure. Am J Physiol 1991;261:E419–E424.
20. Pequignot JM, Peyrin L, Favier R, Flandrois R. Adrenergic response to intense muscular activity in sedentary subjects as a function of emotivity and training. Eur J Appl Physiol 1979;40:117–135.
21. Ferretti G. On maximal oxygen consumption in hypoxic humans. Experientia 1990;46:1188–1194.
22. Brooks GA, Wolfel EE, Butterfield GE, Cymerman A, Roberts AC, Mazzeo RS, et al. Poor relationship between arterial [lactate] and leg net release during exercise at 4,300 m altitude. Am J Physiol 1998;275:R1192–R1201.
23. Mazzeo RS, Brooks GA, Butterfield GE, Cymerman A, Roberts AC, Selland M, et al. Beta-adrenergic blockade does not prevent the lactate response to exercise after acclimatization to high altitude. J Appl Physiol 1994;76:610–615.
24. Mazzeo RS, Wolfel EE, Butterfield GE, Reeves JT. Sympathetic response during 21 days at high altitude (4300 m) as determined by urinary and arterial catecholamines. Metabolism 1994;43: 1226–1232.
25. Mazzeo RS. Pattern of sympathoadrenal activation at altitude. In: Sutton JR, Houston CS, Coates G, eds. Hypoxia and Molecular Medicine. Queen City Printers, Burlington, VT, 1993, pp. 53–61.
26. Wolfel EE, Selland MA, Mazzeo RS, Reeves JT. Systemic hypertension at 4,300 m is related to sympathoadrenal activity. J Appl Physiol 1994;76:1643–1650.
27. Wallin BG, Sundlof G, Eriksson BM, Dominiak P, Grobecker H, Lindblad LE. Plasma noradrenaline correlates to sympathetic muscle nerve activity in normotensive man. Acta Physiol Scand 1981;111: 69–73.
28. Seals DR, Victor RG, Mark AL. Plasma norepinephrine and muscle sympathetic discharge during rhythmic exercise in humans. J Appl Physiol 1988;65:940–944.
29. Rowell LB, Johnson DG, Chase PB, Comess KA, Seals DR. Hypoxemia raises muscle sympathetic activity but not norepinephrine in resting humans. J Appl Physiol 1989;66:1736–1743.
30. Seals DR, Johnson DG, Fregosi RF. Hypoxia potentiates exercise-induced sympathetic neural activation in humans. J Appl Physiol 1991;71:1032–1040.

31. Saito M, Mano T, Iwase S, Koga K, Abe H, Yamazaki Y. Responses in muscle sympathetic activity to acute hypoxia in humans. J Appl Physiol 1988;65:1548–1552.
32. Manhem P, Lecerof H, Hokfelt B. Plasma catecholamine levels in the coronary sinus, the left renal vein and peripheral vessels in healthy males at rest and during exercise. Acta Physiol Scand 1978;104: 364–369.
33. Favier RJ, Desplanches D, Pequignot JM, Peyrin L, Flandrois R. Effects of hypoxia on catecholamine and cardiorespiratory responses in exercising dogs. Respir Physiol 1985;61:167–177.
34. Pequignot JM, Favier R, Desplanches D, Peyrin L, Flandrois R. Free dopamine in dog plasma: lack of relationship with sympathoadrenal activity. J Appl Physiol 1985;58:763–769.
35. Peronnet F, Nadeau RA, de Champlain J, Magrassi P, Chatrand C. Exercise plasma catecholamines in dogs: role of adrenals and cardiac nerve endings. Am J Physiol 1981;241:H243–H247.
36. Henley W, Bellush L. Time-dependent changes in catecholamine turnover in spontaneously hypertensive rats exposed to hypoxia. Proc Soc Exp Biol Med 1995;208:413–421.
37. Braunwald E, Harrison, DC, Chidsey CA. The heart as an endocrine organ. Am J Med 1964;36:1–4.
38. Johansson M, Rundqvist B, Eisenhofer G, Friberg P. Cardiorenal epinephrine kinetics: evidence for neuronal release in the human heart. Am J Physiol 1997;273:H2178–H2185.
39. Hesse B, Kanstrup IL, Christensen NJ, Ingemann-Hansen T, Hansen J.F, HalKjær-Kristensen J, et al. Reduced norepinephrine response to dynamic exercise in human subjects during O_2 breathing. J Appl Physiol 1981;51: 176–178.
40. Seals DR, Johnson DG, Fregosi RF. Hyperoxia lowers sympathetic activity at rest but not during exercise in humans. Am J Physiol 1991;260:R873–R878.
41. Seals DR. Influence of muscle mass on sympathetic neural activation during isometric exercise. J Appl Physiol 1989;67:1801–1806.
42. Claybaugh JR, Brooks DP, Cymerman A. Hormonal control of fluid and electrolyte balance at high altitude in normal subjects. In: Sutton JR, Coates G, Houston CS, eds. Hypoxia and Mountain Medicine, Queen City Printers, Burlington, VT, 1992, pp. 61–72.
43. Claybaugh JR, Wade CE, Cucinell SA. Fluid and electrolyte balance and hormonal response to the hypoxic environment. In: Claybaugh JR, Wade CE, eds. Hormonal Regulation of Fluid and Electrolytes, Environmental Effects. Plenum, New York, NY, 1989, pp. 187–214.
44. Walker JEC, Wells RE Jr. Heat and water exchange in the respiratory tract. Am J Med 1961;30: 259–267.
45. Hoyt RW, Honig A. Body fluid and energy metabolism at high altitude. In: Fregly MJ, Blatteis CM, eds. Handbook of Physiology: Environmental Physiology. Oxford University Press, New York, NY, 1996, pp. 1277–1289.
46. Gisolfi CV, Lamb DR, eds. Fluid Homeostasis During Exercise. In: Perspectives in Exercise Science and Sports Medicine, vol. 3. Cooper Publishing Group, Carmel, IN, 1990.
47. Francesconi RP, Sawka MN, Hubbard RW, Pandolf KB. Hormonal regulation of fluid and electrolytes: effects of heat exposure and exercise in the heart. In: Claybaugh JR, Wade CE, eds. Hormonal Regulation of Fluid and Electrolytes: Environmental Effects. Plenum, New York, NY, 1989, pp. 45–85.
48. Bouissou P, Guezennec CY, Galen FX, Defer G, Fiet J, Pesquies PC. Dissociated response of aldosterone from plasma renin activity during prolonged exercise under hypoxia. Horm Metab Res 1988;20:517–521.
49. Bouissou P, Peronnet F, Brisson G, Helie R, Ledoux M. Fluid-electrolyte shift and renin-aldosterone responses to exercise under hypoxia. Horm Metab Res 1987;19:331–334.
50. Rock PB, Kraemer WJ, Fulco CS, Trad LA, Malconian MK, Rose MS, et al. Effects of altitude acclimatization on fluid regulatory hormone response to submaximal exercise. J Appl Physiol 1993;75:1208–1215.
51. Butterfield GE, Gates J, Fleming S, Brooks GA, Sutton JR, Reeves JT. Increased energy intake minimizes weight loss in men at high altitude. J Appl Physiol 1992;72:1741–1748.
52. Gloster J, Heath D, Harris P. The influence of diet on the effects of a reduced atmospheric pressure in the rat. Environ Physiol Biochem 1972;2:117–124.
53. Hilderman T, McKnight K, Dhalla KS, Rupp H, Dhalla NS. Effects of long-term dietary restriction on cardiovascular function and plasma catecholamines in the rat. Cardiovasc Drugs Ther 1996;10 Suppl 1:247–250.
54. Weiner N. Norepinephrine, epinephrine and the sympathomimetic amines. In: Goodman Gilman A, Goodman LS, Gilman A, eds. The Pharmacological Basis of Therapeutics. MacMillan, New York, NY, 1980, pp. 138–175.

55. Grover RF, Weil JV, Reeves JT. Cardiovascular adaptation to exercise at high altitude. Exerc Sport Sci Rev 1986;14:269–302.
56. Vogel JA, Hartley LH, Cruz JC, Hogan R.P. Cardiac output during exercise in sea-level residents at sea level and high altitude. J Appl Physiol 1974;36:169–172.
57. Kontos HA, Levasseur JE, Richardson DW, Mauck HP Jr, Patterson JL Jr. Comparative circulatory responses to systemic hypoxia in man and in unanesthetized dog. J Appl Physiol 1967;23:381–386.
58. Wolfel EE, Selland MA, Cymerman A, Brooks GA, Butterfield GE, Mazzeo RS, et al. O_2 extraction maintains O_2 uptake during submaximal exercise with beta-adrenergic blockade at 4300 m. J Appl Physiol 1998;85:1092–1102.
59. Ward MP, Milledge JS, West JB. High Altitude Medicine and Physiology. University Press. Cambridge, 1989.
60. Fishman AP. Hypoxia on the pulmonary circulation. How and where it acts. Circ Res 1976;38:221–231.
61. Eldridge MW, Podolsky A, Richardson RS, Johnson DH, Knight DR, Johnson EC, et al. Pulmonary hemodynamic response to exercise in subjects with prior high-altitude pulmonary edema. J Appl Physiol 1996;81:911–921.
62. Favier RJ, Desplanches D, Pagliari R, Sempore B, Mayet MH, Simi B, et al. Effect of almitrine administration on pulmonary arterial pressure in resting and exercising dogs. Respir Physiol 1990;82:75–87.
63. Brooks GA, Butterfield GE, Wolfe RR, Groves BM, Mazzeo RS, Sutton JR, et al. Increased dependence on blood glucose after acclimatization to 4300 m. J Appl Physiol 1991;70:919–927.
64. Roberts AC, Reeves JT, Butterfield GE, Mazzeo RS, Sutton JR, Wolfel EE, et al. Altitude and beta-blockade augment glucose utilization during submaximal exercise. J Appl Physiol 1996;80:605–615.
65. Sutton JR. Effect of acute hypoxia on the hormonal response to exercise. J Appl Physiol 1977;42:587–592.
66. Bloom SR, Johnson RH, Park DM, Rennie MJ, Sulaima WR. Differences in the metabolic and hormonal response to exercise between racing cyclists and untrained individuals. J Physiol (Lond), 1976;258:1–18.
67. Karlsson S, Ahren B. Insulin and glucagon secretion in swimming mice: effects of autonomic receptor antagonism. Metabolism 1990;39:724–732.
68. Larsen JJ, Hansen JM, Olsen NV, Galbo H, Dela F. The effect of altitude hypoxia on glucose homeostasis in men. J Physiol (Lond), 1997;504: 241–249.
69. Ahlborg G, Felig P. Influence of glucose ingestion on fuel-hormone response during prolonged exercise. J Appl Physiol 1976;41:683–688.
70. Raff H, Brickner RC, Jankowski B. The renin-angiotensin-aldosterone system during hypoxia: is the adrenal an oxygen sensor? In: Sutton JR, Coates G, Houston CS, eds. Hypoxia and Mountain Medicine. Queen City Printers, Burlington, VT, 1992, pp. 42–49.
71. Lawrence DL, Shenker Y. Effect of hypoxic exercise on atrial natriuretic factor and aldosterone regulation. Am J Hypertens 1991;4:341–347.
72. Vuolteenaho O, Koistinen P, Martikkala V, Takala T, Leppaluoto J. Effect of physical exercise in hypobaric conditions on atrial natriuretic peptide secretion. Am J Physiol 1992;263:R647–R652.
73. Wade CE, Freund BJ, Claybaugh JR. Fluid and electrolyte homeostasis during and following exercise: hormonal and non-hormonal factors. In: Claybaugh JR, Wade CE, eds. Hormonal Regulation of Fluid and Electrolytes: Environmental Effects. Plenum, New York, NY, 1989, pp. 1–44.
74. Maresh CM, Wang BC, Goetz KL. Plasma vasopressin, renin activity, and aldosterone responses to maximal exercise in active college females. Eur J Appl Physiol 1985;54:398–403.
75. Claybaugh JR, Hansen JE, Wozniak DB. Response of antidiuretic hormone to acute exposure to mild and severe hypoxia in man. J Endocrinol 1978;77:157–160.
76. Griffen SC, Raff H. Vasopressin responses to hypoxia in conscious rats: interaction with water restriction. J Endocrinol 1990;125:61–66.
77. Meehan RT. Renin, aldosterone, and vasopressin responses to hypoxia during 6 hours of mild exercise. Aviat Space Environ Med 1986;57:960–965.
78. Hornbein TF. Adrenal cortical response to chronic hypoxia. J Appl Physiol 1962;17:246–248.
79. Bouissou P, Fiet J, Guezennec CY, Pesquies PC. Plasma adrenocorticotrophin and cortisol responses to acute hypoxia at rest and during exercise. Eur J Appl Physiol 1988;57:110–113.
80. Raynaud J, Drouet L, Martineaud JP, Bordachar J, Coudert J, Durand J. Time course of plasma growth hormone during exercise in humans at altitude. J Appl Physiol 1981;50:229–233.

81. VanHelder WP, Casey K, Radomski MW. Regulation of growth hormone during exercise by oxygen demand and availability. Eur J Appl Physiol 1987;56:628–632.
82. Gawel MJ, Park DM, Alaghband-Zadeh J, Rose FC. Exercise and hormonal secretion. Postgrad Med J 1979;55:373–376.
83. Struder HK, Hollmann W, Donike M, Platen P, Weber K. Effect of O_2 availability on neuroendocrine variables at rest and during exercise: O_2 breathing increases plasma prolactin. Eur J Appl Physiol 1996;74:443–449.
84. Bouissou P, Brisson GR, Peronnet F, Helie R, Ledoux M. Inhibition of exercise-induced blood prolactin response by acute hypoxia. Can J Sport Sci 1987;12:49–50.
85. Cunningham WL, Becker EJ, Kreuzer F. Catecholamines in plasma and urine at high altitude. J Appl Physiol 1965;20:607–610.
86. Young PM, Sutton JR, Green HJ, Reeves JT, Rock PB, Houston CS, et al. Operation Everest II: metabolic and hormonal responses to incremental exercise to exhaustion. J Appl Physiol 1992;73:2574–2579.
87. Sharma SC, Hoon RS, Balasubramanian V, Chadha KS. Urinary catecholamine excretion in temporary residents of high altitude. J Appl Physiol 1978;44:725–727.
88. Favier R, Desplanches D, Hoppeler H, Caceres E, Grunenfelder A, Koubi H, et al. Hormonal and metabolic adjustments during exercise in hypoxia or normoxia in highland natives. J Appl Physiol 1996;80:632–637.
89. Sawka MN, Young AJ, Rock PB, Lyons TP, Boushel R, Freund BJ, et al. Altitude acclimatization and blood volume: effects of exogenous erythrocyte volume expansion. J Appl Physiol 1996;81: 636–642.
90. Mazzeo RS, Brooks GA, Butterfield GE, Podolin DA, Wolfel EE, Reeves JT. Acclimatization to high altitude increase muscle sympathetic activity both at rest and during exercise. Am J Physiol 1995;269:R201–R207.
91. Schmitt P, Garcia C, Soulier V, Pujol JF, Pequignot JM. Influence of long-term hypoxia on tyrosine hydroxylase in the rat carotid body and adrenal gland. J Auton Nerv Syst 1992;40:13–19.
92. Schmitt P, Soulier V, Pequignot JM, Pujol JF, Denavit-Saubie M. Ventilatory acclimatization to chronic hypoxia: relationship to noradrenaline metabolism in the rat solitary complex. J Physiol (Lond), 1994;477:331–337.
93. Olson EB Jr, Vidruk EH, Dempsey JA. Carotid body excision significantly changes ventilatory control in awake rats. J Appl Physiol 1988;64:666–671.
94. Wolfel EE, Groves BM, Brooks GA, Butterfield GE, Mazzeo RS, Moore LG, et al. Oxygen transport during steady-state submaximal exercise in chronic hypoxia. J Appl Physiol 1991;70:1129–1136.
95. Bender PR, Groves BM, McCullough RE, McCullough RG, Huang SY, Hamilton AJ, et al. Oxygen transport to exercising leg in chronic hypoxia. J Appl Physiol 1988;65:2592–2597.
96. Kacimi R, Richalet JP, Corsin A, Abousahl I, Crozatier B. Hypoxia-induced downregulation of beta-adrenergic receptors in rat heart. J Appl Physiol 1992;73:1377–1382.
97. Richalet JP, Mehdioui H, Rathat C, Vignon P, Keromes A, Herry JP, et al. Acute hypoxia decreases cardiac response to catecholamines in exercising humans. Int J Sports Med 1988;9:157–162.
98. Bouissou P, Richalet JP, Galen FX, Lartigue M, Larmignat P, Devaux F, et al. Effect of beta-adrenoceptor blockade on renin-aldosterone and alpha-ANF during exercise at altitude. J Appl Physiol 1989;67:141–146.
99. Savard GK, Areskog NH, Saltin B. Cardiovascular response to exercise in humans following acclimatization to extreme altitude. Acta Physiol Scand 1995;154:499–509.
100. Richalet JP. The heart and adrenergic system in hypoxia. In: Sutton JR, Coates G, Remmers, JE, eds. Hypoxia: The Adaptations. Decker BC, Philadelphia, PA, 1990, pp. 231–240.
101. Sawhney RC, Malhotra AS, Singh T. Glucoregulatory hormones in man at high altitude. Eur J Appl Physiol 1991;62:286–291.
102. Santiago JV, Clarke WL, Shah SD, Cryer PE. Epinephrine, norepinephrine, glucagon, and growth hormone release in association with physiological decrements in the plasma glucose concentration in normal and diabetic man. J Clin Endocrinol Metab 1980;51:877–883.
103. Maher JT, Jones LG, Hartley LH, Williams GH, Rose LI. Aldosterone dynamics during graded exercise at sea level and high altitude. J Appl Physiol 1975;39:18–22.
104. Milledge JS, Catley DM, Ward MP, Williams ES, Clarke CR. Renin-aldosterone and angiotensin-converting enzyme during prolonged altitude exposure. J Appl Physiol 1983;55:699–702.

105. Martin IH, Baulan D, Basso N, Taquini AC. The renin-angiotensin-aldosterone system in rats of both sexes subjected to chronic hypobaric hypoxia. Arch Int Physiol Biochim 1982;90:129–133.
106. Martin IH, Basso N, Sarchi MI, Taquini AC. Changes in the renin-angiotensin-aldosterone system in rats of both sexes submitted to chronic hypobaric hypoxia. Arch Int Physiol Biochim 1987;95: 255–262.
107. Bärtsch P, Maggiorini M, Schobersberger W, Shaw S, Rascher W, Girard J, Weidmann P, et al. Enhanced exercise-induced rise of aldosterone and vasopressin preceding mountain sickness. J Appl Physiol 1991;71, 136–143.
108. Ou LC, Tenney SM. Adrenocortical function in rats chronically exposed to high altitude. J Appl Physiol 1979;47:1185–1187.
109. Maresh CM, Noble BJ, Robertson KL, Harvey JS Jr. Aldosterone, cortisol, and electrolyte responses to hypobaric hypoxia in moderate-altitude natives. Aviat Space Environ Med 1985;56:1078–1084.
110. Maresh CM, Noble BJ, Robertson KL, Seip RL. Adrenocortical responses to maximal exercise in moderate-altitude natives at 447 Torr. J Appl Physiol 1984;56:482–488.
111. Nelson ML, Cons JM. Pituitary hormones and growth retardation in rats raised at simulated high altitude (3800 m). Environ Physiol Biochem 1975;5:273–282.
112. Basu M, Pal K, Prasad R, Malhotra AS, Rao KS, Sawhney RC. Pituitary, gonadal and adrenal hormones after prolonged residence at extreme altitude in man. Int J Androl 1997;20:153–158.
113. Knudtzon J, Bogsnes A, Norman N. Changes in prolactin and growth hormone levels during hypoxia and exercise. Horm Metab Res 1989;21:453,454.
114. Gonzales GF, Carrillo CE. Low serum prolactin levels in native women at high altitude. Int J Gynaecol Obstet 1993;43:169–175.
115. Basu M, Pal K, Malhotra AS, Prasad R, Sawhney RC. Free and total thyroid hormones in humans at extreme altitude. Int J Biometeorol 1995;39:17–21.
116. Stock MJ, Chapman C, Stirling JL, Campbell IT. Effects of exercise, altitude, and food on blood hormone and metabolite levels. J Appl Physiol 41978;5:350–354.
117. Jelkmann W. Erythropoietin: structure, control of production, and function. Physiol Rev 1992;72:449–489.
118. Eckardt KU, Dittmer J, Neumann R, Bauer C, Kurtz A. Decline of erythropoietin formation at continuous hypoxia is not due to feedback inhibition. Am J Physiol 1990;258:F1432–F1437.
119. De Paoli Vitali E, Guglielmini C, Casoni I, Vedovato M, Gilli P, Farinelli A, et al. Serum erythropoietin in cross-country skiers. Int J Sports Med 1988;9:99–101.
120. Schmidt W, Eckardt KU, Hilgendorf A, Strauch S, Bauer C. Effects of maximal and submaximal exercise under normoxic and hypoxic conditions on serum erythropoietin level. Int J Sports Med 1991;12:457–461.
121. Banfi G, Marinelli M, Roi GS, Colombini A, Pontillo M, Giacometti M, et al. Growth hormone and insulin-like growth factor I in athletes performing a marathon at 4000 m of altitude. Growth Regul 1994;4:82–86.
122. Schmidt W, Spielvogel H, Eckardt KU, Quintela A, Penaloza R. Effects of chronic hypoxia and exercise on plasma erythropoietin in high-altitude residents. J Appl Physiol 1993;74:1874–1878.
123. Favier R, Spielvogel H, Desplanches D, Ferretti G, Kayser B, Hoppeler H. Maximal exercise performance in chronic hypoxia and acute normoxia in high-altitude natives. J Appl Physiol 1995;78: 1868–1874.

22 Exercise, Circadian Ryhthms, and Hormones

Thomas Reilly, DSC, Greg Atkinson, PHD, and Jim Waterhouse, DPHIL

CONTENTS

INTRODUCTION
CHRONOBIOLOGY—THE STUDY OF RHYTHMIC CHANGES IN THE BODY
CIRCADIAN RHYTHMS IN SPORTS PERFORMANCE
CIRCADIAN RHYTHMS IN SUBJECTS AT REST
CIRCADIAN RHYTHMS IN THE FACTORS DIRECTLY ASSOCIATED
   WITH EXERCISE
PHYSIOLOGICAL RESPONSES TO EXERCISE
FURTHER IMPLICATIONS OF CIRCADIAN RHYTHMS FOR EXERCISE
DISRUPTIONS CAUSED BY TRAVEL
SUMMARY
REFERENCES

INTRODUCTION

It is important for human health and efficiency to maintain physiological and biochemical processes within narrow bands in spite of external influences. This homeostasis is achieved by means of negative feedback control loops, and superimposed on the "constancy" produced by it, there are rhythmic changes. The main rhythms can have a period—the length of time that elapses until the cycle is repeated—of a day, week, month, or year. Ultradian rhythms refer to cycles with a period of <20 h and that recur within a single day. With regard to those rhythms with a period of a day, which are therefore known as circadian rhythms, there is now good evidence that an internal "body clock" contributes to their control.

In this chapter, the evidence for and properties of this body clock are first outlined, before indicating how it influences those physiological and biochemical variables, both at rest and during exercise, that are relevant to sports performance. Some implications of rhythms to sports persons are considered, and advice on "jet lag" is presented.

From: *Contemporary Endocrinology: Sports Endocrinology*
Edited by: M. P. Warren and N. W. Constantini © Humana Press Inc., Totowa, NJ

CHRONOBIOLOGY—THE STUDY OF RHYTHMIC CHANGES IN THE BODY

Endogenous and Exogenous Components of a Rhythm

There are daily changes in core temperature, with higher values in the daytime and lower values at night (Fig. 1). Similarly timed rhythms, with higher values in the daytime and lower values during nocturnal sleep, are found in other variables, such as heart rate, blood pressure, and concentrations of adrenaline. By contrast, for many hormones—melatonin and prolactin, for instance—the observed rhythm is in antiphase, that is, with nocturnal concentrations being higher than those in the daytime.

Cortisol values in the evening are roughly half those observed in the early morning, and adrenocorticotrophic hormone also has its highest levels in the morning. Thyroid-stimulating hormone is low in the daytime with its peak during the night, and the rhythm in plasma testosterone is low in the afternoon with a peak at 06:00–07:00 h. Hormones, such as insulin and glucagon, peak during the daytime, however, since their secretion is responsive to food intake.

The body responds to the demands of our environment and lifestyle; it is physiologically primed for activity in the daytime and for relaxation and recuperation via hormonal activity during sleep. Such an explanation can be seen to be inadequate, however, when individuals are studied during a "constant routine." In this, the subject is required: to stay awake and sedentary for at least 24 h in an environment of constant temperature, humidity, and lighting; to engage in similar activities throughout, generally reading or listening to music; and to take identical meals at regularly spaced intervals. In such conditions, any rhythmicity owing to the environment and lifestyle has been removed.

Under such circumstances, the rhythm of core temperature is still evident, but decreases in amplitude (Fig. 1). Three deductions can be made from this result, which applies to all variables that have been tested by this protocol.

1. The rhythm that remains cannot be attributed to an external cause, but must arise instead from within the body; it is described as an endogenous rhythm and its generation is attributed to some form of "body clock."
2. There is some effect of the environment and lifestyle as can be deduced from the finding that the two temperature curves differ; this component of the rhythm is termed "exogenous." In the case of core temperature, values will be increased by light, noise, meals, and mental and physical activities during daytime waking, and will be decreased by darkness, quiet, sleep, and inactivity during the night.
3. In subjects living a conventional lifestyle—daytime activity and nocturnal sleep—these two components are in phase. During the daytime, the core temperature is raised by the body clock acting in synchrony with the environment and lifestyle; during the night, the clock, the environment, and lifestyle all act in concert to reduce core temperature.

Such results apply to all physiological and biochemical variables, though the relative contributions of the endogenous and exogenous components, and the nature of the exogenous component are characteristics of a particular variable. For example, the secretion of plasma melatonin is much more affected by bright light (which inhibits its secretion) than by activity, and in dim light, such as that found domestically, shows a strong endogenous component. The rhythm of cortisol is decreased slightly by sleep, but otherwise has a strong endogenous component. By contrast, the rhythm of heart rate is dominated

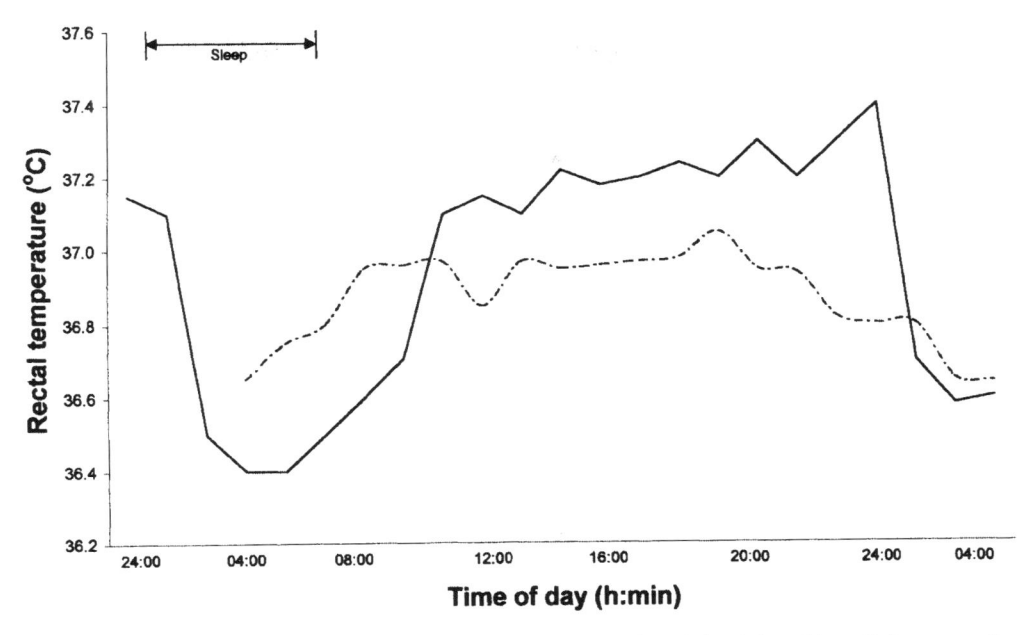

Fig. 1. Mean circadian changes in rectal temperature measured hourly in eight subjects living normally (solid line) and then awoken at 04:00 and spending the next 24 h undergoing a "constant routine" (dashed line).

by exogenous factors, particularly physical activity (which raises it) and sleep (which lowers it), but has a small endogenous, clock-driven component. Likewise, the rhythm of growth hormone is affected mainly by the first hour or so of a sleep, regardless of when this is taken.

The Site of the Body Clock

Humans have paired nuclei in the base of the hypothalamus, the suprachiasmatic nuclei or SCN (1,2). These nuclei represent the site of the body clock in mammals. Thus, slices of brain containing the SCN show rhythmicity of function, whether this be of neuronal firing rates or of neurotransmitter release, when the slices are cultured in vitro in constant conditions. No other region of the brain shows autonomous activity in such circumstances. When the SCN cells are removed surgically in rodents, activity in constant dim light continues to show the same total over the course of a 24-h period, but it is now randomly rather than rhythmically distributed.

Individual human subjects studied in an environment in which there are no time cues—in an underground cave, for example—continue to show rhythmicity in their sleep-activity cycle and in physiological and biochemical variables. Although this confirms the endogenous origins of such rhythms, in the great majority of individuals the rhythms all run slow with a period closer to 25 than 24 h. For this reason, the rhythms are called circadian ("about a day").

Adjustment of the Body Clock

Such a circadian rhythmicity of the body clock implies that it needs to be continually adjusted for the endogenous component of a rhythm to remain synchronized to a solar

(24-h) d. Synchrony is achieved by zeitgebers (German for "time-givers"), rhythms resulting, directly or indirectly, from the environment *(3)*.

In different mammals, rhythms of the light/dark cycle, of food availability/ unavailability, of activity/inactivity, and of social influences are all used, singly or in combination. In humans, the position is not yet fully resolved, but some combination of these zeitgebers is normally present.

LIGHT

Important among possible zeitgebers in humans is the light–dark cycle. The effect of light as a signal depends on the time at which it is presented. The first systematic studies *(4–6)* used bright light (>5000 lx) and showed that light pulses of 3 h or more in length and centred immediately after the trough of the body temperature rhythm (using this rhythm as a marker of the body clock) produced a phase advance, pulses centred immediately before the temperature minimum produced a phase delay, and those centred away from it by more than a few hours (the "dead zone") had little effect. This relationship between the timing of the pulse of light and the phase shift of the body clock that it produces is termed a "phase–response curve." More recent work has shown that light pulses that are much weaker (500 lx or less) also affect the clock and can produce phase shifts of up to about 1 h/d *(7,8)*. Even though most humans are exposed mainly to domestic lighting, which is much weaker than natural daylight, such artificial light–dark cycles can act as a zeitgeber.

MELATONIN

In the presence of dim light, serotonin *N*-acetyl transferase, the rate-limiting enzyme of the pathway within the pineal gland, which synthesises melatonin from serotonin, displays its highest activity nocturnally. As a result, there is a robust circadian rhythm of melatonin secretion, starting at about 21:00 and ending about 08:00 *(9)*. In humans, this is controlled by the sympathetic adrenergic input to the pineal gland that originates from the SCN.

Melatonin ingestion has been shown to adjust the phase of the body clock; according to the time of ingestion, it can cause a phase advance, phase delay, or no effect. The results are the inverse of the effects of light, and so melatonin in the afternoon tends to advance the body clock and in the early morning tends to delay it *(10)*. The exact mechanism by which this is achieved is unknown, but receptors for melatonin are present in the SCN and they would seem to be strong candidates for one of the links in a chain by which the pineal gland influences the SCN *(11)*. Light inhibits melatonin secretion, the amount of inhibition being dependent on light intensity *(12)*. The mechanism for this inhibition appears to be that during the daytime, the retinal photoreceptor cells are hyperpolarized and noradrenaline release is suppressed, as a result of which melatonin is not secreted. This makes the effects on the SCN of light and melatonin reinforce each other *(10)*. Thus, bright light in the early morning, just after the temperature minimum, advances the body clock directly, as described by the phase–response curve to light; bright light is indirectly effective also—by suppressing melatonin secretion, and so preventing the phase-delaying effect that melatonin would exert at this time.

OTHER POSSIBLE ZEITGEBERS

Other zeitgebers have been proposed for humans, such as the feeding–fasting and physical activity–inactivity cycles. The current evidence for them is weak. The "feeding hypothesis" *(13,14)* proposes that a high–protein breakfast raises plasma tyrosine levels and that this promotes the synthesis and release of the neurotransmitters noradrenaline and dopamine, which would activate the body's arousal system. Also, a high-carbohydrate evening meal will raise plasma tryptophan levels, thereby promoting the synthesis and release of serotonin, a major neurotransmitter of the raphe nucleus with an important role in sleep regulation and a precursor of melatonin. According to this hypothesis, adjustment of the body clock to a new time zone would be promoted by the appropriate timing and composition of meals.

The feeding hypothesis was tested on a group of military personnel undergoing an eastward flight across nine time zones *(13,14)*. This group showed small improvements in sleep and performance at mental tasks compared with the control group. However, the control group was allowed to eat ad libitum rather than being subjected to a feeding regimen that was comparable, except for timing and composition, to the experimental group. Therefore, the differences between the groups cannot be ascribed unambiguously to the timing and composition of the diet. Also, experiments on rodents have not substantiated that part of the hypothesis that requires plasma levels of tyrosine or tryptophan to be rate-limiting stages for the release of the neurotransmitters *(15)*.

If hamsters act as a model for humans, then physical activity should promote adjustment of the body clock *(16)*, though whether it is activity *per se* rather than the central nervous system (CNS) arousal produced by it that is effective is not resolved *(17)*. Results with humans have not yet proven conclusive *(18)*, though whether this is because such a mechanism is inoperative in humans, the amount of activity needs to be greater, or subjects are not sufficiently "excited" by exercise remains to be established.

The Inputs and Outputs of the SCN

There are two inputs from the retina to the CNS, one affecting circadian rhythms and the other involved in conscious visual perception. There is a direct pathway from the retina to the SCN, the retinohypothalamic tract *(1)*, which acts via acetylcholine and the induction of immediate early genes *(19)*. The retina contains a subgroup of receptors, whose visual pigment is based on vitamin B_2 rather than the more conventional vitamin A-based opsins *(20)*, and they might be the means by which photic information reaches the SCN.

Another input pathway to the SCN via the intergeniculate leaflet is probably important for nonphotic (activity) zeitgeber inputs in hamsters *(1)*. It is possible, but not yet established, that in humans such a pathway would act as a means for enabling a general rhythmic flux of "excitement," whether derived from mental, physical, or social rhythms, to act as a zeitgeber. As described above, receptors for the hormone melatonin have been found in the SCN *(11)*, and it is suggested that melatonin acts as an "internal zeitgeber."

Outputs from the SCN are widespread and distributed throughout the body *(1)*. There are connections with the raphe system that will influence the sleep–activity cycle, and also outputs to the autonomic nervous system and to the thermoregulatory and neuroendocrine nuclei of the hypothalamus. By such pathways, the endogenous, clock-driven component of circadian rhythms can pass throughout the body via rhythmic changes to the nervous system, hormones, and core temperature.

Mathematical Description of Circadian Rhythms

The conventional description of a circadian rhythm has been to use a sine-wave and to determine its characteristics by cosinor analysis (Fig. 2). The midpoint between the highest

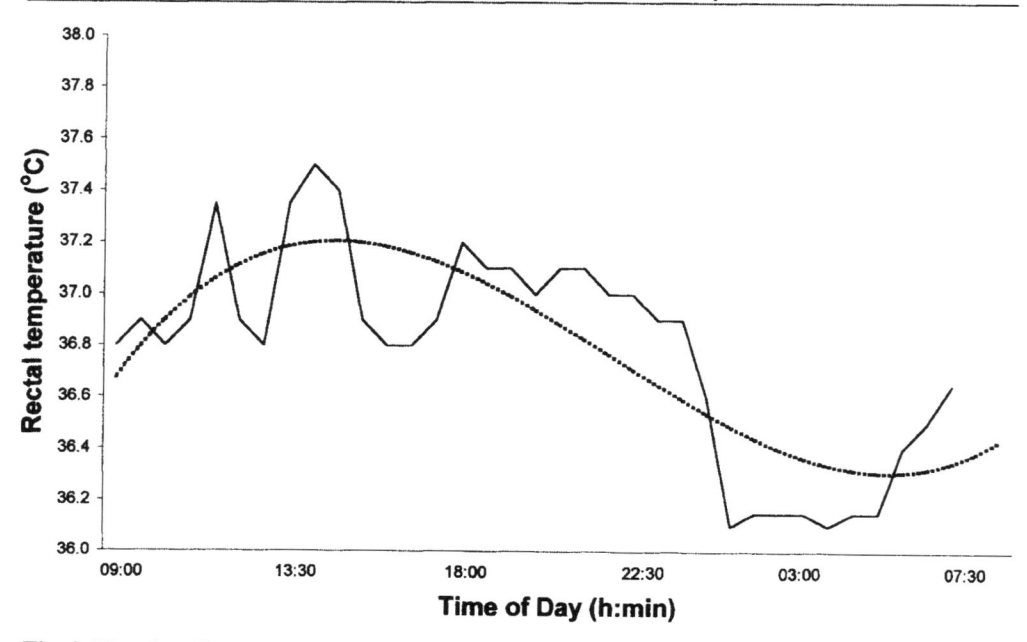

Fig. 2. The circadian rhythm in rectal temperature under nychthemeral conditions (continuous line) and with the rhythm "purified" by removing the effects of habitual activity and described with cosinor analysis (broken line).

and lowest values of a rhythm is the "mesor" (midline estimating statistic of a rhythm). The amplitude of a rhythm is half the difference between the highest and lowest point of the fitted cosine curve; the range of a rhythm is the difference between the maximum and minimum values. The location in time of the peak is termed the acrophase, which is expressed in angular degrees (1 period = 360°) or in absolute units of time, e.g., hours and minutes. In many instances, the cyclical variation may be best fitted by alternative statistical models (such as analysis of variance), which have the advantage over cosinor analysis that they do not assume a sinusoidal rhythm. There may also be substantial subharmonics within a 24-h cycle, in which case the term "peak time" rather than acrophase should be used (21).

CIRCADIAN RHYTHMS IN SPORTS PERFORMANCE

Athletes prefer evening contests and consistently achieve their top performances at this time of day. For example, the work rate of soccer players reflected this preference during indoor five-a-side games sustained for 4 d (22). The pace of play reached its highest intensity at about 18:00 h and a trough at 05:00–06:00 h on each day. Subjective fatigue was correlated negatively with activity level. The self-paced level of activity conformed closely to the curves in body temperature and in heart rate, a relationship that persisted throughout successive days.

The types of interventions demanded by experimental designs are not feasible in sports competitions. Consequently, researchers have tended to consider the effects of time of day on performance in time trials or simulated contests. Six runners, three weight-throwers, and three oarsmen were found to perform better in the evening than in the morning (23), and the speed of running in a 5-min test varied in close correspondence to

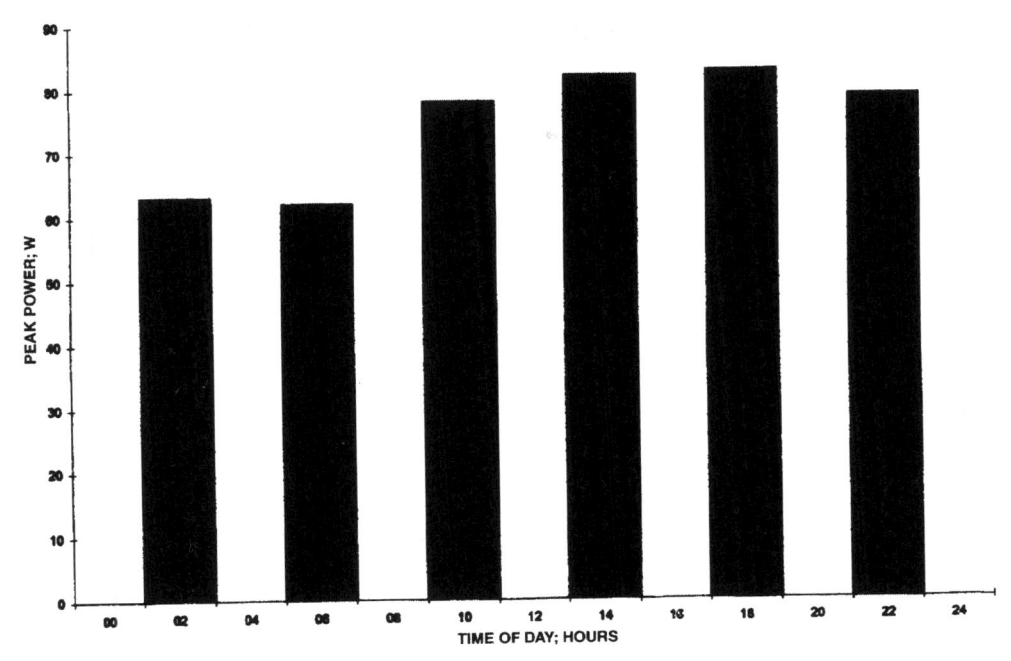

Fig. 3. Peak power output in maximal efforts on a swim-bench simulator at different times of day (from ref. 28).

the circadian curve in body temperature (24). Swimmers produced faster times over 100 m at 17:00 h compared with 07:00 h in three out of four strokes studied (25), and performances in front crawl were 3.6 and 1.9% faster for 400-m and repeated 50-m swim trials, respectively, at 17:30 h than at 06:30 h (26). This time-of-day effect was also observed through three successive days of partial sleep deprivation (27). The superiority of evening time for swim time trials "in the pool" is likely to be physiological in origin rather than owing to changes in water temperature, since mean and peak power outputs recorded on a swim bench under controlled conditions vary with time of day (28). The higher amplitude than normal (Fig. 3) is owing to the complexity of the simulated arm action of swimming, compared to a grosser movement, such as arm cranking.

It is clear that evening is best for sprint swimmers, particularly if time trial results are important, such as in achieving championship-qualifying standards. There is a time band close to the acrophase of body temperature in which optimal performance in sports involving gross movements can be attained. This probably extends to a plateau lasting 4–6 h provided that meals and rests are suitably fitted in during the daily routine. Sports requiring fast "explosive" efforts tend to peak earlier, and performance might be influenced more by "arousal" and so more closely related to an early part of the sleep–wake cycle than to the body temperature rhythm. In the last 50 yr, only in men's shot putt and women's javelin have world records been set before noon in track and field events.

CIRCADIAN RHYTHMS IN SUBJECTS AT REST

Exercise induces responses in many physiological and biochemical processes. The physiological systems involved show circadian rhythms in resting subjects and possibly also in the response to exercise.

The Body Temperature Rhythm

Body temperature has been used as a marker of circadian rhythms (see Figs. 1 and 2). Generally, it is measured by means of a rectal probe, but more reliable infrared thermometry has made it possible to monitor tympanic temperature safely (29). In field conditions, social circumstance may dictate the use of oral temperature, which is less satisfactory, since drinks and talking will affect it. Midstream urine can provide a reliable means for indicating core temperature, but suffers from similar social constraints to those when obtaining measurements of rectal temperature.

The circadian rhythm in core temperature at rest results mainly from fluctuations in heat loss mechanisms—vasomotor and insensible sweating—rather than heat production—metabolic rate (30). The set point of thermoregulation, determined by the thresholds for sweating and changes in vasomotor tone, varies with time of day. Noradrenergic activity and plasma adrenaline might contribute to this; they rise during the hours before noon (31), and the dissipation of body heat would be counteracted by the resultant vasoconstriction, core temperature rising as a consequence. Melatonin lowers body temperature (32), possibly through an action on peripheral vasculature (33), the onset of its secretion from the pineal gland coinciding with a sharp fall in core temperature.

Rhythms in Metabolic Variables

The oxygen consumption (VO_2) at rest displays a circadian rhythm, with a minimum at around 04:00 h. The VO_2 rhythm is partly a result of the body temperature rhythm, the circadian change in core temperature explaining about one-third of the range observed in VO_2 (34). The circadian rhythm in VO_2 is not attributable to changes in thyroid-stimulating hormone, since this variable peaks at the same time as VO_2 drops to its nadir (35), though levels of circulating catecholamines might have some influence.

The blood glucose level is relatively stable over 24 h, though a few authors (e.g., ref. 36) have detected rhythmicity in this variable, albeit with a very low amplitude. It is usual to find a small amplitude ultradian rhythm in blood glucose with peak levels corresponding to the three diurnal meals and a fourth increase at the end of sleep (37). The body's tolerance to a glucose load is less in the evening and at night, owing to decreases then in insulin release in response to a glucose load and the sensitivity of tissues to this hormone (38). Insulin is also less effective during nocturnal sleep, since the release of growth hormone (the "diabetogenic factor") opposes its actions at the level of the cell membrane.

At night, therefore, particularly when fasting (as is generally the case), there is a tendency to metabolize fats rather than glucose, and plasma free fatty acids are higher than during the day (39). The increased metabolism of fat has a hormonal basis; the decreased effectiveness of insulin means that lipogenesis is reduced, and the raised plasma cortisol promotes the breakdown of excess amino acids by gluconeogenesis (40). These circadian rhythms in the hormone associated with metabolism contribute to the "lipogenic–lipolytic" cycle of daily metabolism (41).

Rhythms in Ventilation

The forced expiratory volume and peak expiratory flow both vary with time of day, falling to minima between 03:00 and 08:00 h (42). These two variables are indicators of pulmonary airway resistance. Asthmatic patients exhibit markedly greater amplitudes in airway rhythms depending on the severity of the disease (43). Symptoms of asthma are exacerbated at night and in the early morning, giving rise to the debilitating complaint of "nocturnal asthma" *(44)*. For this reason, asthmatic athletes are advised against performing strenuous training in the early hours of the morning.

The circadian rhythm of pulmonary airway resistance is probably caused by neural and endocrine factors, and these rhythms help explain the potential problems arising in the evening in asthmatics. In the evening, there is a decease in bronchodilatation owing to falling output from the sympathetic nervous system, increasing vagal tone (to promote nocturnal bradycardia), and decreasing plasma adrenaline levels. There is also an increased risk of histamine release from mast cells in response to allergens owing to low levels of the immunosuppressant hormone, cortisol *(45)*.

Cardiovascular Rhythms

Heart rate varies with an amplitude of 5–15% of the 24-h mean depending on the extent of the exogenous influences: its acrophase usually occurs around 15:00 h when activity is controlled *(34)*. Similar rhythm characteristics are found for stroke volume, cardiac output, blood flow, and blood pressure *(46)*. Zulch and Hossman *(47)* reported that blood pressure showed an ultradian rhythm with a "postlunch dip" followed by a secondary peak in the afternoon. This phenomenon is clearly evident if individuals nap and tends to be more marked in aged individuals *(48)*.

Given the numerous exogenous influences on heart rate and blood pressure (activity, sleep, food intake), their fluctuations over 24 h can be extremely complicated. Nevertheless, a small endogenous component is present, probably owing to the combined effects of core temperature and plasma adrenaline, both of which will raise heart rate and blood pressure during the daytime. The changes at night are caused by changes in sympathetic (decreases) and vagal (increases) tone at this time *(49)*; these changes are dominated by sleep, but probably have a small endogenous component also.

Rhythms in Gastrointestinal Function and Urinary Excretion

There are circadian rhythms in gastrointestinal motility patterns, intestinal absorption rates, and the secretion of gastric acid, gastrointestinal enzymes, and hormones *(41,50)*. Peak rates are nearly always in the daytime. Goo et al. *(51)* reported that rates of gastric emptying for meals administered at 20:00 h were over 50% slower than emptying rates for the same meal taken at 08:00 h. There are some obvious implications when the uptake of drugs from the gastrointestinal tract into the bloodstream is considered. It is not known whether the gastric emptying of carbohydrate drinks during exercise varies with time of day.

Touitou et al. *(52)* reported the peak levels of urinary electrolytes occur in the afternoon at around 16:00 h (exceptions being urinary phosphates and 17-ketosteroids, which peak soon after waking, and urea, which peaks in the evening). Circadian changes in urinary pH mirror those of the excretion of most urinary electrolytes, with the most acidic urine (pH = 5.0) observed during the period of sleep, rising to a maximum (pH = 8.0) in the afternoon *(53)*. Circadian rhythms in urinary pH and excretion of electrolytes should be acknowledged in laboratories concerned with drug testing, since the excretion of acidic or basic drugs is passive and determined by urine pH *(54)*. Chronopharmacological studies are needed to ascertain whether an ingested drug would be detected in an athlete's urine at one time of day more than another.

The causes of the circadian rhythms in many aspects of renal function have proven difficult to elucidate (55); antidiuretic hormone and hormones of the hypothalamo–pituitary–adrenal axis are implicated, but details remain unclear. There is stronger evidence, however, to implicate cortisol in the control of potassium excretion (56), the circadian rhythm of this hormone producing a rhythm of potassium flux between the intra- and extracellular fluid compartments. Since the circadian rhythms in excretion of water and several electrolytes are in phase with those of blood pressure, glomerular filtration rate, and renal plasma flow, it has been assumed that they are linked causally in some way (55); the recent demonstration of normally phased circadian rhythms of renal function in transgenic rats—in whom the blood pressure rhythm is inverted—has cast some doubt on this (57). The circadian changes in renal blood supply are likely to have only a marginal influence on sports performance (owing to the relative shutdown of the blood supply to the kidneys that takes place in exercise).

Rhythms in Hormonal Secretions

Clearly, hormones have an important role in contributing to circadian rhythms at rest—*see also* reviews by Krieger (58) and Van Cauter (59). Three more general points need to be added:

1. Hormones differ in the relative importance of their endogenous and exogenous components; some, like cortisol and melatonin, have strong endogenous components, whereas others, such as adrenaline and antidiuretic hormone, are dominated by exogenous influences. This difference will become important when changes in the sleep–activity schedule—as after a time zone transition—are considered.
2. The circadian rhythms of most hormones originate from within or close to the hypothalamus, readily explaining the origin of their circadian rhythmicity.
3. With age, there is a tendency for the amplitude of circadian rhythms to decrease. This probably has exogenous—the individuals become less active by day and sleep less well at night—and endogenous—there is a deterioratin in function of the body clock—causes. There is also some evidence to indicate that the phasing of circadian rhythms becomes earlier by an hour or so (60,61). Many hormones show these changes, and not only those associated with reproduction.

CIRCADIAN RHYTHMS IN THE FACTORS DIRECTLY ASSOCIATED WITH EXERCISE

Sports performance results from a combination of processes, some of which are unimportant except in exercise, and others are engaged to a far greater extent than at rest. In both cases, the presence of circadian rhythms might go some way toward explaining rhythmicity in sports performance.

Rhythms in Subjective States and Mental Performance

Subjective states of "arousal" or its inverse, "fatigue," have been studied using simple visual-analog scales, inventories, such as the Stanford Sleepiness Scale (62)—for the measurement of sleepiness—or a questionnaire, the Profile of Mood States (63). Alertness and positive mood states peak in the waking hours, usually the afternoon (64); conversely, mood disturbance is lowest in the afternoon and early evening (Fig. 4). Mood and subjective alertness are important, since such states can alter an individual's motiva-

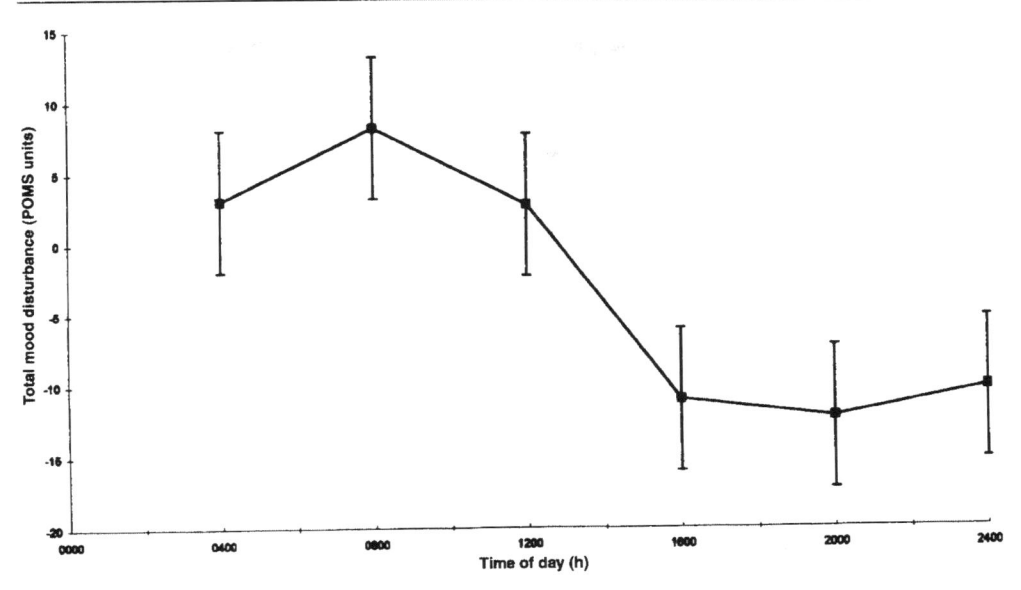

Fig. 4. Mood factors vary with circadian rhythms, disturbances being greatest at night-time and in the morning (from ref. 65).

tion for strenuous physical exercise. Circadian variations in mood states may also affect the "team cohesion" of a sports squad.

"Mental performance" covers a huge range of tasks, included among which are reaction time, vigilance, and tasks making particular demands on the sensory input of information, decision making, manipulative dexterity, long-term memory, or short-term memory. These aspects of mental performance differ in the relative importance of a circadian component (generally in phase with the temperature rhythm) and a deterioration owing to the time awake or spent carrying out a particular task. Such differences will alter the time of day when a particular task is performed best. Most sports require a combination of several of these tasks.

Simple reaction time (either to auditory or visual stimuli) is a major component of performances in sprint events. It is an element also of many games' skills, such as goalkeeping in soccer or hockey. Reaction time peaks in the early evening at the same time as the maximum in body temperature. This is partly because nerve conduction velocity increases by 2.4 m/s for every 1°C rise in body temperature.

Often, there is an inverse relation between the speed and the accuracy with which a simple repetitive test is performed. Therefore, accuracy may be worse in the early evening. There are many sports that demand accuracy without speed (e.g., golf, darts), and others where there are opportunities to emphasize power (e.g., the first serve in tennis). Although the effects of time of day on actual performances in these sports have rarely been examined (but *see* ref. 66), their complexity probably means that they are susceptible to the effects of time awake and so performed best before the late afternoon. As a further example, the ability to balance while standing represents a task demanding fine motor control, which is performed better in the morning.

Cognitive operations and short-term memory also peak in the morning rather than in the evening *(64)*. Rhythms in cognitive variables have relevance to sport in that they influence competitive strategies, decisions, and the delivery and recall of complex coaching instructions.

Circadian rhythms in psychomotor performance, particularly tasks that entail cognitive operations, also seem prone to the "postlunch dip." Some aspects of performance deteriorate at this time without a corresponding decrease in body temperature, and decrements occur even if no food is ingested at lunchtime. This time of day is best avoided when the coach is trying to impart new skills or tactics to a group of athletes.

A model of arousal, based on the combination of a circadian component in phase with the circadian rhythm of core temperature and an exponential decline owing to time awake, has been used to predict circumstances when alertness might fall to values that are low enough to jeopardize sufficient awareness of the environment for effective responses *(67)*. Investigations of other mood and mental performance variables suggest that their rhythms also can be described as the sum of a circadian component and a component that changes with time awake (*see* ref. *68*, for example). It seems that the basic model could, with suitable adjustment of its parameters, be adapted to these other variables.

Joint Flexibility and Stiffness

Joint flexibility (range of movement) shows marked rhythmicity across a wide range of human movements. Gifford *(69)* noted circadian variation in lumbar flexion and extension, glenohumeral lateral rotation, and whole-body forward flexion, but there are large interindividual differences in the peak times for flexibility. Amplitudes of these rhythms can be as high as 20% of the 24-h mean value. The normal rest–activity rhythm imposes compressive loading on the spine during the waking day, leading to the extrusion of water through the invertebral disk wall and a consequent loss of disk height. The resultant loss of stature is known as "spinal shrinkage" and there is an increase in the stiffness of the intervertebral disks. This shrinkage is reversed at night during the recumbency of sleeping. Reilly et al. *(70)* provided a comprehensive characterisation of the circadian rhythm in human stature. Using a stadiometer accurate to 0.01 mm, they reported that the diurnal variation was 1.1% of overall stature. The circadian variation in the data was better fitted by a power function than by cosinor analysis *(71)*. Peak stature was measured at 07:30 h with the greatest rate of shrinkage occurring in the hours immediately after getting up from bed. A period of rest prior to training or competing in the evening helps to unload the spine and restore its normal responses to compressive loads. The circadian variation in human stature was attributed to exogenous, rather than endogenous, neural, or endocrinological variables.

Muscle Strength

Muscle strength, independent of the muscle group measured or the speed of contraction, consistently peaks in the early evening. Grip strength is measured by means of a portable dynamometer, and so it has been frequently used as a marker of the circadian rhythm of physical performance. The rhythm in isometric grip strength peaks between 15:00 and 19:00 h with an amplitude of about 6% of the 24-h mean. The grip strength rhythm is partly endogenously controlled, since it persists during sleep deprivation and adjusts slowly to changes in sleep–wake regimens. The peak-to-trough variation in grip strength can be three times higher than normal in rheumatoid arthritic patients.

There may be a subharmonic within a main circadian rhythm in muscle strength. For example, when the isometric strength of the knee extensors was measured repeatedly during the waking hours of the solar day, two daytime peaks were noted, one at the end of the morning and another in the late afternoon/evening *(72)*. Performance transiently declined between these times of day. Similarly, there can be a drop in grip strength between 13:00 and 14:00 h, the "postlunch dip," when the variable is measured every hour for a 24-h period.

With respect to the isometric strength of other muscle groups, elbow flexion strength varies with time of day, peaking in the early evening. Back strength is also higher in the evening than in the morning, with an amplitude of around 6% of the 24-h mean *(73)*. Circadian rhythms in both concentric (while the muscle is shortening) and eccentric (while the muscle is lengthened) strength values have been found. Peak isokinetic torque values occurred in the early evening, when measured at slow (between 1.05 and 3.14 rad/s) angular velocities of movement. The test–retest variation of measurements made with computer-controlled isokinetic dynamometers may be as high as 20% at fast angular velocities of >6 rad/s. Unless this error is reduced through multiple trials, any circadian variation may go undetected *(74)*. This inadequate test–retest repeatability of measuring equipment is a more general problem in this area of chronobiological research.

Short-Term Power Output

Circadian rhythms have been identified in laboratory measures of anaerobic power and conventional tests of short-term dynamic activity. Hill and Smith *(75)* measured power and capacity with a modified version of the Wingate 30-s cycle ergometry test at 03:00, 09:00, 15:00, and 21:00 h. Peak power in the evening was 8% higher than at 03:00 h. Similar results were found for mean power over the 30-s test period. Vigorous warm-up procedures, which raise both arousal and muscle temperature, may "swamp" any existing rhythm in short-term power output.

The results of studies that have examined the effects of time of day on fixed-intensity work rates close to maximal oxygen uptake (VO_2max) seem more conclusive than those that have employed "supramaximal exercise," such as is required for the Wingate test. Hill et al. *(76)* reported that total work in high-intensity exercise on a cycle ergometer at a constant work rate was higher in the afternoon compared with the morning. Reilly and Baxter *(77)* similarly reported longer work times and higher blood lactate levels when a set high-intensity exercise was performed at 22:00 h compared with 06:30 h.

With respect to short-term explosive activity, Reilly and Down *(78)* reported significant circadian rhythmicity for standing broad jump, with an acrophase of 17:45 h and an amplitude of 3.4% of the 24-h mean value. Similar rhythm characteristics have been reported *(79)* for anaerobic power output on a stair-run test (*see* Table 1, which summarizes the circadian characteristics of several fitness tests).

As margins of victory in competitive sports events are usually only a few centimeters, time of day should be recognized as an important factor in competitive attempts or in the ability to meet certain performance standards to qualify for major championships.

PHYSIOLOGICAL RESPONSES TO EXERCISE

Having already established the existence of circadian rhythms in a wide range of variables at rest and associated directly and indirectly with exercise, the existence of rhythms in physiological responses to exercise is now considered. Some circadian rhythms in responses to exercise are maintained in amplitude, some disappear, or are undetect-

Table 1
Circadian Characteristics of Fitness Tests, Including Acrophase of the Standard Rhythms[a]

Fitness test	Acrophase	Amplitude, % of 24-h mean	Reference
Whole-body flexibility	20.12	21.6	(65)
PWC$_{150}$	0.49	5.2	(73)
Standing broad jump	17.45	3.4	(78)
Anaerobic power (stair-run)	17.26	2.1	(79)
Leg strength	18.20	9.0	(80)
Back strength	16.53	10.6	(80)
Grip strength	20.00	6.0	(73)

[a]PWC$_{150}$ = physical working capacity at a heart rate of 150 beats/min. The times for the acrophase are in decimal clock hours.

able, whereas others become more marked during exercise. Some of these differing effects of exercise on circadian rhythms could be owing to experimental errors, such as failure to control prior activity and diet of the participants. The intensity of exercise and fitness of the individuals involved in the study may also affect the results.

Temperature

Fluctuations in body temperature mediate many circadian rhythms in performance. Reilly and Brooks *(81,82)* found that the acrophase and amplitude of the rhythm in rectal temperature remained unchanged during exercise despite the exercise-induced elevation in the mean value. Rhythms in skin temperature during exercise were generally in phase with their corresponding resting rhythms (as described in ref. *30*), but depended on the site of measurement—skin temperature of the exercising limb did not evidence rhythmicity, for example. Similar results were obtained in a more recent study *(83)*. Circadian changes in the thresholds to the cutaneous vasodilatation and sweating occur in response to the heat load produced by exercise. These thresholds change in phase with the circadian rhythm of resting core temperature *(84,85)*.

Aldemir et al. *(86)* described the time-courses of the changes in core temperature and forearm skin blood flow during 30-min bouts of exercise of equal intensity taken at 08:00 and 18:00. There was a more rapid rise of core temperature, coupled with a slower rise of cutaneous blood flow, in the morning compared with the evening exercise (Fig. 5). This time dependence of the thermoregulatory response to exercise can be explained in terms of the mechanisms accounting for the circadian rhythm of core temperature at rest *(30)*. Namely, in the morning when the resting temperature is rising, the body loses less heat than it produces and, while in such a "heat-gain" mode, responds less readily to imposed thermal loads. In the late afternoon, by contrast, when the phase of falling resting temperature is approaching, heat loss is promoted, as a result of which exercise will produce a smaller rise in core temperature and a more rapid increase in forearm skin flow.

Cardiovascular and Ventilatory Variables

Wahlberg and Astrand *(87)* studied responses of 20 men to both submaximal and maximal exercise at 03:00 h and 15:00 h. Heart rates during exercise were consistently

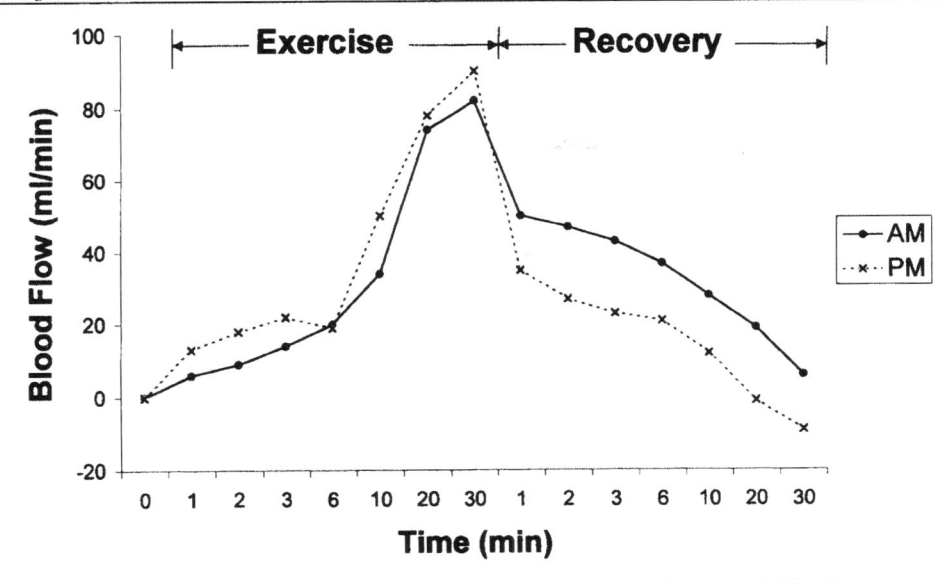

Fig. 5. Changes from baseline (B) during 30 min exercise at 70% VO_2max and 30-min recovery, the exercise being taken at 08:00 AM and 18:00 PM. Top, rectal temperature; bottom, blood flow (from ref. *86*).

lower at night, irrespective of work rate, the day–night difference amounting to 3–5 beats/min. Cohen and Muehl *(88)* measured heart rate at rest, during exercise on a rowing ergometer, and in the recovery period of this exercise at seven times during the solar day. The lowest heart rates occurred between 04:00 and 08:00 h. This temporal pattern was evident both during and following exercise. Whereas Cohen *(89)* found no circadian rhythm in heart rate during maximal exercise, Reilly et al. *(90)* found that the rhythm in heart rate persisted during maximal exercise, but with a reduced amplitude compared with the resting rhythm.

Both systolic and diastolic blood pressure, measured for 5 min after a set exercise regimen, were reported by Reilly et al. *(90)* to be unaffected by time of day. While emphasizing the measurement errors associated with conventional sphygmomanometry, these authors suggested that their pre-exercise conditions may have swamped any variations in blood pressure. Cable and coworkers *(91)* concentrated on the phenomenon of postexercise hypotension and reported that the fall in blood pressure during recovery from exercise was more pronounced in the morning. Cabri et al. *(92)* measured blood pressure before and after leg exercise on an isokinetic dynamometer at six times of the solar day. Although systolic blood pressure responses did not exhibit rhythmicity before or after exercise, diastolic blood pressure (postexercise) did vary with time of day. The greater perturbation of blood pressure in the morning compared to the evening led the authors to promote a "shock theory of exercise" when intensive activity is performed in the morning.

The amplitude of the rhythm in minute ventilation (V_E) is increased during light or moderate exercise. Reilly and Brooks *(93)* found that the V_E response to exercise displayed rhythmicity that was phased similarly to the resting rhythm, but 20–40% higher in terms of amplitude. The rhythm in V_E may explain the reports of mild dyspnoea when exercise is performed in the early morning.

Metabolism

The studies of circadian variations in metabolic responses to submaximal exercise are not conclusive. Reilly *(94)* performed a longitudinal study involving one person in order to control for intersubject variability. Circadian rhythmicity was observed in VO_2 (expressed in mL/kg/min) at a power output of 150 W, peaking at 14:40 h, but this rhythm could be explained by the circadian variations in body mass (values were slightly lighter in the afternoon). However, rhythmicity in VO_2 responses to a lighter work rate than 150 W was evident irrespective of changes in body mass. The time required for VO_2 to reach steady state (expressed as the fifth minute value) did not vary with time of day. No circadian variations were found for expired carbon dioxide (VCO_2) or the respiratory exchange ratio during exercise. This suggests there is no selective use of energy sources for exercise that is dependent on time of day rather than meal times.

The metabolic responses to exercise at maximal intensities do not demonstrate a circadian rhythm. In both longitudinal and cross-sectional studies, it has been found that VO_2max is a stable function, independent of the time of day of measurement (*see* ref. *34*). The amplitude of the resting rhythm in VO_2 if maintained during maximal exercise, would be <0.5% of VO_2max. Such a small amplitude would be difficult to detect, in light of the insensitivity of equipment used to measure VO_2max (*see* Fig. 6). This is not the conclusion that would be drawn if VO_2max had been estimated from heart rate *(34)*.

Perceived Exertion—The Psychological Connection

Circadian variations in the subjective reactions to exercise may be an alternative explanation for rhythms in maximal exercise performance *(95)*. Faria and Drummond *(96)* employed a crossover-treatment and reverse-sequence design to examine the effects of time of day on ratings of perceived exertion (RPE) during graded exercise on a treadmill. The strength of the relationship between RPE and heart rate depended on the time of day. The RPE values were higher during exercise carried out in the early hours of the morning (02:00–04:00 h) than in the evening (20:00–22:00 h). In this study, work rates were set to elicit heart rates of 130, 150, and 170 beats/min. The higher subjective ratings reported at nighttime would accord with the higher exercise intensities that were needed at this time to keep heart rate at the required value, irrespective of any circadian variation in RPE for a given workload.

FURTHER IMPLICATIONS OF CIRCADIAN RHYTHMS FOR EXERCISE

The effects of circadian rhythmicity permeate almost every aspect of exercise physiology, and a consideration of these factors goes a considerable way toward explaining rhythms in sports performance. There are further implications, however, which will be described in the following sections.

Endurance Races and Environmental Temperature

Endurance athletes frequently have to compete in hot environments, with their body temperatures above the level conducive to optimal performance and close to temperatures normally indicative of heat injury. In training for an attempt at the 1-h world record, cyclist Chris Boardman's core temperature after a simulation of the effort required for the whole hour was 40°C. If endurance exercise is carried out in the afternoon or evening, there may be a greater risk that such body temperatures are attained, since the rhythm in

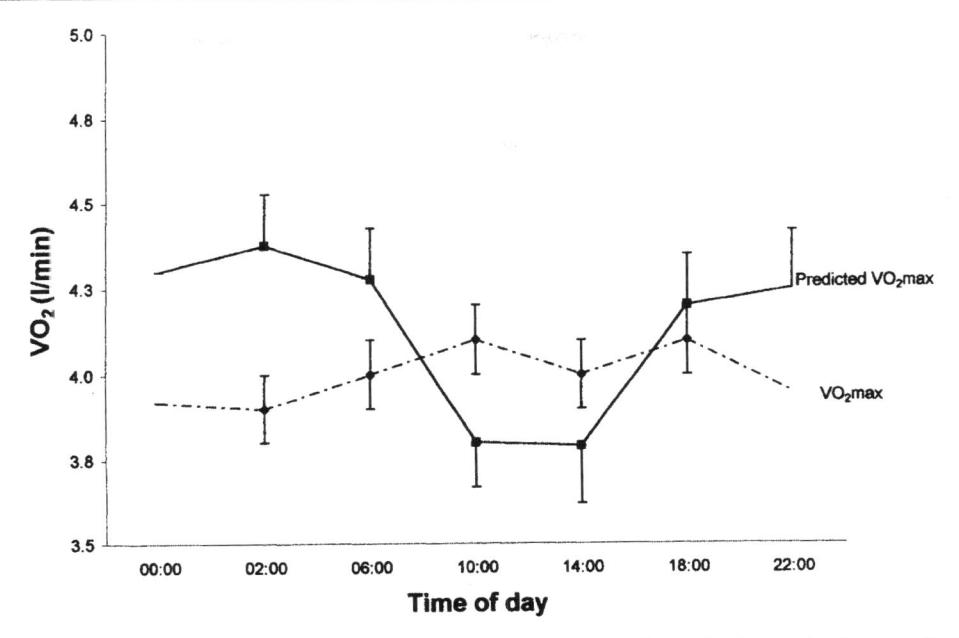

Fig. 6. The contrast between results measured for VO_2max throughout the day and values predicted from heart rate response to submaximal exercise (from ref. *24*).

the body temperature persists during exercise (*see* Temperature section). Although a set body temperature threshold for heat injury has yet to be confirmed, the margin of safety for heat injury can be calculated to be 0.5 to 0.8°C greater in the morning than the afternoon when a constant threshold is assumed to apply throughout the day.

Two sources support the hypothesis that in fit individuals, performance in sustained exercise is improved by lowered body temperatures. First, precooling body temperature before 1 h of submaximal exercise by an amount that corresponds to the amplitude of the circadian rhythm causes a significant increase in work rate *(97)*. Second, there is an interaction between self-selected work rate measured every 10 min during 80 min of submaximal exercise and the time of day *(98,99)*. In the evening, when body temperature was highest, individuals chose greater work rates at the beginning of the exercise period compared with exercise level chosen in the morning. However, as body temperature rose above optimal levels during the evening exercise, the work rate dropped. In the morning, by contrast, work rate gradually increased as body temperature rose toward optimal levels until, at the end of the exercise period, individuals chose higher work rates in the morning than in the afternoon.

Environmental temperature may be more favorable for athletes in marathon races in the early morning. Consequently, in hot and humid cities (e.g., Hong Kong, Singapore, and Penang), marathon races start at 05:00–06:00 h. In recent years, various competitive marathons have been scheduled at later times of day to coincide with the demands of television audiences. Such scheduling may be disastrous to athletes if environmental temperature is high.

In cold and wet conditions, however, athletes exercising at very low intensities (e.g., charity runners in marathon races) might be at greater risk of hypothermia in the morning. Their low work rate could be insufficient to maintain heat balance due to the high loss of heat to the cold environment. In such conditions there is a need for appropriate clothing to safeguard against a dangerous drop in core temperature.

Training and Time of Day

Research on the circadian variation in the efficacy of endurance training programs is equivocal. In one study, the circadian effects of an aerobic training program in three groups of men who exercised in the morning (09:00–09:30), afternoon (15:00–15:30), or evening (20:00–20:30) were investigated *(100)*. Each group performed exercise for 30 min on a cycle ergometer at 60% VO_2max—that is, the training stimulus was the same irrespective of time of day—for 4 d/wk over a 4-wk period. The VO_2max was estimated, and adaptive responses of heart rate and blood lactate levels to the training program were recorded. The afternoon group showed the greatest increase in estimated VO_2max after 4 wk, suggesting that aerobic training in the afternoon was the most effective. By contrast, other researchers found no significant differences in the training responses to morning and evening exercise. In another study, improvements in muscle strength following training sessions scheduled at 21:00 h were 20% higher than those following training carried out at 09:00 h *(101)*, although this was with maximal isometric contractions as the training stimulus, which can themselves vary with time of day. Moreover, the responses to training of each group of subjects were examined only at the times of day when training had taken place. Plasma levels of somatotrophin and testosterone are significantly higher following training in the evening compared with the morning *(102)*.

There is some evidence that the learning of motor skills is faster when tasks are performed in the morning; the greatest improvement in the performance of a pursuit rotor task was evident when the task was performed at 09:00 h *(103)*. Like the studies on strength, it is difficult to separate a true time of day effect on learning/training (the response) from the ability to execute the task (the stimulus) better at certain times of the day.

The interpretation of these types of study is complicated also by the circadian rhythms of perceived exertion in response to a training stimulus and of general mood. In future, investigators should not only take these factors into account, but also employ sport-specific skills and examine the effect of long-term training in the morning and afternoon on responses measured at both times of day. It seems unlikely that habitual training in the morning over many weeks (carried out by swimmers, for example) would fully reverse the evening superiority of self-selected training stimuli.

Current evidence suggests that practices where skills have to be acquired should be conducted early in the day or around midday, but more severe training drills and "pressure training" practices are best scheduled later in the day. Appropriate warm-ups are needed when athletes train or prepare for competitions earlier in the day than they are accustomed to.

Estimates of Performance

The existence of circadian rhythms in many of the variables associated with sports performance leads to complications when interpreting exercise tests conducted at different times of the day. For example, if an exercise test that raises heart rate to 160 beats/min is performed, since the resting heart rate shows a circadian rhythm with a peak and a minimum at about 18:00 and 06:00 h, respectively, the exercise will be slightly greater when it takes place at night or in the early morning. It is precisely this effect that is responsible for the circadian rhythm of estimated VO_2max (Fig. 6). If the exercise intensity is made equal at all times of testing—by making equal the increases in heart rate that are produced, or even by making equal the power output on a cycle ergometer—then the perceived exertion (and motivation needed to maintain the required rate of exercising) will be elevated in the night and early morning.

For clinical and training purposes, the effect of circadian rhythmicity should be taken into account when determining maximal voluntary contraction strength (MVC) at different times of the day. For such a correction, the cosinor characteristics of the curve relating MVC to time of day must be known. The $MVC._{corr}$ (MVC corrected for time of day) can be estimated from:

$$MVC._{corr} = MVC._t / [1 + A. \cos(15t + 15p)] \qquad (1)$$

where: $MVC._t$ is the value measured at time t (decimal clock hours), A is the amplitude of MVC (as a fraction of the mean), and p is the acrophase or peak time (decimal clock hours).

The correction was originally proposed for tests of isometric leg strength, but the equation is a general one. It can be employed for other variables that display time-of-day fluctuations in a cosinor manner *(104)*.

Injury, Soreness, and Medical Problems

As has been mentioned previously, particular care should be taken with warming up before heavy exercise taken in the morning (*see* Training and Time of Day section), and it is desirable to unload the spine before evening exercise, by lying down for at least 30 min, so that the compressibility of the spine can be restored (*see* Joint Flexibility and Stiffness section).

Delayed-onset muscle soreness (DOMS) is a transient condition of musculoskeletal trauma that can follow vigorous exercise, particularly that involving eccentric muscle contractions. Soreness ratings reach their peak 2–3 d after exercise, although any circadian variation within this period has not been researched. The plasma level of creatine kinase (following its leakage from the muscle cell) increases during DOMS, and so this enzyme has been employed as a marker of muscle damage. Lowest ratings of soreness and plasma levels of creatine kinase have been found after exercise performed in the evening *(102)*. The mechanisms responsible for this finding are unknown.

Exercise in the evening may be safer than morning workouts. Willich et al. *(105)* reported that the risk of acute coronary events triggered by physical activity is increased threefold in the morning compared with other times of day. There was a separate effect of physical exertion on cardiac events, the risk being slightly greater in inactive individuals who suddenly perform physical activity. Although there may be an interaction between these two effects, it would seem to be good advice for cardiac patients not to schedule their exercise bouts in the morning. For reasons discussed earlier (*see* Rhythms in Ventilation), asthmatic athletes should be discouraged from exercising before or soon after breakfast. Caution should also be exerted by them in the midafternoon if they train in urban areas, since this is usually the peak time of day for photochemical smog.

DISRUPTIONS CAUSED BY TRAVEL

Travel Fatigue

Travel fatigue linked with long-distance air flights poses a unique range of problems for athletes and team management. These travel stresses apply to all visitors to overseas countries. They include the procedures associated with obtaining and presenting the necessary travel documents, having enough money, checking in and getting through security, passport and customs screening, and so on. These stresses are independent of the direction or distance of travel and can be compounded by delay in boarding at takeoff. They call for a positive psychological approach to the problems and overriding any negative feelings.

Travel fatigue in long-haul flights may be linked with a gradual dehydration as a result of ambient conditions on board. This is owing to the water vapor content of the cabin air, which is low in comparison with fresh air. Headaches may also be linked to a combination of low air pressure and the loss of body water to the dry air within the airplane (106). Caffeine and alcohol are diuretics, and so are unsuitable for rehydration purposes.

Spending a long time in a cramped posture can cause stiffness, which can be relieved by simple stretching or by isometric contractions of the muscles affected. These exercises should help to eliminate residual stiffness at the end of the journey. Exercise can also be protective against deep vein thrombosis, which occurs as a result of being inactive in a constrained posture for a prolonged period.

The Problem of Jet Lag

Flights eastward or westward that entail travel across time zones additionally lead to a disturbance of the circadian body clock. This desynchronization of biological rhythms is the cause of "jet lag." This is a general malaise and a sense of feeling and acting "below par." Physical exercise will appear to be more difficult, and fine skills are likely to be executed less well until the symptoms abate (107). The most common of these symptoms are shown in Table 2.

Jet lag affects individuals differently, but in general it is more pronounced (that is, it is more severe and lasts longer) after a flight to the east than one to the west through the same number of time zones. It is more pronounced the more time-zones that are crossed rather than by the amount of change in culture that might be experienced. Younger and fitter people tend to suffer less than do older persons.

Women may be affected more than men. Disruptions of the menstrual cycle in female travelers have been linked to disturbances in melatonin secretion. In Scandinavia, it has been found that higher melatonin levels in the winter compared with summer values have an inhibiting effect on lutenizing hormone. As a result, ovulation might not occur during that cycle (108).

Although the symptoms will be exacerbated by all the general hassle of travel, the essential difference from travel fatigue is that jet lag does not wear off by the next day and the problems continue, because it can be difficult to sleep well for the first nights in the new time zone. The origin of the problem is a disturbance of the body clock.

JET LAG AND THE ATHLETE

Circadian rhythms must be taken into account when traveling across multiple time zones to compete in sport. Deleterious effects of jet lag will be exacerbated if there are

Table 2
Symptoms Associated with the Phenomenon of Jet Lag

Fatigue during the new daytime, and yet inability to sleep at night
Decreased mental performance, particularly if vigilance is required
Decreased physical performance, particularly with regard to events that require stamina or precise movement
A loss of appetite, coupled with indigestion and even nausea
Increased irritability, headaches, mental confusion, and disorientation

additional environmental stressors, such as heat or altitude, to be encountered. Performance can be adversely affected even when flights are within one country, coast to coast in the United States, for example *(109–111)*, though this has not been a universal conclusion (*see*, for example, ref. *112*).

For the first few days in the new time zone, all-out exercise should be avoided. Skills requiring fine coordination are likely to be impaired, which could lead to accidents or injuries if, for example, athletes conducted training sessions or matches too strenuously. While jet lag symptoms persist, even if only periodically during the day, it is recommended that training be light in intensity to reduce possibilities of accidents and injuries occurring. Individuals may be more vulnerable to defeat in the early rounds of tournaments at the hands of home-based players, unless the need for adjustment to the new time zone is considered in the timetable of the "tour." Where a series of tournament engagements is scheduled, it is useful to have at least one friendly match during the initial period, that is, before the end of the first week in the overseas country. Subject to these caveats, exercise for sports participants is recommended; it helps mental preparations for competition and prevents detraining.

The sleep loss that is part of the difficulties resulting from jet lag is unlikely to have a major adverse effect on exercise performance, even though the effects of substantial sleep disturbances are more pronounced on complex tasks than on gross measures, such as muscle strength *(113)*. Indeed the circadian variation in sports performances was found to be greater than that induced by partial sleep deprivation over three consecutive nights *(27)*. Difficulties in sleeping after crossing multiple time zones are eventually self-correcting, but disturbances may last longer following eastward compared to westward flights.

Secondary amenorrhea is common in air flight attendants *(108)* and occurs also among athletes who frequently travel across multiple time zones. Disturbance of the normal balance between estrogen and melatonin in females inhibits the surge in luteinizing hormone, which triggers ovulation. The extent to which the menstrual disturbances accompanying traveling across multiple time-zones in themselves alter athletic performance is uncertain.

THE BODY CLOCK AND JET LAG

The body clock is normally in harmony with the 24-h changes between daylight and darkness (that is, the endogenous and exogenous components of a circadian rhythm are in phase; *see* Fig.1). Since the earth spins on its axis, the sun is at its maximum height above the horizon at any point on the earth's surface once in every 24-h period. This time is called local noon. The world's 24 time zones effectively standardize all of these times.

The time zone that all others are related to passes through England, i.e., Greenwich Mean Time (GMT). Countries to the east of the UK have clocks that are ahead of this, because the sun rises earlier, whereas time to the west appears delayed with respect to this reference.

Adjusting to a new local time on flying to a new time zone presents difficulties for the endogenous body clock *(106)*. The body clock is slow to adjust to the change in schedule that is required on traveling to a new country with its own local time. Before adjustment takes place, the athlete might train or compete at a time when the body's signal denotes a preference to be asleep, and attempt to sleep when the body clock is directing wakefulness. It is during this period that jet lag is experienced. Once the body clock has adjusted, jet lag disappears.

It takes on average about 1 d for every time zone crossed to recover fully from the effects of jet lag *(114)*, although the recovery is nonlinear. The effects can be more intense at particular times of the day. The athlete may not recognize any adverse effects, unless he/she has to do something quickly, take decisions, or perform sports skills.

Local environmental factors can also influence the effects of jet lag symptoms. Dehydration associated with heat stress, for example, may accentuate difficulties in concentration and mental fatigue. A program of heat acclimatization prior to departure across multiple time zones can benefit sports participants *(115)*.

Procedures That Can Be Adopted Before and During the Flight

Ultimately, the aim of any procedures designed to alleviate the effects of jet lag must be to promote adjustment of its timing to coincide with new local time. This will require strengthening of appropriately timed zeitgebers in the new time zone. Additional procedures can be implemented before the new time zone has been reached.

A practice frequently adopted by athletes prior to flying overseas in a westward direction is to go to bed 1–2 h later than normal each night and get up 1–2 h later each morning. In contrast, those going eastward bring forward getting to bed and getting up by 1–2 h. It might not always be possible to do this, but its main benefit is to promote thinking ahead about times in the country of destination. It is not useful to try to adjust fully to the time zone transition before the journey, since this will interrupt training schedules and lifestyles too much, and will not, anyway, alter the body clock very much *(116)*.

Where there is a choice of flight times and airports, a schedule that makes planning the process of adjustment easier could be aimed for. A flight that gets the European traveler to a US destination in the evening, for example, would be helpful. For trips that entail crossing eight time zones or more, it can be beneficial to plan an overnight stopover midway, since this has been reported to reduce the symptoms experienced in comparison with a journey done without a break *(117)*. The ideal travel schedule is seldom available, but at least alternatives that are on offer can be consulted.

Taking naps and even sleeping pills for more prolonged sleep is an important issue. Naps and sleep should be avoided during the flight unless they coincide with night at the destination, or unless individuals have been chronically deprived of sleep.

Procedures That Can Be Adopted After the Flight

Complete adjustment so that local time and the body clock are in synchrony will take several days. It is only when fully adjusted to the new time zone that the athlete's performance will return to its peak. This applies to training as well as to competition. Until that time, it will be more difficult for an individual to produce maximal effort, both physically and mentally. While adjustment is taking place, the shape of a circadian rhythm is changed, generally displaying a lower amplitude, a lower peak value, and a lower average value overall *(65)*. The individual might choose to be helped during this time by the use of sleeping pills and pills to promote alertness.

SLEEPING PILLS

Disturbance of sleep is one of the unwanted corollaries of jet lag. Resynchronizing the normal sleep–wakefulness cycle seems to occur first, prior to restoration of physiological and performance measures to their normal circadian rhythm *(29)*.

Sports teams traveling on long-haul flights have used sleeping pills to induce sleep while on board *(34)*. Minor tranquilizers (e.g., temazepam) have been employed to help get travelers to sleep in order to be refreshed for immediate activities on arrival. Although drugs, such as benzodiazepines, are effective in getting people to sleep, they do not guarantee a prolonged period asleep. Also, they have not been satisfactorily tested for subsequent residual effects on motor performance, such as sports skills. They may be counterproductive if given at the incorrect time. A prolonged sleep at the time an individual feels drowsy (presumably when he or she would have been asleep in the time zone departed from) anchors the rhythms at their former phases and so operates against adjustment to the new time zone *(65)*. The administration of temazepam was found to have little influence on subjective, physiological, and performance measures following a westward flight across five time zones *(29)*. The circadian rhythms of athletes differed from those of sedentary subjects, although neither group benefited from the sleeping pill. Whether short-acting hypnotics, such as Zolpiden, which has a shorter half-life than most benzodiazepines, would be effective, remains to be clarified.

Jet lag and sleep disturbances may be more severe in members of the team management than in athletes. The former are generally older and less fit than the latter.

PROMOTING ALERTNESS

One approach towards combating the effects of loss of sleep arising from jet lag is to use pharmacological means for promoting and maintaining alertness. Such drugs include amphetamines, caffeine, Modafinil (an α-adrenoceptor antagonist), and Pemoline (a drug with dopamine-like properties). Although these drugs improve performance in several tasks, they adversely affect the ability to initiate and sustain sleep *(118)*. These effects could be counterproductive following time zone transitions. In addition, their effects on physical performance relevant to sport have not been adequately addressed, and their use could contravene doping regulations.

Promoting Adjustment of the Body Clock

Athletes and coaches must acknowledge the disturbance of the body's circadian rhythms following rapid travel across time zones and can then take steps to promote adjustment to the new time zone. Several methods have been suggested (*see* refs. *119,120*), differing in their practicality and in their potential side-effects. They encompass nutritional, environmental, and behavioral measures. In effect, they amount to strengthening the zeitgebers than normally adjust the body clock. Attention here will be directed to the two methods that seem to be most effective, melatonin and bright light.

Melatonin

In normal circumstances, melatonin from the pineal gland is secreted into the bloodstream between about 21:00 and 07:00 h (*see* Rhythms in Hormonal Secretions). It can be regarded as a "dark pulse" or "internal zeitgeber" for the body clock *(121)*. Studies have shown that melatonin capsules taken in the evening by local time in the new time zone reduce the symptoms of jet lag (*see*, for example, ref. *122*). The value of melatonin has been confirmed in both sexes, after flights in both directions, and at whatever time the flight itself takes place (*see*, for example, refs. *123–126*). These are important findings, but there are some caveats:

1. Jet lag, as defined in these studies, has concentrated on subjective symptoms; it is not known if there would also be improvements in mental and physical performance, and in motivation to train hard—or even if there would be further decrements.
2. It is not clear if melatonin produces its effect by promoting adjustment of the body clock or by some other means (increasing a sense of well-being or the ability to sleep, for example). Although recent work suggests that melatonin can adjust the body clock, this requires careful timing of ingestion according to whether the need is to advance or delay the clock *(10)*.
3. Melatonin has a lowering effect on body temperature, and this may account for its hypnotic action.
4. Melatonin is only just becoming commercially available (largely in the United States), and the results from clinical trials are still awaited.

In summary, more information is required before melatonin can be recommended and the Position Statement of the British Olympic Association was guarded about its use *(127)*. Systematic monitoring of athletes voluntarily taking melatonin (freely available in the US, but not licenced for Australia or Europe) during long-haul flights and days afterward would help provide a rationale for giving advice.

Bright Light Exposure and Exercise

Bright light (that is, of an intensity found naturally, but not normally indoors) can adjust the body clock. The timing of exposure is crucially important *(119)* and is the opposite of that for melatonin ingestion; thus, bright light in the morning "body time" (05:00–11:00 h) advances the clock on, and bright light in the evening (21:00–03:00 h) delays body time. Light should be avoided at those times that produce a shift of the body clock in a direction opposite to that desired. Table 3 gives times when light should be sought or avoided on the first day after different time zone transitions.

Adjusting sleep as fully as possible to the lifestyle and habits in the new zone would seem to be the best remedy. This is not always the case on the first day or so after the flight. Consider a westward flight through eight time zones. To delay the clock requires bright light at 21:00–03:00 h body time and its avoidance at 05:00–11:00 h. By new local time, this becomes equal to 13:00–19:00 h for bright light and 21:00–03:00 h for dim light (*see* Table 3). Natural daylight and night would provide this. By contrast, a flight to the east through eight time zones requires light at 05:00–11:00 h body time (13:00–19:00 h local time) and should be avoided at 21:00–03:00 h body time (05:00–11:00 h local time). That is, morning light for the first day or so would be unhelpful and tend to make the clock adjust in the wrong direction (though afternoon and evening light are fine).

Table 3
The Use of Bright Light to Adjust the Body Clock After Time Zone Transitions

	Bad local times for exposure to bright light	Good local times for exposure to bright light
Time zones to the west		
4 h	01:00–07:00[a]	17:00–23:00[b]
8 h	21:00–03:00[a]	13:00–19:00[b]
12 h	17:00–23:00[a]	09:00–15:00[b]
Time zones to the east		
4 h	01:00–07:00[b]	09:00–15:00[a]
8 h	05:00–11:00[b]	13:00–19:00[a]
10–12 h	Treat this as 12–14 h to the west[c]	

[a]Will advance the body clock.
[b]Will delay the body clock.
[c]Note that this is because the body clock adjusts to delays more easily than advances (see ref. 128).

After a couple of days, when partial adjustment has occurred, it is then advised to alter the timing of the light exposure toward that of the local inhabitants, so that the visitors' habits become synchronized with those of locals.

Even though the "bright light" required by these regimens is of an intensity normally not achieved in domestic or interior lighting, light boxes and visors are now available commercially that produce a light source of sufficient intensity. Light visors, in particular, might prove useful.

The question of whether physical exercise and inactivity can, in some way, add to the effects of light and dark, respectively, has not yet been answered. There is very little research evidence to suggest that exercise by itself will alter the speed of adjustment of the body clock in humans. Nevertheless, to combine exposure to bright light and exercise outdoors, and to combine dim light exposure (bright light avoidance) and relaxation indoors would seem a practicable way of combining training sessions and appropriate light exposure.

SUMMARY

In normal circumstances, circadian rhythms exert their effects throughout the body, preparing us for daytime activity and nocturnal sleep and rest. There is, in addition, an impact on athletic performance and on the inclination or ability to train hard.

The body clock, which is responsible for these rhythms, is normally adjusted each day by the very regularity of our lifestyle and the ways in which this will expose us to the environmental rhythms. Recent research has begun to reveal some of the properties of this clock, together with the ways in which it is controlled and exerts its effects throughout the body.

Mostly we are aware of our circadian rhythms only when pushing our body physically or mentally, or when the various timekeeping mechanisms underlying them are desynchronized, as happens in the case of long-haul flights. After such a flight, the general malaise known as "jet lag" arises, due to the transient mismatching between the timing of our body clock and the environment. Sports performance and the desire and ability to train effectively are compromised. Knowledge of the properties of the body clock enables advice to be given to a traveler so that these undesirable side effects can be alleviated.

REFERENCES

1. Moore R. Organization of the mammalian circadian system. In: Circadian Clocks and Their Adjustment. Ciba Foundation Symposium 183, John Wiley, Chichester, 1995, pp. 88–106.
2. Weaver D. The suprachiasmatic nucleus: a 25-year retrospective. J Biol Rhythms 1998;13:100–112.
3. Aschoff J. Circadian rhythms in man. Science 1965;148:1427–1432.
4. Honma K, Honma S. A human phase response curve for bright light pulses. Jpn J Psychiat 1988;42:167–168.
5. Czeisler C, Kronauer R, Allen J. Bright light induction of strong (Type 0) resetting of the human circadian pacemaker. Science 1989;244:1328–1333.
6. Minors D, Waterhouse J, Wirz-Justice A. A human phase-response curve to light. Neurosci Lett 1991;133:36–40.
7. Boivin D, Duffy J, Kronauer R, Czeisler C. Dose–response relationships for resetting of human circadian clock by light. Nature 1996;379:540–542.
8. Waterhouse J, Minors D, Folkard S, Owens D, Atkinson G, Macdonald I, et al. Light of domestic intensity produces phase shifts of the circadian oscillator in humans. Neurosci Lett 1998;245:97–100.
9. Arendt J. The pineal. In: Touitou Y, Haus E, eds. Biological Rhythms in Clinical and Laboratory Medicine. Springer-Verlag, Berlin, 1992, pp. 348–362.
10. Lewy A, Bauer V, Ahmed S, Thomas K, Cutler N, Singer C, et al. The human phase response curve (PRC) to melatonin is about 12 hours out of phase with the PRC to light. Chronobiol Int 1998;15:71–83.
11. Reppert S, Weaver D, Rivkees S, Stopa E. Putative melatonin receptors in a human biological clock. Science 1988;242:78–81.
12. Lewy A, Wehr T, Goodwin F, Newsome D, Markey S. Light supresses melatonin secretion in humans. Science 1980;210:1267–1269.
13. Graeber R, Sing H, Cuthbert B. The impact of transmeridian flight on deploying soldiers. In: Johnson L, Tepas D, Colquhoun P, eds. Biological Rhythms, Sleep and Shiftwork. MTP, Lancaster, 1981, pp. 513–537.
14. Graeber R. Jet lag and sleep disruption. In: Krugger M, Roth T, Dement C, eds. Principles and Practice in Sleep Medicine. Saunders, Philadelphia, 1989, pp. 324–331.
15. Leathwood P. Circadian rhythms of plasma amino acids, brain neurotransmitters and behaviour. In: Arendt J, Minors D, Waterhouse J, eds. Biological Rhythms in Clinical Practice. Butterworth, Guildford, 1989, pp. 131–159.
16. Reebs S, Mrosovsky N. Effects of induced wheel-running on the circadian activity rhythm of Syrian hamsters: entrainment and phase response curve. J Biol Rhythms 1989;4:39–48.
17. Mistlberger R, Marchant E, Sinclair S. Nonphotic phase-shifting and the motivation to run. Cold-exposure reexamined. J Biol Rhythms 1996;11:208–215.
18. Redlin U, Mrosovsky N. Exercise and human circadian rhythms: what we know and need to know. Chronobiol Int 1997;14:221–229.
19. Hastings M. Resetting the circadian cycle. Nature 1995;376:296,297.
20. Miyamoto Y, Sancar A. Vitamin B_2 based blue-light photoreceptors in the retinohypothalamic tract as the photoactive pigments for setting the circadian clock in mammals. Proc Natl Acad Sci USA 1998;95:6097–6102.
21. Atkinson G, Reilly T. Circadian variations in sports performance. Sports Med 1996;21:292–312.
22. Reilly T, Walsh T. Physiological, psychological and performance measures during an endurance record for 5-a-side soccer play. Brit J Sports Med 1981;15:122–128.
23. Conroy R, O'Brien M. Diurnal variation in athletic performance. J Physiol 1974;236:51P.
24. Reilly T. Circadian rhythms and exercise. In: McLeod D, Maughan RJ, Nimmo M, Reilly T, Williams C, eds. Exercise: Benefits, Limits, and adaptations. E. and F. Spon, London, 1987, pp. 346–366.

25. Rodahl A, O'Brien M, Firth P. Diurnal variation in performance of competitive swimmers. J Sports Med Physic Fitness 1976;16:72–76.
26. Baxter C, Reilly T. Influence of time of day on all-out swimming. Brit J of Sports Med 1983;17:122–127.
27. Sinnerton S, Reilly T. Effects of sleep loss and time of day in swimmers. In: MacLaren D, Reilly T, Lees A, eds. Biomechanics and Medicine in Swimming: Swimming Science VI. E. and F.N. Spon, London: 1992, pp. 399–405.
28. Reilly T, Marshall S. Cireadian rhythms in power output on a swim bench. J Swimming Res 1991; 7:11–13.
29. Reilly T, Atkinson G, Budgett R. Effects of temazepam on physiological and performanc variables following a westerly flight across five time zones. J Sports Sci 1997;15:62.
30. Aschoff J, Heise A. Thermal conductance in man: its dependence on time of day and on ambient temperature. In: Itoh S, Ogata K, Yoshimura H, eds. Advances in Climatic Physiology. Igaku Shoin, Tokyo, 1972, pp. 334–348.
31. Akerstedt T. Altered sleep/wake patterns and circadian rhythms. Acta Physiol Scand 1979; Suppl 469.
32. Cagnacci A. Influences of melatonin on human circadian rhythms. Chronobiol Int 1997;14:205–220.
33. Brezezinska A. Melatonin in humans. New Eng Med J 1997;336:186–195.
34. Reilly T. Human circadian rhythms and exercise. Crit Rev Biomed Eng 1990;18:165–180.
35. Veldhuis J, Johnson M, Iranmanesh A. Rhythmic and non-rhythmic modes of anterior pituitary hormone release in man. In: Touitou Y, Haus E, eds. Biological Rhythms in Clinical and Laboratory Medicine. Springer-Verlag, Berlin, 1992, pp. 277–291.
36. Swoyer J, Haus E, Lakatua D. Chronobiology in the clinical laboratory. In: Haus H, Kabat H, eds. Chronobiology 1982–1983. Karger, New York, 1984, pp. 533–543.
37. Mejean L, Kolopp M, Drouin P. Chronobiology, nutrition and diabetes mellitus. In Touitou Y, Haus E, eds. Biological Rhythms in Clinical and Laboratory Medicine. Springer-Verlag, Berlin, 1992, pp. 375–385.
38. Van Cauter E, Blackman I, Roland D, Spire J-D, Refetoff S, Polonsky K. Modulation of glucose regulation and insulin secretion by circadian rhythmicity and sleep. J Clin Invest 1991;88:934–942.
39. Schlierf G. Diurnal variations in plasma substrate concentration. Eur J Clin Invest 1978;8:59–60.
40. Van Cauter E, Shapiro E, Tillil H, Polonsky K. Circadian modulation of glucose and insulin responses to meals; relationship to cortisol rhythm. Am J Physiol 1992;262:E467–E475.
41. Waterhouse J, Akerstedt T, Lennernas M, Arendt J. Chronobiology and nutrition; internal and external factors. Canad J Diabet Care 1999;23(Suppl2):82–88.
42. Gaultier C, Reinberg A, Girard F. Circadian rhythms in lung resistance and dynamic lung compliance of healthy children. Effect of two bronchodilators. Resp Physiol 1977;31:169–182.
43. Smolensky M, Scott P, Barnes P. The chronopharmacology and chronotherapy of asthma. Ann Rev Chronopharmacol 1986;2:229–273.
44. Smolensky M, Alonzo G. Nocturnal asthma: mechanisms and chronotherapy. In Touitou Y, Haus E, eds. Biological Rhythms in Clinical and Laboratory Medicine. Springer-Verlag, Berlin, 1992, pp. 453–469.
45. Barnes P. Circadian rhythms in the respiratory system. In: Arendt J, Minors D, Waterhouse J, eds. Biological Rhythms in Clinical Practice. Butterworth, Guildford, 1989, pp. 71–82.
46. Smolensky M, Tatar S, Bergman S. Circadian rhythmic aspects of human cardiovascular function: a review by chronobiologic statistical methods. Chronobiologia 1976;3:337–371.
47. Zulch K, Hossman V. 24-hour rhythm of human blood pressure. Ger Med Monthly 1967;12:513–518.
48. Atkinson G, Coldwells A, Reilly T, Waterhouse J. Effects of age on diurnal variations in prolonged physical performance and physiological responses to exercise. J Sports Sci 1994;12:127.
49. Mancia G. Autonomic modulation of the cardiovascular system during sleep. New Eng J Med 1993;328:347–349.
50. Moore J. Chronobiology of the gastrointestinal system. In Touitou Y, Haus E, eds. Biological Rhythms in Clinical and Laboratory Medicine. Springer-Verlag, Berlin, 1992, pp. 210–217.
51. Goo R, Moore J, Greenberg E. Circadian variation in gastric emptying of meals in man. Gastroenterol 1987;93:515–518.
52. Touitou Y, Touitou C, Bogdan A. Circadian and seasonal variations of electrolytes in ageing humans. Clin Chim Acta 1989;180:245–254.

53. Robertson W, Hodgkinson A, Marshall,D. Seasonal variations in the composition of urine from normal subjects during a longitudinal study. Clin Chim Acta 1977;80:34–55.
54. Moore-Ede M. Circadian rhythms of drug effectiveness and toxicity. Clin Pharmacol Ther 1973; 14:925–935.
55. Koopman M, Minors D, Waterhouse J. Urinary and renal circadian rhythms. In: Arendt J, Minors D, Waterhouse J, eds. Biological Rhythms in Clinical Practice. Butterworth, Guildford, 1989, pp. 83–98.
56. Moore-Ede M, Brennan M, Ball M. Circadian variation of inter-compartmental potassium fluxes in man. J Appl Physiol 1975;38:163–170.
57. Pons M, Schnecko A, Witte K, Lemmer B, Waterhouse J, Cambar J. Circadian rhythms in renal function in hypertensive TGR (mRen2)27 rats and their normotensive controls. Am J Physiol 1996; 271:R1002–R1010.
58. Krieger D. Endocrine rhythms. Raven Press, New York, 1979.
59. Van Cauter E. Endocrine rhythms. In: Arendt J, Minors D, Waterhouse J, eds. Biological Rhythms in Clinical Practice. Butterworth, Guildford, 1989, pp. 23–50.
60. Minors D, Atkinson G, Bent N, Rabitt P, Waterhouse J. The effects of age on some aspects of lifestyle and implications for studies on circadian rhythmicity. Age Ageing 1998;27:67–72.
61. Reilly T, Waterhouse J, Atkinson G. Ageing, rhythms of physical performance and adjustment to changes in the sleep-activity cycle. Occup Environ Med 1997;54:812–816.
62. Hoddes E, Zarcone V, Smythe H, Dement W. Quantification of sleepiness: a new approach. Psychophysiology 1973;10:431–436.
63. McNair D, Lorr M, Droppleman L. EITS Manual for the Profile of Mood States. San Diego: Educational and Industrial Testing Service, 1971.
64. Folkard S. Circadian performance rhythms: some practical and theoretical implications. Phil Trans R Soc Lond 1990;327:543–553.
65. Reilly T, Atkinson,G, Waterhouse J. Biological Rhythms and Exercise. Oxford: Oxford University Press, 1997.
66. Atkinson G, Speir, L. Diurnal variation in tennis service. Percept Motor Skills 1998;86:1335–1338.
67. Folkard S, Akerstedt T. A three process model of the regulation of alertness and sleepiness. In: Ogilvie R, Broughton R, eds. Sleep, Arousal and Performance: Problems and Promises. Birkhauser, Boston, 1991, pp. 11–26.
68. Johnson M, Duffy J, Dijk J, Ronda J, Dyal C, Czeisler C. Short-term memory, alertness and performance: a reappraisal of their relationship to body temperature. J Sleep Res 1992;1:24–29.
69. Gifford L. Circadian variation in human flexibility and grip strength. Aust J Physiother 1987;33:3–9.
70. Reilly T, Tyrrell A, Troup J. Circadian variations in human stature. Chronobiol Int 1984;1:121–126.
71. Wilby J, Linge K, Reilly T, Troup J. Spinal shrinkage in females: circadian variation and the effects of circuit weight-training. Ergonomics 1987;30:47–54.
72. Wit A. Zagadnienia regulacji w procesic rozwoju sily miesnionej na przykladzi zawodnikow uprawiajacych podnoszenie ciezarow [in Polish]. Institute of Sport, Warsaw, 1980.
73. Atkinson G, Coldwells A, Reilly T, Waterhouse J. A comparison of circadian rhythms in work performance between physically active and inactive subjects. Ergonomics 1993;36:273–281.
74. Atkinson G, Greeves J, Reilly T, Cable T. Day-to-day and circadian variability of leg strength measured with the LIDO isokinetic dynamometer. J of Sports Sci 1995;13:18,19.
75. Hill D, Smith J. Circadian rhythm in anaerobic power and capacity. Can J Sports Sci 1991;16:30–32.
76. Hill D, Borden D, Darnaby K. Effect of time of day on aerobic and anaerobic responses to high intensity exercise. Can J Sports Sci 1992;17:316–319.
77. Reilly T, Baxter C. Influence of time od day on reactions to cycling at a fixed high intensity. Br J Sports Med 1983;17:128–130.
78. Reilly T, Down A. Circadian variation in the standing broad jump. Percept Motor Skills 1986;62:830.
79. Reilly T, Down A. Investigation of circadian rhythms in anaerobic power and capacity of the legs. J Sports Med Phys Fitness 1992;32:342–347.
80. Coldwells A, Atkinson G, Reilly,T. Sources of variation in back and leg dynamometry. Ergonomics 1993;37:79–86.
81. Reilly T, Brooks G. Investigation of circadian rhythms in metabolic responses to exercise. Ergonomics 1982;25:1093–1107.
82. Reilly T, Brooks G. Exercise and the circadian variation in body temperature measures. Int J Sports Med 1986;7:358–362.

83. Aoki K, Shiojiri T, Shibasaki M, Takano T, Kondo N, Iwata A. The effect of diurnal variation on the regional differences in sweating and skin blood flow during exercise. Eur J Appl Physiol 1995;71:276–280.
84. Marrotte J, Timbal J. Circadian rhythm of thermoregulating responses in man exposed to thermal stimuli. Chronobiologia 1982;9:375–387.
85. Stephenson L, Wenger C, O'Donovan B, Nadel E. Circadian rhythm in sweating and cutaneous blood flow. Amer J Physiol 1984;246:R321–R324.
86. Aldemir H, Atkinson G, Cable T, Edwards B, Waterhouse J, Reilly,T. Immediate effects of moderate exercise on core temperature and cutaneous thermoregulatory mechanisms. Chronobiol Int 1999, in press.
87. Wahlberg I, Astrand I. Physical work capacity during the day and at night. Work Environ Health 1973;10:65–68.
88. Cohen C, Muehl G. Human circadian rhythms in resting and exercise pulse rates. Ergonomics 1977;20:475–479
89. Cohen C. Human circadian rhythms in heart rate response to a maximal exercise stress. Ergonomics 1980;23:591–595.
90. Reilly T, Robinson G, Minors D. Some circulatory responses to exercise at different times of day. Med Sci Sports Exerc 1984;16:477–482.
91. Cable T, Reilly T, Winterburn S, Atkinson G. Circadian variation in post-exercise hypotension. Med Sci Sports Exerc 1995;27:566 (Abstract).
92. Cabri J, Clarys J, De Witte,B, Reilly T, Strass D. Circadian variation in blood pressure responses to muscular exercise. Ergonomics 1988;31:1559–1566.
93. Reilly T, Brooks G. Selective persistence of circadian rhythms in physiological responses to exercise. Chronobiol Int 1990;7:59–67.
94. Reilly T. Circadian variation in ventilatory and metabolic adaptations to submaximal exercise. Brit J Sports Med 1982;16:115–116.
95. Atkinson G, Coldwells A, Reilly T, Waterhouse J. Circadian rhythmicity in self-chosen work-rate. In: Gutenbrunner C, Hildebrandt G, Moog R, eds. Chronobiology and Chronomedicine. Peter Lang, Frankfurt, 1993, pp. 478–484.
96. Faria I, Drummond B. Circadian changes in resting heart rate and body temperature, maximal oxygen consumption and perceived exertion. Ergonomics 1982;25:381–386.
97. Hessemer V, Langusch D, Bruck K, Bodeker R, Breidenbach T. Effects of slightly lowered body temperature on endurance performance in humans. J Appl Physiol Resp Environ Exerc Physiol 1984;57:1731–1737.
98. Atkinson G, Reilly T. Effects of age and time of day on preferred work-rates during prolonged exercise. Chronobiol Int 1995;12:121–129.
99. Reilly T, Garrett R. Effects of time of day on self-paced performances of prolonged exercise. J Sports Med Phys Fitness, 1995;35:99–102.
100. Torii J, Shinkai S, Hino S, Kurokawa Y, Tomita N, Hirose M, et al. Effect of time of day on adaptive response to a 4-week aerobic exercise program. J Sports Med Phys Fitness 1992;32:348–352.
101. Hildebrandt G, Gutenbrunner C, Reinhart C. Circadian variation of isometric strength training in man. In: Morgan E, ed. Chronobiology and Chronomedicine. Vol II. Peter Lang, Frankfurt, 1990, pp. 322–329.
102. Gutenbrunner C. Circadian variations in physical training. In Gutenbrunner C, Hildebrandt G and Moog R, eds. Chronobiology and chronomedicine. Frankfurt, Peter Lang, 1993;665–680.
103. Hildebrandt G, Strempel H. Chronobiological problems of performance and adaptional capacity. Chronobiologia 1974;4:103–105.
104. Taylor D, Gibson H, Edwards R, Reilly T. Correction of isometric leg strength tests for time of day. Eur J Exp Musculoskeletal Res 1994;3:25–27.
105. Willich S, Lewis M, Lowel H. Physical exertion as a trigger of acute myocardial infarction. N Engl J Med 1993;329:1684–1690.
106. De Looy A, Minors D, Waterhouse J, Reilly T, Tunstall Pedoe, D. The coach's guide to competing abroad. National Coaching Foundation, Leeds, 1988.
107. Winget C, De Roshia C, Markley C, Holley D. A review of human physiological performance changes associated with desynchronosis of biological rhythms. Aviat Space Environ Med 1984; 54:132–137.

108. Harma M, Laitinen J, Partinen M, Suvanto S. The effect of four-day round trip flights over 10 time zones on the circadian variation in salivary melatonin and cortisol in air-line flight attendants. Ergonomics 1994;37:1479–1489.
109. Jehue R, Street D, Huizenga R. Effect of time zone and game time changes on team performance. National Football League. Med Sci Sports Exerc 1993;25:127–131.
110. Smith R, Guilleminault C, Efron B. Circadian rhythms and enhanced athletic performance in the National Football League. Sleep 1997;20:362–365.
111. Steenland K, Deddens J. Effects of travel and rest on performance of professional basketball players. Sleep 1997;20:366–369.
112. O'Connor P, Morgan W, Koltyn K, Raglin J, Turner J, Kalin N. Air travel across four time zones in college swimmers. J Appl Physiol 1991;70:756–763.
113. Reilly T, Piercy M. The effects of partial sleep deprivation in weight-lifting performance. Ergonomics 1994;37:107–115.
114. Reilly T, Mellor S. Jet lag in student Rugby League players following a near-maximal time-zone shift. In: Reilly T, Lees A, Davids K, Murphy W, eds. Science and Football. E. and F.N. Spon, London, 1988, pp. 249–256.
115. Reilly T, Maughan R, Budgett R, Davies B. The acclimatisation of international athletes. In: Robertson S, ed. Contemporary Ergonomics. Taylor and Francis, London, 1997, pp. 136–140.
116. Reilly T, Maskell P. Effects of altering the sleep-wake cycle in human circadian rhythms and motor performance. Proceedings of the First IOC Congress on Sport Science, Colorado Springs, 1989, pp. 106,107.
117. Tsai T-H, Okumura M, Yamasaki M, Sasaki T. Simulation of jet lag following a trip with stopovers by intermittent schedule shifts. J Interdiscipl Cycle Res 1988;19:89–96.
118. Akerstedt T, Ficca G. Alertness-enhancing drugs as a countermeasure to fatigue in irregular work hours. Chronobiol Int 1997;14:145–158.
119. Waterhouse J, Atkinson G, Reilly T. Jet lag. Lancet 1997a;350:1611–1616.
120. Waterhouse J, Reilly T, Atkinson G. Travel and body clock disturbances. Sports Exerc Injury 1997; 3:9–14.
121. Atkinson G, Reilly T, Waterhouse J, Winterburn S. Pharmacology and the travelling athlete. In: Reilly T, Orme M, eds. The Clinical Pharmacology of Sports and Exercise. Elsevier, Amsterdam, 1997, pp. 293–301.
122. Arendt J, Aldhous M, Marks V. Alleviation of jet lag by melatonin: preliminary results of controlled double blind trial. Brit Med J 1986;292:1170.
123. Arendt J, Deacon S, English J, Hampton S, Morgan L. Melatonin and adjustment to phase shift. J. Sleep Res. 1995;4(Suppl 2):74–79.
124. Comperatore C, Lieberman H, Kirby A, Adams B, Crowley, J. Melatonin efficacy in aviation missions requiring rapid deployment and night operations. Aviat Space Environ Med 1996;67:520–524.
125. Petrie K, Dawson A, Thompson L, Brook R. A double-blind trial of melatonin as a treatment for jet lag in international cabin crew. Biol Psychiatr 1993;33:526–530.
126. Suhner A, Schlagenhauf P, Johnson R, Tschopp A, Steffef R. Comparative study to determine the optimal dosage form for the alleviation of jet lag. Chronobiol Int 1998;15:655–666.
127. Reilly T, Maughan R, Budgett R. Melatonin: a position statement of the British Olympic Association. Br J Sports Med 1998;32:99,100.
128. Gundel A, Wegmann H. Transition between advance and delay responses to eastbound transmeridian flights. Chronobiol Int 1989;6:147–156.

23 Physical Activity and Mood
The Endocrine Connection

Gal Dubnov, MD, MSC
and Elliot M. Berry, MD, FRCP

CONTENTS
    INTRODUCTION
    PHYSICAL ACTIVITY, HORMONES, AND MOOD
    SUMMARY
    REFERENCES

INTRODUCTION

Physical Activity Causes Mood Changes

Various researchers have pointed out the affective changes brought about by physical activity (PA) *(1–5)*. The mood changes documented are generally an increase in "positive" mood states, such as calmness and pleasantness, and a decrease in "negative" mood states, such as depression and anger. The improvement in overall mood scores is seen after most types of exercise, both aerobic and anaerobic, that last for a minimal period of time or intensity.

It has been demonstrated that the regular participation in PA is more important in enhancing mood than the overall fitness *(3)*. This study shows that even in subjects with high fitness levels, inactivity is associated with decreased mood scores, suggesting an advantage of regular activity on fitness in influencing mood. In the group of regularly active subjects, a higher fitness level did not lead to a better mood, and affective scores remained independent of it. Fitness level would obviously be important in the physical benefits of PA, whereas the mental effects might be related to other chronic and repeated mechanisms. Further, PA deprivation in habitual exercisers increased mood disturbance scores, which improved when exercise was later resumed *(6)*. This suggests that repeated exercising might cause some degree of "addiction."

PA affects many different systems in the body and in various ways. Following PA, there is a rise in core temperature, a temporary lack of oxygen to some organ systems, and the secretion of different hormones and neurotransmitters is changed. These effects of PA are difficult to isolate, since they all occur together. Additionally, they may all lead to mood changes.

Several theories exist regarding the mechanism by which PA might cause mood changes, as reviewed by Yeung (5). The "thermogenic hypothesis" regards the elevation in the body's temperature as the cause for mood effects following PA. The "distraction hypothesis" posits that the distraction of one's mind from everyday stressors by PA is a major cause of mood elevation. The "mastery hypothesis" associates the mood changes with the achievement sensation in sport. The "endorphin hypothesis," which relates the affective changes to β-endorphin (βE), is the major hypothesis discussed here. Thus, we see that enjoyment from sport can be owing to a combination of changes brought on by PA, where are not all fully understood.

In a study comparing groups of volunteers before, and after, a PA class or a hobby class, several differences in mood changes were observed (1). Although the hobby class group showed less tension and depression as compared to preclass measurements, the PA group also exhibited less tension and depression, but also less anger, less fatigue, and a higher measure of pleasantness after the exercise. For several mood indices, PA had a greater effect than a hobby class. However, seeing that the part of the mood enhancement in the PA group was also seen in the hobby class, these results provide some support for the distraction hypothesis. The difference between PA and hobby groups can be related to additional mechanisms besides distraction. Other differences between groups were seen in some preclass measurements. The PA group was less sad, angry, and depressed than the contrasting hobby group, and this could be related to the chronic effects of PA on mood.

Another connection between two hypotheses—the thermogenic and the endorphin—was seen in a further study (7). It suggested that the increase in plasma βE, together with a breakdown of the blood–brain barrier following PA-induced heat load, led to higher opioid levels in the cerebrospinal fluid (CSF). This enabled the thermogenic hypothesis to "enhance" the endorphin response and to increase the cerebral action of plasma βE.

Mood Assessment: The Profile of Mood Scores

The most common test used to quantify mood changes following PA is the Profile of Mood States (POMS) (8). Other tests for specific measures of cognition, anxiety, frustration, fatigue, and others may also be used, but provide narrower spectra of mood indices. When taken together with the POMS, these tests generally give similar results (1,4,6). The POMS is a list of 65 adjectives describing various affective states, which the subject grades on a five-point scale. The test is then used to calculate six measures of mood: tension–anxiety, depression–dejection, confusion–bewilderment, vigor–activity, anger–hostility, and fatigue–inertia. The six scores may be combined to yield a "total mood disturbance" score.

One major methodological drawback of this kind of questionnaire is its subjectiveness, since it relies on self-rated, rather than observer-related mood scores. Perhaps in the future, biomarkers that assess mood levels, such as neurotransmitter metabolites, will allow for a more objective measurement of "mood" to enable comparison.

PHYSICAL ACTIVITY, HORMONES, AND MOOD

Hormones Can Cause Mood Changes

Many hormones are found to respond to PA (9). Hormones that could participate in affective changes are thyroxine (T4), cortisol, reproductive hormones, growth hormone (GH), βE, leptin, and more. Endocrine effects may modulate neurotransmitter synthesis, metabolism, and release, or they may alter the amount of receptors present on target neurons. Several hormones, which may influence mood states following PA, will be discussed in this section.

THYROID HORMONE

It is well documented that thyroid diseases may be associated with mood disturbances. The mechanism is not clear, but could be owing to the influence of thyroid hormone on synthesis of adrenergic receptors *(10)*. β-adrenergic receptors are also found as postsynaptic receptors for noradrenaline in the brain, so rises in thyroid hormone levels might elevate the brain adrenergic "tone."

Free T4 levels in plasma may rise following PA *(9,11)*. The reason for this increase is probably owing to an elevated level of free fatty acids in plasma, which displaces T4 from its binding protein. Since free T4 is the active hormone, this displacement has a functional effect. However, there is no correlation between the rise in free T4 levels and the rise in thyroid-stimulating hormone (TSH), which is the releasing hormone for T4 *(11)*. TSH levels have been reported previously to remain unchanged following exercise *(9)*, so total T4 levels should also remain constant. The increase in free hormone levels does not appear to have a physiological function. Otherwise, we would expect an activation of the releasing axis and higher TSH levels. The hormonal changes might be related to the increased energy requirements of the exercising body. The effect of repeatedly higher free T4 levels in the exercising person could add to the arousal sensation originating from noradrenergic brain activity.

CORTISOL

Cortisol is secreted from the adrenal cortex following stimulation by the adrenocorticotropic hormone (ACTH). ACTH, like βE, is derived from the large precursor protein proopiomelanocortin (POMC). These two hormones are secreted together in response to stress situations. Although ACTH activates the hormonal stress system, βE counterregulates it through its relaxing effect, discussed below. Receptors for cortisol are found in various brain areas and are associated with emotions and mood *(12)*.

Circulating plasma cortisol levels rise following aerobic and strenuous anaerobic types of PA *(13,14)*. Even though ACTH levels rise during short bouts of PA *(13,15)*, it takes about 20 min for cortisol to reach a higher and statistically significant level as compared to pre-exercise levels. This could be owing to the fact that steroid hormones are not stored, but require synthesis following the appropriate stimulus.

When cortisol and peripheral catecholamines were measured in relation to self-expressed mood, urinary cortisol levels correlated positively with the reported level of "alertness" by the subjects *(16)*. However, does cortisol cause arousal, or does the aroused state activate the stress pathway? An infusion of pharmacological levels of cortisol did not cause any significant changes in the measured affective states of healthy subjects *(17)*. Therefore, perhaps acute changes in cortisol levels, such as after PA, do not affect mood. Nevertheless, it should be noted that the cortisol effects on mood are probably more chronic and dose-dependent, as sometimes seen in patients on prolonged treatment with systemic steroids; short-term infusions may not be able to mimic the exact action of endogenous cortisol in the brain.

THE REPRODUCTIVE HORMONES

PA has been shown to affect levels of reproductive hormones in men and in women *(9)*. In women, moderate exercise during the midluteal phase can raise estrogen and progesterone levels. However, exercising during the follicular phase does not seem to influence estrogen levels *(18)*. Therefore, exercise-induced mood changes, which could be caused by estrogen, are expected to be dependent upon basal estrogen levels. Different conclusions may be reached with varying fertility status (prepubertal, premenopausal [amenorrheic/eumenorrheic], postmenopausal) and in different stages of the menstrual cycle *(9,18)*. The interaction between the reproductive hormones and the stress system *(19)* may also contribute to the response of estrogen levels to PA. Frequent activation of the stress hormone cascade might cause menstrual difficulties. Additionally, estrogen itself can elevate ACTH and cortisol levels *(19)*. Another interaction of estrogen and progesterone with cortisol may be through the competition between the different steroid hormones and free fatty acids on plasma binding proteins during PA.

The mood effects of the female sex hormones can be inferred from conditions in which estrogen levels decline, such as the late-luteal phase ("premenstrual syndrome"), following child delivery and entering menopause *(19,20)*. In these estrogen withdrawal states, mood can be enhanced by estrogen therapy, so estrogen is regarded as a mood-elevating hormone. The mechanism by which estrogen influences mood is probably through enhancement of monoamine neurotransmitter action by adding noradrenaline (NA) and serotonin (5-hydroxytryptamine [5-HT]) receptors to neural cell membranes *(21)*.

The counterregulatory hormone progesterone can be considered as a mood-destabilizing hormone *(20)* by reducing estrogen effects. Additionally, progesterone can act directly on GABA receptors as a neuroactive steroid, producing sedative or hypnotic actions *(12)*.

In trained men, acute aerobic or anaerobic exercise may induce a rise in plasma testosterone concentrations *(14)*. However, when testing for mood changes following infusion of supraphysiologic doses of testosterone, no such changes were found *(22)*.

INSULIN

Insulin concentrations are also affected by PA. After a single bout of exercise, plasma insulin levels fall for a day or more. The major effect of this decline on mood would be through the contribution to the higher level of plasma free fatty acids. A lower level of insulin releases the inhibition of the hormone-sensitive lipase in adipose tissue and allows for a higher rate of lipolysis. The rise in free fatty acids in plasma would increase the free fractions of T4 and steroid hormones, as discussed previously. Another metabolite affected by this mechanism is the amino acid tryptophan, precursor of 5-HT, which might elevate 5-HT levels in the brain.

As for the effects of glucose on mood, it has been shown that lower levels of glucose are associated with more negative affective states *(23)*. In this regard, a possible lower glucose availability to the brain during PA might be expected to depress mood. In a study in which a carbohydrate supplementation drink was given to participants in a training camp, the increased availability of carbohydrates had a limited effect on mood *(24)*. The only variable that changed was the measure of central fatigue, which according to the POMS was only slightly lower on some occasions in the supplemented group.

The effect of glucose on mood during or following PA is probably a minor one, since glucose levels in the brain could remain sufficient for its activity during PA. The mechanism of reduced fatigue might also be via the effect of slightly higher insulin levels on free fatty acids in plasma and the consequent lower tryptophan availability to the brain.

Leptin

Another hormone affected by PA is the adipose tissue-derived leptin. Leptin levels may decline in physically active people owing to a decline in fat mass *(25–27)*. Acute bouts of moderate intensity PA were not shown to influence its mean plasma levels *(25,28,29)*, although sample sizes were small and changes varied among individual subjects. Only an exercise as strenuous as a marathon run could alter its levels by reducing them only a little more than 10% *(27)*. Additionally, as with other hormones, there may be a diurnal variation in leptin levels, which may confound exercise-induced results *(30)*.

Leptin inhibits the action of neuropeptide Y (NPY), a ubiquitous peptide neurotransmitter, thus regulating food intake. Antagonism of the NPY-Y1 receptor caused anxiety in the rat as assessed by behavior in a specific maze *(31)*. Although the food-regulatory receptor seems quite different from the NPY-Y1 receptor, a connection between leptin and anxiety may be suggested.

βE and Mood: From POMC to POMS

Biological Roles of βE

βE is a 30 amino acid peptide that is derived from the large precursor protein POMC. This protein is synthesized mainly in the anterior pituitary gland on activation of the stress system and also produces ACTH. βE binds to opioid receptors in various tissues, especially relevant for this discussion, to the brain and skeletal muscle. In the brain, activation of μ opioid receptors in the locus ceruleus inhibits noradrenergic activity *(32)*, which might be part of the anxiolytic effect of βE. The diffuse and para-synaptic distribution of the μ opioid receptors on these cells implies that βE reaches the neurons mostly as a hormone, and not as a neurotransmitter *(33)*.

In the nucleus accumbens, opioids cause the release of dopamine (DA), which may explain the mood elevation and exercise dependence brought about by βE *(34)*. This dopaminergic excitatory effect is indirect, since the action of opioids is actually on GABA containing neurons synapsing with the dopaminergic cells *(35)*. Activation of μ receptors hyperpolarizes GABA neurons, thus releasing their inhibition from the dopaminergic neurons. The DA-containing cells, which originate from the ventral tegmental area to end in the nucleus accumbens, are believed to play a major role in opioid rewarding effects, along with additional nondopaminergic pathways *(35)*.

A metabolic role of βE is suggested to be owing to its effect on glucose levels during PA *(36)*. βE enhances glucose uptake by skeletal muscles. This effect could be in the muscle tissue by activation of local opioid receptors, as can be seen by a βE-induced glucose uptake by isolated muscle *(37)*, or by increasing the levels of the glucose counterregulatory hormones *(38)*.

Therefore, βE may have two distinct roles in exercise. The first is the cessation of the stress response, since βE is excreted together with ACTH perhaps as an intended counterregulator. βE has a longer half-life and, therefore, will terminate the stress response after ACTH is degraded. This mechanism will allow PA to be calming and relaxing. The stress response is not fully shut down, so the levels of alertness and vigor may remain elevated. The second role of βE may be the delivery of glucose fuel into the working muscle.

βE LEVELS AND MOOD CHANGES

Several clues regarding the involvement of opioid receptors in PA-induced mood changes have led to the discovery of the βE connection. The increased feeling of "pleasantness" after running *(2)* resembles that of the opioid drugs and is frequently termed the "runner's high." Cessation of habitual exercise results in withdrawal symptoms in mice *(39)*, and in humans—the POMS reveals increased tension, anxiety, depression, confusion, and total mood disturbance *(6)*. After observing that βE rises following acute exercise and correlates with mood improvement, a direct blocking of opioid receptors showed that PA-associated mood elevation is indeed opioid-mediated *(4)*. In this study, subjects were given naltrexone (an opioid receptor antagonist) or placebo prior to a high-intensity aerobics class. As expected, subjects that ingested the placebo exhibited mood improvements after class for most indices, whereas subjects given naltrexone did not. The total mood disturbance score decreased in the placebo group, but not in the naltrexone group.

Various stimuli elevate βE levels in plasma. These range from mental stressors, such as public speaking *(40)* or listening to techno-music *(41)*, to acute pain signals, such as 90 s of coronary balloon angioplasty *(42)*. Different types of PA can elevate plasma βE levels, as elaborated elsewhere in this volume. In brief—regarding aerobic exercise, a minimal duration of activity, lasting for about 60 min below the anaerobic threshold (the level of exercise in which the muscles require an anaerobic metabolism), has been suggested *(43)*. Regarding incremental exercise, the rise in βE appears after the anaerobic threshold is breached *(13)*. In this study, Schwartz and Kindermann *(13)* showed that the rise in βE parallels the rise in lactate levels. βE levels differed significantly from baseline at lactate concentrations of about 10 mmol/L. During resistance exercise, a very specific and intense workout is needed. In a study that employed six different combinations of intensity and rest, only one raised βE levels above baseline *(44)*. This protocol was the most demanding, since it raised lactate levels to peak around 10 mmol/L and also reached the highest levels of plasma creatine kinase (an index of muscle breakdown). Other protocols utilizing lower resistance volumes could not demonstrate βE elevations *(44,45)*.

Taken together, intensities that raise lactate levels as high as 10 mmol/L are not common among leisure time activities. The mechanism causing βE changes in a moderately exercising population would generally be the first one mentioned—a minimal period of aerobic PA, lasting about 60 min. Naturally, large deviations from this prediction might be expected among various exercisers.

The correlation between lactate and βE levels led Taylor et al. *(46)* to examine the importance of acidosis in βE release. Subjects infused with a bicarbonate buffer exhibited a suppressed βE response to exercise, as compared with placebo-infused controls. Therefore, the lowering of blood pH may be a major signal for βE release. βE correlated best with the measure of base excess, implying that the buffer capacity of the individual may determine the threshold for βE release by activity intensity. Various types and intensities of exercise that can lower pH levels below a specific individual threshold will cause βE secretion and its mood elevating effects. Interestingly, other exercise-released pituitary hormones, such as GH, follicle-stimulating hormone (FSH), and luteinizing hormone (LH), do not show this regulation *(47)*. In this study, prolactin exhibited a higher level following exercise combined with base administration as compared to exercise plus saline, suggesting an inhibitory role of acidosis on its release.

We conclude that an exercise load sufficient to lower pH beyond a certain individual level may elevate βE levels and cause mood changes. A possible bias in this cascade could be the choice of subjects. It could be that certain individuals who do not benefit from this mechanism are the ones who dislike PA, since most studies employ trained volunteers, who willingly engage in sports. Another issue is that variations in mood states before exercise could possibly alter the positive affective response, such as if the subject did not want to perform the exercise or vice versa: athletes who want to participate in the trial could be prone to easier mood enhancements.

Monoamine Neurotransmitters

Eventually, all the hormones previously discussed as modulating mood have been shown to alter neurotransmitter action. This is trivial, since "mood" itself is a product of interaction among neurons, although complex and spanning several brain regions. We shall briefly review the exercise-induced affective roles of the classic transmitters of the monoamine family—noradrenaline (NA), dopamine (DA), and serotonin (5-HT).

NORADRENALINE (NA) AND DOPAMINE (DA)

The production of NA and DA is derived from the amino acid tyrosine. The key enzyme in their synthesis is tyrosine hydroxylase, whose activity increases following stress, including PA *(48)*. The regulation of this enzyme is very complex, since it affects the levels of these very important neurotransmitters *(49)*. Cortisol may elevate enzyme levels by increasing transcription rate, although much more in NA-containing cells than in dopaminergic ones. An increase in the rate of synthesis and metabolism of NA and DA could influence mood. The higher levels of arousal and alertness following PA may be affiliated with higher NA levels. On the contrary, activation of opioid receptors on NA-containing cells of the locus ceruleus would inhibit their activity, suppress the arousal level and stress, and produce calmness *(32)*. The rewarding effect of βE in the nucleus accumbens is mainly through DA action *(34,35)* via a common pathway for most addicting agents.

SEROTONIN (5-HT)

5-HT is a neurotransmitter involved in appetite regulation, pain perception, mood, and sleep; it is possible that 5-HT plays a role in central fatigue during PA *(50)*. The synthesis of 5-HT is also based on an amino acid precursor—tryptophan. Once again, cortisol may play an important part in the regulation of the key synthetic enzyme, tryptophan hydroxylase *(51)*. Additionally, and in contrast to NA and DA synthesis, which is not enhanced by elevated tyrosine levels, 5-HT synthesis is affected by altering tryptophan levels *(52)*. This is owing to the fact that the enzyme is not saturated with its substrate tryptophan. Elevation of free tryptophan levels in plasma might therefore raise 5-HT levels in the appropriate neurons. Indeed, in brains of exercising rats, higher levels of free tryptophan raised 5-HT concentrations by 35% *(53)*.

The carrier protein for large neutral amino acids introduces several amino acids across the blood–brain barrier, including tryptophan. During PA, branched chain amino acids are utilized by the active muscle *(54)*, therefore allowing more tryptophan to enter the brain owing to decreased competition. In this case, would ingestion of branched chain amino acids influence central fatigue? A study in which supplementation of these amino

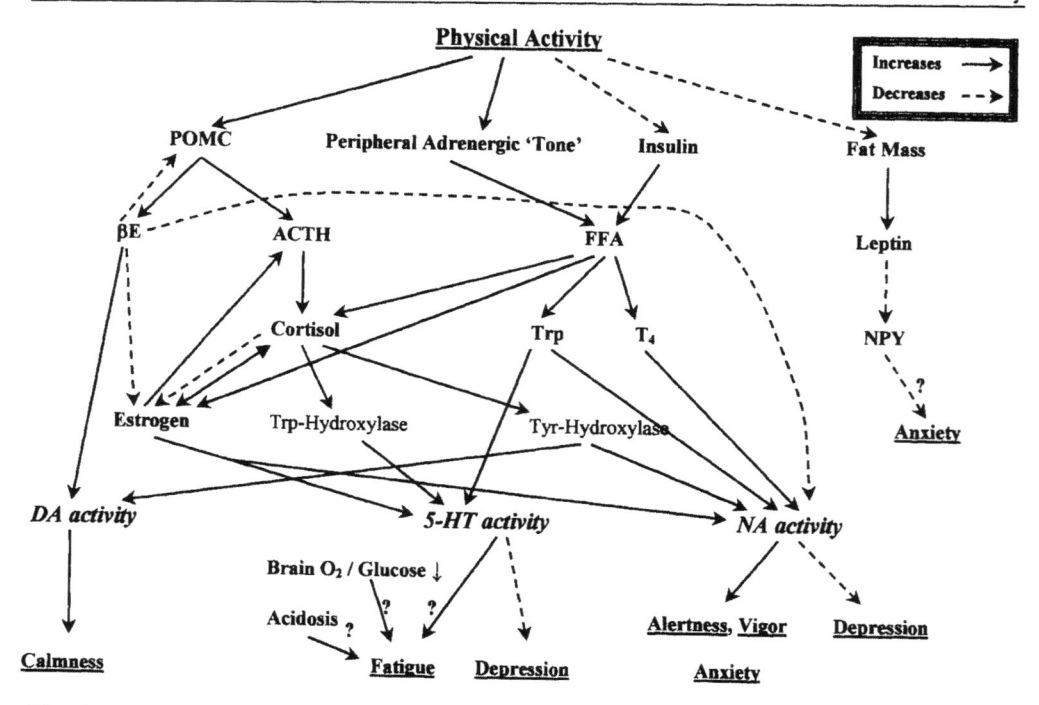

Fig. 1. Summary of the complex interrelationships among exercise, neurohumoral, and metabolic activity and their possible influences on mood states. Activation of the stress system during physical activity initiates several metabolic cascades, resulting in changes in neurotransmitter action. Both transmitter concentrations and receptor activity may be affected. Although neurotransmitters are considered, for simplicity, to be responsible for the different mood changes, the latter is probably a resultant of their combined actions.

A solid arrow indicates stimulatory, and a broken one, inhibitory effects. POMC—proopiomelanocortin; βE—β-endorphin; ACTH—adrenocorticotropic hormone; FFA—free fatty acids; T4—free thyroid hormone; Trp—tryptophan; Tyr—tyrosine; NPY—neuropeptide Y; DA—dopamine; 5-HT—serotonin; NA—noradrenaline.

acids was given to runners revealed only slight mood changes (55). For the measure of fatigue, one part of the study revealed a trend for slightly less fatigue in the supplemented group. Another part revealed no influence of the amino acid supplementation, and in both experimental and control groups, fatigue measures were higher postrace. Some positive effect of the supplementation was found—a better coping with complex cognitive tasks.

Another reason for higher tryptophan levels in plasma during PA is the lipolytic effect of exercise. The higher level of free fatty acids being mobilized in plasma displaces albumin-bound tryptophan and raises the free fraction of tryptophan, which is now available for entry into the brain.

In whole, both mechanisms may contribute to central fatigue during exercise. Another reason for fatigue could be merely energetic: slightly lower glucose or oxygen levels might also affect brain metabolism during PA, although for glucose this is unlikely (24).

SUMMARY

Moderate physical activity is widely accepted as a "recipe" for maintaining good health. Its beneficial action on delaying the onset or preventing many common diseases of western culture, such as ischemic heart disease *(56–58)*, diabetes *(59)*, stroke *(60)*, and cancer *(61,62)*, is widely accepted. However, an additional benefit emerges—one of psychological well-being and of a better ability to cope with modern-day stress. It too has its mechanisms, although not fully demystified at the present. Future research will certainly expand our perception of brain pathways involved in emotion and mood state.

The acute effects of exercise include hormonal changes, mainly involving the activation of the stress system, as summarized in Fig. 1. Among the substances released is the neurohormone βE, the levels of which seem to correlate best with indicators of effort, such as blood acidosis. Its calming and anxiolytic effects are mediated mostly through modifying DA and NA neurotransmission in defined brain areas.

REFERENCES

1. Lichtman S, Poser EG. The effects of exercise on mood and cognitive functioning. J Psychosom Res 1983;27:43–52.
2. Wildmann J, Kruger A, Schmole M, Niemann J, Matthaei H. Increase of circulating β-endorphin-like immunoreactivity correlates with the change in feeling of pleasantness after running. Life Sci 1986;38:997–1003.
3. Thirlaway K, Benton D. Participation in physical activity and cardiovascular fitness have different effects on mental health and mood. J Psychosom Res 1992;36:657–665.
4. Daniel M, Martin AD, Carter J. Opiate receptor blockade by naltrexone and mood state after acute physical activity. Br J Sports Med 1992;26:111–115.
5. Yeung RR. The acute effects of exercise on mood state. J Psychosom Res 1996;40:123–141.
6. Mondin GW, Morgan WP, Piering PN, Stegner AJ, Stotesbery CL, Trine MR, et al. Psychological consequences of exercise deprivation in habitual exercisers. Med Sci Sports Exerc 1996;28:1199–1203.
7. Appenzeller O, Wood SC. Peptides and exercise at high and low altitudes. Int J Sports Med 1992;13:S135–S140.
8. McNair DM, Lorr M, Droppleman LF. Profile of Mood States Manual. Educational and Industrial Testing Service, San Diego, 1971.
9. Howlett TA. Hormonal responses to exercise and training, a short review. Clin Endocrinol 1987;26:723–742.
10. Lazar-Wesley E, Hadcock JR, Malbon CC, Kunos G, Ishac EJ. Tissue–specific regulation of alpha 1B, beta 1 and beta 2 adrenergic receptor mRNAs by thyroid state in the rat. Endocrinol 1991;129:1116–1118.
11. Liewendahal K, Helenius T, Naveri H, Tikkanen H. Fatty acid-induced increase in serum dialyzable free thyroxine after physical exercise: implication for nonthyroidal illness. J Clin Endocrinol Metab 1992;74:1361–1365.
12. Holsboer F. Neuroendocrinology of mood disorders. In: Bloom, FE, Kupfer DJ, eds. Psychopharmacology: The Fourth Generation of Progress. Raven, New York, NY, 1995, pp. 957–969.
13. Schwarz L, Kindermann W. β-endorphin, adrenocorticotropic hormone, cortisol and catecholamines during aerobic and anaerobic exercise. Eur J Appl Physiol 1990;61:165–171.
14. Hackney AC, Premo MC, McMurray RG. Influence of aerobic versus anaerobic exercise on the relationship between reproductive hormones in men. J Sports Sci 1995;13:305–311.
15. Gerra G, Volpi R, Delsignore R, Caccavari R, Gaggiotti MT, Montani G, et al. ACTH and β-endorphin responses to physical exercise in adolescent women tested for anxiety and frustration. Psychiatry Res 1992;41:179–186.

16. Fibiger W, Singer G, Miller AJ, Armstrong S, Datar M. Cortisol and catecholamines changes as functions of time-of-day and self-reported mood. Neurosci Biobehav Rev 1984;8:523–530.
17. Goodwin GM, Muir WJ, Seckl JR, Bennie J, Carroll S, Dick H, et al. The effects of cortisol infusion upon hormone secretion from the anterior pituitary and subjective mood in depressive illness and in controls. J Affective Disord 1992;26:73–84.
18. Arena B, Maffulli N, Maffulli F, Morleo MA. Reproductive hormones and menstrual changes with exercise in female athletes. Sports Med 1995;19:278–285.
19. Chrousos GP, Torpy DJ, Gold PW. Interactions between the hypothalamic-pituitary-adrenal axis and the female reproductive system: clinical implications. Ann Intern Med 1998;129:229–240.
20. Stahl SM. Basic psychopharmacology of antidepressants, part 2: Estrogen as an adjunct to antidepressant treatment. J Clin. Psychiatry 1998;59(Suppl 4):15–24.
21. Biegon A, Reches A, Snyder L, McEwen BS. Serotonergic and noradrenergic receptors in the rat brain: modulation by chronic exposure to ovarian hormones. Life Sci 1983;32:2015–2021.
22. Bhasin S, Storer TW, Berman N, Callegari C, Clevenger B, Phillips J, et al. The effects of supraphysiological doses of testosterone on muscle size and strength in normal men. N Engl J Med 1996;335:1–7.
23. Taylor LA, Rachman SJ. The effects of blood sugar level changes on cognitive function, affective state and somatic symptoms. J Behav Med 1988;11:279–291.
24. Kreider RB, Hill D, Horton G, Dowens M, Smith S, Anders B. Effects of carbohydrate supplementation during intense training on dietary patterns, psychological status, and performance. Int J Sports Nutr 1995;5:125–135.
25. Perusse L, Collier G, Gagnon J, Leon AS, Rao DC, Skinner JS, et al. Acute and chronic effects of exercise on leptin levels in humans. J Appl Physiol 1997;83:5–10.
26. Kohrt WM, Landt M, Birge SJ Serum leptin levels are reduced in response to exercise training, but not hormone replacement therapy in older women. J Clin Endocrinol Metab 1996;81:3980–3985.
27. Leal-Cerro A, Garcia-Luna PP, Astorga R, Parejo J, Peino R, Dieguez C, et al. Serum leptin levels in male marathon athletes before and after the marathon run. J Clin Endocrinol Metab 1998;83:2376–2379.
28. Racette SB, Coppack SW, Landt M, Klein S. Leptin production during moderate–intensity aerobic exercise. J Clin Endocrinol Metab 1997;82:2275–2277.
29. Hickey MS, Considine RV, Israel RG, Mahar TL, McCammon MR, Tyndall GL, et al. Leptin is related to body fat content in male distance runners. Am J Physiol 1996;271:E938–E940.
30. Koistinen HA, Tuominen JA, Ebeling P, Heiman ML, Stephens TW, Koivisto VA. The effect of exercise on leptin concentration in healthy men and in type 1 diabetic patients. Med Sci Sports Exerc 1998;30:805–810.
31. Wahlestedt C, Pich EM, Koob GF, Yee F, Heilig M. Modulation of anxiety and Neuropeptide Y-Y1 receptors by antisense oligonucleotide. Science 1993;259:528–531.
32. Williams JT, North RA, Tokimasa T. Inward rectification of resting and opiate activated potassium currents in rat locus coeruleus neurons. J Neurosci 1988;8:4299–4306.
33. Moyse E, Marcel D, Leonard K, Beaudet A. Electron microscopic distribution of Mu opioid receptors on noradrenergic neurons of the locus coeruleus. Eur J Neurosci 1997;9:128–139.
34. Spyraki C, Fibiger HC, Phillips AG. Attenuation of heroin reward in rats by disruption of the mesolimbic dopamine system. Psychopharmacology 1983;79:278–283.
35. Di Chiara G, North RA. Neurobiology of opiate abuse. Trends Pharmacol Sci 1992;13:185–193.
36. Goldfarb AH, Jamurtas AZ. β-endorphin response to exercise: An update. Sports Med 1997;24:8–16.
37. Evans AAL, Khan S, Smith ME. Evidence for a hormonal action of β-endorphin to increase glucose uptake in resting and contracting skeletal muscle. J Endocrinol 1997;155:387–392.
38. Hickey MS, Trappe SW, Blostein AC, Edwards BA, Goodpaster B, Craig BW. Opioid antagonism alters blood glucose homeostasis during exercise in humans. J Appl Physiol 1994;76:2452–2460.
39. Christie MJ, Chesher GB. Physical dependence on psychologically released endogenous opiates. Life Sci 1982;30:1173–1177.
40. Miller PF, Light KC, Bragdon EE, Ballenger MN, Herbst MC, Maixner W, et al. Beta endorphin response to exercise and mental stress in patients with ischemic heart disease. J Psychosom Res 1993;37:455–465.
41. Gerra G, Zaimovic A, Franchini D, Palladino M, Giucastro G, Reali N, et al. Neuroendocrine responses of healthy volunteers to techno-music, relationships with personality traits and emotional state. Int J Psychophysiol 1998;28:99–111.

42. Hikita H, Etsuda H, Takase B, Satomura K, Kurita A, Nakamura H. Extent of ischemic stimulus and plasma β-endorphin levels in silent myocardial ischemia. Am Heart J 1998;135:813–818.
43. Schwartz L, Kindermann W. β-endorphin, catecholamines and cortisol during exhaustive endurance exercise. Int J Sports Med 1989;2:160–165.
44. Kraemer WJ, Dziados JE, Marchitelly LJ, Gordon SE, Harman EA, Mello R, et al. Effects of different heavy–resistance exercise protocols on plasma β-endorphin concentrations. J Appl Physiol 1993;74:450–459.
45. Kraemer RR, Acevedo EO, Dzewaltowski D, Kilgore JL, Kraemer GR, Castracane VD. Effects of low-volume resistive exercise on beta-endorphin and cortisol concentrations. Int J Sports Med 1996;17:12–16.
46. Taylor DV, Boyajian JG, James N, Woods D, Chicz-Demet A, Wilson AF, et al. Acidosis stimulates β-endorphin release during exercise. J Appl Physiol 1994;77:1913–1918.
47. Elias AN, Wilson AF, Naqvi S, Pandian MR. Effects of blood pH and blood lactate on growth hormone, prolactin, and gonadotropin release after acute exercise in male volunteers. Proc Soc Exp Biol Med 1997;214:156–160.
48. Chaouloff F. Physical exercise and brain monoamines: a review. Acta Physiol Scand 1989;137:1–13.
49. Vrana KE. Intricate regulation of tyrosine hydroxylase activity and gene expression. J Neurochem 1996;67:443–462.
50. Blomstrand E, Celsing F, Newsholme EA. Changes in plasma concentrations of aromatic and branched chain amino acids during sustained exercise in man and their possible role in fatigue. Acta Physiol Scand 1988;133:115–121.
51. Sze PY, Neckers L, Towle AC. Glucocorticoids as a regulatory factor for brain tryptophan hydroxylase. J Neurochem 1976;26:169–173.
52. Fernstrom JD, Wurtman RJ. Brain serotonin content: Physiological dependence on plasma tryptophan levels. Science 1971;173:149–152.
53. Blomstrand E, Perrett D, Parry-Billings M, Newsholme EA. Effect of sustained exercise on plasma amino acid concentrations and on 5-hydroxytryptamine metabolism in six different brain regions in the rat. Acta Physiol Scand 1989;136:473–481.
54. Wagenmakers AJM, Brookes JH, Coakley JH, Reilly T, Edwards RHT. Exercise induced activation of the branched-chain-2-oxo-acid dehydrogenase in human muscle. Eur J Appl Physiol 1989;59:159–167.
55. Hassmen P, Blomstrand E, Ekblom B, Newsholme EA. Branched chain amino acid supplementation during 30-km competitive run: mood and cognitive performance. Nutrition 1994;10:405–410.
56. Lakka TA, Venalainen JM, Rauramaa R, Salonen R, Tuomilehto J, Salonen JT. Relation of leisure-time physical activity and cardiorespiratory fitness to the risk of acute myocardial infarction. N Engl J Med 1994;330:1549–1554.
57. Haapanen N, Miilunpalo S, Vuori I, Oja P, Pasanen M. Characteristics of leisure time physical activity associated with decreased risk of premature all-cause and cardiovascular disease mortality in middle-aged men. Am J Epidemiol 1996;143:870–880.
58. Pols MA, Peeters PH, Twisk JW, Kemper HC, Grobbee DE. Physical activity and cardiovascular disease risk profile in women. Am J Epidemiol 1997;146:322–328.
59. Lynch J, Helmrich SP, Lakka TA, Kaplan GA, Cohen RD, Salonen R, et al. Moderately intense physical activities and high levels of cardiorespiratory fitness reduce the risk of non-insulin-dependent diabetes mellitus in middle-aged men. Arch Intern Med 1996;156:1307–1314.
60. Gillum RF, Mussolino ME, Ingram DD. Physical activity and stroke incidence in women and men. Am J Epidemiol 1996;143:860–869.
61. Thune I, Brenn T, Lund E, Gaard, M. Physical activity and the risk of breast cancer. N Engl J Med 1997;336:1269–1275.
62. Thune I, Lund E. The influence of physical activity on lung-cancer risk. A prospective study of 81,516 men and women. Int J Cancer 1997;70:57–62.

24 Hormones as Performance-Enhancing Drugs

Mark Myhal, PhD and David R. Lamb, PhD

CONTENTS

    INTRODUCTION
    ANABOLIC-ANDROGENIC STEROIDS
    GROWTH HORMONE AND INSULIN-LIKE GROWTH FACTOR I
    CLENBUTEROL AND OTHER BETA AGONISTS
    INSULIN
    THYROID HORMONES
    DEHYDROEPIANDROSTERONE
    $\Delta D^{4/5}$-ANDRO- AND NOR-$\Delta^{4/5}$-ANDROSTENE- DIONE/DIOL
    TAMOXIFEN
    CLOMIPHENE
    HUMAN CHORIONIC GONADOTROPIN
    TESTOLACTONE
    FINASTERIDE
    GAMMA-HYDROXY-BUTYRATE
    EPHEDRINE
    ANTICORTISOL DRUGS
    ERYTHROPROTEIN
    DOPING CONTROL
    CONCLUSIONS
    REFERENCES

INTRODUCTION

Numerous publications have addressed the medical, ethical, and legal issues surrounding nonmedical hormone use by healthy individuals. The ethical and legal implications of hormone use in sports to enhance performance are clear—it is unethical and illegal. However, the medical implications surrounding this practice are far less certain, particularly when hormones are used to enhance appearance or performance in noncompetitive athletic settings. A considerable amount of misinformation exists among both users and

From: *Contemporary Endocrinology: Sports Endocrinology*
Edited by: M. P. Warren and N. W. Constantini © Humana Press Inc., Totowa, NJ

their primary-care physicians. Many in the medical/scientific community are unaware of why some of these drugs are used, their basic mechanisms of action, and differences among agents within a class of drugs, such as anabolic-androgenic steroids. In addition, sensationalistic media coverage and anecdotal case reporting have further clouded our understanding of performance-enhancing drugs, has impeded research, and has suppressed potentially important clinical applications of these agents. Therefore, the purpose of this chapter is to

1. Provide an overview of hormones and related drugs commonly used to enhance performance and/or physical appearance;
2. Provide a critique of the various rationales given by individuals to support their use of performance-enhancing drugs; and
3. Discuss the basis for the prevailing dogmas surrounding the nonmedical use of hormones, particularly those involving side effects and overall risk.

Because anabolic-androgenic steroids remain the most controversial and widely used class of drugs for enhancing athletic enhancement and/or physical appearance and because they are widely used to enhance fat-free mass and alter body fat content and distribution in otherwise healthy individuals, a large portion of this chapter will be devoted to their use, especially for enhancing lean body mass. Topics will include an overview of commonly used anabolic-androgenic steroids, the rationale for their use, information on types of steroids used, effective doses, and adverse side effects. In addition, the use and medical implications of other nonsteroidal hormones and drugs, such as insulin, growth hormone, thyroid hormone, ephedrine, clenbuterol, and gamma-hydroxy butyrate, will be discussed.

Although a considerable amount of information presented in this chapter is based on published data, it also includes anecdotal information derived from users of various ergogenic drugs. The anecdotal information will focus primarily on user rationale, dosing, and perceived effects/side effects of compounds that have not been well studied in an athletic population.

It is important to note that although a considerable amount of drug and dose information will be presented in this chapter, it is for illustrative and educational purposes only. This information is not intended as a guide for ergogenic drug use or treatment. Much of this information is anecdotal and has not been adequately evaluated scientifically or medically. In addition, the authors do not condone the use of any drugs to enhance athletic performance.

ANABOLIC-ANDROGENIC STEROIDS

Rationale for Use

Anabolic-androgenic steroids, i.e., steroid hormones or synthetic analogs of steroid hormones that promote both tissue growth and masculinization, have been used in sport for almost 50 yr; the historical background of steroid use in sport has been thoroughly reviewed by others *(1–4)*. Although estrogenic steroid hormones can also promote anabolism, it is the androgenic compounds that are widely used to enhance lean body mass and to improve sport performance. Hereafter, the terms "anabolic steroids" and "steroids" will be used as synonyms for anabolic-androgenic steroids.

Both scientifically and anecdotally, there is little doubt that the use of anabolic steroids can cause significant decreases in body fat, increases in lean body mass, and improvements in muscular strength. The anabolic-androgenic activity of each steroid compound is a function of its chemical structure and/or metabolites, and this activity can vary considerably *(5–8)*. The most widely used anabolic steroids and some of their characteristics are described in Table 1.

In addition to those described in Table 1, numerous other anabolic-androgenic steroids are available on the world market. Some are designer steroids produced in clandestine laboratories for top athletes attempting to circumvent current drug testing methods *(27)*, whereas others are obscure foreign steroids that have had little clinical use so that far less is known about their actions and potential toxicity. Furthermore, many steroids obtained on the black market contain either little or no anabolic steroids, or the container may be labeled as a highly sought after agent, such as methenolone or oxandrolone, but actually contain a testosterone ester or methyltestosterone, respectively.

According to anecdotal reports, some athletes are using "anabolic" pellets designed for use in cattle. These pellets contain a mixture of either testosterone/estrogens or trenbolone/estrogens, and are purportedly used in one of three ways. The first two methods involve crushing the pellets and then either mixing the resulting powder with dimethylsulfoxide (DMSO) and applying it to the skin or mixing the powder with sterile sesame oil and injecting the suspension intramuscularly. The third method involves attempting to remove the estrogen component with methanol and/or diethyl ether and then mixing what is assumed to be the anabolic steroid component with either DMSO or sesame oil for transdermal or intramuscular use, respectively *(26)*. Apparently these athletes are willing to tolerate the potentially deleterious side effects associated with high doses of estrogens, nonsterile products, and contamination with toxic organic compounds in order to obtain relatively small amounts of anabolic steroids.

Mechanism of Action of Anabolic Steroids

A complete review of the mechanisms by which anabolic steroids elicit their anabolic, anticatabolic, and performance-enhancing effects is beyond the scope of this chapter. In brief, these drugs may act by binding with androgen and glucocorticoid receptors *(8,23,28)*, by exerting central *(29–31)* and peripheral *(32,33)* effects on neurotransmitters, and by interacting with and perhaps regulating the amount or activity of insulin-like growth factor I (IGF-I) or its binding proteins in the circulation and/or in the muscles *(34–37)*.

Demographics of Anabolic Steroid Users

It has been estimated that there are more than 1 million users of anabolic steroids in the United States *(38)*. Although it is not known with certainty the extent to which top male and female athletes use steroids, in some sports the striking level of muscularity, very low body fat percentages, frank virilization in women, gynecomastia in men, and acne in both genders are certainly suggestive of anabolic steroid use. In one study, the average estimated ratio of fat-free mass (FFM) to height (Ht) in a group of professional women bodybuilders was 0.40 kg/cm (range: 0.36–0.46 kg/cm) *(39)*. In contrast, a group of elite Australian male athletes exhibited an average FFM/Ht ratio of 0.37 kg/cm (range: 0.29–0.51 kg/cm), and for elite female Australian athletes this value was 0.29 kg/cm (range: 0.17–0.37 kg/cm) (K. Norton, personal communication). In addition to possessing a greater average FFM/HT ratio than the elite male athletes, the competitive women bodybuilders averaged 4.5% body fat, in comparison to an average of 10% in the elite

Table 1
Overview of Anabolic-Androgenic Steroids Purportedly Used for Athletic Enhancement

Drug brand name (Generic)	Route of administration	General structure	Common side effects	Anecdotal reports of efficacy	Comments
Delatestryl® Depo-Testosterone® Androderm® *Testosterone enanthanate, cypionate, and numerous other esters* (US)	IM aqueous suspension and oil-based esters, sublingual, and transdermal	17-β esters; all potent androgens that aromatize and 5 α-reduce to estradiol and dihydrotestosterone (DHT), respectively	17-β esterified forms exert minimally hepatotoxic and few adverse effects on blood lipids in low to moderate doses (600 mg/wk) (9). All forms cause dose-related androgenic side effects (PDR)	Effective for increasing skeletal muscle mass and strength (10).	Commonly used by male and female athletes; some forms are difficult to detect with current drug-testing methods
Testred® *Methyltestosterone* (US)	Oral	C-17 α-alkylated form of testosterone; aromatizable	Hepatotoxic, adversely affects blood lipids, causes common androgen related side effects, and has been associated with adverse psychological events (10)	Perceived by athletes to be ineffective for skeletal muscle mass and strength (10)	Rarely used by athletes because of toxicity and lack of perceived efficacy
Halotestin® *Fluoxymesterone* (US)	Oral	C-17 α-alkylated compound; fluoride ion at the 9-α position reduces aromatization potential (11)	Same as methyltestosterone	A few strength athletes use the drug short-term to increase aggressiveness (10,11); some female bodybuilders use it in low doses (10 mg/d) 2–3 wk prior to a competition to "harden" the physique	Short-term use only because of toxicity and limited anabolic properties
Anadrol® *Oxymetholone* (US)	Oral	C-17 α-alkylated compound; a potent aromatizable androgen	Implicated in numerous fatal hepatic events, including peliosis hepatis and hepatocellular carcinoma (11,12). Androgen related side effects, such as water retention, acne, balding, and gynecomastia are likely with higher doses (PDR)	Perceived to be most effective steroid for promoting size and strength gains	A 9-mo study of AIDS patients using oxymetholone in relatively high doses failed to demonstrate any adverse side effects (13).

Winstrol® Winstrol-V® *Stanozolol* (US)	Oral (humans) Oral and injectable (veterinary)	C-17 α-alkylated compound with a heterocyclic ring fused to ring A of the steroid. Nonaromatizable with reduced androgenic properties	Reduced hepatotoxic potential in comparison to other oral C-17 α-alkylated compounds (11)	More women than men perceive stanozolol to be an effective anabolic agent. Used by physique competitors because it causes little water retention. IM suspension perceived to be more effective mg for mg than the oral form	Use of IM suspension may elicit a positive drug test long after the last injection
Oxandrin® *Oxandrolone* (US)	Oral	C-17 α-alkylated steroid reduced in the 5-α position. Does not aromatize (11) and undergoes little hepatic metabolism (14)	Minimal hepatotoxicity; minimal androgenic effects in low to moderate doses (14). Did not cause virilization in women in doses up to 80 mg/d for 30 d (14). Use in children for up to 6 yr to promote linear growth did not cause significant side effects (15)	Very popular among female bodybuilders because it can increase muscle mass with little virilization. Popular for pre-contest use because it does not promote water retention or acne in moderate doses. Thought to be one of the safest and most potent oral anabolic agents available	Use (15 mg/d) increases skeletal muscle androgen receptor mRNA (292).
Deca-Durabolin® Durabolin® *Nandrolone phenylpropionate, decanoate,* and numerous other esters (US)	Injectable oil-based esters	A testosterone derivative lacking a C-19 methyl group. Undergoes less aromatization (16) than testosterone and has reduced androgenic potential (17–19)	Minimally hepatotoxic (20) with effects on blood lipids (21) similar to those of testosterone. The 5-α reduced form is 10 times less androgenic than dihydrotestosterone (18,19,22), thus reducing its androgenic activity in such tissues as the prostate, skin, and scalp.	Probably the most commonly used anabolic steroid by male and female physique competitors. Causes less water retention than testosterone esters. Thought to be among the safest steroids available	Urinary metabolites may be detectable for well over 1 yr following the last injection; the use of nandrolones has resulted in numerous positive drug tests (12)
Primobolan *Methenolone*	Injectable oil-based ester	1-α methyl derivative of dihydrotestosterone. Does not aromatize (12)	Minimal hepatotoxicity and androgenicity; causes little water retention (11)	Used by bodybuilders as a pre-contest drug to spare fat-free mass during dieting with little water retention and few side effects	This drug is also popular among women steroid users (11) but is not currently marketed in the US

(continued)

Table 1 (*continued*)
Overview of Anabolic-Androgenic Steroids Purportedly Used for Athletic Enhancement

Drug brand name (Generic)	Route of administration	General structure	Common side effects	Anecdotal reports of efficacy	Comments
Masteron Proviron *Dromostanolone propionate* *Mesterolone Androstanolone*	Injectable oil-based solution	Analogs of dihydrotestosterone (DHT); like DHT, these analogs do not aromatize *(12)*	Minimal hepatotoxicity; potent androgens *(12)*	Thought to "harden" the appearance of an already lean physique by some unknown mechanism. Because 5α-reductase is not present in skeletal muscle *(23)*, it is unclear what effects, if any, these drugs exert in muscle.	Because dihydrotestosterone upregulates androgen receptor mRNA in skeletal tissue *(24)*, a similar mechanism may exist in muscle. Thus, these compounds may potentiate the effects of circulating androgens
Dianabol® *Methandienone or methandrostenolone*	Oral	C-17 α-alkylated derivative of methyltestosterone	Side effects similar to those of methyltestosterone, although methandienone is significantly more anabolic *(11)*	Methandienone (Dianabol®) was the drug of choice for athletes through the late 1970s. It is no longer sold in the US legally, but is available on the black market	Counterfeits of this drug have been shown to contain methyltestosterone and clenbuterol *(25)*
Esiclene *Formebolone*	Injectable	Unknown	Purportedly painful to inject and contains a small quantity of lidocaine *(10)*	An anabolic steroid with inflammatory properties; used to swell a small muscle group immediately prior to a physique contest	There is no information available on the physiologic properties of these drugs in humans
Finajet Parabolan *Trenbolone acetate* Equipoise *Boldenone*	Injectable veterinary anabolic steroids	17-β acetoxyestra-trienone 1-dehydrotestosterone (17-β hydroxy-1,4-androstadien-3-one)	Trenbolones are purportedly renal toxic and mood-altering drugs *(10)* Users of boldenone describe effects/side effects similar to nandrolones	Used because human drugs are difficult to obtain	
Revalor-S/H/G® Synovex-Plus® *Trenbolone/ estradiol (livestock implants)*	Crushed pellets are mixed with oil and injected, or DMSO and applied to the skin *(26)*	Trenbolone and estradiol	Same as trenbolone plus increased risk of thrombosis, gynecomastia, and depression because of the estrogen component (PDR)	Used because human or common veterinary drugs are difficult to obtain	Some users attempt to extract the estradiol prior to administration using methanol and diethyl ether

male athletes. However, even though bodybuilders are often cited for their steroid use, they represent only a small fraction of the athletic population that uses anabolic steroids *(27)*.

Positive drug tests for anabolic steroids in athletes who exhibit some of the cosmetic characteristics described above *(27,40,41)* are consistent with the hypothesis of anabolic steroid use. (However, neither the absence of cosmetic effects nor negative drug tests necessarily prove that the athlete is "clean.") Furthermore, lightly muscled endurance athletes may utilize steroids for their anticatabolic and protein synthesizing properties. Thus, almost any sport that places an inordinate level of physical and psychological stress on an athlete could theoretically benefit from anabolic steroid use *(42)*.

Androgenic-anabolic steroids are also used by a growing number of nonathletes. For example, women with gynoid fat distributions exhibit greater body dissatisfaction than women with android fat distributions, and women are often dissatisfied with the appearance of their gluteal-femoral and triceps body regions *(43)*. Because anabolic-androgenic steroids are lipolytic and shift body fat from gynoid to android fat patterns *(44)*, some women who are distraught over their genetic fat patterning may use steroids in the hope of altering their fat distribution. Although interest in competitive women's bodybuilding is on the decline, some women seem to find a lean and muscular look attractive, and this could in part explain recent data showing increasing use of anabolic steroids in high-school women *(45)*. Similarly, the use of steroids for cosmetic purposes is presumably appealing to young males who grow up in a society that associates a lean, muscular physique with economic and social success.

Effects of Steroid Use on Body Composition and Sport Performance

BODY COMPOSITION

The positive effects of steroids on body composition include increased fat-free mass, decreased total body fat *(9,46–49)*, and a decrease in the percentage of body fat located in the gluteal, femoral, and triceps regions in women *(44)*. The effects of anabolic steroids on lipolysis and skeletal muscle mass are potentiated by caloric restriction *(44,50)* and mechanical loading *(9)*, respectively, and are evident in clinically relevant doses *(44,50)*. Thus, for those who participate in sports that demand a high degree of strength and skeletal muscle mass and/or a low percentage of body fat, the use of steroids could be of benefit.

In postmenopausal women undergoing caloric restriction, administration of 30 mg nandrolone decanoate every 2 wk for 9 mo increased fat-free mass, decreased body fat, redistributed abdominal body fat from subcutaneous to visceral stores, and increased thigh muscle cross-sectional area in comparison to a control group *(44)*. Also, in a cross-sectional study comparing steroid-using vs nonsteroid-using female bodybuilders, the steroid group displayed greater fat-free mass (58.2 ± 2.0 vs 46.1 ± 2.3 kg), decreased percent body fat (13.8 ± 0.9% vs 18.7 ± 2.3%), and greater cross-sectional area of the fibers of the biceps brachii than did the nonsteroid group. The steroid group consumed a combination of nandrolone decanoate, stanozolol, and testosterone enanthate intermittently over a 4.2-yr period, with an average dose of 175 ± 15 mg/wk *(46)*.

In men, treatment with 600 mg/wk of testosterone enanthate for 10 wk increased muscle mass, and this effect was augmented with resistance exercise *(9)*. Mean increases in lean mass were 6.1 and 3.2 kg in the steroid-treated groups with and without resistance exercise, respectively. In another study, increases of 7.5 kg of fat-free mass were observed following the weekly administration of 3 mg/kg of testosterone enanthate over a 12-wk period *(48)*. In addition, steroids with greater anabolic/androgenic ratios, such as nandrolone, stanozolol, boldenone, and oxandrolone, can elicit 5–7 kg increases in lean mass in as little as 6–8 wk, with doses totaling <300 mg/wk in some highly trained male and female physique athletes (personal observations).

Evidence for the effects of anabolic steroids on body fat distribution in young adult females has been accumulated in studies of women undergoing gender reassignment and women physique athletes. Women ingesting high doses of androgens experience a shift in body fat from a gynoid to an android distribution *(51)* and a decrease of subcutaneous body fat in the abdomen, hip, and thigh regions *(52)*. In contrast, postmenopausal women treated with estrogens maintain a gynoid fat pattern *(53)*, suggesting that fat patterning is controlled in large part by the ratio of circulating estrogens to androgens. In addition, some women who use steroids claim that it is easier to lose body fat when it is distributed in an android pattern. This contention is supported by evidence of greater fat loss in energy-restricted women who have android versus gynoid fat distributions *(54)*.

Furthermore, the lipolytic and fat patterning effects of anabolic steroids depend on the type of drug employed *(48)*. Thus, the contention by physique competitors that some anabolic steroids are preferred for precontest preparation because of their lipolytic effects on specific regional body fat stores may be correct.

EXERCISE AND SPORT PERFORMANCE

Investigations into the performance-enhancing effects of anabolic steroids began in the late 1960s and continued into the early 1980s; these reports have been comprehensively reviewed *(1)*. Some of these studies demonstrated a positive effect of steroids on strength when drug use was combined with resistance training *(55–59)*, whereas others did not *(60–66)*. Most of these earlier studies, whether their findings were positive or negative, were fraught with numerous confounding variables. Thus, in general, these investigations provided no definitive evidence to support or refute the purported performance-enhancing effects of anabolic steroids.

During the mid-1980s, antisteroid sentiment began to grow resulting from case reports of serious physical and psychological consequences associated with anabolic steroid use. In addition, the positive drug test of a Canadian sprinter in the 1988 Olympics set the political stage for a landslide of antisteroid legislation that culminated in the Federal Anabolic-Steroid Control Act of 1990, which classified anabolic steroids as Schedule III drugs. These legislative measures and exaggerations in the media of the side effects of steroid use stifled clinical interest in anabolic steroids as a therapeutic modality. In addition, research on steroids during this period was focused on documenting the deleterious effects of these drugs in an effort to dissuade potential users. Thus, until recently, there has been little effort to investigate any potentially positive effects of anabolic steroids.

Beginning in the mid-1990s, several clinicians began to experiment with anabolic steroids in an effort to augment muscle mass in human immunodeficiency virus (HIV) patients. Because the results from early case reports were promising *(67)*, clinicians and scientists began taking a renewed interest in this class of drugs that could theoretically help preserve muscle mass and strength in patients with wasting syndromes. In addition, since 1994, three papers have documented the performance-enhancing effects of anabolic steroids in athletes and in healthy men. The first study was a cross-sectional comparison of female bodybuilders who used steroids with a group who did not *(46)*. All of these women were highly competitive bodybuilders who had trained for roughly 6 yr with similar exercise regimens. The drugs were self-administered and included a combination of nandrolone decanoate, stanozolol, and testosterone enanthate. The drugs were used intermittently over 4.2 yr for a total average dose of 175 ± 15 mg/wk. The steroid users exhibited greater cross-sectional areas of the biceps brachii fibers, performed more work using concentric muscle actions, and produced greater average power and isokinetic strength when compared to the nonusers. Furthermore, there was less muscle fatigue during a concentric exercise challenge in the steroid users.

The second study reported data from the covert doping program conducted by the German Democratic Republic (GDR) prior to 1990 *(42)*. During this period, anabolic hormones were systematically administered to GDR athletes, with the most popular agents being oral-Turinabol and a variety of testosterone esters. These drugs were administered to both men and women who engaged in a wide variety of sports, including track and field, swimming, gymnastics, handball, kayaking, rowing, and various winter sports. Performance-enhancing effects of these agents were dramatic. For example, a veteran female shot-putter increased her throwing distance by roughly 2 m over a 3-mo period using <15 mg/d oral-Turinabol. Even after prolonged cessation of steroid use, this shot-putter retained a 1-m advantage over her previous best drug-free throws. In other events, increases of 2.5–5 m in the shot-put (men and women), 10–20 m in the discus throw (men and women), 6–10 m in the hammer throw (men), and 8–15 m in the javelin throw could be expected within a 4-yr period of steroid use. In addition, women track athletes who used steroids improved their times by 4–5, 5–10, and 7–10 s in the 400, 800, and 1500 m events, respectively. Striking increases in performance were also noted in women's swimming events *(42)*.

The third study investigated the effects of 600 mg/wk of testosterone enanthate administered for 10 wk to healthy men. The subjects were divided into four groups, two placebo groups with or without resistance training and two testosterone-treated groups with or without resistance training. The testosterone treatment alone increased cross-sectional areas of the triceps brachii and quadriceps femoris muscles and improved strength in the bench-press and squat exercises vs placebo treatment. When combined with resistance exercise, the testosterone-treated group demonstrated further increases in muscle cross-sectional area and strength, documenting a synergistic effect between anabolic steroids and resistance exercise. This study was well controlled, and the investigators administered the anabolic steroids *(9)*. In a similar study by Sattler et al. *(68)*, 30 male HIV patients were given 600 mg/wk of nandrolone decanoate for 12 wk; half of the subjects engaged in resistance exercise, whereas the others were sedentary. The results were similar to those observed by Bhasin et al. *(9)*. The group treated only with nandrolone increased lean body mass, muscle size, and muscle strength, and these effects were augmented with resistance exercise.

In summary, the recent scientific reports are consistent with overwhelming anecdotal evidence, namely that anabolic steroids in low to moderate doses, particularly in combination with resistance exercise, can enhance many types of exercise performance that depend on skeletal muscle function.

UNRESOLVED ISSUES

Several issues remain unresolved regarding the use of anabolic-androgenic steroids for athletic and/or cosmetic enhancement. First, it is unknown what minimal doses of a steroid or combination of steroids are necessary to produce significant increases in strength and muscle mass in healthy, resistance-trained men and women. Although there is anecdotal evidence that in well-trained athletes small therapeutic doses of anabolic steroids in conjunction with adequate dietary intake (total energy and protein) and resistance exercise can produce dramatic increases in strength and muscle mass, there are no well-controlled studies to document this effect. Second, some female physique competitors contend that it is possible to use various hormones to achieve a high degree of leanness and muscle mass without experiencing significant virilizing side effects (personal communications). These women contend that the use of modest doses of steroids, such as oxandrolone and methenolone, in addition to nonsteroidal hormones, such as growth hormone, and β-agonists, are in part responsible for their success as physique competitors while preserving their "femininity" following their competitive careers. Third, the belief that several different anabolic steroids used concurrently will elicit a significantly greater anabolic response than any single drug has not been addressed in controlled studies. Finally, there is speculation that some of the gains in lean mass and strength acquired while using steroids are maintained indefinitely following cessation of drug treatment. For example, in men, significant gains in lean mass may persist for up to 10 wk following cessation of steroid use (48). Whether these gains persist even longer is unclear. Anecdotally, some women physique competitors actually find it difficult to lose the muscle mass they gained while using anabolic steroids despite cessation of resistance training, and find it easy to surpass their presteroid strength and muscle mass if they resume resistance exercise in the absence of further steroid use (personal communications).

Types and Doses of Anabolic-Androgenic Steroids Used by Athletes

It is difficult to obtain accurate drug-use information from athletes because many of them mistrust the scientific community and are aware of potential legal penalties if their drug use is publicized (69). (In the United States, possession and distribution of nonprescribed anabolic-androgenic steroids can result in 1- and 5-yr prison sentences, respectively [70].) Thus, the use of steroids by athletes and nonathletes is probably substantially underreported. A summary of the anabolic-androgenic steroids used by athletes, their side effects, and their purported efficacy for performance enhancement is shown in Table 1.

TYPES OF ANABOLIC STEROIDS USED

Considerable controversy exists over the types of anabolic steroids that are commonly used by athletes. One recent study suggested that the drugs methyltestosterone and norethandrolone were those most commonly used by athletes (71). However, other studies do not support this contention. For example, a survey of over 500 anabolic-steroid users conducted in 1990 reported that the most commonly used steroids were nandrolone and testosterone esters; neither methyltestosterone nor norethandrolone was reported as being employed by those surveyed (10). Testosterone esters were ranked highly for increasing size and strength. Drugs that produced the greatest incidence of side effects included oxymetholone, testosterone suspension, fluoxymesterone, and methyltestosterone, whereas those producing the least side effects included oxandrolone, methenolone, nandrolone, and stanozolol.

In a 1992 survey conducted in Great Britain, the majority of male anabolic steroid users reported that testosterone or nandrolone esters were the drugs of choice, whereas the women preferred oxandrolone, stanozolol, and methandienone; methyltestosterone and norethandrolone were reportedly not used *(72)*.

Results obtained through unannounced drug-testing of 253 male and female bodybuilders at various national and international contests conducted over a 6-yr period in Flanders showed that the most commonly detected anabolic steroids were nandrolones (36.4%), methenolones (29.6%), and testosterones (11.9%), representing 77.9% of the total steroids used *(41)*. Methyltestosterone was detected in only 2.4% of those tested, and norethandrolone use was not detected in any competitor. In addition, the Flanders data showed that the percentage of competitors using more than two steroids concurrently was <15%. Thus, the majority of the competitors in this study used only one anabolic-androgenic steroid at a time, and most were non-C-17 α-alkylated agents *(41)*.

Testing by International Olympic Committee laboratories in 1993 revealed similar findings *(40)*. The most commonly detected steroids were testosterones (32.5%), nandrolones (23.9%), stanozolol (11.4%), metandienone (10.7%), and methenolones (7.7%). Again, methyltestosterone was detected in only 2.4% of the positive samples, and norethandrolone was not detected.

TYPICAL DOSES

The dose of anabolic-androgenic steroids used by athletes varies considerably and is often thought to exceed 10–40 times the recommended therapeutic dose *(71)*. It appears, however, that the average doses of anabolic steroids are generally less than five times the recommended replacement dose in men, which is 100 mg/wk. Data collected in the early 1980s showed that successful advanced-level physique and strength competitors used an average of 300 and 440 mg/wk, respectively, for 10–14 wk cycles *(11)*. The anabolic steroids included mostly testosterones and nandrolones, and a mix of oxandrolone, stanozolol, and methandienone. A survey by Korkia *(72)* reported that men and women used average doses of 385 and 143 mg/wk, respectively. Alway *(46)* reported that the average dose consumed by national-level women physique competitors was 175 mg/wk and that the drugs of choice were mostly testosterones, nandrolones, and, to a lesser extent, stanozolol. Even in studies documenting doses reportedly exceeding 1000 mg/wk, the overall percentage of those consuming >1000 mg/wk was <29% of the total, and these data were obtained from populations known for a high prevalence of anabolic steroid use *(73)*.

In addition to a limited supply of unadulterated black-market steroids, the cost of most pharmaceutical-grade anabolic steroids places further restraints on their use. For example, a conservative precontest drug array for a bodybuilder might include 10 mg/d of both stanozolol and oxandrolone and 150 mg/wk of nandrolone decanoate. The total drug dose would be <300 mg/wk. Based on 1998 wholesale pharmacy prices, a 12-wk cycle, if prescribed by a physician, would cost $1740. Thus, from a cost standpoint alone, it is unlikely that most steroid users could afford chronic high dosing, even if they could find legitimate access to anabolic steroids. This contention is supported by data from a 5-yr Australian study in which some subjects who had legal access to anabolic steroids chose not to continue with the drug program because they could not afford it *(74)*. Thus, although some athletes believe massive doses are necessary and have the resources to obtain them, it is unlikely that they represent the majority of current anabolic steroid users.

Side Effects of Anabolic-Androgenic Steroids

The side effects associated with anabolic-androgenic steroids use are numerous and involve multiple organ systems *(1,75)*; however, over the past 40 yr, the overall incidence of life-threatening events caused by the nonmedical use of steroids is believed to be low *(1)*. Nevertheless, sporadic case reports of morbidity and mortality in young athletes using steroids have spurred predictions that most users will inevitably experience serious consequences of steroid use *(76)*. The classification of anabolic-androgenic steroids as Schedule III drugs in 1990 seems to have had little effect on the nonmedical use of steroids *(38,77)*. In addition, because of criminalization, the distribution of anabolic steroids has been driven further underground, resulting in a thriving black market of counterfeit drugs. Furthermore, users are now more reluctant to seek, or are sometimes refused, medical supervision. Thus, the risks involving the use of anabolic-androgenic steroids have increased well beyond those of the drugs themselves.

A comprehensive review of the potential side effects of anabolic steroid use in apparently healthy individuals is beyond the scope of this chapter. Some of the more commonly reported adverse effects are listed in Table 1, and a brief summary of some recent reports on human subjects is included below.

POTENTIAL FLAWS IN CLINICAL CASE REPORTS

With the exception of the association between hepatic dysfunction and the use of some oral anabolic-androgenic steroids *(78)*, many of the reports of serious side effects in otherwise healthy individuals have come from anecdotal case studies *(1,75,79)*. Whether there is an underreporting of serious steroid-related side effects in such case reports is unclear. Although some of these isolated reports are disconcerting, the occurrence of serious adverse effects reported in case studies is many times in direct contrast to the lack of such effects reported during controlled clinical studies. For example, a recent case report describes a 25-yr-old male athlete who suffered an acute myocardial infarction attributed to the use of the steroid nandrolone decanoate *(80)*. However, over the past 20 yr, there have been no reports of adverse circulatory events during clinically controlled administration of nandrolone decanoate, including doses identical to those administered to the aforementioned athlete *(16,20,81–84)*.

Authors of case reports are often quick to underscore the association between an adverse medical event and anabolic steroid use, but they often gloss over or fail to account for other potential contributing factors. In addition, these case reports cannot be evaluated statistically, so their true significance remains unclear. For example, in 1995, it was estimated that for every 100,000 North American males aged 25–44, roughly 20 will die of cardiovascular disease *(85)*. Considering there are an estimated 500,000 past and current anabolic-androgenic steroid users over the age of 26 *(38)*, it is therefore likely that about 100 users will suffer from premature cardiovascular mortality independent of steroid use. Thus, it is unclear if the occurrences of some medical events in users of steroids are significantly greater than those normally observed in the general population. The concerns raised about steroid use that are based on case reports may be akin to the continuing hysteria, government regulation, and litigation that have evolved as a result of anecdotal case reports of morbidity in women with silicone breast implants, despite the preponderance of evidence that now suggests little, if any cause-and-effect relationship *(86,87)*.

Confounding factors, such as undiagnosed pre-existing conditions, family history, and concurrent use of other drugs (knowingly or unknowingly), further dampen the credibility of case reports. Because most anabolic steroids are obtained on the black market and are of dubious quality *(25,88)*, there is considerable potential for adverse medical events to occur independent of steroid use. In addition, numerous other black market drugs are often used in conjunction with anabolic steroids to alter body composition. These include thyroid hormones, a variety of stimulants, β-agonists, and peptide hormones, such as growth hormone and insulin *(89–91)*. Viral, bacterial, and/or chemical contaminants may be present in counterfeit and/or adulterated steroids and may play a role in some of the complications associated with the nonmedical use of anabolic steroids. Furthermore, without a baseline evaluation prior to steroid use (i.e., blood work, electrocardiogram [ECG], general physical examination, and review of family history), it is problematic to infer a cause-and-effect relationship between steroid use and an adverse medical event.

Two case studies illustrate the doubtful nature of some of these case reports. The first describes an acute myocardial infarction in a 22-yr-old male weight lifter who used anabolic steroids. Upon admission to the hospital, the patient weighed 330 lb with total high-density lipoprotein (HDL) and low-density lipoprotein (LDL) cholesterol values of 14 and 513 mg/dL, respectively. He had been using intramuscular and oral anabolic-androgenic steroids for 6 wk prior to his heart attack. He had no family history and denied cocaine use, although no urinalysis was performed. The authors stated that this athlete developed hypercholesterolemia, platelet hyperaggregability, and a myocardial infarction while taking anabolic steroids, and suggested that the hypercholesterolemic state contributed to a coronary artery spasm. Twelve days following this patient's infarction, there was no evidence of platelet hyperaggregation, and 24 d after infarction, his LDL cholesterol dropped to 220 mg/dL *(92)*. What brings into question the association between steroid use and this subject's infarction was the rapid resolution of platelet hyperaggregation and elevated circulating cholesterol levels. Because androgen-induced increases in platelet hyperaggregation remain significant 2 wk following an intramuscular dose of testosterone enanthate *(93)*, it is questionable whether this subject's platelet hyperaggregation was dependent on his ingestion of anabolic-androgenic steroids. Furthermore, because parenteral anabolic steroids have long half-lives, it is unlikely that the steroid-related cholesterol changes would have been resolved in 24 d. In addition, the effects of oral anabolic steroids on LDL cholesterol persist for at least 2 wk *(94)*, and increases in LDL cholesterol associated with anabolic steroid use average roughly 30% *(94,95)*. Because this patient's LDL concentration was increased by at least 270%, it is likely that other factors, such as his myocardial infarction, may have influenced his circulating cholesterol concentrations.

A second case involved a 29-yr-old bodybuilder who developed systemic lupus erythematosus following a 6 wk cycle of oral nandrolone (75 mg/d) *(96)*. It was speculated that his ingestion of nandrolone suppressed endogenous testosterone levels and, in conjunction with pre-existing hyperprolactinemia, triggered the lupus. This was the only case report of this nature; nevertheless, the authors suggested that, "drug induced systemic lupus erythematosus may represent a new addition to the growing list of health hazards associated with anabolic steroid use *(96)*." There are several potential flaws with this conclusion. First, the only oral nandrolone derivative (ethylestrenol) manufactured in the United States was discontinued years ago, and was available only in 2-mg tablets. Thus, it is very unlikely that this subject was actually consuming oral nandrolone. Second, his circulating testosterone was within normal limits at admission and remained unchanged during an 8-mo follow-up. Because nandrolones suppress circulating testosterone levels *(82,84)*, it is unlikely that this individual was actually consuming an active steroid hormone. Third, his anabolic steroid use was not verified by urinalysis.

In summary, if case reports are to be scientifically credible, a concerted effort must be made to collect enough data to suggest a sound cause-and-effect relationship. Prior to the mid-1980s, clinicians could rely on drug use information provided by the user, but today even the user often has no idea what he or she is ingesting. Therefore, the following guidelines should be followed when an athlete presents with a serious medical condition in which anabolic steroid use is suspected.

1. Conduct a urinalysis screening for anabolic steroids, stimulants (including ephedrine), and beta-agonists (particularly clenbuterol). This is especially important when the subject is presenting with cardiovascular and/or psychological complications.
2. Assess the patient's current endocrine status, especially thyroid (including thyroid-stimulating hormone [TSH]) and gonadal hormones (testosterone and luteinizing hormone [LH]). Because high doses of exogenous thyroid could lead to serious cardiovascular complications, its use should be ruled out. In addition, the level of gonadal dysfunction would give some indication if an active hormone were actually used.
3. If possible, obtain a sample of the drug(s) ingested for analysis. Because many black-market agents are "cut," the actual dosing may be far less than that reported by the user. Thus, even though the subject's urine may be positive for a certain drug, the actual dose of the drug in question may be so low that a physiological effect (or side effect) is unlikely. In addition, the possibility of viral, bacterial, and/or chemical contamination of parenteral agents should be investigated.

POTENTIAL PSYCHOLOGICAL SIDE EFFECTS

Numerous studies have suggested that anabolic steroid use may lead to significant psychological morbidity. Psychological pathologies associated with anabolic steroids include anxiety, psychosis, irritability, increased aggression, and antisocial and violent behavior *(69,73,97,98)*. Based on these studies, some have suggested that anabolic steroid users represent a serious public health threat *(73)*. However, with the exception of one small study employing methyltestosterone, an anabolic steroid rarely used by athletes *(99)*, many adverse effects have been documented solely in free-living populations and have not been observed in controlled clinical settings *(9,100,101)*. Although some of the free-living studies show an association between steroid use and abnormal behavior, they fail to take into account numerous confounding variables that may occur in conjunction with drug use.

It is clear that not all anabolic steroids elicit the same behavioral effects in mammalian models *(102)*, and it is unknown what steroids or combinations of steroids, if any, are more likely to cause adverse psychological events. Furthermore, most, if not all, subjects in steroid studies are using drugs of unknown origin and purity *(70,88)*; thus, it is quite possible that other psychoactive substances are being consumed unbeknownst to the user. For example, several bodybuilders were recently admitted to a hospital for ingesting 25 mg methandrostenolone (Dianabol®) manufactured in Thailand. Their symptoms included palpitations, tachycardia, tremor, nausea, vomiting, chest pain, and muscle cramps. Tablets were obtained for analysis, and results showed that each tablet contained 30 µg clenbuterol and 5 mg methyltestosterone. Thus, these individuals were suffering from an acute overdose of clenbuterol (25). The tablets were exact counterfeits of "Thai Dianabol" and further illustrate the problems with case reports.

Because anabolic steroids are often used during a preparatory phase of an athletic event, it is important that control groups be subjected to the same psychological and physiological stressors as the steroid group. For example, when bodybuilders are chosen for steroid studies, factors that occur in conjunction with contest preparation can adversely affect behavior independent of steroids, but these factors are often overlooked. During an average 12-wk contest preparation phase, bodybuilders undergo extreme restriction of energy intake and often carbohydrate intake. They also typically attempt to sequester themselves from many aspects of life to focus on intense training. These behaviors in themselves can produce many of the adverse psychological symptoms observed in anabolic steroid users (103–107). Furthermore, it is unclear what behavioral changes may occur in an individual engaged in a socially unacceptable and illegal activity, i.e., the use of black-market steroids (108), particularly when an attempt is made to conceal this activity from family members and friends. Because of the sensationalistic media coverage directed at bodybuilding and drug use, many bodybuilders, particularly women, are viewed as freaks and social outcasts (109). Thus, their sometimes paranoid and antisocial behavior may well be a reaction to societal pressures. In addition, steroid use, unlike recreational drug use, is difficult to conceal; steroid users can achieve dramatic changes in body composition in relatively short periods of time, making the use of these illegal drugs readily discernable.

Only recently have the psychological effects of suprahysiologic doses of androgens been examined in controlled settings in human beings. In one study, subjects were administered testosterone enanthate in doses of 600 mg/wk (roughly six times the replacement dose) for 10 wk (9). There were no changes in behavior or aggressiveness as assessed by the both the investigators and family members (110). Interestingly, in another steroid study, a control subject given placebo (oil) injections demonstrated increased aggressiveness (111). This supports the hypothesis that some anabolic-androgenic steroids users actually believe they are going to become more aggressive and act accordingly, or perhaps steroid use gives them an excuse to behave in an antisocial fashion (112).

In addition to behavioral problems, dependence (113), withdrawal symptoms (114), and depression (115) have been reported with and following the nonmedical use of anabolic steroids. However, these are isolated case reports, and controlled studies have not been undertaken to evaluate these phenomena or potential treatment protocols (114).

In summary, current evidence is not sufficient to draw cause-and-effect conclusions about adverse psychological side effects of using anabolic steroids, particularly in doses totaling <1000 mg/wk. Although it is likely that a small percentage of anabolic steroids users who employ massive steroid doses, i.e., >1000 mg/wk, particularly those with preexisting psychopathologies, may experience adverse behavioral problems, there is no justification to conclude that the nonmedical use of anabolic steroids represents a significant public health threat.

Possible mechanisms for the psychological side effects associated with anabolic steroid use include changes in neurotransmitter systems, hypogonadism following steroid use, direct effects of steroids or their metabolites on the brain, and interactions with glucocorticoid receptors. In animal models, high doses of anabolic steroids can affect brain neurotransmitter systems *(116)* and beta-endorphin levels *(117)*. The behavioral effects of anabolic steroids appear to be dependent on gender and on the type of anabolic steroid administered *(29)*. In humans, clinically relevant doses of anabolic-androgenic steroids can elicit antidepressant effects *(31,118)* and improve the overall mood of hypogonadal men and women *(119,120)*. In addition, fluoxetine is effective in resolving depression following steroid use, suggesting possible involvement of serotonergic pathways *(115)*.

Recent data from a transgenic mouse model suggests that estrogens, and not androgens, may be responsible for aggressive behavior, since male mice devoid of estrogen receptors lacked normal aggressive behavior *(121)*. Because many anabolic-androgenic steroids can be aromatized to estrogens, and estrogen administration elicits aggressive behavior *(122)*, it is possible that the aromatization of anabolic-androgenic steroids in the brain may be responsible for the adverse behavioral problems observed in some anabolic steroid users. Furthermore, the *de novo* synthesis of different estrogenic metabolites may be responsible for the contrasting behavioral effects observed among androgen analogs *(102)*.

What is unusual about reports of steroid withdrawal syndromes is that they seem to be predominant in physique athletes. Clinically, it is rare for other athletes to encounter problems with anabolic steroid cessation following their competitive careers *(123)*. In addition, clinical studies fail to describe depressed moods or withdrawal symptoms following supraphysiologic doses of anabolic-androgenic steroids *(9,82,84,101,111,124)*. Thus, the exact cause of mood disturbances following the use of steroids in some individuals, particularly physique athletes, remains unclear.

DYSLIPIDEMIA AND THE CARDIOVASCULAR SYSTEM

In general, the ingestion of oral C-17 α-alkylated anabolic steroids will cause an average 30% decrease in HDL, particularly the HDL_2 subfraction, and an average 30% increase in LDL *(125)*. The mechanisms for this effect are unknown, but apparently include an increase in the activity of hepatic triglyceride lipase that catabolizes HDL particles *(126,127)*. Most studies suggest that injectable non-C-17 α-alkylated anabolic steroids, such as testosterone and nandrolone esters, exert minimal adverse effects on blood lipids *(9,83,84,125,128)*. However, this is not a universal finding *(118)*. Possible mechanisms for this relatively benign effect of some androgens include their avoidance of degradation during the first pass through the hepatic portal system, the more extensive aromatization of these particular androgens to estrogens, which decrease hepatic triglyceride lipase activity *(94)*, and the lack of a C-17 α-alkyl group. However, it is unclear if the adverse changes in blood lipids as a function of testosterone use actually lead to an increase in the incidence of coronary artery disease among steroid users. For example, long-term treatment of transsexual women with high doses of testosterone results in significant adverse changes in blood lipids *(129)*, but does not increase the incidence of coronary artery disease in comparison to normal women *(130)*. Moreover, in animal models, treatment with high doses of testosterone does not necessarily lead to atherogenesis and may, in fact, be beneficial. In male rabbits fed an atherogenic diet, high doses of testosterone (25 mg/kg/wk) with or without estrogen elicited atheroprotective effects by reducing plaque formation in the aortic arch. In female rabbits, the administration of testosterone to the estrogen-treated group did not alter the atheroprotective effect of estrogen. These effects were independent of changes in blood lipids *(131)*.

Another potential factor in the development of heart disease in steroid users is their use of aromatase inhibitors or nonaromatizing androgens. Because many athletes perceive estrogen to be an ergolytic hormone, they either use aromatase inhibitors to decrease circulating estrogen concentrations when using aromatizable androgens, or they use nonaromatizable androgens, such as stanozolol. However, because estrogen has multiple cardiovascular protective effects *(132–135)*, these athletes may be increasing their risk of an ischemic event by decreasing circulating estrogen concentrations for prolonged periods of time.

OTHER POTENTIAL EFFECTS ON THE CARDIOVASCULAR SYSTEM

The effects of anabolic-androgenic steroids on platelet aggregation and the myocardium, and the relationship between any such effects and cardiovascular disease are unclear. Although some reports suggest a link between anabolic steroid use, platelet hyperaggregation, and changes in the myocardium, the relationship is far from conclusive *(136,137)*. Some studies have demonstrated left ventricular dysfunction in anabolic steroid users *(138)*, and others have not *(139,140)*. Occasional reports of cardiomyopathies and arrhythmias associated with steroid use have been published, and numerous mechanisms have been proposed *(75,89,136,141)*. However, such adverse effects have yet to be observed during clinical treatment with anabolic-androgenic steroids. This disparity may in part be caused by the use of contaminated counterfeit parenteral anabolic steroids by those who use steroids for nonmedical purposes *(142)*. Because intravenous drug use is an independent risk factor for the development of myocarditis *(143)*, case reports of cardiac pathologies and arrhythmias in some steroid users may be a function of the immunologic consequences of a past bout of myocarditis or healed myocarditis *(144)* caused by chemical or infectious contaminants present in counterfeit drugs, rather than by anabolic steroids.

Hypertension is perhaps the most overstated side effect associated with anabolic steroid use. It is not commonly observed in steroid users *(75)*, even those ingesting massive doses *(89)*. One recent study did find altered nocturnal blood pressure patterns in otherwise normotensive anabolic steroid users *(145)*; the clinical significance of this is unknown.

Overall, it is unclear what role anabolic-androgenic steroids may play in the development of cardiovascular disease. Considering that perhaps 10–20% of 1 million anabolic steroids users have ingested large doses over relatively long periods of time, only 30 life-threatening circulatory events have been linked to anabolic steroid use over the past 20 yr *(136)*, representing a very small percentage of steroid users. In addition, numerous factors, such as gender, type and dose of steroid, diet and antioxidant supplementation, percent and distribution of body fat, activity level, family history, and concurrent use of additional drugs or hormones, may either attenuate or augment any possible deleterious effects of anabolic-androgenic steroids on the cardiovascular system. Therefore, without adequate longitudinal data, it cannot be stated unequivocally that anabolic steroid users, particularly those who maintain low levels of body fat and total circulating cholesterol and have no family history or other predisposing factors, are actually increasing their risk of coronary artery disease, particularly with low to moderate dosing of certain anabolic steroids.

POTENTIAL EFFECTS ON HEPATIC FUNCTION

Liver disease is a well-documented side effect of most, but not all, C-17 α-alkylated anabolic-androgenic steroids, the exception being oxandrolone. In contrast, most non-C-17 α-alkylated steroids exert minimal hepatoxicity. Documented liver pathologies associated with anabolic steroids include cholestasis, peliosis hepatis, hepatocellular adenoma and carcinoma, and hepatic angiosarcoma and cholangiocarcinoma *(78)*.

The mechanisms by which steroids elicit their effects on the liver depend on their chemical structures. Alkylation at the C-17 position, particularly methylation, leads to the greatest risk of dysfunction, regardless of the route of administration. A keto group at the C-3 position can lead to greater dysfunction than a hydroxyl group in the same position. A saturated A ring appears to attenuate the hepatotoxic effects of the anabolic steroids *(78)*, which explains the lack of hepatotoxicity with chronic oxandrolone therapy *(14)*.

Overall, even with chronic anabolic steroid use, life-threatening hepatic events in otherwise healthy individuals are rare. Mild or moderate hepatic dysfunction generally resolves following the cessation of anabolic steroid use or by substituting a parenteral non-C-17 α-alkylated steroid for an oral C-17 α-alkylated drug *(146)*. Life-threatening hepatic events, such as hepatoma and ruptured peliosis hepatis, carry a less optimistic prognosis, but full recovery is possible with early detection and intervention *(78)*. Thus, chronic users of anabolic steroids, particularly those who consume large doses of oral agents, should undergo a periodic liver ultrasound examination because routine blood chemistries may not detect potentially life-threatening hepatic lesions in early stages. In fact, intense exercise and the resulting muscle damage can markedly elevate the blood levels of various enzymes typically associated with liver function *(147,148)*, and this can confound the interpretation of blood chemistry results.

POTENTIAL EFFECTS ON THE REPRODUCTIVE SYSTEM IN MEN AND WOMEN

Infertility and testicular atrophy have long been cited as potential adverse side effects of anabolic steroid use in men. Although all anabolic-androgenic steroids will suppress the hypothalamic-pituitary axis to some extent, the resulting infertility is generally reversible *(82)*, even in those who ingest high doses of steroids for long periods of time *(149,150)*. In addition, during an 8–10-yr follow-up of adolescent boys treated for excessively tall stature with high doses of testosterone (500 mg/2 wk for up to 3 yr), there was no evidence of impaired fertility *(151,152)*. For those steroid users who find testicular atrophy psychologically disturbing, the concurrent use of hCG can maintain both testicular size and normal spermatogenesis during high-dose testosterone treatment *(153)*.

Benign prostatic hypertrophy and prostate cancer are also cited as side effects of anabolic steroid use, but this has been reported only once in otherwise healthy steroid users *(75)*. In addition, clinical studies employing supraphysiologic doses of anabolic-androgenic steroids have not detected adverse effects on the prostate *(9,20,82,111)*. It is also important to note that not all anabolic steroids are metabolized to potent androgens; thus, the effects of anabolic-androgenic steroids on the prostate likely depend on the chemical structure *(19,154)* and androgenicity of the drugs.

The effect of anabolic-androgenic steroid use on fertility in women is unknown. High doses of androgens decrease circulating follicle-stimulating hormone (FSH) and sex-hormone-binding globulin (SHBG) concentrations in eugonadal women *(155)*, whereas no changes are observed in mean nadir and LH pulse amplitude and in circulating concentrations of estradiol, estrone, and adrenal steroids *(156,157)*. Menstruation is either diminished or absent in steroid users *(158)*, but ovulation may occur *(159)*. In addition, high circulating concentrations of testosterone cause marked changes in genital tract histology *(159)*, an upregulation of ovarian androgen receptor expression *(160)*, and pathological criteria consistent for the diagnosis of polycystic ovaries *(157)*. What effects these changes may have on fertility following steroid cessation is unknown, but former steroid users who tested positive at competitions have conceived apparently normal healthy children. Because ovulation may occur during a steroid cycle, it is imperative that the female user minimize the risk of pregnancy during this period with nonhormonal contraception methods.

ACNE

All anabolic-androgenic steroids may cause some degree of acne if taken in a high enough dose *(75)*. This is especially true with strong androgen preparations, which may cause severe scarring acne; however, more conservative doses of steroids, such as oxandrolone or methenolone, may produce little or no acne. Anecdotally, many bodybuilders use tretinoin and, more recently, adapalene gel for mild to moderate acne during anabolic steroid use. Adapalene gel is less irritating to the skin, which is especially important to bodybuilders as contest time approaches because peeling dry skin can cause a discernable mottling effect following the application of artificial tanning dyes. A few bodybuilders have used isotretinoin, but this agent can be hepatotoxic, and the hepatotoxicity may be augmented with oral steroid use.

VIRILIZATION IN WOMEN

With the exception of oxandrolone *(14)* and perhaps methenolone, if used intermittently in conservative doses, most women will experience some form of permanent virilization if they use anabolic steroids *(158,161)*. The degree of virilization depends on the drug, the dose, the duration of use, and the individual's response. Body composition changes during steroid use are similar to those experienced in young boys during puberty *(162)*. In addition to irreversible side effects, such as a deepened voice, increased terminal facial hair, and a hypertrophied clitoris, some of the hypertrophic effects of anabolic steroids on skeletal muscle in women may be permanent.

HAIR LOSS

Balding is common in those who use anabolic-androgenic steroids that undergo 5-α reduction to potent androgens. Anecdotally, the most common offenders in both men and women are testosterone and oxymetholone *(163)*. Some male and female bodybuilders use finasteride and/or ketoconazole 2% shampoo with some success to attenuate hair loss.

GYNECOMASTIA

In some male steroid users, gynecomastia may be caused by increased circulating estrogen associated with the use of aromatizable androgens and/or hCG, with decreased clearance of circulating estrogens as a result of impaired hepatic function, and/or with a temporary state of hypotestosteronemia following anabolic-androgenic steroid use *(11,12)*.

Tamoxifen can be used in an attempt to antagonize the effects of increased circulating estrogens *(164)*, but in many cases the gynecomastia does not regress, and surgical resection is necessary. Once the lesion has formed, even low doses of aromatizable androgens can stimulate further growth. Gynecomastia is generally an esthetic problem, but it is unclear if these lesions could become malignant at some point.

MUSCULOSKELETAL INJURIES

Ruptured tendons have been associated with steroid use in bodybuilders and powerlifters *(165)*, although there is no evidence that the incidence is greater in anabolic steroid users in comparison to nonsteroid-using athletes *(75)*. Although animal studies suggest a deleterious effect of anabolic steroids on the biomechanical and histological properties of tendons *(165)*, there are no human data to support this observation. In fact, a recent study by Evans et al. *(166)* found no ultrastructural differences in the ruptured tendons from athletes who did or did not use steroids. Nonetheless, it is possible that during high-dose steroid use, the tendon's ability to compensate for the rapid increase in muscle mass and force-generating capacity may be compromised. Therefore, the use of more conservative doses of steroids (allowing for a gradual increase in strength) and a reduction of training intensity and loads following a steroid cycle may minimize the risk of a tendon rupture.

IMMUNE FUNCTION

Sex steroids play a role in immune function in both humans and animals *(167)*. Some anabolic steroids are immunostimulatory, whereas others are immunosuppressive *(168–173)*, so the effects of various anabolic steroids on immune function may vary dramatically. Furthermore, the effects of steroids on the host immune response may be dependent on gender *(174)*. To date, only one study has investigated the effects of steroid use on immune function in resistance-trained men *(175)*. The steroid-using group had lower serum immunoglobulin levels, increased natural killer cell activity, and enhanced proliferative ability to the B-cell mitogen and *Staphylococcus aureus* Cowan strain I *(175)*. No changes were observed in T-cell subsets, and several subjects from both groups had detectable antinuclear antibodies. The clinical ramifications of these findings are unknown. Clearly, further research is warranted in this area, particularly because anabolic steroids are becoming an important tool for maintenance of lean mass in patients infected with HIV *(13,68,81,176)*.

HIV AND OTHER BLOOD-BORNE DISEASES

Because of the criminalization of anabolic steroids, needle sharing and the use of contaminated black-market drugs have become commonplace. This has resulted in HIV infection *(75)* and the potential for hepatitis and other blood-borne diseases. In addition, a growing number of localized and/or systemic bacterial infections are being reported with illegal steroid use *(142,143,177)*.

SUMMARY OF STEROID-RELATED SIDE EFFECTS

In summary, it appears that:

1. With short-term administration (several months to 2 yr), steroid-related side effects are generally mild and reversible, even with moderate doses of some non-17α-alkylated agents, including doses large enough to promote significant increases in fat-free mass, particularly when combined with resistance exercise.
2. Adverse changes in blood lipid profiles as a result of chronic steroid use are common, but whether these changes necessarily lead to increased cardiovascular disease remains unclear.

3. The long-term health implications of medically supervised anabolic steroid use are unknown. However, given the relatively low incidence of life-threatening side effects among those who have ingested massive doses of black-market steroids *(73)*, it is likely that the risk of serious adverse side effects associated with the medically supervised use of anabolic steroids will be extremely low.
4. Controlled research is needed on the effects of low to moderate doses of single and multiple anabolic steroids in conjunction with resistance training on muscle hypertrophy, body composition, and physiological and psychological side effects. There is widespread speculation in the medical community that high doses of anabolic steroids are necessary to produce dramatic increases in lean tissue mass, and this opinion leads to the conclusion that research using such high doses is unethical. However, it is quite possible that more moderate doses (<500 mg/wk) of single or multiple steroids in conjunction with an adequate diet and resistance training could produce the same results with far less risk.
5. It seems likely that many of the serious side effects associated with the use of steroids could have been prevented with appropriate medical monitoring and education prior to, during, and following the use of these drugs. It is time to evaluate steroids in large-scale, multicenter, long-term (5–10 yr) trials consisting of controlled, medically supervised distribution programs designed to build a database of knowledge regarding the physiological and psychological effects and side effects of anabolic steroids in healthy individuals. These studies should be combined with educational efforts directed at reducing the demand for steroid use by adolescents. Such efforts should emphasize alternatives to anabolic steroid use, such as proper training, diet, and nutritional supplementation, and should strive to instill a sense of ethics and fair play in competitive sports. Furthermore, strict doping control programs and refinements in steroid detection are crucial to minimizing steroid use in competitive sports. However, for those adults who choose to use anabolic steroids for noncompetitive purposes, then perhaps harm-reduction programs should be considered as a less costly and far safer alternative to current public policy.

GROWTH HORMONE AND INSULIN-LIKE GROWTH FACTOR I

Growth Hormone

Growth hormone (GH) is indicated for the treatment of short stature in children and for replacement therapy in GH-deficient adults. Experimentation with GH as an ergogenic aid became popular in the early 1980s when "underground" drug handbooks began touting GH as the "Holy Grail" of anabolic hormones. It was thought that exogenous GH administration could produce dramatic and permanent increases in fat-free mass. This contention was later withdrawn in a 2nd edition of one such handbook in 1989 when it became clear to that author that GH was ineffective as an anabolic agent *(178)*. Nevertheless, because of improved methods of detecting anabolic steroids, the inability of current drug tests to detect GH use, and the availability of recombinant human growth hormone (rhGH), the purported use of GH has increased dramatically.

Although GH administration to GH-deficient adults increases fat-free mass and decreases fat-mass *(179,180)*, only one study has demonstrated this effect in healthy men and women undergoing intense exercise *(181)*. Recent studies conducted on resistance-trained males treated with recombinant human GH (rhGH) did not detect increases in fat-free mass or skeletal muscle protein synthesis beyond those observed with resistance training alone *(182,183)*. Also, earlier studies employing GH as a lipolytic agent in the treatment of obesity have been equally disappointing *(184)*. However, two recent studies in obese men *(185)* and women *(186)* found that GH treatment augmented fat loss in conjunction with dietary restriction and/or exercise. Anecdotally, most physique athletes believe that GH is useless as an anabolic agent, although some find it helpful for augmenting fat loss during caloric restriction.

Insulin-Like Growth Factor I (IGF-I)

Genetically engineered recombinant, human insulin-like growth factor I (rhIGF-I) is considered an experimental drug with no current use indications. There is little information regarding the effects of exogenous rhIGF-I administration on body composition in humans. One study in elderly women showed increased fat-free mass (3.3 kg) and decreased fat mass (1.8 kg) following 4 wk of treatment with rhIGF-I, but side effects were numerous *(187)*. No studies were found examining the effects of exogenous IGF-I in a young, healthy, resistance-trained population. Anecdotally, the use of rhIGF-I appears to be losing popularity because of its ineffectiveness and potential for side effects. In addition, there is a growing concensus among researchers that circulating IGF-I plays a relatively minor role in the modulation of muscle mass during mechanical loading *(188)*.

Growth Hormone Plus Insulin-Like Growth Factor I

There is some evidence from human and animal studies that combining GH and IGF-I will result in an enhanced anabolic effect *(189–191)*. However, these studies did not include healthy people engaging in resistance training. Therefore, it is not known if a GH/IGF-I combination would benefit athletes. In addition to GH, some athletes combine growth factors with anabolic steroids and/or insulin *(89)*. Although there is theoretical support for a synergistic anabolic effect with steroids *(35)*, it is unclear how exogenous insulin would potentiate this hormonal array.

Mechanism of Action of Growth Hormone and/or IGF-I

The mechanisms by which GH and/or IGF-I may alter skeletal muscle mass include an increase in circulating and tissue concentrations of IGF-I *(187,192,193)*, regulation of the expression of GH receptors *(194)*, and alterations of circulating and tissue IGF-binding proteins *(195–197)*. Furthermore, because anabolic-androgenic steroids regulate circulating and intramuscular IGF-I and IGF-binding proteins *(34,36)*, it is certainly possible that a specific combination of steroid and peptide hormones could create an optimal anabolic environment for skeletal muscle, provided an adequate mechanical stimulus is employed and adequate concentrations of circulating amino acids and energy substrate (carbohydrates and fats) are available to support protein synthesis.

Side Effects Associated With Growth Hormone and/or Insulin-Like Growth Factor I

The side effects of high doses of GH can include acromegaly, insulin resistance, and changes in skin texture. Creutzfeld-Jakob disease has been associated with pituitary-derived GH that may be available on the black market *(198)*. Side effects associated with IGF-I use include suppressed GH production, hypoglycemia, headaches, and papilledema *(199)*. Although these hormones are not yet detectable with urinalysis, their use is evident in some top male physique competitors who display visibly distended abdomens (personal observations). In addition, some athletes are purportedly using cell-culture grade IGF-I and variants of IGF-I, such as LR^{3}IGF-I, that do not bind to IGF-binding proteins and therefore exhibit increased bioavailability. Although these variants of IGF-I possess superior anabolic properties in animals (200), they have not been studied in humans and may pose additional risks, including reactions to contaminants from cell-culture media, immune reactions to foreign proteins, development of neutralizing antibodies, and uncontrolled tissue growth as a result of bypassing binding-protein regulation.

In summary, the use of growth factors for athletic enhancement lacks both scientific and anecdotal support. Moreover, high circulating concentrations of free IGF-I may potentiate the growth of certain cancers (201,202).

CLENBUTEROL AND OTHER BETA AGONISTS

Beta-agonists are indicated for the treatment of asthma. Clenbuterol (not available in the United States) is perhaps the most popular β-agonist used by athletes and physique competitors (203). The interest in clenbuterol for use as an anabolic agent in athletes stems from a large body of animal literature that shows it to be an effective nutrient-repartitioning agent. Animals treated with clenbuterol have increased fat-free mass and decreased fat mass (204–209). However, the doses employed in animal studies exceed the maximum human therapeutic dose by 1000-fold. Clenbuterol is acutely toxic in relatively low doses, and symptoms of an overdose include tremor, nausea, vomiting, and headache (25). Despite its noted toxicity, most who use clenbuterol in conservative doses (40–80 μg/d) find the side effects to be mild and transient after continued use (personal communications).

In animals, the anabolic effects of clenbuterol are attenuated following 2 wk of continuous treatment. This effect is probably caused by a rapid downregulation of β-receptors and subsequent decreased responsiveness, but this phenomenon can be prevented with intermittent dosing (210). Although few if any athletes currently use clenbuterol for its anabolic effects, many still find that low intermittent doses augment fat loss while dieting. There appear to be no controlled studies that investigate the effects of clenbuterol on body composition in conjunction with a hypocaloric diet and/or resistance exercise in healthy individuals. In summary, anecdotal reports indicate that clenbuterol and other β-agonists in therapeutic doses are not effective anabolic agents, and their efficacy as lipolytic agents appears to be minimal at best.

Because β-agonists are often combined with thyroid hormones, stimulants (such as ephedrine), and anabolic steroids, athletes should be informed about the potential deleterious interactions of these drugs. Few athletes understand the mechanisms of action of these agents and the potentially serious cardiovascular complications, such as spasms of the coronary arteries and myocardial infarcts, that can occur as a result of combining these drugs (203).

INSULIN

Because insulin increases the uptake of glucose and amino acids into skeletal muscle, a growing number of athletes have begun to experiment with insulin as an anabolic agent (211). Studies have shown increases in muscle protein synthesis with localized insulin infusions (212) and a potentiating effect of insulin on protein synthesis in muscle following a bout of resistance exercise in animals *(213,214)*. However, no evidence exists to support the use of exogenous insulin as an anabolic agent in nondiabetic individuals. Furthermore, adequate circulating amino acids must be present for insulin to increase net protein synthesis *(215)*. Because consuming a large amount of simple carbohydrate in conjunction with protein will simulate large increases in endogenous insulin secretion *(216)* and will increase circulating amino acid concentrations, there is no logical reason for an individual with normal insulin sensitivity and production to use exogenous insulin.

Anecdotally, those who have experimented with insulin alone do not experience any increases in fat-free mass, and they struggle to maintain euglycemia. Furthermore, insulin promotes lipogenesis and inhibits fatty acid release during exercise *(217)*, so its chronic use by physique competitors attempting to stay lean would be counterproductive. Interestingly, many physique competitors avoid high carbohydrate diets to lower daily insulin levels and to minimize gains in fat-mass and/or augment fat loss. Thus, it is unclear why they would then inject exogenous insulin. With the exception of a large intravenous bolus of IGF-I or an overdose of clenbuterol, cocaine, or other stimulant, insulin use probably presents the greatest risk for incurring a life-threatening side effect. Furthermore, the long-term use of insulin in athletes may predispose them to the pathologies observed in the insulin-dependent diabetic population. The use of insulin as an anabolic agent is completely unfounded and dangerous. Few athletes understand insulin's mechanism of action, its interaction with exercise on accelerating the uptake of circulating glucose, and its potential for life-threatening side effects as evidenced by reports of acute overdoses *(211)*.

THYROID HORMONES

Thyroid preparations include tetraiodothyronine (T4; Synthroid®), triiodothyronine (T3; Cytomel®), and lyothyronine acetate (Triacana, a synthetic European T3 with an extended half-life). Because 5′-deiodinase activity is reduced during caloric restriction, thereby limiting the conversion of T4 to T3 *(218)*, many physique competitors feel that supplemental T3 will attenuate the decrease in metabolic rate that occurs during dieting *(219)*. Although supplemental thyroid is contraindicated for use in weight loss, some studies have demonstrated augmented fat loss or an attenuated decrease in resting metabolic rate in obese women supplemented with T3 during caloric restriction *(220,221)*. Also, many contend that mild hyperthyroidism increases protein oxidation, which would prove counterproductive if one is attempting to gain lean mass. However, the decrease in nitrogen balance that occurs as a result of mild pharmacologically induced hyperthyroidism appears to return to baseline within 9 wk, whereas the elevation in total energy expenditure persists *(222)*. Furthermore, recent evidence suggests that altering circulating thyroid hormone concentrations within normal physiologic limits may have significant effects on resting energy expenditure *(223)*. Thus, it may be possible to "fine tune" one's metabolic rate during caloric restriction with conservative doses of thyroid.

Side Effects of Thyroid Preparations

The use of thyroid preparations has not been investigated in otherwise healthy individuals who incorporate severe dietary energy restriction to achieve extremely low percentages of body fat. Accordingly, athletes considering the use of thyroid should be advised of the following consequences of thyroid use. First, their endogenous thyroid hormone production will be suppressed, the long-term implications of which are unknown. Second, high doses of thyroid preparations will accelerate the loss of muscle mass through increased protein oxidation *(222)*, will adversely affect the circulating IGF-I system *(224,225)*, and will increase oxidation of LDL cholesterol *(226)*, which can accelerate atherogenesis. Finally, the use of exogenous thyroid preparations has been associated with various cardiac pathologies, including arrhythmias, cardiac hypertrophy, and congestive heart failure *(227,228)*. Thus, the use of large doses of thyroid preparations may predispose an athlete to a cardiomyopathy that may be potentiated by the use of β-agonists or other stimulants. Furthermore, if the users obtain the thyroid preparations from the black market, and the supply is suddenly cut off, they will become acutely hypothyroid. This will result in the development of hyperhomocystinemia (an independent risk factor for coronary artery disease) *(229)*, increased platelet aggregation *(230)*, increased LDL cholesterol oxidation *(226)*, and marked disruptions in metabolism.

DEHYDROEPIANDROSTERONE

Dehydroepiandrosterone (DHEA) is a weak adrenal androgen that can be converted to either testosterone or estradiol in vivo *(231)*, but ingesting 50 mg/d DHEA for 30 d has only minimal effects on the testosterone-to-epitestosterone ratio (an indicator of testosterone doping) in men *(232)*. Administration of DHEA does not influence body composition in healthy young men *(233)*. Currently, DHEA is under investigation for use in the elderly as a means to restore physical and psychological well-being *(231,234)* and immune function *(235)*. Treatment with 50 mg/d DHEA in older men and women increased their sense of well-being and circulating IGF-I *(231)*, and treatment with 100 mg/d increased strength and decreased fat mass in older men, but not in women *(234)*. In contrast, recent work by Flynn et al. *(236)* did not find any effect of DHEA supplementation (100 mg/d) on body composition or feelings of well-being in older men. Moreover, although increases in circulating concentrations of free (but not total) testosterone are observed with DHEA treatment in aging men, serum concentrations of both estradiol and estrone are also elevated *(237)*. Although DHEA supplementation may have positive effects in the elderly and in other individuals who have low concentrations of DHEA in the blood, the effects of supplementation in individuals with normal levels of DHEA are unknown.

Because DHEA has a short half-life (30 min) and is released episodically, measurement of circulating DHEA-sulfate (half-life ~ 24 h) provides a better assessment of DHEA production or supplementation. Although side effects have not been noted in clinical studies, a recent case report described a 55-yr-old man who developed premature atrial and ventricular contractions while ingesting 50 mg/d DHEA *(238)*. However, because this individual purchased his DHEA over the counter, and a recent analysis of 16 different brands of DHEA found that only 44% contained what was specified on the label *(239)*, it is possible that the palpitations were a result of contamination with ephedrine or another stimulant, not the DHEA itself. This underscores the importance of medical supervision and blood DHEA analysis to ensure proper dosing if over-the-counter products are used.

$\Delta^{4/5}$-ANDRO- AND NOR-$\Delta^{4/5}$-ANDROSTENE- DIONE/DIOL

Androstenedione is an adrenal androgen, a precursor to both epitestosterone and testosterone *(12)*, and it is one of the primary sources of circulating testosterone in women *(3)*. Androstenedione and other androgen precursors have recently become popular over-the-counter supplements. They are available as preparations to be orally ingested, used sublingually (cyclodextrin formulations), or applied topically (sterile aqueous suspensions). The various forms of andro- and nor-androstene- ($\Delta^{4/5}$, dione/diol) can be converted by either 3 or 17β-hydroxysteroid dehydrogenase and/or by Δ^5-isomerase into testosterone or nandrolone, respectively. In addition, androstenedione can be converted into epitestosterone by 17α-dehydrogenase *(12)*.

Although lay magazine advertisements describe prohormones as legal anabolic steroids capable of increasing circulating testosterone concentrations and producing ergogenic effects, there is mounting evidence that at least one form of prohormone (oral androstenedione) may actually be ergolytic. Several recent studies have suggested that oral androstenedione ingestion does not increase circulating testosterone concentrations or alter body composition, but does increase blood estradiol, estrone, and dihydrotestosterone and decreases HDL cholesterol *(240–243)*. However, these changes in estrogen, dihydrotestosterone, and HDL were small and similar to those observed with traditional testosterone replacement therapy *(244)*. Thus, given that long-term studies of side effects have not been reported, there is no current evidence that moderate doses (<400 mg/d) of oral androstenedione ingestion cause serious health consequences, particularly with short-term use (<12 wk) in otherwise healthy individuals.

It is unknown if the ingestion of other forms of prohormones, e.g., androstenediol and nor-androstenedione/diol, will elicit effects similar to those observed with moderate doses of androstenedione. In fact, preliminary results from a study by Ziegenfuss et al. (personal communication) indicated that sublingual androstenediol increased blood testosterone concentrations by 98% above baseline, with peak values of 41.3 nmol/L, 40 min following a single dose. These values are similar to those found with sublingual testosterone administration (testosterone cyclodextrin) for replacment therapy *(244)*. In addition, 4 wk of sublingual androstenediol administration (450 mg/d) increased body mass, body water, and vertical leap performance. Unlike oral androstenedione administration, sublingual androstenediol administration did not alter circulating concentrations of LH, HDL, or estrogen.

Nor-androstenedione/diol is a precursor to 19-nortestosterone and is theoretically more anabolic and less androgenic than androstenedione because it is converted to nandrolone rather than to testosterone. However, no evidence suggests that consuming nor-androstenedione/diol products would produce blood concentrations of nandrolone high enough to elicit an anabolic effect. In addition, athletes who are subject to testing for anabolic steroid use should be aware that the ingestion of nor-androstenedione/diol will produce a positive drug test for nandrolone that may persist for up to 8 d *(245)*.

Further research is needed before appropriate conclusions can be drawn regarding the anabolic potential of prohormones. However, clinicians should advise patients that potential androgen-like side effects may occur in some prohomone users. Those at particular risk include men with pre-existing prostate or breast cancer and women who are or could potentially become pregnant.

TAMOXIFEN

Tamoxifen (Nolvadex®) is a mixed estrogen agonist/antagonist used in the treatment of breast cancer in women *(246)* and for some cases of gynecomastia in men *(164)*. Both male and female athletes use this compound to antagonize the effects of circulating estrogen. Males use tamoxifen with aromatizable androgens to minimize or prevent gynecomastia, and many female physique competitors use tamoxifen to "harden" their physiques while dieting. The idea that estrogen is responsible for increased body fat in women is based on the observed changes in girls at puberty *(162,247)* and in transsexual men treated with estrogen for gender reassignment *(52)*. In postmenopausal women, estrogen administration can alter body composition, but its effects are dependent on the route of administration and may involve the circulating GH/IGF-I system. For example, 24 wk of oral estrogen treatment leads to an increase in fat mass and circulating GH, and a decrease in lean body mass and circulating IGF-I concentrations. In contrast, similar treatment with transdermal estrogen did not affect body composition or the GH/IGF-I axis. In addition, when compared to women treated with transdermal estrogen, oral estrogen increased carbohydrate oxidation and decreased lipid oxidation following a mixed meal *(248)*. Taken together, these studies suggest that circulating estrogen concentrations may play a role in nutrient repartitioning, and these effects may involve the GH/IGF-I system. However, it is unknown if an estrogen antagonist, such as tamoxifen, would augment fat loss in women during a period of caloric restriction. Interestingly, some women use tamoxifen for several weeks following anabolic steroid use to reduce the perceived psychological and physiological effects of what they describe as "estrogen rebound." Whether there is any merit to this practice is unknown.

Interactions of Tamoxifen with IGF-I

The tumor growth-inhibiting properties of tamoxifen involve suppression of some aspects of the IGF system *(249–251)*, which is also important in muscle hypertrophy *(252)*. Therefore, the use of tamoxifen could theoretically interfere with muscle growth. Anecdotally, bodybuilders have perceived decrements in the hypertrophic process while using tamoxifen.

CLOMIPHENE

Clomiphene (Clomid®) is used to treat infertility in both men and women. Clomiphene increases gonadotropin production (LH and FSH) by acting directly on the hypothalamus to trigger the release of GnRH *(253)*. Clomiphene possesses mild estrogenic activity and acts as an antiestrogen. Men use this agent to restore the hypothalamic-pituitary axis following an anabolic steroid cycle. When using testosterone as an anabolic agent, men also employ clomiphene to decrease the ratio of circulating testosterone to LH in an attempt to circumvent a positive drug test *(12)*.

HUMAN CHORIONIC GONADOTROPIN

Human chorionic gonadotropin (hCG) is a peptide hormone produced during the early stages of pregnancy and is used for the treatment of hypogonadism and infertility. Men use this hormone to stimulate endogenous testosterone production beyond their normal circulating concentrations, to maintain spermatogenesis during exogenous anabolic steroid use, and to restore testicular function following an anabolic steroid cycle. Women use it in an attempt to confound drug-testing results, i.e., by inducing a false-positive test for pregnancy.

Common side effects of hCG use in men include those associated with androgen excess. Administration of hCG also increases circulating estradiol *(153)* and could exacerbate gynecomastia in some individuals *(11)*. Although hCG administered concurrently with anabolic steroids will maintain fertility, testicular volume, and endogenous testosterone production *(153)*, it is unknown if this use of hCG will shorten the relative hypogonadal state that follows use of anabolic steroids. Administration of hCG following treatment with anabolic steroids will also increase circulating testosterone. However, this increase in testosterone is minimal and is not accompanied by an increase in circulating estradiol, suggesting a suppression of the activity of steroidogenic enzymes *(254)*. In any case, decreases in gonadotropin and testosterone production will still occur following the cessation of hCG treatment.

TESTOLACTONE

Testolactone (Teslac®) is an aromatase inhibitor used clinically as an adjunct for the treatment of breast cancer (PDR). Both male and female athletes might use this agent to reduce circulating concentrations of estrogen. In males prone to gynecomastia, this may reduce the side effects of using aromatizable anabolic steroids. As with tamoxifen, there would be no rationale for its use in women athletes. Testolactone is not an anabolic steroid and possesses no androgenic properties, but it is classified as a Schedule III drug (PDR). The use of testolactone reduces circulating estrogen and HDL concentrations during exogenous testosterone use *(94)*. Thus, although it may offset the side effects of aromatizable androgens, it could reduce the potential cardiovascular benefits of circulating estrogen.

FINASTERIDE

Finasteride (Proscar®) is indicated for the treatment of benign prostatic hypertrophy and baldness in men. Finasteride inhibits the conversion of testosterone to dihydrotestosterone in such tissues as the scalp and prostate *(255)*, but it does not reduce sebum production *(256)*. Because finasteride seems to be effective in the treatment of hirsute women *(257,258)*, some women athletes who use testosterone esters have begun using the drug to reduce the accompanying growth of facial and body hair. Finasteride can also slightly increase circulating testosterone, reduce cortisol, and blunt the cortisol response to corticotropin stimulation *(259)*. Because increasing the testosterone:cortisol ratio might enhance muscle protein synthesis *(260)*, finasteride could theoretically enhance protein synthesis, but there is no evidence that the drug has any noticeable effect on body composition or performance. Furthermore, women should be warned that finasteride use during pregnancy could adversely affect the external genitalia of a male fetus (PDR).

Anecdotally, finasteride is used by some athletes in conjunction with testosterone and nandrolone in the hope of enhancing their anabolic effects. The rationale underlying this regimen is that the drug will presumably increase the ratio of testosterone to dihydrotestosterone or nandrolone to dihydronandrolone, which would theoretically enhance muscle protein synthesis. There is no evidence that this strategy is especially effective in stimulating muscle hypertrophy.

GAMMA-HYDROXY-BUTYRATE

Gamma-hydroxy-butyrate (GHB) was originally sold in health food stores and was subsequently banned in late 1990. In late 1998, precursors of GHB were marketed as food supplements but were also subsequently banned in mid 1999. GHB is thought to effect the dopaminergic and endogenous opioid systems, and has a very short half-life (20–60 min) following ingestion *(261,262)*. GHB has recently gained considerable media attention resulting from reports of toxic side effects and deaths associated with its use. It is also purportedly being used as a recreational and "date rape" drug *(262)*. Anecdotally, athletes initially used GHB to enhance GH release, but this was perceived to be ineffective. They now use about 4 g or 4 mL of GHB primarily as a sedative following an intense workout in an effort to speed recovery. The effects are typically felt in about 20–30 min and last roughly 3 h. Users report feeling refreshed without residual hangover effects after awakening. Side effects noted include dizziness and sweating at the onset of GHB action. There are recent reports of vomiting, bradycardia, seizures, coma, respiratory depression, and death associated with GHB ingestion *(261,262)*. These adverse effects may be caused by the use of large doses, impure products (most GHB is made in clandestine laboratories), and the use of GHB with other agents, such as alcohol, pharmaceutical sedatives, and/or recreational drugs.

EPHEDRINE

Ephedrine is a central nervous system stimulant. The drug is banned by the National Collegiate Athletic Association and the International Olympic Committee. It does not seem to enhance athletic performance *(3)* when consumed alone, but it may enhance performance when combined with caffeine *(263)*. Ephedrine is an effective lipolytic drug with few side effects when used in conservative doses *(264–267)*, so physique competitors have begun using it as a diet aid. To date, no human studies have examined the lipolytic effects of ephedrine in nonobese individuals. However, the treatment of lean rhesus monkeys with ephedrine and caffeine resulted in an increase in 24-h energy expenditure and a decrease in body fat *(268)*. Thus, it is possible that similar effects may be observed in lean humans.

The FDA has released warnings regarding serious adverse effects associated with the use of products containing ephedrine, including insomnia, tremors, anxiety, nausea, tachycardia, arrhythmia, hypertension, dependence, and death *(269)*. However, some side effects may be associated with consuming excessive doses and/or combining ephedrine with other drugs for recreational purposes. Nonetheless, athletes should be informed about potentially deleterious interactions with other commonly used dieting agents, such as clenbuterol, thyroid preparations, and/or other stimulants.

ANTICORTISOL DRUGS

Cortisol elicits catabolic effects on skeletal muscle *(270–272)*, and intense resistance training elevates circulating cortisol concentrations *(273)*. Therefore, some athletes have begun using such drugs as ketoconazole, aminoglutethimide, and RU486 in an attempt to either reduce cortisol production or block glucocorticoid receptors. In rats, the administration of RU486 attenuates the muscle atrophy and myofibrillar protein breakdown caused by glucocorticoid treatment and causes hypertrophy of the levator ani muscle

(274). However, in humans, there is no evidence that reducing circulating cortisol concentrations will augment muscle mass. In addition, both ketoconazole and aminoglutethimide inhibit testosterone synthesis *(275)*, likely making their use counterproductive. Furthermore, all three of these drugs can produce symptoms consistent with an adrenal crisis *(276)*.

ERYTHROPROTEIN

Erythropoietin (EPO) is a peptide hormone produced by the kidneys that stimulates red blood cell production *(277)*. Its recombinant form is used clinically for the treatment of anemia, and it is purportedly the hormone of choice for elite endurance athletes. Although banned, exogenous erythropoietin use is not detectable by urinalysis. Administration of erythropoietin to healthy endurance athletes increases hemoglobin concentration, endurance performance, maximal aerobic power, and arterial pressure during exercise *(278,279)*. Large doses alone or in combination with dehydration may increase blood viscosity to levels that would either impair performance and/or increase the risk of thrombosis.

DOPING CONTROL

For a thorough review of drug-testing methods and issues surrounding doping control, please *see* refs. *27,280–284*. Currently, all known anabolic-androgenic steroids, in addition to nonsteroidal agents, such as clenbuterol, can be detected via urinalysis (gas chromatography-mass spectrometry) for a period of time following the last dose. The detection of these drugs depends on numerous factors, including their chemical structures, metabolism, the form in which they were administered (i.e., oral vs parenteral), pattern of dosing, concurrent use of other drugs, and so forth. The limit of detection for most oral anabolic steroids and clenbuterol is generally about 3 wk and 7 d, respectively (R.C. Kammerer, personal communication). For parenteral drugs such as nandrolone, the limit of detection may extend beyond 1 yr.

Assessment of illegal testosterone use is based on the urinary ratio of testosterone to epitestosterone, with a ratio of six being the upper legal limit. Because testosterone is not readily converted to epitestosterone, exogenous use of testosterone will increase this ratio. This test is fraught with problems, however. For example, in one study, the use of testosterone esters in doses up to 300 mg/wk did not raise the ratio above six *(285)*, but such a dose is sufficient to increase fat-free mass in normal men *(48)*. Furthermore, some athletes inject epitestosterone prior to drug testing in an effort to mask exogenous testosterone use. To combat this, urinary epitestosterone concentrations above 200 ng/mL are considered proof of epitestosterone manipulation. However, this limit may still allow for substantial testosterone use. Furthermore, short lasting forms of testosterone, e.g., sublingual testosterone cyclodextrin, or testosterone patches can raise serum testosterone for only a few hours *(286)*, after which *(287)* the testosterone:epitestosterone ratio may return rapidly to baseline. Detection of testosterone use represents a significant challenge for doping control labs. Testing for other peptides, such as growth hormone, insulin-like growth factor-I, insulin, and erythropoietin, has yet to be implemented, so their covert use continues unchecked.

Many other factors hamper doping control efforts, including cover-ups of positive samples, mishandling of samples, legal challenges, falsification of specimens, deliberate contamination of specimens, use of masking agents, development of designer drugs, outlaw laboratories that assist athletes in establishing drug clearance times, covert state-run doping programs, and the costs associated with large-scale, frequent, random testing *(288)*. Thus, even with flawless collection and analytical procedures, current doping control can at best only reduce the use of some hormones in sports. In addition, it is possible that in the near future, viral-mediated gene-transfer therapy may render current doping control methods obsolete. In animal models, it is already feasible to initiate the expression of sustained levels of proteins, such as IGF-I in skeletal muscle, by a single injection of a recombinant adeno-associated viral vector *(289)*. The production of these proteins and their effects may be limited to the infected skeletal muscle, e.g., increased intramuscular IGF-I may cause localized hypertrophy *(290)*. Other gene transfers may also produce systemic effects by releasing large quantities of a protein, such as EPO, into circulation *(291)*.

CONCLUSIONS

It is surprising that despite their widespread use, many nonsteroidal ergogenic drugs have not been studied in a healthy athletic population. Although clinicians warn of potential side effects and lack of efficacy, in many cases no controlled studies refute anecdotally reported ergogenic benefits or confirm deleterious side effects. Thus, the clinician lacks scientific evidence to support his or her recommendations. By grossly exaggerating side effects and minimizing performance benefits, the medical and scientific communities have already lost considerable credibility in their efforts to discourage steroid use in sports. Thus, it is imperative that properly controlled studies be conducted to support claims that are made. Otherwise, it is likely that medical warnings will fall on deaf ears. This is particularly important with such drugs as insulin, clenbuterol, thyroid preparations, and gamma-hydroxy-butyrate. Because all of these drugs are used for legitimate medical purposes (although not all in the United States), it is hard to convince users that they carry significant risks or, more importantly, that they possess little or no ergogenic value. An effort must be made to educate athletes regarding potential interactions of many alleged ergogenic drugs. For example, thyroid preparations, stimulants, and beta-agonists are often combined for their lipolytic effects, and gamma-hydroxy-butyrate could be combined (perhaps unknowingly) with nalbuphine and other narcotic analgesics. Any of these combinations could prove fatal. Furthermore, few users understand that many of these drugs have a relatively low therapeutic index and a certain safety factor; thus, even a mild overdose could prove lethal.

Word-of-mouth and drug dealers in gyms are coercive elements in athletic circles, but with appropriate educational efforts and well-controlled studies, it should be possible for the clinician to become the primary disseminator of ergogenic drug information.

REFERENCES

1. Lombardo JA, Hickson RC, Lamb DR. Anabolic/androgenic steroids and growth hormone. In: Lamb DR, Williams MH, eds. Perspectives in Exercise Science and Sports Medicine Volume 4: Ergogenics-Enhancement of Performance in Exercise and Sport, Wm. C. Brown, Ann Arbor, MI, 1991, pp. 249–284.
2. Yesalis CE III, Courson SP, Wright JE. History of anabolic steroid use in sport and exercise. In: Yesalis CE III, ed., Anabolic Steroids in Sport and Exercise, Human Kinetics, Champaign, IL, 1993, pp. 35–47.
3. Wadler GI, Hainline B. Anabolic steroids. In: Ryan AS, ed. Drugs and the Athlete. F.A. Davis, Philadelphia, PA, 1989, pp. 55–69.

4. Haupt HA, Rovere GD. Anabolic steroids: a review of the literature. Am J Sports Med 1984;12: 469–484.
5. Rogozkin VA. Anabolic steroid metabolism in skeletal muscle. J Steroid Biochem 1979;11:923–926.
6. Saartok T, Dahlberg E, and Gustafsson JA. Relative binding affinity of anabolic-androgenic steroids: Comparison of the binding to the androgen receptors in skeletal muscle and in prostate, as well as to sex hormone-binding globulin. Endocrinology 1984;114:2100–2106.
7. Liao S, Liang T, Fang S, Castañeda, Shag T-C. Steroid structure and androgenic activity. Specificities involved in the receptor binding and nuclear retention of various androgens. J Biol Chem 1973;248:6154–6162.
8. Carlson KE, Katzenellenbogen JA. A comparative study of the selectivity and efficiency of target tissue uptake of five tritium-labeled androgens in the rat. J Steroid Biochem 1990;36:549–561.
9. Bhasin S, Storer TW, Berman N, Callegari C, Clevenger B, Phillips J, Bunnell TJ, Tricker R, Shirazi A, Casaburi R. The effects of suprapysiological doses of testosterone on muscle size and strength in normal men. N Engl J Med 1996;335:1–7.
10. Phillips WN. Survey says…. In: Phillips WN, ed. Anabolic Reference Guide. Mile High Publishing, Golden, CO, 1991, pp. 213–218.
11. Wright JE. Anabolic steroids. In: Wright JE, ed. Anabolic Steroids and Sports Volume II. Sports Science Consultants, Natick, MA, 1982, pp. 31–116.
12. Di Pasquale MG. Anabolic steroids. In: Di Pasquale MG, ed. Drug Use and Detection in Amateur Sports. M.G.D. Press, Warkworth, Ontario, 1984, pp. 41–65.
13. Hengge UR, Baumann M, Maleba R, Brockmeyer NH, and Goos M. Oxymetholone promotes weight gain in patients with advanced human immunodeficiency virus (HIV-1) infection. Br J Nutr 1996;75:129–138.
14. Henney HR III. Investigator Brochure. Oxandrolone. Bio-Technology General Corp., Iselin, NJ, 1997, pp. 5–56.
15. Rosenfeld RG, Frane J, Attie KM, Brasel J, Burstein S, Cara JF, Chernausek S, Gotlin RW, Kuntze J, Lippe BM, Mahoney PC, Moore WV, Saenger P, Johanson AJ. Six-year results of a randomized, prospective trial of human growth hormone and oxandrolone in Turner syndrome. J Pediatr 1992;121:49–55.
16. Hobbs CJ, Jones RE, Plymate SR. Nandrolone, a 19-nortestosterone, enhances insulin-independent glucose uptake in normal men. J Clin Endocrinol Metab 1996;81:1582–1585.
17. Wijnand HP, Bosch AMG, Donker CM. Pharmacokinetic parameters of nandrolone (19-nortestosterone) after intramuscular administration of nandrolone decanoate (Deca-Durabolin®) to healthy volunteers. Acta Endocrinol (Copenh) 1985;271(Suppl):19–30.
18. Bergink EW, Janssen PSL, Turpijn EW, Van der Vies J. Comparison of the receptor binding properties of nandrolone and testosterone under *in vitro* and *in vivo* conditions. J Steroid Biochem 1985;22: 831–836.
19. Tóth M, Zakár T. Relative binding affinities of testosterone, 19-nortestosterone and their 5α-reduced derivatives to the androgen receptor and to other androgen-binding proteins: A suggested role of 5α-reduced steroid metabolism in the dissociation of "myotropic" and "androgenic" activities of 19-nortestosterone. J Steroid Biochem 1982;17:653–660.
20. Teruel JL, Aguilera A, Avila C, Ortuño J. Effects of androgen therapy on prostatic markers in hemodialyzed patients. Scand J Urol Nephrol 1996;30:129–131.
21. Davis WM, Long SF, Lin TL. Nandrolone decanoate reduces the premature mortality of cardiomyopathic hamsters. Res Commun Chem Pathol Pharmacol 1993;81:21–32.
22. Bergink EW, Geelen JAA, Turpijn EW. Metabolism and receptor binding of nandrolone and testosterone under in vitro and in vivo conditions. Acta Endocrinol (Copenh) 1985;271(Suppl):31–37.
23. Hughes BJ. Steroid receptors and the muscular system. In: Sheridan PJ, Blum K, Trachtenberg MC, eds. Steroid Receptors and Disease, Marcel Dekker, New York, NY, 1988, pp. 415–433.
24. Wiren KM, Zhang X, Chang C, Keenan E, Orwoll ES. Transcriptional up-regulation of the human androgen receptor by androgen in bone cells. Endocrinology 1997;138:2291–2300.
25. Van der Kuy P-H, Stegeman A, Looij BJ Jr, Hooymans PM. Falsification of Thai dianabol. Pharm World Sci 1997;19:208,209.
26. Colescott S. Livestock implants: not just for cattle anymore? Peak Training J 1997;1(4):30–33.
27. Bamberger M, Yaeger D. Over the edge. Sports Illustrated 1997;86(15):60–70.

28. Summerfield AE, Diaz Cruz PJ, Dolenga MP, Smith HE, Trader CD, Toney JH. Tissue-specific pharmacology of testosterone and 5α-dihydrotestosterone analogues: characterization of a novel canine liver androgen-binding protein. Mol Pharmacol 1995;47:1080–1088.
29. Masonis AET, McCarthy MP. Direct effects of the anabolic/androgenic steroids, stanozolol and 17α-methyltestosterone, on benzodiazepine binding to the γ-aminobutyric acid$_A$ receptor. Neurosci Lett 1995;189:35–38.
30. Masonis AET, McCarthy MP. Effects of the androgenic/anabolic steroid stanozolol on GABA$_A$ receptor function: GABA-stimulated ^{36}C$^-$, Influx and [^{35}S] TBPS binding. J Pharmacol Exp Ther 1996;279:186–193.
31. Itil TM, Cora R, Akpinar S, Herrmann WM, Patterson CJ. "Psychotropic" action of sex hormones: computerized EEG in establishing the immediate CNS effects of steroid hormones. Ther Res 1974;16:1147–1170.
32. Vyskocil E, Gutmann E. Electrophysiologic and contractile properties of the levator ani muscle after castration and testosterone administration. Pflügers Arch 1977;368:104–109.
33. Bleisch WV, Harrelson AL, Luine VN. Testosterone increases acetylcholine receptor number in the "levator ani" muscle of the rat. J Neurobiol 1982;13:153–161.
34. Urban RJ, Bodenburg YH, Gilkison C, Foxworth J, Coggan AR, Wolfe RR, Ferrando A. Testosterone administration to elderly men increases skeletal muscle strength and protein synthesis. Am J Physiol (Endocrinol Metab 32) 1995;269:E820–E826.
35. Thompson SH, Boxhorn LK, Kong W, Allen RE. Trenbolone alters the responsiveness of skeletal muscle satellite cells to fibroblast growth factor and insulin-like growth factor I. Endocrinology 1989;124:2110–2117.
36. Hobbs CJ, Plymate SR, Rosen CJ, Adler RA. Testosterone administration increases insulin-like growth factor-I levels in normal men. J Clin Endocrinol Metab 1993;77:776–779.
37. Saggese G, Cesaretti G, Franchi G, Startari L. Testosterone-induced increase in insulin-like growth factor I levels depends upon normal levels of growth hormone. Eur J Endocrinol 1996;135:211–215.
38. Yesalis CE III, Kennedy NJ, Kopstein AN, Bahrke MS. Anabolic-androgenic steroid use in the United States. JAMA 1993;270:1217–1221.
39. Myhal M, Buckworth J, Elsea D, Lamb DR. Anthropometric characteristics of elite female bodybuilders, fitness competitors, and fit college women. Med Sci Sports Exerc 1998;30:S237.
40. Catlin DH. Androgen abuse by athletes. In: Bhasin S, Gabelnick HL, Spieler JM, Swerdloff RS, Wang C, Kelly C, eds. Pharmacology, Biology, and Clinical Applications of Androgens. Wiley-Liss, New York, NY, 1996, pp. 289–295.
41. Delbeke FT, Desmet N, Debackere M. The abuse of doping agents in competing body builders in Flanders (1988–1993). Int J Sports Med 1995;16:66–70.
42. Franke WW, Berendonk B. Hormonal doping and androgenization of athletes: a secret program of the German Democratic Republic government. Clin Chem 1997;43:1262–1279.
43. Kay S. The psychology and anthropometry of body image. In: Norton K, Olds T, eds. Anthropometrica. University of New South Wales Press, Marrickville, New South Wales, Australia, 1996, pp. 236–258.
44. Lovejoy JC, Bray GA, Bourgeois MO, Macchiavelli R, Rood JC, Greeson C, Partington C. Exogenous androgens influence body composition and regional body fat distribution in obese postmenopausal women—A clinical research center study. J Clin Endocrinol Metab 1996;81:2198–2203.
45. Yesalis CE III, Barsukiewicz CK, Kopstein AN, Bahrke MS. Trends in anabolic-androgenic steroid use among adolescents. Arch Pediatr Adolesc Med 1997;151:1197–1206.
46. Alway SE. Characteristics of the elbow flexors in women bodybuilders using androgenic-anabolic steroids. J Strength Cond Res 1994;8:161–169.
47. Yeater R, Reed C, Ullrich I, Morise A, Borsch M. Resistance trained athletes using or not using anabolic steroids compared to runners: effects on cardiorespiratory variables, body composition, and plasma lipids. Br J Sports Med 1996;30:11–14.
48. Forbes GB, Porta CR, Herr BE, Griggs RC. Sequence of changes in body composition induced by testosterone and reversal of changes after drug is stopped. JAMA 1992;267:397–399.
49. Arslanian S, Suprasongsin C. Testosterone treatment in adolescents with delayed puberty: changes in body composition, protein, fat, and glucose metabolism. J Clin Endocrinol Metab 1997;82:3213–3220.

50. Lovejoy JC, Bray GA, Greeson C, Klemper M, Morris J, Partington C, Tulley R. Oral anabolic steroid treatment, but not parenteral androgen treatment, decreases abdominal fat in obese, older men. Int J Obesity 1995;19:614–624.
51. Elbers JMH, Asscheman H, Seidell JC, Megens JAJ, Gooren LJG. Long-term testosterone administration increases visceral fat in female to male transsexuals. J Clin Endocrinol Metab 1997;82:2044–2047.
52. Elbers JMH, Asscheman H, Seidell JC, Gooren LJG. Effects of sex steroid hormones on regional fat depots as assessed by magnetic resonance imaging in transexuals. Am J Physiol (Endocrinol Metab 39): 1999;276:E317–E325.
53. Reubinoff BE, Wurtman J, Rojansky N, Adler D, Stein P, Schenker JG, Brzezinski A. Effects of hormone replacement therapy on weight, body composition, fat distribution, and food intake in early postmenopausal women: a prospective study. Fertil Steril 1995;64:963–968.
54. Gaal LV, Vansant G, Moeremans M, Leeuw ID. Lipid and lipoprotein changes after long-term weight reduction: the influence of gender and body fat distribution. J Am Coll Nutr 1995;14:382–386.
55. O'Shea JP. The effects of an anabolic steroid on dynamic strength levels of weightlifters. Nutr Rep Internat 1971;4:363–370.
56. Ward P. The effect of an anabolic steroid on strength and lean body mass. Med Sci Sports Exerc 1973;5:277–283.
57. Stamford BA, Moffatt R. Anabolic steroid: effectiveness as an ergogenic aid to experienced weight trainers. J Sports Med Phys Fitness 1974;14:191–197.
58. Hervey GR, Knibbs AV. Effects of methandienone on the performance and body composition of men undergoing athletic training. Clin Sci 1981;60:457–461.
59. Alen MK, Hakkinen K, Komi PV. Changes in neuromuscular performance and muscle fiber characteristics of elite power athletes self-administering androgenic and anabolic steroids. Acta Physiol Scand 1984;122:535-544.
60. Fowler WM Jr, Gardner GW, Egstrom GH. Effect of an anabolic steroid on physical performance in young men. J Appl Physiol 1965;20:1038–1040.
61. Fahey TD, Brown CH. The effects of an anabolic steroid on strength, body composition and endurance of college males when accompanied by a weight training program. Med Sci Sports Exerc 1973;5:272–276.
62. Golding LA, Freydinger JE, Fishel SS. The effect of an androgenic-anabolic steroid and a protein supplement on size, strength, weight and body composition in athletes. Physician Sports Med 1974;2:39–45.
63. Stromme SB, Meen HD, Aakvaag A. Effects of an androgenic-anabolic steroid on strength development and plasma testosterone levels in normal males. Med Sci Sports Exerc 1974;6:203–208.
64. Hervey GR, Knibbs AV, Burkinshaw L, Jones PRM, Norgan NG, Levell MJ. Anabolic effects of methandienone in men undergoing athletic training. Lancet 1976;2:702.
65. Loughton S, Ruhling R. Human strength and endurance responses to anabolic steroid and training. J Sports Med Phys Fitness 1977;17:285–296.
66. Crist DM, Stackpole PJ, Peake GT. Effects of androgenic-anabolic steroids on neuromuscular power and body composition. J Appl Physiol 1983;54:366–370.
67. Berger JR, Pall L, Winfield D. Effect of anabolic steroids on HIV-related wasting myopathy. South Med J 1993;86:865,866.
68. Sattler FR, Jaque SV, Schroeder ET, Olson C, Dube MP, Martinez C, Briggs W, Horton R, Azen S. Effects of pharmacological doses of nandrolone decanoate and progressive resistance training in immunodeficient patients infected with human immunodeficiency virus. J Clin Endocrinol Metab 1999;84:1268–1276.
69. Cooper CJ, Noakes TD, Dunne T, Lambert MI, Rochford K. A high prevalence of abnormal personality traits in chronic users of anabolic-androgenic steroids. Br J Sports Med 1996;30:246–250.
70. Bahrke MS, Yesalis CE III, Wright JE. Psychological and behavioural effects of endogenous testosterone and anabolic-androgenic steroids: an update. Sports Med 1996;22:367–390.
71. Bronson FH, Matherne CM. Exposure to anabolic-androgenic steroids shortens life span of male mice. Med Sci Sports Exerc 1997;29:615–619.
72. Korkia P, Stimson GV. Indications of prevalence, practice and effects of anabolic steroid use in Great Britain. Int J Sports Med 1997;18:557–562.
73. Pope HG, Katz DL. Psychiatric and medical effects of anabolic-androgenic steroid use. Arch Gen Psychiatry 1998;51:375–382.

74. Millar AP. Licit steroid use—hope for the future. Br J Sports Med 1994;28:79–83.
75. Freidl KE. Effects of anabolic steroids on physical health. In: Yesalis CE III, ed. Anabolic Steroids in Sport and Exercise. Human Kinetics, Champaign, IL, 1993, pp. 107–150.
76. Goldman B. Death in the Locker Room. Icarus Press, South Bend, IN, 1984, pp. 93–94.
77. Yesalis CE III, Wright JE. Societal alternatives. In: Yesalis CE III, ed. Anabolic Steroids in Sport and Exercise. Human Kinetics, Champaign, IL, 1993, pp. 309–315.
78. Ishak KG, Zimmerman HJ. Hepatotoxic effects of the anabolic/androgenic steroids. Semin Liver Dis 1987;7:230–236.
79. Street C, Antonio J, Cudlipp D. Androgen use by athletes: a reevaluation of the health risks. Can J Appl Physiol 1996;21:421–440.
80. Huie MJ. An acute myocardial infarction occuring in an anabolic steroid user. Med Sci Sports Exerc 1997;26:408–413.
81. Gold J, High HA, Li Y, Michelmore H, Bodsworth NJ, Finlayson R, Furner VL, Allen BJ, Oliver CJ. Safety and efficacy of nandrolone decanoate for treatment of wasting in patients with HIV infection. AIDS 1996;10:745–752.
82. Schürmeyer T, Knuth UA, Belkien L, Nieschlag E. Reversible azoospermia induced by the anabolic steroid 19-nortestosterone. Lancet 1984;1:417–420.
83. Hassager C, Riis BJ, Pødenphant J, Christiansen C. Nandrolone decanoate treatment of postmenopausal osteoporosis for 2 years and effects of withdrawal. Maturitas 1989;11:305–317.
84. Knuth UA, Behre HM, Belkien L, Bents H, Nieschlag E. Clinical trial of 19-nortestosterone-hexoxyphenylpropionate (Anadur) for male fertility regulation. Fertil Steril 1985;44:814–821.
85. Rosenburg HM, Ventura SJ, Maurer JD, et al. Births and deaths. United States. 1995. Monthly Vital Statistics Report 1995;45:31.
86. Angell M. Shattuck Lecture—Evaluating the health risks of breast implants: the interplay of medical science, the law, and public opinion. N Engl J Med 1996;334:1513–1518.
87. Connell EB. Silicone breast implants: the impact of litigation on women's health care. Women's Health Digest 1996;2:102–105.
88. Musshoff F, Daldrup T, Ritsch M. Anabole steroide auf dem deutschen schwarzmarkt. Arch Kriminol 1997;199:152–158.
89. Nieminen MS, Rämö MP, Viitasalo M, Heikkilä P, Karjalainen J, Mäntysaari M, Heikkilä J. Serious cardiovascular side effects of large doses of anabolic steroids in weight lifters. Eur Heart J 1996;17:1576–1583.
90. Phillips WN. Future vogue. In: Phillips WN, ed. Anabolic Reference Guide. Mile High Publishing, Golden, CO, 1991, pp. 243–245.
91. Duchaine D. The drugs in particular. In: Underground Steroid Handbook II. HLR, Venice, CA, 1989, pp. 27–59.
92. McNutt RA, Ferenchick GS, Kirlin PC, Hamlin NJ. Acute myocardial infarction in a 22-year-old world class weight lifter using anabolic steroids. Am J Cardiol 1988;62:164.
93. Ajayi AAL, Mathur R, Halushka PV. Testosterone increases human platelet thromboxane A_2 receptor density and aggregation responses. Circulation 1995;91:2742–2747.
94. Friedl KE, Hannan CJ, Jones RE, Plymate SR. High-density lipoprotein cholesterol is not decreased if an aromatizable androgen is administered. Metabolism 1990;39:69–74.
95. Kleiner SM, Calabrese LH, Fielder KM, Naito HK, Skibinski CI. Dietary influences on cardiovascular disease risk in anabolic steroid-using and nonusing bodybuilders. J Am Coll Nutr 1989;8:109–119.
96. Radis CD, Callis KP. Systemic lupus erythematosus with membranous glomerulonephritis and transverse myelitis associated with anabolic steroid use. Arthritis Rheum 1997;40:1899–1902.
97. Pope HG, Katz DL. Homicide and near-homicide by anabolic steroid users. J Clin Psychiatry 1990;51:28–31.
98. Choi PYL, Pope HG. Violence toward women and illicit androgenic-anabolic steroid use. Ann Clin Psychiatry 1994;6:21–25.
99. Su T-P, Pagliaro M, Schmidt PJ, Pickar D, Wolkowitz O, Rubinow R. Neuropsychiatric effects of anabolic steroids in male normal volunteers. JAMA 1993;269:2760–2764.
100. Anderson RA, Bancroft J, Wu FCW. The effects of exogenous testosterone on sexuality and mood of normal men. J Clin Endocrinol Metab 1992;75:1503–1507.
101. Bagatell CJ, Heiman JR, Matsumoto AM, Rivier JE, Bremner WJ. Metabolic and behavioral effects of high-dose exogenous testosterone in healthy men. J Clin Endocrinol Metab 1994;79:561–567.

102. Clark AS, Fast AS. Comparison of the effects of 17α-methyltestosterone, methandrostenolone, and nandrolone decanoate on the sexual behavior of castrated male rats. Behav Neurosci 1996;110: 1478–1486.
103. Fry RW, Grove JR, Morton AR, Zeroni PM, Gaudieri S, Keast D. Psychological and immunological correlates of acute overtraining. Br J Sports Med 1994;28:241–246.
104. Nindl BC, Friedl KE, Frykman PN, Marchitelli LJ, Shippee RL, Patton JF. Physical performance and metabolic recovery among lean, healthy men following a prolonged energy deficit. Int J Sports Med 1997;18:317–324.
105. Young SN. The use of diet and dietary components in the study of factors controlling affect in humans: a review. J Psychiatr Neurosci 1993;18:235–244.
106. Morgan WP, Costill DL, Flynn MG, Raglin JS, O'Conner PJ. Mood disturbance following increased training in swimmers. Med Sci Sports Exerc 1988;20:408–414.
107. Fry RW, Morton AR, Keast D. Overtraining in athletes. Sports Med 1991;12:32–65.
108. Bahrke MS, Wright JE, O'Connor JS, Strauss RH, Catlin DH. Selected psychological characteristics of anabolic-androgenic steroid users. N Engl J Med 1990;323:834,835.
109. Dayton L. What price glory? Women's Sports and Fitness (March), 1990;52–55.
110. Tricker R, Casaburi R, Storer TW, Clevenger B, Berman N, Shirazi A, Bhasin S. The effects of supraphysiological doses of testosterone on angry behavior in healthy engonadal men—A clinical research study. J Clin Endocrinol Metab 1996;81:3754–3758.
111. Matusmoto AM. Effects of chronic testosterone administration in normal men: safety and efficacy of high dosage testosterone and parallel dose-dependent supression of luteinizing hormone, follicle-stimulating hormone, and sperm production. J Clin Endocrinol Metab 1990;70:282–287.
112. Bjorkqvist K, Nygren T, Bjorklund A-C. Testosterone intake and aggressiveness: real effect or anticipation. Aggressive Behav 1994;20:17–26.
113. Brower KJ, Eliopulos GA, Blow FC, Catlin DH, Beresford TP. Evidence for physical and psychological dependence on anabolic androgenic steroids in eight weight lifters. Am J Psychiatry 1990;147:510–512.
114. Brower KJ. Withdrawal from anabolic steroids. In: Krieger DT, Bardin CW, eds. Current Therapy in Endocrinology and Metabolism. Mosby, Philadelphia, PA, 1997, pp. 339–343.
115. Malone DA, Dimeff RJ. The use of fluoxetine in depression associated with anabolic steroid withdrawal: a case series. J Clin Psychiatry 1992;53:130–132.
116. Bitran D, Kellogg CK, Hilvers RJ. Treatment with an anabolic-androgenic steroid affects anxiety-related behavior and alters the sensitivity of cortical $GABA_A$ receptors in the rat. Horm Behav 1993;27:568–583.
117. Johansson P, Ray A, Zhou Q, Huang W, Karlsson K, Nyberg F. Anabolic androgenic steroids increase beta-endorphin levels in the ventral tegmental area in the male rat brain. Neurosci Res 1997;27:185–189.
118. Vogel W, Klaiber EL, Broverman DM. A comparison of the antidepressant effects of a synthetic androgen (mesterolone) and amitriptyline in depressed men. J Clin Psychiatry 1985;46:6–8.
119. Alexander GM, Swerdloff RS, Wang C, Davidson T, McDonald V, Steiner B, Hines M. Androgen-behavior correlations in hypogonadal men and eugonadal men. I. Mood and response to auditory sexual stimuli. Horm Behav 1997;31:110–119.
120. Sherwin BB. Androgen use in women. In: Bhasin S, Gabelnick HL, Spieler JM, Swerdloff RS, Wang C, Keey C, eds. Pharmacology, Biology, and Clinical Applications of Androgens. Wiley-Liss, New York, NY, 1996, pp. 319–332.
121. Ogawa S, Washburn TF, Taylor J, Lubahn DB, Korach KS, Pfaff DW. Modifications of testosterone-dependent behaviors by estrogen receptor-alpha gene disruption in male mice. Endocrinology 1998;139:5058–5069.
122. Finkelstein JW, Susman EJ, Chinchilli VM, Kunselman SJ, D'Arcangelo MR, Schwab J, Demers LM, Liben LS, Lookingbill G, Kulin HE. Estrogen or testosterone increases self-reported aggressive behaviors in hypogonadal adolescents. J Clin Endocrinol Metab 1997;82:2423–2438.
123. Malone DA, Dimeff RJ, Lombardo JA, Barry Sample RH. Psychiatric effects and psychoactive substance use in anabolic-androgenic steroid users. Clin J Sport Med 1995;5:25–31.
124. Wu FCW, Farley TMM, Peregoudov A, Waites GMH. Effects of testosterone enanthate in normal men: experience from a multicenter contraceptive efficacy study. Fertil Steril 1996;65:626–636.
125. Thompson PD, Cullinane EM, Sady SP, Chenevert C, Saritelli AL, Herbert PN. Contrasting effects of testosterone and stanozolol on serum lipoprotein levels. JAMA 1989;261:1165–1168.

126. Zmuda JM, Fahrenbach MC, Younkin BT, Bausserman LL, Terry RB, Catlin DH, Thompson PD. The effect of testosterone aromatization on high-density lipoprotein cholesterol level and postheparin lipolytic activity. Metabolism 1993;42:446–450.
127. Bausserman LL, Saritelli AL, Herbert PN. Effects of short-term stanozolol administration on serum lipoproteins in hepatic lipase deficiency. Metabolism 1997;46:992–996.
128. Glazer G, Suchman AL. Lack of demonstrated effect on nandrolone on serum lipids. Metabolism 1994;43:204–210.
129. Goh HH, Loke DF, Ratnam SS. The impact of long-term testosterone replacement therapy on lipid and lipoprotein profiles in women. Maturitas 1995;21:65–70.
130. Van Kesteren PJM, Asscheman PJM, Megens AJ, Gooren LLG. Mortality and morbidity in transsexual subjects treated with cross-sex hormones. Clin Endocrinol 1997;47:337–342.
131. Bruck B, Brehme U, Gugel N, Hanke S, Finking G, Lutz C, Benda N, Schmahl FW, Haasis R, Hanke H. Gender-specific differences in the effects of testosterone and estrogen on the development of atherosclerosis in rabbits. Arterioscler Thromb Vasc Biol 1997;17:2192–2199.
132. Williams JK, Adams MR, Klopfenstein S. Estrogen modulates responses of atherosclerotic coronary arteries. Circulation 1990;81:1680–1687.
133. Knopp RH. Editorial: multiple beneficial effects of estrogen on lipoprotein metabolism. J Clin Endocrinol Metab 1997;82:3952–3954.
134. McCrohon JA, Walters WAW, Robinson JTC, McCredie RJ, Turner L, Adams MR, Handelsman DJ, Celermajer DS. Arterial reactivity is enhanced in genetic males taking high dose estrogens. J Am Coll Cardiol 1997;29:1432–1436.
135. New G, Timmins KL, Duffy SJ, Tran BT, O'Brien RC, Harper RW, Meredith IT. Long-term estrogen therapy improves vascular function in male to female transsexuals. J Am Coll Cardiol 1997;29:1437–1444.
136. Rockhold RW. Cardiovascular toxicity of anabolic steroids. Ann Rev Pharmacol Toxicol 1993;33:497–520.
137. Pratico D, FitzGerald GA. Testosterone and thromboxane. Of muscles, mice and men. Circulation 1995;91:2694–2698.
138. Urhausen A, Holpes R, Kindermann W. One- and two-dimensional echocardiography in bodybuilders using anabolic steroids. Eur J Appl Physiol 1989;58:633–640.
139. Dickermen RD, Schaller F, Zachariah NY, McConathy WJ. Left ventricular size and function in elite bodybuilders using anabolic steroids. Clin J Sport Med 1997;7:90–93.
140. Thompson PD, Sadaniantz A, Cullinane EM, Bodziony KS, Catlin DH, Torek-Both G, Douglas PS. Left ventricular function is not impaired in weight-lifters who use anabolic steroids. J Am Coll Cardiol 1992;19:278–282.
141. Ferrera PC, Putnam DL, Verdile VP. Anabolic steroid use as the possible precipitant of dilated cardiomyopathy. Cardiology 1997;88:218–220.
142. Rich JD, Dickinson BP, Flanigan TP, Valone SE. Abscess related to anabolic-androgenic steroid injection. Med Sci Sports Exerc 1999;31:207–209.
143. Turnicky RP, Goodin J, Smialek JE, Herskowitz A, Beschorner WE. Incidental myocarditis with intravenous drug abuse: the pathology, immunopathology, and potential implications for human immunodeficiency virus-associated myocarditis. Hum Pathol 1992;23:138–143.
144. Zeppilli P, Santini C, Dello Russo A, Picani C, Giordano A, Frustaci A. Brief report: healed myocarditis as a cause of ventricular repolarization abnormalities in athlete's heart. Int J Sports Med 1997;18:213–216.
145. Palatini P, Giada F, Garavelli G, Sinisi F, Mario L, Michieletto M, Baldo-Enzi G. Cardiovascular effects of anabolic steroids in weight-trained subjects. J Clin Pharmacol 1996;36:1132–1140.
146. Lowdell CP, Murray-Lyon IM. Reversal of liver damage due to long term methyltestosterone and safety of non-17 α-alkylated androgens. Br Med J 1985;291:637.
147. Nosaka K, Clarkson PM. Variability in serum creatine kinase response after eccentric exercise of the elbow flexors. Int J Sports Med 1996;17:120–127.
148. Nosaka K, Clarkson PM, Apple FS. Time course of serum protein changes after stenuous exercise of the forearm flexors. J Lab Clin Med 1992;119:183–188.
149. Knuth UA, Maniera H, Nieschlag E. Anabolic steroids and semen parameters in bodybuilders. Fertil Steril 1989;52:1041–1047.
150. Garzvani MR, Buckett W, Luckas MJM, Aird IA, Hipkin LJ, Lewis-Jones DI. Conservative management of azoospermia following steroid abuse. Hum Reprod 1997;12:1706–1708.

151. Lemcke B, Zentgraf J, Behre HM, Kleisch S, Bramswig JH, Neischlag E. Long-term effects on testicular function of high-dose testosterone treatment for excessively tall stature. J Clin Endocrinol Metab 1996;81:296–301.
152. De Wall WJ, Vreeburg JTM, Bekkering F, De Jong FH, De Muinck KS, Drop SLS, Weber RFA. High dose testosterone therapy for reduction of final height in consitutionally tall boys: Does it influence testicular function in adulthood? Clin Endocrinol 1995;43:87–95.
153. Matsumoto AM, Paulsen CA, Hopper BR, Rebar RW, Bremner WJ. Human chorionic gonadotropin and testicular function: Stimulation of testosterone, testosterone precusors, and sperm production despite high estradiol levels. J Clin Endocrinol Metab 1983;56:720–728.
154. Sundaram K, Kumar N, Monder C, Bardin CW. Different patterns of metabolism determine the relative anabolic activity of 19-norandrogens. J Steroid Biochem Mol Biol 1995;53:253–257.
155. Malarkey WB, Strauss RH, Leizman DJ, Liggett M, Demers LM. Endocrine effects in female weight lifters who self-administer testosterone and anabolic steroids. Am J Obstet Gynecol 1991;165:1385–1390.
156. Futterweit W, Green G, Tarlin N, Dunaif A. Chronic high-dose androgen administration to ovulatory women does not alter adrenocortical steroidogenesis. Fertil Steril 1992;58:124–128.
157. Spinder T, Spijkstra JJ, Van Den Tweel JG, Burger CW, Van Kessel H, Hompes PGA, Gooren LJG. The effects of long term testosterone administration on pulsatile luteinizing hormone secretion and on ovarian histology in eugonadal female to male transsexual subjects. J Clin Endocrinol Metab 1989;69:151–157.
158. Strauss RH, Liggett M, Lanese RR. Anabolic steroid use and perceived effects in ten weight-trained women athletes. JAMA 1985;253:2871–2873.
159. Miller N, Bédard YC, Cooter NB, Shaul DL. Histological changes in the genital tract in transsexual women following androgen therapy. Histopathology 1985;10:661–669.
160. Chadha S, Pache TD, Huikeshoven JM, Brinkmann AQ, Van der Kwast TH. Androgen receptor expression in human ovarian and uterine tissue of long-term androgen-treated transsexual women. Hum Pathol 1994;25:1198–1204.
161. Strauss RH, Yesalis CE III. Additional effects of anabolic steroids on women. In: Yesalis CE III, ed. Anabolic Steroids in Sport and Exercise. Human Kinetics, Champaign, IL, 1993, pp. 151–160.
162. Vliet GV. Clinical aspects of normal pubertal development. Horm Res 1991;36:93–96.
163. Duchaine D. Side effects. In: Underground Steroid Handbook II. HLR, Venice, CA, 1989, pp. 60–68.
164. Parker LN, Gray DR, Lai MK, Levin ER. Treatment of gynecomastia with tamoxifen: a double-blind crossover study. Metabolism 1986;35:705–708.
165. Miles JW, Grana WA, Egle D, Min KW, Chitwood J. The effect of anabolic steroids on the biochemical and histological properties of rat tendon. J Bone Joint Surg Am 1992;74-A:411–422.
166. Evans NA, Bowrey DJ, Newman DR. Ultrastructural analysis of ruptured tendon from anabolic steroid users. Injury 1998;29:769–773.
167. Kumar N, Shan L-X, Hardy MP, Bardin CW. Mechanism of androgen-induced thymolysis in rats. Endocrinology 1995;136:4887–4893.
168. Mendenhall CL, Grossman CJ, Roselle GA, Hertelendy Z, Ghosn SJ, Lamping K, Martin K. Anabolic steroid effects on immune function: differences between analogues. J Steroid Biochem Mol Biol 1990;37:71–76.
169. Bizzarro A, Valentini G, Di Martino G, Daponte A, De Bellis A, Iacono G. Influence of testosterone therapy on clinical and immunological features of autoimmune diseases associated with Klinefelter's syndrome. J Clin Endocrinol Metab 1987;64:32–36.
170. Kovacs WJ, Olsen NJ. Androgen receptors in human thymocytes. J Immunol 1987;139:490–493.
171. Ahmed SA, Dauphinée MJ, Talal N. Effects of short-term administration of sex hormones on normal and autoimmune mice. J Immunol 1985;134:204–210.
172. Cutolo M, Balleari E, Giusti M, Intra E, Accardo S. Androgen replacement therapy in male patients with rheumatoid arthritis. Arthritis Rheum 1991;34:1–5.
173. Bruley-Rosset M, Dardeene M, Schuurs A. Functional and quantitative changes of immune cells of ageing NZB mice treated with nandrolone decanoate. I. Effect on survival and autoantibody development. Clin Exp Immunol 1985;62:630–638.
174. Lahita RG, Cheng CY, Monder C, Bardin CW. Experience with 19-nortestosterone in the therapy of systemic lupus erythematosus: worsened disease after treatment with 19-nortestosterone in men and lack of improvement in women. J Rheumatol 1992;19:547–555.

175. Calabrese LH, Kleiner SM, Barna BP, Skibinski CI, Kirkendall DT, Lahita RG, Lombardo JA. The effects of anabolic steroids and strength training on the human immune response. Med Sci Sports Exerc 1989;21:386–392.
176. Berger JR, Pall L, Hall CD, Simpson DM, Berry PS, Dudley R. Oxandrolone in AIDS-wasting myopathy. AIDS 1996;10:1657–1662.
177. Graves MK, Soto L. Left-sided endocarditis in parenteral drug abusers: recent experience at a large community hospital. South Med J 1992;85:378–380.
178. Duchaine D. Human growth hormone. In: Underground Steroid Handbook II. HLR, Venice, CA, 1989, p. 74.
179. Hwu C-M, Kwok CF, Lai T-Y, Shih K-C, Lee T-S, Hsiao L-C, Lee S-H, Fang VS, Ho L-T. Growth hormone (GH) replacement reduces total body fat and normalizes insulin sensitivity in GH-deficient adults: a report of one-year clinical experience. J Clin Endocrinol Metab 1997;82:3285–3292.
180. Cuneo RC, Salomon F, Wiles CM, Hesp R, Sönksen PH. Growth hormone treatment in growth hormone-deficient adults. I. Effects on muscle mass and strength. J Appl Physiol 1991;70:688–694.
181. Crist DM, Peake GT, Egan PA, Waters DL. Body composition response to exogenous GH during training in highly conditioned adults. J Appl Physiol 1988;65:579–584.
182. Yarasheski KE, Zachwieja JJ, Bier DM. Short-term growth hormone treatment does not increase muscle protein synthesis in experienced weight lifters. J Appl Physiol 1993;74:3073–3076.
183. Deyssig R, Frisch H, Blum WF, Waldhör T. Effect of growth hormone treatment on hormonal parameters, body composition and strength in athletes. Acta Endocrinol (Copenh) 1993;128:313–318.
184. Yarasheski KE. Growth hormone effects on metabolism, body composition, muscle mass, and strength. In: Holloszy JO, ed. Exercise and Sports Science Reviews. Williams and Wilkins, Baltimore, MD, 1994, pp. 285–312.
185. Johannsson G, Mårin P, Lönn L, Ottosson M, Stenlöf K, Björntorp P, Sjöström L, Bengtsson B-A. Growth hormone treatment of abdominally obese men reduces abdominal fat mass, improves glucose and lipoprotein metabolism, and reduces diastolic blood pressure. J Clin Endocrinol Metab 1997;82:727–734.
186. Thompson JL, Butterfield GE, Gylfadottir UK, Yesavage J, Marcus R, Hintz RL, Pearman A, Hoffman AR. Effects of human growth hormone, insulin-like growth factor I, and diet and exercise on body composition of obese postmenopausal women. J Clin Endocrinol Metab 1998;83:1477–1484.
187. Thompson JL, Butterfield GE, Marcus R, Hintz RL, Van Loan M, Ghiron L, Hoffman AR. The effects of recombinant human insulin-like growth factor-I and growth hormone on body composition in elderly women. J Clin Endocrinol Metab 1995;80:1845–1852.
188 Adams GR. Role of insulin-like growth factor-I in the regulation of skeletal muscle adaptation to increased loading. In: Holloszy JO, ed. Exercise and Sports Science Reviews. Williams and Wilkins, Baltimore, MD, 1998, pp. 31–60.
189. Lo H-C, Hinton PS, Peterson CA, Ney DM. Simultaneous treatment with IGF-I and GH additively increases anabolism in parenterally fed rats. Am J Physiol (Endocrinol Metab 32) 1995;269:E368–E376.
190. Berneis K, Ninnis R, Girard J, Frey BM, Keller U. Effects of insulin-like growth factor I combined with growth hormone on glucocorticoid-induced whole-body protein catabolism in man. J Clin Endocrinol Metab 1997;82:2528–2534.
191. Kupfer SR, Underwood LE, Baxter RC, Clemmons DR. Enhancement of the anabolic effects of growth hormone and insulin-like growth factor I by use of both agents simultaneously. J Clin Invest 1993;91:391–396.
192. Ramsey TG, Chung IB, Czerwinski SM, McMurtry JP, Rosenbrough RW, Steele NC. Tissue IGF-I protein and mRNA responses to a single injection of somatotropin. Am J Physiol (Endocrinol Metab 32) 1995;269:E627–E635.
193. Taaffe DR, Pruitt L, Reim J, Hintz RL, Butterfield GE, Hoffman AR, Marcus R. Effect of recombinant human growth hormone on the muscle strength response to resistance exercise in elderly men. J Clin Endocrinol Metab 1994;79:1361–1366.
194. Butler AA, Funk B, Breier BH, LeRoith D, Roberts CT Jr, Gluckman PD. Growth hormone (GH) status regulates GH receptor and GH binding protein mRNA in a tissue- and transcript-specific manner but has no effect on insulin-like growth factor-I mRNA in the rat. Mol Cell Endocrinol 1996;116:181–189.

195. Lemmey AB, Glassford J, Flick-Smith HC, Holly JMP, Pell JM. Differential regulation of tissue insulin-like growth factor-binding protein (IGFBP)-3, IGF-I and IGF type 1 receptor mRNA levels, and serum IGF-I and IGFBP concentrations by growth hormone and IGF-I. J Endocrinol 1997;154:319–328.
196. Gosteli-Peter MA, Winterhalter KH, Schmid C, Froesch ER, Zapf J. Expression and regulation of insulin-like growth factor-I (IGF-I) and IGF-binding protein messenger ribonucleic acid levels in tissues of hypophysectomized rats infused with IGF-I and growth hormone. Endocrinology 1994;135:2558–2567.
197. Tapanainen J, Rönnberg L, Martikainen H, Reinilä M, Koistinen R, Seppälä M. Short and long term effects of growth hormone on circulating levels of insulin-like growth factor-I (IGF-I), IGF-binding protein-1, and insulin: a placebo-controlled study. J Clin Endocrinol Metab 1991;73:71–74.
198. Sturmi JE, Diorio DJ. Anabolic agents. Clin Sports Med 1998;17:261–282.
199. Jabri N, Schalch DS, Schwartz SL, Fischer JS, Kipnes MS, Radnik BJ, Turman NJ, Marcsisin VS, Guler HP. Adverse effects of recombinant human insulin-like growth factor I in obese insulin resistant type II diabetic patients. Diabetes 1994;43:369–374.
200. Tomas FM, Lemmey AB, Ballard FJ. Superior potency of infused IGF-I analogues which bind poorly to IGF-binding proteins is maintained when administered by injection. J Endocrinol 1996;150:77–84.
201. Torring N, Vinter-Jensen L, Pedersen SB, Sorensen FB, Flybjerg A, Nexo E. Systemic administration of insulin-like growth factor I (IGF-I) causes growth of the rat prostate. J Urol 1997;158:222–227.
202. Jungwirth A, Schally AV, Pinski J, Halmos G, Groot K, Armatis P. Inhibition of in vivo proliferation of androgen-independent prostate cancers by an antagonist of growth hormone-releasing hormone. Br J Cancer 1997;75:1585–1592.
203. Prather ID, Brown DE, North PE, Wilson JR. Clenbuterol: a substitute for anabolic steroids? Med Sci Sports Exerc 1995;27:1118–1121.
204. Cartañà J, Segués T, Yebras M, Rothwell NJ, Stock MJ. Anabolic effects of clenbuterol after long-term treatment and withdrawal in the rat. Metabolism 1994;43:1086–1092.
205. Yang YT, McElligott MA. Review article. Multiple actions of β-adrenergic agonists on skeletal muscle and adipose tissue. Biochem J 1989;261:1–10.
206. Eadara JK, Dalrymple RH, DeLay RL, Ricks CA, Romsos DR. Effects of cimaterol, a beta-adrenergic agonist, on lipid metabolism in rats. Metabolism 1989;38:522–529.
207. Choo JJ, Horan MA, Little RA, Rothwell NJ. Anabolic effects of clenbuterol on skeletal muscle are mediated by β_2-adrenoceptor activation. Am J Physiol (Endocrinol Metab 26) 1992;263:E50–E56.
208. Belahsen R, Deshaies Y. Modulation of lipoprotein lipase activity in the rat by the β_2-adrenergic agonist clenbuterol. Can J Physiol Pharmacol 1992;70:1555–1562.
209. Carter WJ, Lynch ME. Comparison of the effects of salbutamol and clenbuterol on skeletal muscle mass and carcass composition in senescent rats. Metabolism 1994;43:1119–1125.
210. McElligott MA, Barretto A Jr, Chaung L-Y. Effect of continuous and intermittent clenbuterol feeding on rat growth rate and muscle. Comp Biochem Physiol A Physiol 1989;92C:135–138.
211. Dawson RT, Harrison MW. Use of insulin as an anabolic agent. Br J Sports Med 1997;31:259.
212. Biolo G, Fleming RYD, Wolfe RR. Physiologic hyperinsulinemia stimulates protein synthesis and enhances transport of selected amino acids in human skeletal muscle. J Clin Invest 1995;95:811–819.
213. Fluckey JD, Vary TC, Jefferson LS, Evans WJ, Farrell PA. Insulin stimulation of protein synthesis in rat skeletal muscle following resistance exercise is maintained with advancing age. J Gerontol A Biol Sci Med Sci 1996;51A:B323–B330.
214. Fluckey JD, Vary TC, Jefferson LS, Farrell PA. Augmented insulin action on rates of protein synthesis after resistance exercise in rats. Am J Physiol (Endocrinol Metab 33) 1996;270:E313–E319.
215. Jacob R, Hu X, Niederstock D, Hasan S, McNulty PH, Sherwin RS, Young LH. IGF-I stimulation of muscle protein synthesis in the awake rat: permissive role of insulin and amino acids. Am J Physiol (Endocrinol Metab 33) 1996;270:E60–E66.
216. Zawadzki KM, Yespelkis BB III, Ivy JL. Carbohydrate–protein complex increases the rate of muscle glycogen storage after exercise. J Appl Physiol 1992;72:1854–1859.
217. Capaldo B, Napoli R, Di Marino L, Guida R, Pardo F, Sacca L. Role of insulin and free fatty acid (FFA) availability on regional FFA kinetics in the human forearm. J Clin Endocrinol Metab 1994;79:879–882.

218. Loucks AB, Heath EM. Induction of low-T_3 syndrome in exercising women occurs at a threshold of energy availability. Am J Physiol (Regulatory Integrative Comp Physiol 35) 1994;266:R817–R823.
219. Ferner RE, Burnett A, Rawlins MD. Tri-iodothyroacetic acid abuse in a female bodybuilder. Lancet 1986;1:383.
220. Welle SL, Campbell RG. Decrease in resting metabolic rate during rapid weight loss is reversed by low dose thyroid hormone treatment. Metabolism 1986;35:289–291.
221. Rozen R, Abraham G, Falcou R, Apfelbaum M. Effects of a 'physiological' dose of triiodothyronine on obese subjects during a protein-sparing diet. Int J Obesity 1986;10:303–312.
222. Lovejoy JC, Smith SR, Bray GA, DeLany JP, Rood JC, Gouvier D, Windhauser M, Ryan DH, Macchiavelli R, Tulley R. A paradigm of experimentally induced mild hyperthyroidism: effects on nitrogen balance, body composition, and energy expenditure in healthy young men. J Clin Endocrinol Metab 1997;82:765–770.
223. Al-Adsani H, Hoffer LJ, Silva JE. Resting energy expenditure is sensitive to small dose changes in patients on chronic thyroid hormone replacement. J Clin Endocrinol Metab 1997;82:1118–1125.
224. Frystyk J, Grønbæk H, Skjærbæk, Flyvbjerg A. Effect of hyperthyroidism on circulating levels of free and total IGF-I and IGFBPs in rats. Am J Physiol (Endocrinol Metab 32) 1995;269:E840–E845.
225. Miell JP, Taylor AM, Zini M, Maheshwari HG, Ross RJM, Valcavi R. Effects of hypothyroidism and hyperthyroidism on insulin-like growth factors (IGFs) and growth hormone- and IGF-binding proteins. J Clin Endocrinol Metab 1993;76:950–955.
226. Sundaram V, Hanna AN, Koneru L, Newman HAI, Falko JM. Both hypothyroidism and hyperthyroidism enhance low density lipoprotein oxidation. J Clin Endocrinol Metab 1997;82:3421–3424.
227. Piepho R, Whelton A, Mayor G, Neu H, Laddu A. Excess synthroid ingestion as CHF. J Clin Pharmacol 1992;32:18–23.
228. Ching GW, Franklyn JA, Stallard TJ, Daykin J, Sheppard MC, Gammage MD. Cardiac hypertrophy as a result of long-term thyroxine therapy and thyrotoxicosis. Heart 1996;75:363–368, 1996.
229. Nedrebø BG, Ericsson U-B, Nygård O, Refsum H, Ueland PM, Aakvaag A, Aanderud S, Lien EA. Plasma total homocysteine levels in hyperthyroid and hypothyroid patients. Metabolism 1998; 47:89–93.
230. Masunaga R, Nagasaka A, Nakai A, Kotake M, Sawai Y, Oda N, Mokuno T, Shimazaki K, Hayakawa N, Kato R, Hirano E, Hagiwara M, Hidaka H. Alteration of platelet aggregation in patients with thyroid disorders. Metabolism 1997;46:1128–1131.
231. Morales AJ, Nolan JJ, Nelson JC, Yen SC. Effects of replacement dose of dehydroepiandrosterone in men and women of advancing age. J Clin Endocrinol Metab 1994;78:1360–1367.
232. Bosy TZ, Moore KA, Poklis A. The effect of oral dehydroepiandrosterone (DHEA) on the urine testosterone/epitestosterone (T/E) ratio in human volunteers. J Anal Toxicol 1998;22:455–459.
233. Welle S, Jozefowicz R, Statt M. Failure of DHEA to influence energy and protein metabolism in humans. J Clin Endocrinol Metab 1990;71:1259–1264.
234. Morales AJ, Haubrich RH, Hwang JY, Asakura H, Yen SC. The effect of six months treatment with a 100 mg daily dose of dehydroepiandrosterone (DHEA) on circulating sex steroids, body composition and muscle strength in age-advanced men and women. Clin Endocrinol 1998;49:421–432.
235. Khorram O, Vu L, Yen SSC. Activation of immune function by dehydroepiandrosterone (DHEA) in age-advanced men. J Gerontol A Biol Sci Med Sci 1998;52A:M1–M7.
236. Flynn MA, Weaver-Osterholtz D, Sharpe-Timms KL, Allen S, Krause G. Dehydroepiandrosterone replacement in aging humans. J Clin Endocrinol Metab 1999;84:1527–1533.
237. Arlt W, Haas J, Callies F, Reincke M, Hübler D, Oettel M, Ernst M, Schulte HM, Allolio B. Biotransformation of oral dehydroepiandrosterone in elderly men: significant increase in circulating estrogens. J Clin Endocrinol Metab 1999;84:2170–2176.
238. Sahelian R, Borken S. Dehydroepiandrosterone and cardiac arrhythmia. Ann Intern Med 1998;129:588.
239. Parasrampuria J, Schwartz K, Petesch R. Quality control of dehydroepiandrosterone dietary supplement products. JAMA 1998;280:1565.
240. King DS, Sharp RL, Brown GA, Reifenrath TA, Uhl NL. Oral anabolic-androgenic supplements during resistance training: effects on serum testosterone and estrogen concentrations. Med Sci Sports Exerc 1999;31:S266.
241. Reifenrath TA, Sharp RL, Brown GA, Uhl NL, King DS. Oral anabolic-androgenic supplements during resistance training: effects on body composition and muscle strength. Med Sci Sports Exerc 1999;31:S266.

242. Brown GA, Reifenrath TA, Uhl NL, Sharp RL, King DS. Oral anabolic-androgenic supplements during resistance training: effects on glucose tolerance, insulin action, and blood lipids. Med Sci Sports Exerc 1999;31:S266.
243. King DS, Sharp RL, Vukovich MD, Brown GA, Reifenrath TA, Uhl NL, Parsons KA. Effect of oral androstenedione on serum testosterone and adaptations to resistance training in young men. JAMA 1999;281:2020–2028.
244. Salehian B, Wang C, Alexander G, Davidson T, McDonald V, Berman N, Dudley RE, Ziel F, Swerdloff RS. Pharmacokinetics, bioefficacy, and safety of sublingual testosterone cyclodextrin in hypogonadal men: comparison to testosterone enanthate—A clinical research center study. J Clin Endocrinol Metab 1995;80:3567–3575.
245. Kintz P, Cirimele V, Ludes B. Norandrostenolone and noretiocholanolone: metabolite markers. Acta Clin Belg Suppl 1999;1:68–73.
246. Powles TJ, Tillyer CR, Jones AL, Ashley SE, Treleaven J, Davey JB, McKinna JA. Prevention of breast cancer with tamoxifen—an update on the Royal Marsden hospital pilot programme. Eur J Cancer 1990;26:680–684.
247. Wheeler MD. Physical changes of puberty. Endocrinol Metab Clin North Am 1991;20:12,13.
248. O'Sullivan AJ, Crampton LJ, Freund J, Ho KKY. The route of estrogen replacement therapy confers divergent effects on substrate oxidation and body composition in postmenopausal women. J Clin Invest 1998;102:1035–1040.
249. Guvakova MA, Surmacz E. Tamoxifen interferes with the insulin-like growth factor I receptor (IGF-IR) signaling pathway in breast cancer cells. Cancer Res 1997;57:2606–2610.
250. Tannenbaum GS, Gurd W, LaPointe M, Pollak M. Tamoxifen attenuates pulsatile growth hormone secretion: mediation in part by somatostatin. Endocrinology 1992;130:3395–3401.
251. Lien EA, Johannessen DC, Aakvaag A, Lonning PE. Influence of tamoxifen, aminoglutethimide and goserelin on human plasma IGF-I levels in breast cancer patients. J Steroid Biochem Mol Biol 1992;41:541–543.
252. Florini JR, Ewton DZ, Coolican SA. Growth hormone and the insulin-like growth factor system in myogenesis. Endocr Rev 1996;17:481–517.
253. Guay AT, Bansal S, Heatley GJ. Effect of raising endogenous testosterone levels in impotent men with secondary hypogonadism: double blind placebo-controlled trial with clomiphene citrate. J Clin Endocrinol Metab 1995;80:3546–3552.
254. Martikainen H, Markku A, Rahkila P, Vihko R. Testicular responsiveness to human chorionic gonadotrophin during transient hypogonadotrophic hypogonadism induced by androgenic/anabolic steroids in power athletes. J Steroid Biochem 1986;25:109–112.
255. Dallob AL, Sadick NS, Unger W, Lipert S, Geissler LA, Gregoire SL, Nguyen HH, Moore EC, Tanaka WK. The effect of finasteride, a 5α-reductase inhibitor on scalp skin testosterone and dihydrotestosterone concentrations in patients with male pattern baldness. J Clin Endocrinol Metab 1994;79:703–706.
256. Imperato-McGinley J, Gautier T, Cai LQ, Yee B, Epstein J, Pochi P. The androgen control of sebum production. Studies of subjects with dihydrotestosterone deficiency and complete androgen insensitivity. J Clin Endocrinol Metab 1993;76:524–528.
257. Wong E, Morris RS, Chang L, Spahn M-A, Stanczyk FZ, Lobo RA. A prospective randomized trial comparing finasteride to spironolactone in the treatment of hirsute women. J Clin Endocrinol Metab 1995;80:233–238.
258. Castello R, Negri C, Tosi F, Muggeo M, Perrone F, Moghetti P. Outcome of long-term treatment with the 5α-reductase inhibitor finasteride in idiopathic hirsutism: clinical and hormonal effects during a 1-year course of therapy and 1-year follow-up. Fertil Steril 1996;66:734–740.
259. Fruzzetti F, De Lorenzo D, Parrini D, Ricci C. Effects of finasteride, a 5α-reductase inhibitor, on circulating androgens and gonadotropin secretion in hirsute women. J Clin Endocrinol Metab 1994;79:831–835.
260. Crowley MA, Matt KS. Hormonal regulation of skeletal muscle hypertrophy in rats: the testosterone to cortisol ratio. Eur J Appl Physiol 1996;73:66–72.
261. CDC. Gamma hydroxy butyrate use—New York and Texas, 1995–1996. JAMA 1997;277:1511.
262. Marwick C. Coma-inducing drug GHB may be reclassified. JAMA 1997;277:1505,1506.
263. Bell DG, Jacobs I, Zamecnik J. Effects of caffeine, ephedrine and their combination on time to exhaustion during high-intensity exercise. Eur J Appl Physiol 1998;77:427–433.

264. Pasquali R, Casimirri F, Melchionda N, Grossi G, Bortoluzzi L, Morselli Labate AM, Stefanini C, Raitano A. Effects of chronic administration of ephedrine during very-low-calorie diets on energy expenditure, protein metabolism and hormone levels in obese subjects. Clin Sci 1992;82:85–92.
265. Astrup A, Lundsgaard C, Madsen J, Christensen NJ. Enhanced thermogenic responsiveness during chronic ephedrine treatment in man. Am J Clin Nutr 1985;42:83–94.
266. Astrup A, Madsen J, Holst JJ, Christensen NJ. The effect of chronic ephedine treatment on substrate utilization, the sympathoadrenal activity, and energy expenditure during glucose-induced thermogenesis in man. Metabolism 1986;35:260–265.
267. Astrup A, Toubro S, Cannon S, Hein P, Madsen J. Thermogenic synergism between ephedrine and caffeine in healthy volunteers: a double-blind, placebo-controlled study. Metabolism 1991;40:323–329.
268. Ramsey JJ, Colman RJ, Swick AG, Kemnitz JW. Energy expenditure, body composition, and glucose metabolism in lean and obese rhesus monkeys treated with ephedrine and caffeine. Am J Clin Nutr 1999;68:42–51.
269. Chase SL. The FDA warns of the dangers of ephedrine. RN 1996;59:67.
270. Seene T, Viru A. The catabolic effect of glucocorticoids on different types of skeletal muscle fibres and its dependence upon muscle activity and interaction with anabolic steroids. J Steroid Biochem 1982;16:349–352.
271. Kayali AG, Young VR, Goodman MN. Sensitivity of myofibrillar proteins to glucocortiocoid-induced muscle proteolysis. Am J Physiol (Endocrinol Metab 15) 1987;252:E621–E626.
272. Simmons PS, Miles JM, Gerich JE, Haymond MW. Increased proteolysis. An effect of increases in plasma cortisol within the physiologic range. J Clin Invest 1984;73:412–420.
273. Kraemer WJ, Nobel BJ, Clark ML, Culver BW. Physiologic responses to heavy-resistance exercise with very short rest periods. Int J Sports Med 1987;8:247–252.
274. Konagaya M, Max SR. A possible role for endogenous glucocorticoids in orchiectomy-induced atrophy of the rat levator ani muscle: studies with RU 38486, a potent and selective antiglucocorticoid. J Steroid Biochem 1986;25:305–308.
275. Pont A, Williams PL, Azhar S, Reitz RE, Bochra C, Smith ER, Stevens DA. Ketoconazole blocks testosterone synthesis. Arch Intern Med 1982;142:2137–2140.
276. Laue L, Lotze MT, Chrousos GP, Barnes K, Loriaux DL, Fleisher TA. Effect of chronic treatment with the glucocorticoid antagonist RU 486 in man: toxicity, immunological, and hormonal aspects. J Clin Endocrinol Metab 1990;71:1474–1480.
277. Fisher JW. Erythropoietin: physiologic and pharmacologic aspects. Proc Soc Exp Biol Med 1997;216:358–368.
278. Casoni I, Ricci G, Ballarin E, Borsetto C, Grazzi G, Guglielmini C, Manfredini F, Mazzoni G, Patracchini M, De Paoli Vitali E, Rigolin F, Bartalotta S, Franzè GP, Masotti M, Conconi F. Hematological indices of erythropoietin administration in athletes. Int J Sports Med 1993;14:307–311.
279. Ekblom B. Blood doping and erythropoietin. The effects of variation in hemoglobin concentration and other related factors on physical performance. Am J Sports Med 1996;24:S40–S42.
280. Ayotte C, Goudreault D, Charlebois A. Testing for natural and synthetic anabolic agents in human urine. J Chromatogr B Biomed Appl 1996;687:3–25.
281. Catlin DH, Hatton CK, Starcevic SH. Issues in detecting abuse of xenobiotic anabolic steroids and testosterone by analysis of athletes' urine. Clin Chem 1997;43:1280–1288.
282. Bowers LD. Analytical advances in detection of performance-enhancing compounds. Clin Chem 1997;43:1299–1304.
283. Damewood MD, Shen W, Zacur HA, Schlaff WD, Rock JA, Wallach EE. Disappearance of exogenously administered human chorionic gonadotropin. Fertil Steril 1989;52:398–400.
284. Kammerer RC. Drug testing and anabolic steroids. In: Yesalis CE III, ed. Anabolic Steroids in Sport and Exercise. Human Kinetics, Champaign, IL, 1993, pp. 283–308.
285. Friedl KE, Jones RE, Hannan CJ, Plymate SR. The administration of pharmacological doses of testosterone or 19-testosterone to normal men is not associated with increased insulin secretion or impaired glucose tolerance. J Clin Endocrinol Metab 1989;68:971–975.
286. Findlay JC, Place V, Synder PJ. Treatment of primary hypogonadism in men by the transdermal administration of testosterone. J Clin Endocrinol Metab 1989;68:369–373.
287. Dobs AS, Hoover DR, Chen M-C, Allen R. Pharmacokinetic characteristics, efficacy, and safety of buccal testosterone in hypogonadal males: a pilot study. J Clin Endocrinol Metab 1998;83:33–39.

288. Ferstle J. Evolution and politics of drug testing. In: Yesalis CE III, ed. Anabolic Steroids in Sport and Exercise. Human Kinetics, Champaign, IL, 1993, pp. 251–282.
289. Kessler PD, Podsakoff GM, Chen X, McQuiston SA, Colosi PC, Matelis LA, Kurtzman GJ, Byrne BJ. Gene delivery to skeletal muscle results in sustained expression and systemic delivery of a therapeutic protein. Proc Natl Acad Sci U S A 1996;93:14,082–14,087.
290. Barton-Davis ER, Shoturma DI, Musaro A, Rosenthal N, Sweeney HL. Viral mediated expression of insulin-like growth factor I blocks the aging-related loss of skeletal muscle function. Proc Natl Acad Sci USA 1998;95:15,603–15,607.
291. Tripathy SK, Svensson EC, Black HB, Goldwasser E, Margalith M, Hobart PM, Leiden JM. Long-term expression of erythropoietin in the systemic circulation of mice after intramuscular injection of a plasmid DNA vector. Proc Natl Acad Sci USA 1996;93:10,876–10,880.
292. Sheffield-Moore M, Urban RJ, Wolf SE, Jiang J, Catlin DH, Herndon DN, Wolfe RR, Ferrando AA. Short-term oxandrolone administration stimulates net muscle protein synthesis in young men. J Clin Endocrinol Metab 1999;84:2705–2711.

Index

A

Acid-base status,
  confounding variable in hormone analysis, 9
  β-endorphin and exercise, 38
ACTH, see Adrenocorticotropic hormone
Adrenaline, see Epinephrine
Adrenergic response, see Epinephrine; Norepinephrine
Adrenocorticotropic hormone (ACTH), see also Hypothalamo–pituitary–adrenal axis,
  cytokine effects on levels, 288
  diurnal variation, 11
  exercise effects at altitude,
    acute exercise, 377, 378
    chronic exercise, 382
  overtraining effects, 359, 360
Adrenomedullin, exercise response, 214
AFP, see α-Feto protein
Aging, confounding factor in hormone analysis, 6
Alcohol use, effects in hormone analysis, 9
Aldosterone, see Renin–angiotensin–aldosterone system
Altitude,
  acute exercise response,
    adrenocorticotrophic hormone, 377, 378
    arginine vasopressin, 377
    atrial natriuretic peptide, 376, 377
    catecholamines,
      hypohydration effects, 373, 374
      hypoxemia effects, 372–375
      overview, 372, 373
      physiological significance of response, 374, 375
      undernutrition effects, 373, 374
    cortisol, 377, 378
    glucagon, 376
    growth hormone, 378
    insulin, 375, 376
    prolactin, 378
    renin–angiotensin–aldosterone system, 376, 377
  chronic exercise effects,
    adrenocorticotrophic hormone, 382
    arginine vasopressin, 382
    catecholamines,
      hypertension response, 380
      hypoxia stimulation of tyrosine hydroxylase, 379, 380
      maximum heart rate modulation, 380, 381
      overview, 378, 379
      work intensity relationship, 379
    cortisol, 382
    erythropoietin, 384
    glucagon, 381
    growth hormone, 383
    insulin, 381
    prolactin, 383
    renin–angiotensin–aldosterone system, 381, 382
    thyroid hormone, 383
Amenorrhea, athletic,
  body composition hypothesis, 165, 166, 175
  bone,
    density effects on reversal, 264, 265
    effects, 240–242
  carbohydrate availability hypothesis, 176
  definition, 134
  energy availability hypothesis, 166, 167, 175, 191, 192, 240, 241
  exercise stress hypothesis, 167, 175, 241
  hypothalamic adaptations in exercise,
    dose–response, 148, 149
    marathon runners, 151
    molimia prior to ovulation disturbances, 152
    normality of adaptations, 159
    prospective studies of menstrual cycle and luteal length effects, 147–151
    reversibility of adaptation, 153–156, 158
    time-course of ovulatory adaptation, 152, 153
  hypothalamo–pituitary–adrenal axis in exercise-induced disorder, 50
  osteopenia risks, 261, 262
  overview, 133, 134
  prospective studies,
    distinguishing exercise stress from energy availability effects, 168, 169
    luteinizing hormone pulsatility as outcome variable, 168, 177
    luteinizing hormone pulsatility studies,
      Excalibur III, 172–174, 176
      Excalibur IV, 174, 175
    T_3 evaluation studies,
      Excalibur I, 169, 170
      Excaliber II, 170–172
  thyroid hormone response to exercise, 110
  treatment and reversal, 242, 248
Anabolic-androgenic steroids,
  administration routes, 436–438
  demographics of users, 435, 439
  doping control, 462

477

doses, 443, 444
effects,
  body composition, 439, 440, 442, 453
  sport performance, 440, 441
illegality of use, 433, 442
mechanism of action, 435
prevention of use, 453
rationale for use, 434, 435
side effects,
  acne, 451
  blood-borne diseases from needle sharing, 452
  cardiovascular disease, 448, 449, 452
  clinical case report flaws, 444–446
  female fertility, 450, 451
  gynecomastia, 451, 452
  hair loss, 451
  hypertension, 449
  immune function, 452
  liver disease, 450
  low-density lipoprotein effects, 445, 448
  male fertility, 450
  musculoskeletal injury, 452
  prostate disease, 450
  psychological side effects, 446–448
  reversibility of effects, 452
  table, 436–438
  virilization in women, 451
types, 435–438, 442, 443
Androstenedione,
  performance-enhancing use, 458
  precision in assays, 5
Angiotensin, *see* Renin–angiotensin–aldosterone system
Anorexia nervosa, *see* Eating restraint
Anovulatory cycle, definition, 134–136
ANP, *see* Atrial natriuretic peptide
Appetite, hormonal control, 195, 196
Arginine vasopressin (AVP), *see also* Hypothalamo–pituitary–adrenal axis,
  exercise effects at altitude,
    acute exercise, 377
    chronic exercise, 382
  exercise response, 208, 212

Atrial natriuretic peptide (ANP), exercise effects,
  altitude effects, 376, 377
  response, 208, 212, 213
AVP, *see* Arginine vasopressin

B

B-cell, exercise response, 291
Basal metabolic rate (BMR), ovulatory disorders, 143
Basophil, exercise response, 291
Bioassay, hormones, 14
BMD, *see* Bone mineral density
BMR, *see* Basal metabolic rate
BNP, *see* Brain natriuretic peptide
Body composition, *see also* Energy balance,
  anabolic-androgenic steroid effects, 439, 440, 442, 453
  determinant of growth hormone exercise response, 58
  eumenorrhea hypothesis, 165, 166
  hormone analysis confounding factor, 7
Bone,
  modeling and remodeling, 255, 256
  negative effects of exercise on hormones,
    calcitonin, 244
    estrogen, 240–242
    parathyroid hormone, 243, 244
    progesterone, 240–242
    testosterone, 242
    vitamin D, 244
  positive effects of exercise on hormones,
    acute exercise effects on anabolic hormones, 245, 246
    calcitonin, 247–249
    growth hormone, 244, 245
    insulin-like growth factor-1, 244–247
    parathyroid hormone, 247–249
    testosterone, 244–246
    training effects on anabolic hormones, 246, 247
    vitamin D, 248, 249

Bone mineral density (BMD),
  areal versus volumetric, 254, 255
  measurement, 254
  menstrual dysfunction effects,
    amenorrhea and osteopenia risk, 261, 262
    eumenorrhea, 262
    exercise offset of bone loss, 263, 264
    menses resumption effects on bone density, 264, 265
    oligomenorrhea, 262
    risk factors in menstrual dysfunction, 263
    stress fracture, 263
  osteotrophic effect of exercise,
    adult premenopausal women,
      aerobic exercise, 259
      cross-sectional studies, 259
      impact loading, 260, 261
      weight training, 259, 260
    bone shape and strength, 265, 271–273
    intense training effects on immature skeleton, benefits in adulthood, 267, 273
    gymnasts, 266, 267
    tennis players, 266
    loading during growth, effects on bone geometry and strength, 271, 272
    moderate physical activity in active non-athletic children, 267–269
    optimal timing for maximum benefit,
      difficulty of study, 269
      prepuberty, 270, 271
      puberty, 270
  peak bone mass,
    age in females, 192, 256, 257
    genetic determinants, 258
    maintenance, 257
    osteoporosis fracture role, 253, 261
Brain natriuretic peptide (BNP),
  exercise response, 213, 214

Index

C

Caffeine, effects in hormone analysis, 9
Calcitonin,
  exercise effects on bone,
    negative effects, 244
    positive effects, 247–249
  functions, 243
Catecholamines, *see* Epinephrine; Norepinephrine
Chronobiology, *see* Circadian rhythm
Circadian rhythm, *see also specific hormones*,
  body temperature,
    exercise effects, 404
    resting state, 392, 396, 398
  cardiovascular rhythms,
    exercise effects, 404, 405
    resting state, 399
  components, 392, 393
  duration of rhythms, 391
  gastrointestinal function, 399
  hormonal secretions at rest, 400
  jet lag,
    body clock adjustment and recovery time, 411, 412
    gender differences, 410, 411
    management,
      alertness promotion, 413
      exercise timing, 415
      intra-flight, 412
      light therapy, 414, 415
      melatonin therapy, 414
      post-flight, 412, 413
      pre-flight, 412
      sleeping pills, 413
    symptoms, 410, 411
    travel fatigue, 410
  joint flexibility and stiffness, 402
  mathematical description, 395, 396
  maximal voluntary contraction strength, correction for time of day, 409
  mental performance, 400–402
  metabolism,
    exercise effects, 406
    resting state, 398
  muscle strength, 402, 403
  oxygen consumption,
    exercise effects, 406
    resting state, 398
  perceived exertion, 406
  practical implications, delayed-onset muscle soreness, 409
  endurance races and environmental temperature, 406–408
  performance estimate testing, 408, 409
  training, time of day, 408, 409
  short-term power output, 403
  sports performance, 396, 397
  suprachiasmatic nuclei,
    control of rhythms, 393, 394
    inputs and outputs, 395
  urinary excretion, 399, 400
  ventilation,
    exercise effects, 404, 405
    resting state, 398, 399
  zeitgebers,
    feeding hypothesis, 394, 395
    light, 394
    melatonin, 394
Clenbuterol, performance-enhancing use, 455
Clomiphene, performance-enhancing use, 459
Coefficient of variation,
  allowable levels, 4
  calculation, 3
Colorimetric assay, hormones, 14, 15
Confounding variables, hormone analysis, *see also* Variation, hormone analysis,
  controls, 2
  table, 22
Corticotropin-releasing hormone (CRH), *see also* Hypothalamo–pituitary–adrenal axis,
  female reproductive system effects, 141
  testosterone response in exercise, 123, 124, 126
Cortisol, *see also* Hypothalamo–pituitary–adrenal axis,
  circadian rhythm, 392
  exercise effects,
    altitude effects,
      acute exercise, 377, 378
      chronic exercise, 382
    immune system, 287
    pregnancy, 338, 339
  inhibitors as performance-enhancing use, 461, 462
  mood effects, 423
  overtraining effects, 356—358
  precision in assays, 5
  protein binding, 43
CRH, *see* Corticotropin-releasing hormone
Crossreactivity, hormone assays, 16
Cycle disturbance, *see* Menstrual cycle
Cytokines,
  effects on hormone concentrations, 287, 288
  response to exercise, 292

D

Dehydroepiandrosterone (DHEA), performance-enhancing use, 457
Dehydroepiandrosterone sulfate (DHEAS), precision in assays, 5
Delayed-onset muscle soreness (DOMS), time of day effects, 409
DHEA, *see* Dehydroepiandrosterone
DHEAS, *see* Dehydroepiandrosterone sulfate
Diabetes mellitus type 2, exercise benefits,
  cardiovascular disease prevention, 231
  dyslipidemia control, 232
  gestational diabetes, 338
  glycemic control, 228
  hypertension reduction, 231
  mechanisms, 228, 229
  obesity control, 232
  overview, 227, 228, 235, 236
  prescription of exercise,
    intensity and duration, 234
    risks, 235
    type, 234
  prevention studies, 233, 234
  type 1 diabetes benefits, 229–231
Disease, confounding factor in hormone analysis, 8
DOMS, *see* Delayed-onset muscle soreness
Dopamine, mood effects, 427
Doping control, performance-enhancing drugs, 462, 463

E

Eating restraint, effect on female reproductive function, 144, 145, 191

β-Endorphin,
 acute exercise effects on peripheral levels,
  aerobic exercise, 33–35
  anaerobic exercise bouts, 32, 33
  data collection, 31, 32
  incremental graded exercise, 32
  resistance exercise, 34, 35
 effects and mechanisms in sports activity, 38, 39
 factors influencing response to exercise,
  acid-base status, 38
  adrenocorticotropic hormone, 37
  catecholamines, 37, 38
  cortisol, 37
 functions, 425, 429
 immune system, exercise effects, 287, 289, 290
 individual anaerobic threshold, 33, 34
 mood effects, 425–427
 pregnancy, exercise effects, 341, 342
 processing, 425
 training status effects,
  endurance training, 35, 36
  overtraining effects, 361
  resistance training, 36
  study design, 37

Energy balance,
 endocrine effects in premenopausal women, 195, 196
 female reproduction influence,
  menstrual cycle effects,
   diet composition, 198
   energy drain, 196–198
   energy expenditure changes, 196
   weight loss effects in obese women, 198
  overview, 144, 166, 167, 175
  weight regulation in girls, 191, 192
 growth hormone effects, 194, 195
 hypothalamo–pituitary–gonadal axis effects,
  females, 191, 192
  males, 193, 194
 postmenopausal women,
  body composition changes, 198, 199
  caloric restriction effects on aging, 198, 199
  leptin effects, 199, 200
 surplus, 189, 190
 thyroid hormone, effects in exercise, 108–110

Eosinophil, exercise response, 291

Ephedrine, performance-enhancing use, 461

Epinephrine,
 exercise effects,
  acute effects at altitude,
   hypohydration effects, 373, 374
   hypoxemia effects, 372–375
   overview, 372, 373
   physiological significance of response, 374, 375
   undernutrition effects, 373, 374
  acute exercise, 181, 182
  chronic effects at altitude,
   hypertension response, 380
   hypoxia stimulation of tyrosine hydroxylase, 379, 380
   maximum heart rate modulation, 380, 381
   overview, 378, 379
   work intensity relationship, 379
  endurance running, 353
  fat metabolism, 185, 186
  fluid homeostasis, 210–212
  glucose metabolism,
   hepato-splanchic glucose production, 184
   skeletal muscle metabolism, 185
  glycemic control, 229
  immune system, 287, 289
  motor control and reflex influence on response, 182, 183
  pregnancy, 340, 341
 receptor downregulation in overtraining, 354, 355
 training, 183, 184
 synthesis, 373

Erythropoietin,
 exercise effects at altitude, 384
 performance-enhancing use, 462

Estrogen,
 exercise effects,
  bone, negative effects, 240–242
  pregnancy, 339
 menstrual cycle levels,
  disturbed cycle, 137
  normal cycle, 136, 322
 mood effects, 423, 424
 precision in assays, 5

Eumenorrhea,
 body composition hypothesis, 165, 166
 definition, 134, 135
 energy availability hypothesis, 166, 167
 exercise stress hypothesis, 167

F

Female reproductive physiology, see Amenorrhea, athletic; Eumenorrhea; Hypothalamo–pituitary–gonadal axis; Menstrual cycle

α-Feto protein (AFP), precision in assays, 5

Finasteride, performance-enhancing use, 460

Fluid homeostasis, hormonal control,
 exercise response,
  adrenomedullin, 214
  arginine vasopressin, 208, 212
  atrial natriuretic peptide, 208, 212, 213
  brain natriuretic peptide, 213, 214
  duration effects, 208
  epinephrine, 210–212
  modulating factors, 210
  norepinephrine, 210–212
  renal function,
   electrolyte excretion, 220
   glomerular filtration rate, 219, 220

renal blood flow, 219
urine flow rate, 220
renin–angiotensin–aldosterone system, 214, 215
sweat loss, 217
total body water reduction, 216–218
training effects, 208–210
urodilatin, 214
workload dependence, 208
fluid and electrolyte intake during exercise, 217, 218
overview, 207, 208
Fluorescence assay, hormones, 14–16
Follicle-stimulating hormone (FSH), *see also* Hypothalamo–pituitary–gonadal axis,
precision in assays, 5
FSH, *see* Follicle-stimulating hormone

G

Gamma-hydroxy-butyrate, performance-enhancing use, 461
Gas chromatography (GC), hormone assay, 15
Gastrin, precision in assays, 5
GH, *see* Gas chromatography
GH, *see* Growth hormone
Glucagon, exercise effects,
altitude effects,
acute exercise, 376
chronic exercise, 381
pregnancy, 336
GnRH, *see* Gonadotropin-releasing hormone
Gonadotropin-releasing hormone (GnRH), *see also* Hypothalamo–pituitary–gonadal axis,
overtraining effects, 359, 362
pulsatile secretion, 121
regulation of secretion, 121
Growth hormone (GH),
aging effects on levels, 79
axis description, 78, 79, 304
binding protein, training effects, 87
catabolic adaptation, 88—91
cytokine effects on levels, 288
determinants of exercise response,
aging, 62

body composition, 58
confounding factors, 63, 65, 66
duration and intensity of exercise, 79, 80
fitness of subjects, 79, 84–86
gender differences, 59, 60, 63
nutrition, 81
refractory period, 80
species differences, 63
temperature, 81
energy balance effects, 194, 195
exercise effects,
acute exercise in puberty, 307, 308
altitude effects,
acute exercise, 378
chronic exercise, 383
bone, positive effects, 244–247
immune system, 287
feedforward and feedback, 57, 58, 66, 194
interactions with other neuroendocrine axes, 66, 67, 69
metabolic mechanisms in control, 67, 69, 77
overtraining effects, 360
performance-enhancing use,
combination therapy with insulin-like growth factor 1, 454
mechanism of action, 454
rationale, 453, 454
side effects, 454, 455
physiological stimulation testing, 81
practical implications of exercise response, 82
precision in assays, 5
puberty,
acute exercise effects, 307, 308
role, 304, 305
training effects, 309, 310
pulsatile secretion, 63, 65, 79, 194
releasing hormone feedforward, 57, 58, 78
somatostatin inhibition, 78
training,
effects, 84–91
implications, 69

H

hCG, *see* Human chorionic gonadotropin
High-performance liquid chromatography (HPLC), hormone assay, 15
HPA axis, *see* Hypothalamo–pituitary–adrenal axis
HPG axis, *see* Hypothalamo–pituitary–gonadal axis
HPLC, *see* High-performance liquid chromatography
5-HT, *see* Serotonin
Human chorionic gonadotropin (hCG),
performance-enhancing use, 459, 460
precision in assays, 5
Human placental lactogen, exercise effects in pregnancy, 338
Humidity, effects in hormone analysis, 8, 9
17-Hydroxy progesterone, precision in assays, 5
testosterone response in exercise, 123, 126
Hypertension, exercise reduction in diabetes, 231
Hypothalamo–pituitary–adrenal (HPA) axis,
amenorrhea, 50
circadian rhythms, 63
corticotropin-releasing hormone effects, 43, 44
cortisol inhibition, 43
exercise effects,
aging effects, 45, 46, 62
confounding factors, 63, 65, 66
environmental effects, 46
gender differences, 46, 60
glucose levels, 46
intensity, duration, and timing of exercise, 45
mechanisms, 44
steroid effects, 62
type of exercise, 45
feedforward and feedback, 66
interactions with other neuroendocrine axes, 66, 67
metabolic mechanisms in control, 67–69
overreaching and overtraining effects, 49, 50

overtraining effects, 49, 50, 356–358, 364
overview of stress response, 288, 289
training effects, 47, 49
Hypothalamo–pituitary–gonadal (HPG) axis,
energy balance effects,
females, 191, 192
males, 193, 194
exercise effects,
aging effects, 60, 62
confounding factors, 63, 65, 66
gender differences, 58
men,
acute exercise, 121–123
endurance training, 124, 125
mechanisms of exercise-associated testosterone reduction, 125–127
nutritional factors, 126, 127
prolonged exercise, 123, 124
steroid effects, 62
feedforward and feedback, 66
female reproductive physiology, *see also* Amenorrhea, athletic; Eumenorrhea,
body composition hypothesis, 165, 166, 175
documentation of ovulatory function,
duration of sampling, 139
endometrial biopsy, 138
hormone level analysis, 137, 138
quantitative basal temperature, 139, 140
subsequent cycle analysis, 138
ultrasound, 138
energy availability hypothesis, 166, 167, 175, 196–198
exercise effects,
dose—response, 148, 149
marathon runners, 151
molimia prior to ovulation disturbances, 152
normality of adaptations, 159
prospective studies of menstrual cycle and luteal length effects, 147–151
reversibility of adaptation, 153–156, 158
time-course of ovulatory adaptation, 152, 153
exercise stress hypothesis, 167, 175
hypothalamic adaptation to stress,
clinical applications and treatment of ovulatory dysfunction, 156, 157, 176, 177
eating restraint effects, 144, 145
energy balance effects, 144
energy conservation, 143, 144
overview, 140, 141
reproductive maturity effects, 146, 147
stress intensity effects, 147
stress mechanism, 141–143
ovarian hormone levels,
disturbed cycle, 137
normal cycle, 136
terminology, 134–136
interactions with other neuroendocrine axes, 66, 67
male reproductive physiology, 120, 121, 192, 193
puberty,
acute exercise effects,
females, 308, 309
males, 308
role, 304, 305
training effects, 310, 311
Hypoxemia, *see* Altitude

I

IGF-1, *see* Insulin-like growth factor 1
IGF-2, *see* Insulin-like growth factor 2
IGFBPs, *see* Insulin-like growth factor binding proteins
Immune system,
adaptive immunity, 284, 285
anabolic-androgenic steroid effects, 452
clinical implications of exercise,
aging, 294
cancer susceptibility, 293, 294
chronic fatigue syndrome, 294
sepsis, 294, 295
upper respiratory tract infection prevention, 293
components, 282–284
innate immunity, 284, 285
leukocytosis from acute exercise, 281, 285, 286
memory, 285
overview of exercise effects, 281, 282
training effects,
B-cell counts, 291
basophils, 291
catecholamines, 287, 289
cellular responses, overview of studies, 290
cortisol, 287
cytokines,
effects on hormone concentrations, 287, 288
response, 292
β-endorphin, 287, 289, 290
eosinophils, 291
growth hormone, 287
immunoglobulins, 292, 293
lymphocyte proliferation, 291
monocyte/macrophage counts, 291
natural killer cell number and function, 292
neutrophil counts and activity, 290, 291
T-cell counts, 291
Immunoassay, hormones, 15–17
Immunoglobulin, exercise response, 292, 293

Index

Insulin,
    exercise effects,
        altitude effects,
            acute exercise, 375, 376
            chronic exercise, 381
        pregnancy, 336–338, 343
    mood effects, 424
    overtraining effects, 361, 362
    performance-enhancing use, 455, 456
    precision in assays, 5
    resistance, see Diabetes mellitus type 2
Insulin-like growth factor 1 (IGF-1),
    aging effects on levels, 79
    axis description, 78, 79, 304, 305
    bone, positive effects, 244–247
    exercise effects, 82, 83
    functions, 78
    performance-enhancing use,
        combination therapy with growth hormone, 454
        mechanism of action, 454
        rationale, 454
        side effects, 454, 455
    puberty,
        acute exercise effects, 307, 308
        puberty role, 304, 305
        training effects, 309, 310
    receptors, 79
    regulation of secretion, 57, 58
    tamoxifen interactions, 459
    training effects, 85, 87–91
Insulin-like growth factor 2 (IGF-2), exercise effects, 83
Insulin-like growth factor binding proteins (IGFBPs),
    aging effects on levels, 79
    exercise effects on IGFBP-3, 83, 84
    training effects, 85–89
    types, 78, 79

J

Jet lag,
    body clock adjustment and recovery time, 411, 412
    gender differences, 410, 411
    management,
        alertness promotion, 413
        exercise timing, 415
        intra-flight, 412
        light therapy, 414, 415
        melatonin therapy, 414
        post-flight, 412, 413
        pre-flight, 412
        sleeping pills, 413
    symptoms, 410, 411
    travel fatigue, 410

K

Kidney,
    circadian rhythm of urinary excretion, 399, 400
    exercise effects,
        electrolyte excretion, 220
        glomerular filtration rate, 219, 220
        renal blood flow, 219
        urine flow rate, 220

L

LDL, see Low-density lipoprotein
Leptin,
    effects on other hormones, 200
    exercise suppression, 200
    gender differences, 305–307
    gene, 199, 200, 305
    mood effects, 425
    neuropeptide Y antagonism, 425
    obesity association, 200, 305
    puberty,
        acute exercise effects, 309
        role, 305–307
        training effects, 311, 312
LH, see Luteinizing hormone
Lipoprotein lipase, catecholamine effects, 186
Low-density lipoprotein (LDL), anabolic-androgenic steroid effects, 445, 448
Luteinizing hormone (LH), see also Hypothalamo–pituitary–gonadal axis,
    energy balance effects,
        females, 191
        males, 193, 194
    overtraining effects, 359
    precision in assays, 5
    prospective studies of female ovulatory function, distinguishing exercise stress from energy availability effects, 168, 169
    Excalibur III, 172–174, 176
    Excalibur IV, 174, 175
    pulsatility as outcome variable, 168, 177
    pulsatility, 11, 126, 168
    stress response in women, 141–143

M

Male reproductive physiology, see Hypothalamo–pituitary–gonadal axis
Maximal voluntary contraction (MVC) strength, correction for time of day, 409
Medications, confounding factor in hormone analysis, 8
Melatonin,
    circadian rhythm control, 394
    jet lag therapy, 414
Menarche, delay in athletes, 191, 192
Menstrual cycle, see also Amenorrhea, athletic,
    aerobic exercise response,
        aerobic capacity over cycle, 326, 327
        heart rate, 325
        perceived exertion, 325
        thermoregulation, 323–325
    anabolic-androgenic steroid effects, 450, 451
    cycle disturbance, definition, 135
    dysfunction effects on bone,
        amenorrhea and osteopenia risk, 261, 262
        eumenorrhea, 262
        exercise offset of bone loss, 263, 264
        menses resumption effects on bone density, 264, 265
        oligomenorrhea, 262
        risk factors in menstrual dysfunction, 263
        stress fracture, 263
    effects of cycle phase,
        endurance, 327–329
        long duration athletic performance, 329, 330
        muscle strength, 327–329
        short duration athletic performance, 330
    energy balance effects,
        diet composition, 198
        energy drain, 196–198

energy expenditure changes, 196
weight loss effects in obese women, 198
estradiol levels,
  disturbed cycle, 137
  normal cycle, 136, 322
hormone analysis effects, 10
oral contraceptive effects on performance, 330, 331
prospects for research, 331
studies of athletes,
  confounding factors, 322, 323
  overview, 321, 322
Mental health, confounding factor in hormone analysis, 7, 8
Mood,
  hormone effects,
    cortisol, 423
    dopamine, 427
    β-endorphin, 425–427
    estrogen, 423, 424
    insulin, 424
    leptin, 425
    norepinephrine, 427
    progesterone, 424
    serotonin, 427, 428
    thyroid hormone, 423
  physical activity and mood changes,
    distraction hypothesis, 422
    endorphin hypothesis, 422
    mastery hypothesis, 422
    overview, 421, 422
    thermogenic hypothesis, 422
  Profile of Mood States battery, 422
MVC strength, see Maximal voluntary contraction strength

N

Natural killer cell, number and function with exercise, 292
Neutrophil, exercise response, 290, 291
Noradrenaline, see Norepinephrine
Norandrostenedione, performance-enhancing use, 458
Norepinephrine,
  exercise effects,
    acute effects at altitude,
      hypohydration effects, 373, 374
    hypoxemia effects, 372–375
    overview, 372, 373
    physiological significance of response, 374, 375
    undernutrition effects, 373, 374
  acute exercise, 181, 182
  chronic effects at altitude,
    hypertension response, 380
    hypoxia stimulation of tyrosine hydroxylase, 379, 380
    maximum heart rate modulation, 380, 381
    overview, 378, 379
    work intensity relationship, 379
  endurance running, 353
  fat metabolism, 185, 186
  fluid homeostasis, 210–212
  glucose metabolism,
    hepato-splanchic glucose production, 184
    skeletal muscle metabolism, 185
  immune system, 287, 289
  motor control and reflex influence on response, 182, 183
  pregnancy, 340, 341
  receptor downregulation in overtraining, 354, 355
  training, 183, 184
mood effects, 427
synthesis, 373
Nutrition, see Energy balance

O

Opioids, see β-Endorphin
Oral contraceptives, effects on performance, 330, 331
Overtraining,
  effects on hormones,
    adrenocorticotropic hormone, 359, 360
    cortisol, 356–358
    β-endorphin, 361
    epinephrine, 353–355
    gonadotropin-releasing hormone, 359, 362
    growth hormone, 360
    hypothalamo–pituitary–adrenal axis effects, 49, 50, 356–358, 364
    insulin, 361, 362
    luteinizing hormone, 359
    norepinephrine, 353–355
    prolactin, 361
    testosterone, 355–357
    thyroid hormone, 362
  syndrome,
    diagnosis, 348, 349
    features, 347, 348
    forms, 348
    pathogenesis, 348, 362–364
    studies of blood hormone levels, 349–353
    study design, 349, 364, 365
    tryptophan and serotonin levels, 364
    variable in hormone analysis, 19, 348
Ovulatory adaptation, see Hypothalamo–pituitary–gonadal axis
Oxygen consumption, circadian rhythm,
  exercise effects, 406
  resting state, 398

P

Parathyroid hormone (PTH),
  exercise effects in bone,
    negative effects, 243, 244
    positive effects, 247–249
  functions, 242, 243
  precision in assays, 5
Peak bone mass, see Bone mineral density
Plasma volume, correction for exercise, 20, 21
PMS, see Premenstrual syndrome
POMS, see Profile of Mood States,
Precision, see Variation, hormone analysis
Pregnancy,
  circulatory adaptation,
    fetal, 343
    maternal, 340
  confounding factor in hormone analysis, 7
  exercise effects,
    catecholamines, 340, 341
    cortisol, 338, 339

β-endorphin, 341, 342
estrogen, 339
gestational diabetes, 338
glucagon, 336
human placental lactogen, 338
insulin, 336–338, 343
plasma renin activity, 341
progesterone, 339
prolactin, 339, 340
relaxin, 341
study design, 335, 336
maximal aerobic capacity effects, 335
metabolism,
 fetal, 342
 maternal, 336
prevalence of exercise, 335
Premenstrual syndrome (PMS), food intake, 196
PRL, see Prolactin
Profile of Mood States (POMS), mood evaluation, 422
Progesterone,
 exercise effects,
  bone, negative effects, 240–242
  pregnancy, 339
  mood effects, 424
  precision in assays, 5
Prolactin (PRL),
 exercise effects,
  altitude effects,
   acute exercise, 378
   chronic exercise, 383
  pregnancy, 339, 340
  overtraining effects, 361
  precision in assays, 5
PTH, see Parathyroid hormone
Puberty,
 exercise effects on bone density, 270
 growth hormone,
  acute exercise effects, 307, 308
  puberty role, 304, 305
  training effects, 309, 310
 hypothalamo–pituitary–gonadal axis,
  acute exercise effects,
   females, 308, 309
   males, 308
  puberty role, 304, 305
  training effects, 310, 311
 leptin,
  acute exercise effects, 309
  puberty role, 305–307

training effects, 311, 312
training effects, confounding factors, 313, 314
growth, 312, 313

Q

QBT, see Quantitative basal temperature
Quantitative basal temperature (QBT), ovulatory function monitoring, 139, 140

R

Racial background, confounding factor in hormone analysis, 6, 7
Radioimmunoassay (RIA), hormones, 15–17
Receptor, hormones, 15
Relaxin, exercise effects in pregnancy, 341
Renal function, see Kidney
Renin–angiotensin–aldosterone system,
 exercise effects,
  altitude effects,
   acute exercise, 376, 377
   chronic exercise, 381, 382
  pregnancy, plasma renin activity, 341
  exercise response, 214, 215
  precision in assays, 5
  thirst stimulation, 218
RIA, see Radioimmunoassay

S

SCN, see Suprachiasmatic nuclei
Serotonin (5-HT),
 estrogen effects, 424
 mood effects, 427, 428
 overtraining effects, 364
Sex hormone-binding globulin (SHBG),
 exercise effects, 122
 precision in assays, 5
SHBG, see Sex hormone-binding globulin
Shin splint, testosterone reduction in etiology, 125
Significant difference, calculation, 4
Sleep deprivation, effects in hormone analysis, 9, 10

Specificity, hormone assays, 16, 17
Specimen collection, hormone analysis,
 circadian and rhythmic variation, 11
 experimental intrusion considerations, 14
 hemolysis in blood specimens, 13, 14
 posture, 10, 11
 saliva, 12, 13
 sampling frequency, 14
 serum, 12
 storage, 11, 12
 technique for collection, 11, 12
 urine, 12
Standardized testing conditions, hormone analysis,
 acid/base balance, 9
 alcohol use, 9
 altitude, 8, 9
 caffeine, 9
 humidity, 8, 9
 hypoxia, 8, 9
 menstruation, 10
 nutritional status and hydration, 9
 previous exercise, 10
 sleep deprivation, 9, 10
 stress level, 9, 10
 temperature, 8, 9
Suprachiasmatic nuclei (SCN),
 control of rhythms, 393, 394
 inputs and outputs, 395
Surgery, confounding factor in hormone analysis, 8

T

T-cell, exercise response, 291
Tamoxifen, performance-enhancing use, 459
TBG, see Thyroxine binding globulin
TBW, see Total body water
Testolactone, performance-enhancing use, 460
Testosterone, see also Anabolic-androgenic steroids; Hypothalamo–pituitary–gonadal axis,
 circannual rhythm, 11, 121
 exercise effects in men,
  acute exercise, 121–123
  bone,
   negative effects, 242
   positive effects, 244–246

endurance training, 124, 125
  mechanisms of exercise-associated reduction, 125–127
  prolonged exercise, 123, 124
  overtraining effects, 355–357
  precision in assays, 5
Thyroid hormone,
  abnormalities and athletic performance, 97, 98
  biosynthesis, 98
  cytokine effects on levels, 288
  dietary carbohydrate effects on secretion, 190
  effects,
    cardiac performance and output,
      hyperthyroidism, 101–103
      hypothyroidism, 100, 101
    muscle function,
      hyperthyroidism, 105, 106
      hypothyroidism, 103–105
    overview, 98, 99
    pulmonary effects, 106
  exercise effects,
    altitude, 383
    amenorrheic athletes, 110
    chronic effects, 108
    cold effects, 108, 109, 113
    distance runners, 107
    energy balance effects, 108–110
    ergometry studies, 107
    evaluation considerations, 106, 107, 110, 113, 190, 191
    fitness effects, 108
    summary of studies, table, 111, 112
  inactivating pathway, 98
  mood effects, 423
  overtraining effects, 362
  performance-enhancing use, preparations, 456
  side effects, 456, 457
  precision in assays, 5
  prospective studies of female ovulatory function, distinguishing exercise stress from energy availability effects, 168, 169
    Excaliber II, 170–172
    Excalibur I, 169, 170
  regulation of secretion, 98, 190
  resting metabolic rate effects on secretion, 190
  types, 98, 190
Thyrotropin (TSH),
  diurnal variation, 11
  exercise effects, see Thyroid hormone
  precision in assays, 5
Thyroxine binding globulin (TBG), precision in assays, 5
Total body water (TBW), exercise reduction, 216–218
TSH, see Thyrotropin

U

Upper respiratory tract infection, prevention follopwing exercise, 293
Urodilatin, exercise response, 214

V

Variation, hormone analysis,
  circadian and rhythmic variation, 11
  coefficient of variation,
    allowable levels, 4
    calculation, 3
  data manipulation,
    area under the curve analysis, 21, 22
    individual responses, 22, 23
    net change versus relative change in concentration, 20, 21
    plasma volume correction for exercise, 20, 21
    repeated measures analysis, 21, 22
  exercise variables,
    duration, 17, 18
    frequency of training, 19
    initial training, 19
    intensity, 17
    length of training intervention, 19, 20
    mode, 18, 19
    overtraining, 19
    volume, 18
  impact on study data, 4
  internal validity of assays, 4, 5
  secular trends and evolution effects, 20
  significant difference calculation, 4
  sources,
    analytical variation, 3, 4
    biological variation, 3
  specimen collection, see Specimen collection, hormone analysis
  standardized testing conditions, see Standardized testing conditions, hormone analysis
  state-of-the-art precision, 4, 5
  statistical considerations, 23
  subject profile differences,
    age and maturation status, 6
    body composition, 7
    disease, 8
    gender, 6
    medications, 8
    mental health, 7, 8
    pregnancy, 7
    racial background, 6, 7
    species, 5, 6
    surgery, 8
Vitamin D,
  exercise effects on bone,
    negative effects, 244
    positive effects, 248, 249
  functions, 243
  receptor mutations, 258

Made in the USA
Middletown, DE
12 March 2016